Disorders of Myelin in the Central and Peripheral Nervous Systems

Disorders of Myelin in the Central and Peripheral Nervous Systems

Fernando Dangond, M.D.

Assistant Professor of Neurology, Harvard Medical School,
Brigham and Women's Hospital, Boston

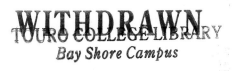
with 26 contributing authors

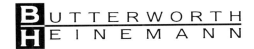

BUTTERWORTH
HEINEMANN

An Imprint of Elsevier Science

Amsterdam • Boston • London • Oxford • New York • Paris
San Diego • San Francisco • Singapore • Sydney • Tokyo

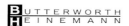

An imprint of Elsevier Science

225 Wildwood Avenue
Woburn, MA 01801

Disorders of Myelin in the Central and Peripheral Nervous Systems
Copyright © 2002, Elsevier Science, Inc. All rights reserved.

Notice

Neurology is an ever-changing field. Standard safety precautions must be followed, but as new research and clinical experience broaden our knowledge, changes in treatment and drug therapy may become necessary or appropriate. Readers are advised to check the most current product information provided by the manufacturer of each drug to be administered to verify the recommended dose, the method and duration of administration, and contraindications. It is the responsibility of the treating physician, relying on experience and knowledge of the patient, to determine dosages and the best treatment for each individual patient. Neither the Publisher nor the author assume any liability for any injury and/or damage to persons or property arising from this publication.

The Publisher

Library of Congress Cataloging-in-Publication Data

Disorders of myelin in the central and peripheral nervous systems / edited by Fernando Dangond.
    p. cm.
  Includes bibliographical references and index.
  ISBN 0-7506-7253-6
  1. Demyelination. I. Dangond, Fernando.

  RC366 .D55 2002
  616.8'3—dc21

                2001056686

The cover illustration shows an oligodendrocyte precursor cell stained with anti-NG2 antibodies (kindly provided by Drs. Samia Khoury and Jaime Imitola, Center for Neurologic Diseases, Brigham and Women's Hospital) on a background depicting a human brain specimen.

Acquisitions Editor: Susan F. Pioli
Assistant Editor: Andrea Sherman

SSC/MVY

Printed in the United States of America.

Last digit is the print number: 9 8 7 6 5 4 3 2 1

To my wife Monica and my children Daniel and David, for their love and support

In the cerebral hemispheres periventricular distribution of plaques is often seen . . . axons are spared within the initial lesions, but are later destroyed.

Jean-Martin Charcot

Contents

Contributing Authors

Barry G. W. Arnason, M.D.
James Nelson and Anna Louise Raymond Professor of Neurology, University of Chicago Pritzker School of Medicine

Fernando Dangond, M.D.
Assistant Professor of Neurology, Harvard Medical School, Brigham and Women's Hospital, Boston

David M. Dawson, M.D.
Professor of Neurology, Harvard Medical School, Brigham and Women's Hospital, Boston

Umberto De Girolami, M.D.
Professor of Pathology, Harvard Medical School, Boston; Director of Neuropathology, Brigham and Women's Hospital, Boston

Suzanne Gartner, Ph.D.
Associate Professor of Neurology, The Johns Hopkins University School of Medicine, Baltimore

Bonnie I. Glanz, Ph.D.
Instructor, Department of Neurology, Harvard Medical School, Boston; Research Associate, Department of Neurology, Brigham and Women's Hospital, Boston

Steven A. Greenberg, M.D.
Instructor in Neurology, Harvard Medical School, Boston; Associate Neurologist, Brigham and Women's Hospital, Boston

David A. Hafler, M.D.
Jack, Sadie, and David Breakstone Professor of Neurology, Harvard Medical School, Brigham and Women's Hospital, Boston

Jaime Imitola, M.D.
Research Fellow in Neurology, Harvard Medical School, Brigham and Women's Hospital, Boston

Reinhard Kiefer, M.D.
Senior Physician, Westfälische Wilhelms-Universitat, Münster, Germany

Shahram Khoshbin, M.D.
Associate Professor of Neurology, Harvard Medical School, Brigham and Women's Hospital, Boston

Samia J. Khoury, M.D.
Associate Professor of Neurology, Harvard Medical School, Boston; Co-Director, Partners Multiple Sclerosis Center, Brigham and Women's Hospital, Boston

Edwin H. Kolodny, M.D.
Bernard A. and Charlotte Marden Professor and Chairman, Department of Neurology, New York University School of Medicine

Igor J. Koralnik, M.D.
Associate Professor of Neurology, Harvard Medical School, Boston; Director, HIV/Neurology Center, Beth Israel Deaconess Medical Center, Boston

Sharon Lefebvre
Research Fellow, Department of Neurology, Beth Israel Deaconess Medical Center, Boston

Karim Makhlouf, M.D.
Research Fellow, Multiple Sclerosis Unit, Center for Neurologic Diseases, Harvard Medical School, Boston; Research Fellow, Brigham and Women's Hospital, Boston

David Margolin, M.D., Ph.D.
Instructor in Neurology, Harvard Medical School, Massachusetts General Hospital, Boston

Allison E. Morgan, M.D.
Clinical Faculty, Partners Multiple Sclerosis Center, Brigham and Women's Hospital, Boston

Michael J. Olek, D.O.
Assistant Professor of Neurology, Harvard Medical School, Boston; Attending, Department of Neurology, Brigham and Women's Hospital, Massachusetts General Hospital, Boston

Carlos A. Pardo, M.D.
Assistant Professor of Neurology, The Johns Hopkins University School of Medicine, Baltimore

Donald W. Paty, M.D.
Professor of Neurology, University of British Columbia, Vancouver; Director, Multiple Sclerosis Research Program, Vancouver Hospital and Health Sciences Center

Gustavo C. Román, M.D., F.A.C.P., F.R.S.M.(Lond.)
Professor of Neurology, University of Texas Health Science Center, San Antonio; Neurologist, Audie Murphy Veterans Affairs Hospital, San Antonio

Derek Smith, M.D.
Assistant Professor of Neurology, Harvard Medical School, Boston; Assistant Professor of Neurology, Partners Healthcare System, Boston

Anthony Traboulsee, M.D.
Clinical Fellow, Multiple Sclerosis Research Program, University of British Columbia, Vancouver; Clinical Fellow, Vancouver Hospital and Health Sciences Center

Timothy Vartanian, M.D., Ph.D.
Assistant Professor of Neurology, Harvard Medical School, Beth Israel Deaconess Medical Center, Boston

Howard L. Weiner, M.D.
Robert L. Kroc Professor of Neurology, Harvard Medical School, Brigham and Women's Hospital, Boston

Preface

This book has a wide scope and an ambitious goal: to comprehensively explain disorders of myelin in the human central and peripheral nervous systems. However, it is not a trivial task to concisely organize a field that by its own complexity and breadth continues to puzzle researchers and clinicians. Much debate still exists about the proper classification of demyelinating and dysmyelinating syndromes, and endless discussions still abound regarding the autoimmune versus neurodegenerative nature of some of these diseases. Having realized that it is not possible to please all readers with a definitive classification, our purpose has been to initiate *Disorders of Myelin in the Central and Peripheral Nervous Systems* with a description of basic science aspects of myelin research. With this background, the discussion then branches out to involve disorders that are either characterized by myelin destruction with and without inflammation or processes that mimic such injury. Hopefully, recent data and some arguments set forth in the chapters will help enlighten new avenues of research for individuals interested in these complex human disorders.

This book's aim is, therefore, to educate the physician neuroscientists, the neurologists, the neurology residents, and the primary care physicians on these constantly evolving issues, with emphasis on the mechanistic details that potentially make these disorders treatable. Hypothetic arguments about potential etiologies for some disorders are exposed with the sole purpose of stimulating controversy and creating a framework of reference, not to reaffirm preconceived notions. A special effort to include the most up-to-date references and factual information should be of aid to the readers wanting to expand their understanding of recent advances. The text incorporates the latest views on pathophysiology, molecular biology, biochemistry, and clinical treatment of disorders of myelin. A glimpse at future approaches of treatment is provided in several chapters, and, therefore, I believe this book provides a starting point, more than a retrospective view, for the interested reader.

The development of new technologies and treatments for human disease has entered a new phase as the new millennium has begun. Owing to an unprecedented rate of discoveries in the neurosciences, we are at the verge of major leaps in our ability to treat complex disorders, including those involving the human nervous system. Consequently, the impact on society at large and how individuals relate to that society are likely to suffer major transformations. For example, knowledge of genetic polymorphisms that might predispose a person to develop a demyelinating disease may soon be generated in a large scale with modern techniques of molecular biology. Issues related to privacy of genetic information, accessibility to this information by employers, and the implications for society will need to be confronted politically and individually by us all. It may indeed become a brave new world, and physicians must recognize the challenges of keeping abreast with new knowledge of diagnostic and therapeutic interventions, taking a basic science, conceptual approach to their fields of interest amid the rapid growth of this new practice of medicine.

Writing a book with a primarily clinical orientation in the setting of the genomics revolution is certainly a challenge, because maintaining the focus on clinical decision making and discussions about up-to-date therapeutic options is not an easy task in a rapidly transforming basic science field. However, the importance of the bedside clinician must never be minimized, because it is this group of professionals who discover the true applications and effectiveness of new treatments in humans. We have therefore attempted to provide information in a descriptive manner that reaches the clinician and the bench scientist in nearly equal terms. We also trust that the book will be of value to students and teachers following this challenging field, and that it will help advance the day-to-day practice of neurology.

Many thanks are given to individuals, too numerous to mention, who steadfastly encouraged me to pursue this project and who, over the years, have provided the leadership and environment necessary for my intellectual growth and training. Special thanks are in order to Drs. Edwin H. Kolodny, Martin A. Samuels, and Howard L. Weiner.

Fernando Dangond

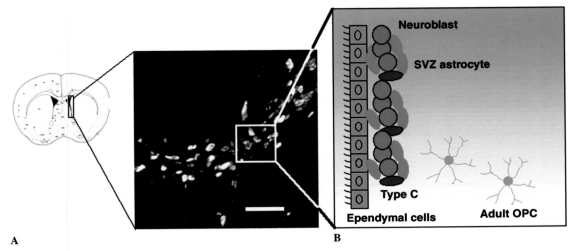

A

B

Color Plate 1. Topology and proliferation of the subventricular zone (SVZ). **A.** Confocal laser microscopy of BRDU incorporation from cells in the SVZ of adult mice demonstrating active proliferation of SVZ precursor cells. **B.** Representation of the types of cellular architecture in the SVZ; the ventricles are lined by the ependymal cell layer, and these cells have been shown to be neural stem cells. The SVZ is composed of a heterogenous population of neuronal progenitors (*red*); SVZ astrocytes or type B cells, which are also neural stem cells; type C multipotent precursor cells (*blue*); and the adult oligodendrocyte progenitor cells (OPCs) that exhibit neural stem cell properties in vivo and in vitro. Scale bar: 25 µm in **A.**

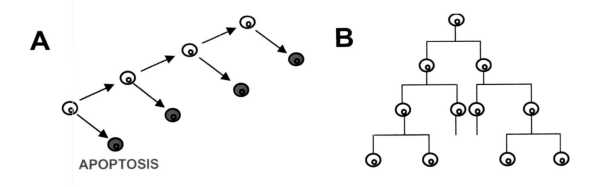

Color Plate 2. Representation of the types of cell division of the neural stem cells (NSCs) and progenitor cells. Representation of the types of cell division that NSCs undergo in vivo. NSCs from the subventricular zone maintain the relative amount of cell number by asymmetric division with apoptosis of one daughter cell (**A**). During development or after injury, the daughter cells proliferate and migrate out to the cortex or the olfactory bulb (**B**). Types of cell division that NSCs exhibit in vitro: One NSC can undergo symmetric cellular division, producing two identical NSCs, and these cells can undergo further symmetric cell division, leading to clonal expansion and producing a clonal neurosphere (**C**). As the time in culture increases, NSCs undergo asymmetric division, wherein an NSC produces daughter stem cells (*white*) and uncommitted progenitor cells (*blue*) that will give rise to more differentiated progenitor cells (*black*).

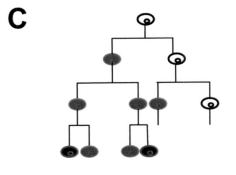

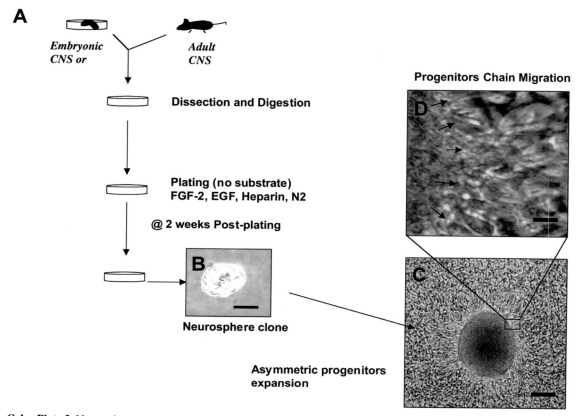

Color Plate 3. Neurosphere assay. Neural stem cells can be isolated from adult and embryonic tissues by digestion with proteases from dissected regions from the central nervous system (CNS). **A.** These cells can be plated without substrate; most mature cells die, and a few cells survive. In the presence of fibroblast growth factor (FGF) and epidermal growth factor (EGF), these cells proliferate and generate neurospheres (**B**). These neurospheres can be passaged, and, if new neurospheres arise from individual plated cells, this demonstrates self-renewal. **C.** After the initial symmetric expansion, rapidly proliferating migratory progenitor cells migrate out of a neurosphere (**C**, center). These migrating progenitors exhibit the typical behavior of chain migration as in **D**, where radially arranged cells appear to migrate out from a neurosphere in an orderly longitudinal fashion. Chain migrating cells (*arrows*) from a neurosphere from adult neural stem cells. Scale bars: 5 μm (**B**), 30 μm (**C**), 5 μm (**D**).

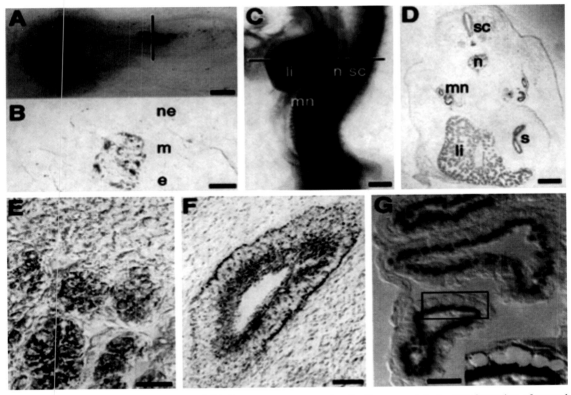

Color Plate 4. Adult neural stem cells (NSCs) from a mouse expressing *lacZ* gene contribute with formation of several organs in chick embryos. **A.** Adult NSCs (*blue*) integrate with chick embryo development, demonstrated by X-Gal staining to show the product of the *lacZ* gene from mouse NSCs. The line indicates the plane of section of the same embryo shown in **B**. Neuroectoderm (ne), mesoderm (m), and endoderm (e) are indicated. **C.** The trunk region of a chimeric chick embryo (*blue*) X-Gal staining from mouse NSCs. A cross section of the embryo in **C** (plane of section indicated by line) is shown in **D**. Adult mouse NSCs contribute to liver (li), mesonephros (mn), notochord (n), and spinal cord (sc). **E.** NSC-derived cells visualized with an antibody against the mouse-specific epitope H-2Kb intermingled with host cells in the liver of a chick embryo. **F.** The epithelium of the stomach shows H-2Kb immunoreactivity (*brown*) and X-Gal staining (*blue*). **G.** Cytoplasmic expression of *lacZ* derived from adult mouse NSCs in mesonephric tubule cells (*blue*) show renal-specific Pax2 immunoreactivity (*red nucleus high magnification of area in box*). Scale bars: 250 μm (**A** and **D**), 50 μm (**B**), 500 μm (**C**), and 25 μm (**E–G**). (Reprinted with permission from DL Clarke, CE Johansson, J Wilbertz, et al. Generalized potential of adult neural stem cells. Science 2000;288:1660.)

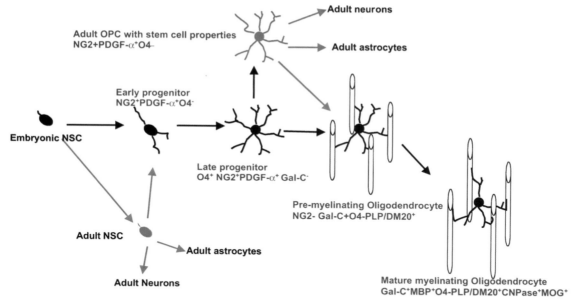

Color Plate 5. Oligodendrocyte developmental lineage. Developmental stages of oligodendrocytes from neural stem cells (NSCs) are shown. Oligodendrocyte progenitor cells (OPCs) undergo several distinct stages defined by antigenic profiles and biologic characteristics (see Chapter 3 text for details). Adult OPCs (*blue*) persist in the adult central nervous system as a cycling population postulated to be NSCs. (CNPase = 2,3 cyclic nucleotide 3-phosphohydrolase; GalC = galactocerebrosidase; MBP = myelin basic protein; MOG = myelin oligodendrocyte glycoprotein; PDGF = platelet-derived growth factor; PLP = proteolipid protein.)

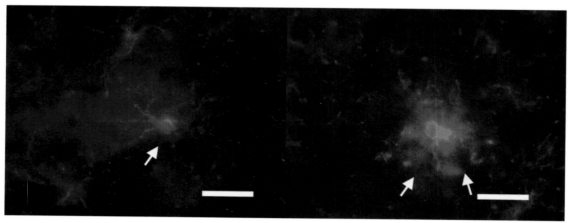

Color Plate 6. Oligodendrocyte progenitor cell in vivo. NG2-positive adult oligodendrocyte progenitors (*green*) from the corpus callosum showing typical morphology with radially oriented processes (*arrows*). Scale bar: 20 μm.

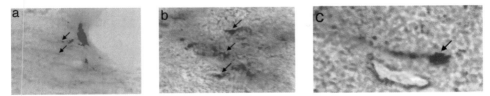

Color Plate 7. Remyelination from subcortical precursor cells in experimental demyelination. A proliferating population of endogenous precursors was labeled by a retrovirus during chemically induced demyelination by lysolecithin injection. The progeny of these cells was followed up. **A.** Retrovirus-labeled myelinating oligodendrocyte (*blue*) arising from precursors is shown in **A** with delineated myelin sheaths (*arrows*). **B, C.** Myelin basic protein expression (*arrows*; *black/purple*) in BAG-labeled myelin (*blue*). (Reprinted with permission from JM Gensert, J Goldman. Endogenous progenitors remyelinate demyelinated axons in the adult CNS. Neuron 1997;19:197–203.)

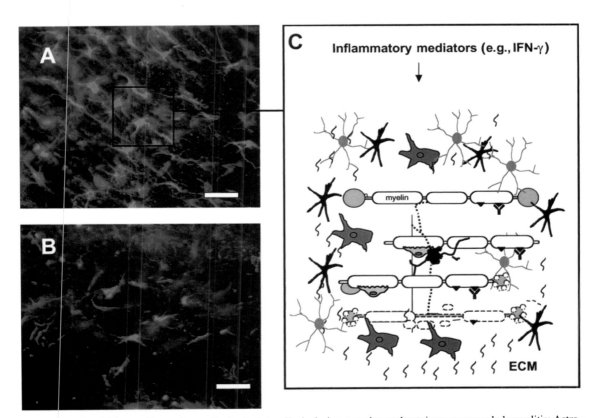

Color Plate 8. Inhibitory effects of astrogliosis. **A.** Astrogliosis during experimental autoimmune encephalomyelitis: Astrocytes exhibit thick processes and increase glial fibrillary acidic protein immunoreactivity (*green*), as compared with the normal central nervous system (**B**). Scale bar: 20 μm. Astrogliosis has been shown to limit remyelination in experimental autoimmune encephalomyelitis. **C.** Diagram showing how reactive astrocytes or interferon (IFN)-γ–stimulated cells (*black and gray cells*) can generate a dense extracellular matrix (ECM) with molecules (*curved lines*) that alter migration, perturb differentiation of oligodendrocyte progenitor cells, or block axonal regeneration.

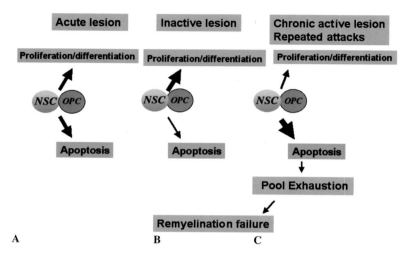

Acute lesion Inactive lesion Chronic active lesion Repeated attacks

Proliferation/differentiation Proliferation/differentiation Proliferation/differentiation

NSC OPC NSC OPC NSC OPC

Apoptosis Apoptosis Apoptosis

Pool Exhaustion

Remyelination failure

A B C

Color Plate 9. "Nonpermissive environment" model for precursor pool during demyelination. A dynamic model of the role of endogenous precursor cells during demyelinating diseases is proposed. The inflammatory environment may influence the kinetics of endogenous precursor cells during autoimmune demyelination by altering a balance between apoptosis and proliferation/differentiation. **A.** An acute lesion may exhibit apoptotic cell death and some proliferation demonstrated by models of experimental autoimmune encephalomyelitis. **B.** Inactive lesions or a change toward a Th2 environment by immunologic treatment (e.g., glatiramer acetate) may help to increase proliferation and differentiation of the endogenous pool. **C.** Chronic active lesions and relapses over time may induce endogenous pool exhaustion and remyelination failure. (NSC = neural stem cell; OPC = oligodendrocyte progenitor cell.)

Color Plate 10. Inflammation in multiple sclerosis. Hematoxylin and eosin stain shows perivascular infiltration of inflammatory cells. These infiltrates are composed of activated T cells, B cells, and macrophages. The cellular infiltrates can be fairly small histologically, and it is thus possible that some may not be detected in vivo by conventional magnetic resonance imaging techniques. (Reproduced with permission from F Dangond. Multiple sclerosis. eMedicine Web site: Neurology. Available at: http://www.emedicine.com. Accessed February 2, 2002. Multimedia image courtesy of eMedicine.com, Inc. Copyright © 2001.)

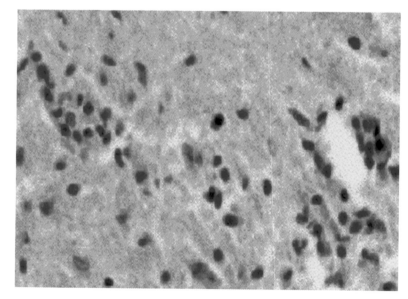

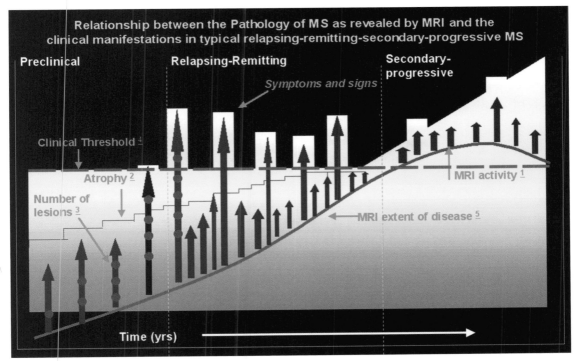

Color Plate 11. This illustration summarizes the relationship between clinical attacks, magnetic resonance imaging (MRI) activity, and MRI-determined burden of disease and atrophy. There is evidence of T_2 lesions before diagnosis of multiple sclerosis (MS) (presymptomatic phase). MRI (1) activity includes gadolinium-enhancing lesions, new lesions, or enlarging lesions. Patients have multiple silent attacks, and atrophy begins early in the course of the disease and continues slowly as axonal loss and shrinkage develop (2). The number of lesions (3) increases with each activity event (only preclinical phase lesions shown). The clinical threshold (4) is the point at which pathologic activity produces recognizable clinical symptoms. The MRI measure of the extent of disease (5) reflects the advancing pathology of the disease. (Prepared by J Oger, D Li, W Moore, et al. Based on ideas from J Wolinsky, B Trapp, D Paty.)

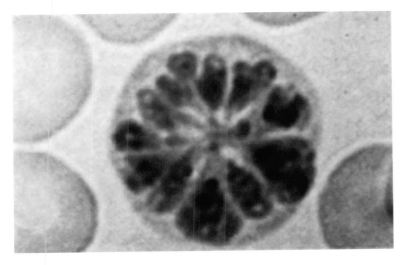

Color Plate 12. T-cell lobulation in human T-cell lymphotropic virus type I infection. Flower-like appearance of a multilobulated T-cell nucleus is shown. This finding suggests adult T-cell leukemia-lymphoma or a pre-adult T-cell leukemia-lymphoma phase. (Courtesy of K Takatsuki, Kumamoto University Medical School, and G Roman, University of Texas at San Antonio; Reprinted with permission from F Dangond, DA Hafler. Neuroimmunology. In R Ransohoff [ed], Continuum Series, vol. 7. American Academy of Neurology, 2001.)

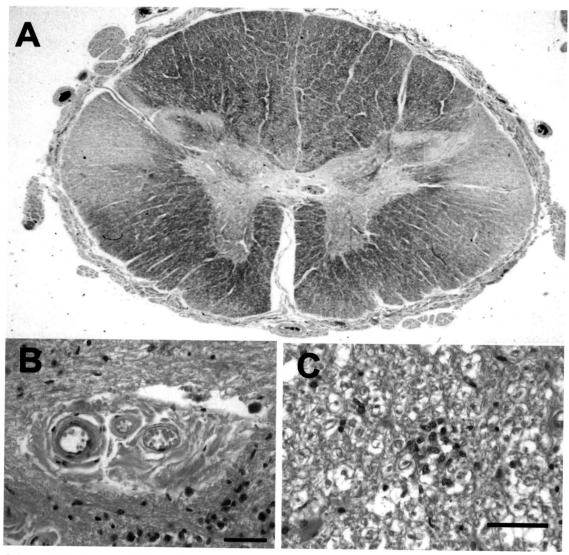

Color Plate 13. Histologic findings in human T-cell lymphotropic virus type I–associated myelopathy/tropical spastic paraparesis. **A.** Spinal cord stained with Luxol fast blue—a myelin stain—demonstrating the presence of demyelination of the lateral corticospinal tracts. **B.** Thickening and fibrosis of the adventitia of blood vessels (hematoxylin and eosin; scale bar: 50 μm). **C.** Cluster of lymphocytes in the white-matter tract (hematoxylin and eosin; scale bar: 50 μm).

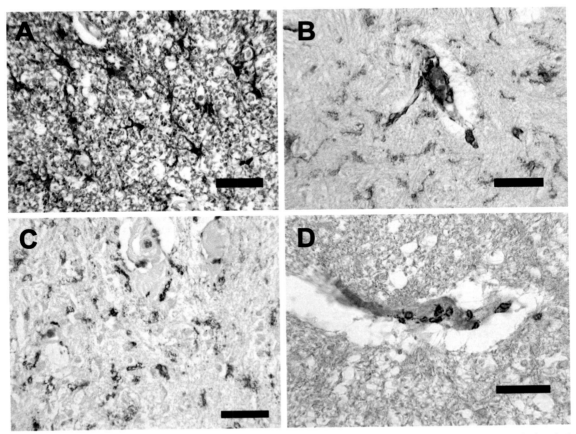

Color Plate 14. Immunocytochemical findings in human T-cell lymphotropic virus type I–associated myelopathy/tropical spastic paraparesis (scale bar: 50 μm) **A.** Astroglial reaction in white-matter tracts is prominent, as visualized by immunocytochemistry with glial fibrillary acidic protein. **B, C.** Perivascular macrophages and activated microglia in the anterior horn, as visualized with the macrophage marker human leukocyte antigen–DR. **D.** Perivascular lymphocytes that are positive for CD8[+], as seen by immunostaining with anti-CD8 antibodies.

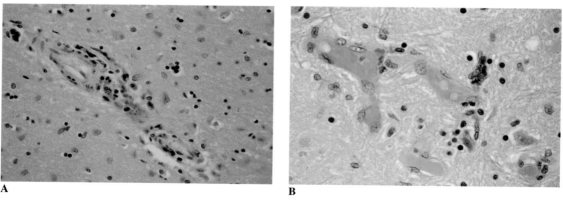

A   B

Color Plate 15. Acute human immunodeficiency virus type 1 encephalitis. **A.** Perivascular collection of chronic inflammatory cells and prominence of endothelial cells (hematoxylin and eosin). **B.** Scattered multinucleated giant cells and chronic inflammatory cells around a blood vessel (hematoxylin and eosin). (Reprinted with permission from U De Girolami, TW Smith, D Henin, J-J Hauw. Neuropathology and Ophthalmologic Pathology of the Acquired Immunodeficiency Syndrome. A Color Atlas. Boston: Butterworth–Heinemann, 1992.)

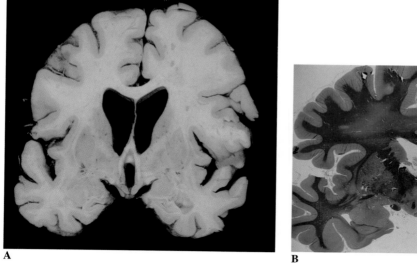
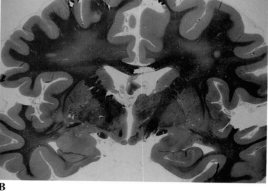

A   B

Color Plate 16. Macroscopic views of human immunodeficiency virus type 1 encephalitis. **A.** Coronal section through formalin-fixed brain at level of anterior commissure showing some ventricular dilatation. **B.** Whole-brain section of paraffin-embedded brain at level of mammillary body showing some pallor of myelin staining in the centrum semiovale and mild ventricular dilatation (Luxol fast blue stain for myelin). (Reprinted with permission from U De Girolami, TW Smith, D Henin, J-J Hauw. Neuropathology and Ophthalmologic Pathology of the Acquired Immunodeficiency Syndrome. A Color Atlas. Boston: Butterworth–Heinemann, 1992.)

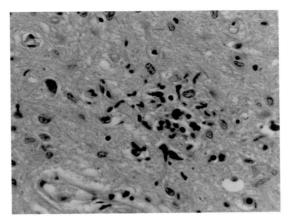

Color Plate 17. Subacute human immunodeficiency virus type 1 encephalitis. Microglial nodule. Note cluster of elongated irregular nuclei (hematoxylin and eosin). (Reprinted with permission from U De Girolami, TW Smith, D Henin, J-J Hauw. Neuropathology and Ophthalmologic Pathology of the Acquired Immunodeficiency Syndrome. A Color Atlas. Boston: Butterworth–Heinemann, 1992.)

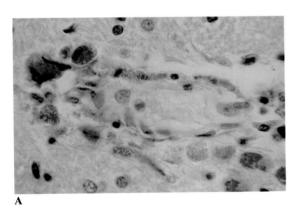

A

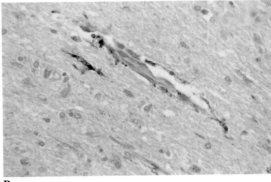

B

Color Plate 18. Subacute human immunodeficiency virus type 1 encephalitis. **A.** Immunoperoxidase method for macrophages (brown staining) demonstrating the nature of perivascular cells. **B.** Immunoperoxidase for human immunodeficiency virus type 1 (glycoprotein 41) to demonstrate the presence of virus within brain tissue, particularly well demonstrated in microglial cells (elongated brown-staining cells). (Reprinted with permission from U De Girolami, TW Smith, D Henin, J-J Hauw. Neuropathology and Ophthalmologic Pathology of the Acquired Immunodeficiency Syndrome. A Color Atlas. Boston: Butterworth–Heinemann, 1992.)

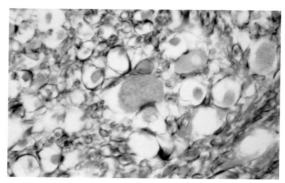

Color Plate 19. Acute infarct in white-matter tract. Note axonal swellings and lack of inflammatory response (hematoxylin and eosin). (Reprinted with permission from U De Girolami, TW Smith, D Henin, J-J Hauw. Neuropathology and Ophthalmologic Pathology of the Acquired Immunodeficiency Syndrome. A Color Atlas. Boston: Butterworth–Heinemann, 1992.)

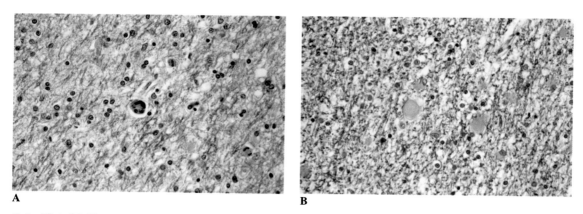

A   **B**

Color Plate 20. Human immunodeficiency virus type 1 leukoencephalitis. **A.** Note patch of pallor of myelin staining, reduction in number of myelinated fibers, gliosis, and single multinucleated giant cell (Luxol fast blue stain for myelin). **B.** Note axonal swellings in region of injured white matter (Luxol fast blue stain for myelin). (Reprinted with permission from U De Girolami, TW Smith, D Henin, J-J Hauw. Neuropathology and Ophthalmologic Pathology of the Acquired Immunodeficiency Syndrome. A Color Atlas. Boston: Butterworth–Heinemann, 1992.)

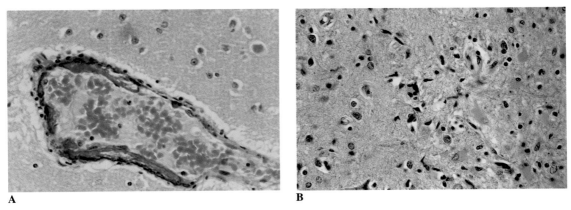

A

B

Color Plate 21. Pediatric human immunodeficiency virus type 1 encephalitis. **A.** Plate-like mineralization in large vessel of basal ganglion (hematoxylin and eosin). **B.** Myelin loss associated with microglial nodule, multinucleated giant cell, and gliosis (Luxol fast blue stain for myelin). (Reprinted with permission from U De Girolami, TW Smith, D Henin, J-J Hauw. Neuropathology and Ophthalmologic Pathology of the Acquired Immunodeficiency Syndrome. A Color Atlas. Boston: Butterworth–Heinemann, 1992.)

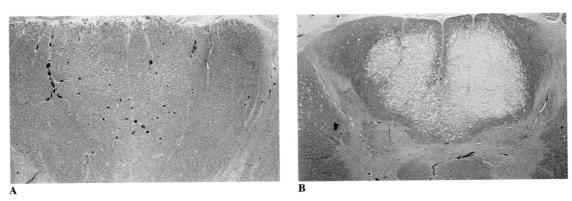

A

B

Color Plate 22. Vacuolar myelopathy of acquired immunodeficiency syndrome. **A.** Horizontal section through thoracic cord showing the posterior columns. Note fine vacuolization of myelin (Luxol fast blue stain for myelin). **B.** Horizontal section through high lumbar cord showing posterior columns and partially lateral columns. Extensive vacuolization of myelin is found in posterior columns and elsewhere in more severe cases. (Reprinted with permission from U De Girolami, TW Smith, D Henin, J-J Hauw. Neuropathology and Ophthalmologic Pathology of the Acquired Immunodeficiency Syndrome. A Color Atlas. Boston: Butterworth–Heinemann, 1992.)

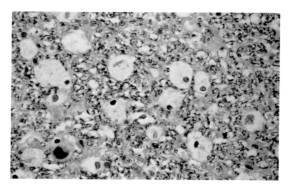

Color Plate 23. Vacuolar myelopathy of acquired immuno-deficiency syndrome. High magnification view of posterior column abnormality showing numerous macrophages (Luxol fast blue stain for myelin). (Reprinted with permission from U De Girolami, TW Smith, D Henin, J-J Hauw. Neuropathology and Ophthalmologic Pathology of the Acquired Immunodeficiency Syndrome. A Color Atlas. Boston: Butterworth–Heinemann, 1992.)

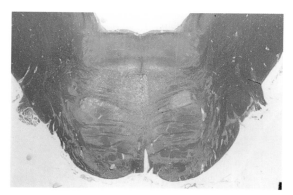

Color Plate 24. Multifocal pontine leukoencephalopathy. Horizontal section through midpons showing multiple areas of vacuolated destruction of pontine myelinated fibers (Luxol fast blue stain for myelin). (Reprinted with permission from U De Girolami, TW Smith, D Henin, J-J Hauw. Neuropathology and Ophthalmologic Pathology of the Acquired Immunodeficiency Syndrome. A Color Atlas. Boston: Butterworth–Heinemann, 1992.)

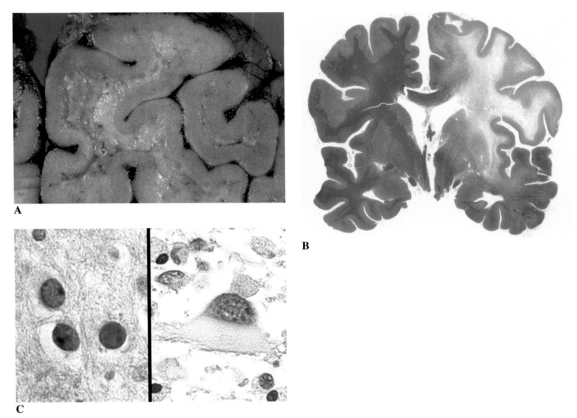

Color Plate 25. Pathologic features of progressive multifocal leukoencephalopathy. **A.** Coronal section of the brain of a human immunodeficiency virus–positive patient with progressive multifocal leukoencephalopathy through the right occipital lobe shows extensive liquefactive necrosis of the white matter and an unaffected cortical ribbon. **B.** Whole-brain coronal section demonstrating massive demyelination (hematoxylin and eosin/Luxol fast blue). This giant coronal section at the level of the globus pallidus illustrates that the myelin of most of the right hemisphere white matter has been destroyed. **C.** Immunoperoxidase staining with an antibody directed to the polyomavirus group antigen was strongly positive in oligodendrocyte nuclei (*left panel*) as well as in the nuclei of some astrocytes (*right panel*) at the periphery of the lesions, consistent with polyomavirus JC infection. (Special thanks to JT Joseph, MD, PhD, Beth Israel Deaconess Medical Center, and U De Girolami, MD, Brigham and Women's Hospital, Boston, for histologic preparation and diagnosis of samples shown.)

Chapter 1

Immunology of Central Nervous System Demyelination: The First Century

Barry G.W. Arnason

Immunologic research in demyelinating diseases has moved in parallel with developments in general immunology. Thus, neuroimmunologists have taken advantage of the increased understanding of immune mechanisms that has occurred in recent decades, including the delineation of the steps involved in immune system development; the characterization of B cells, T cells, natural killer (NK) cells, monocytes, dendritic cells, and their sundry subsets; the discovery of mechanisms involved in the generation of immunologic diversity; the delineation of the roles of cytokines, chemokines, and other reactive molecules both in host defense and in tissue destructive processes; and the recognition that the normally tight regulation of the immune system somehow goes awry in autoimmunity.

This chapter treads lightly on developments in immunology in general, despite their profound influence in shaping thought about demyelinating diseases. Rather, the focus is on developments that, in the opinion of the author, uniquely contributed in some way, particularly in the early years, to a better understanding of demyelinating diseases.

The field of neuroimmunology of demyelinating diseases is vast, but the scope of this chapter is restricted. Accordingly, the reference list must be selective, so it is a certainty that major contributions by those—yet alive—who I hope will remain my friends will not be cited. Additional hazards in an undertaking of this sort are that contributions by the author's collaborators may receive more emphasis than others might give them and that

idiosyncratic views of the author are likely to surface. I take solace in the fact that many major truths began as idiosyncratic or minority opinions. I am also mindful that most minority opinions remain just that.

I have chosen to skirt topics of recent interest that will be covered in detail by others and to emphasize early developments that may have been lost in the mists of time. In the final section, I have taken the liberty of offering speculations involving some possible future developments based on my interpretation of what has gone before and some recent work from my laboratory.

Central Nervous System– Demyelinating Diseases

Rabies Vaccination–Induced Encephalomyelitis

Our story begins on July 6, 1885, when Joseph Meister, age 9, was brought to Louis Pasteur by his mother. The lad had been bitten 14 times by a rabid dog the day before. Pasteur bravely treated Meister using a technique with which he had been experimenting in dogs. Pasteur knew that the spinal cord from rabies-infected rabbits that was desiccated for 2 weeks lost infectivity. Pasteur administered 12 injections of desiccated cord over the next 10 days. As the injections progressed, he administered fresher material. The final injections contained live virus. Rabbits injected with the material given to

Meister as his final injection died of rabies. Meister survived. Meister, in a "beau geste," spent his final years tending to Pasteur's tomb and died by suicide on the day in June 1940 on which the German army entered Paris.

Rabies vaccination spread quickly throughout the world. Within 3 years, the first report of an untoward reaction to vaccination had appeared, and it soon became apparent that neuroparalytic accidents constituted a genuine hazard of the treatment (extremely well reviewed in reference 1). There was confusion for a time whether the reactions were a breakthrough of frank rabies despite vaccination, an attenuated nonfatal rabies caused by the effete rabies virus strain passaged in rabbits, or some other process linked to a nonviral component of the vaccine. The first postulate was discarded promptly when neuroparalytic accidents were observed in vaccinated persons bitten by animals that proved not to be rabid, and neuroparalytic accidents, with their distinct pathology, were observed superimposed on the distinctive pathology of rabies itself in instances in which vaccination had failed to protect against the disease.[1] The second postulate became untenable when brain material from persons with fatal neuroparalytic accidents failed to cause rabies when injected into rabbits. That something else in the brain material had to be implicated became clear when neuroparalytic accidents surfaced in persons receiving injections of uninfected brain material.[2]

In central Europe in the 1950s, there was a fad for injecting extracts of animal organs into recipients who thought that the function of this or that organ was failing. Somehow, the injections were supposed to restore function. Numerous neuroparalytic accidents were documented in recipients of uninfected brain material.[2] When duck embryo and tissue culture rabies vaccines were introduced in developed countries, neuroparalytic accidents became increasingly rare, although, surprisingly, a few cases have been put on record,[3–5] albeit none in recent years. In less developed parts of the world, rabies vaccines prepared from infected animal brains continue to be used because they are cheap to prepare, and neuroparalytic accidents still occur.

What then in brain material is responsible? The factor in cause was shown early on to be remarkably heat stable, a point to which I return when I consider myelin basic protein (MBP). It resisted

phenol used to kill the rabies virus as well as numerous other solvents.[6]

Rabies vaccine was traditionally given as a series of 14–20 daily subcutaneous injections forming a ring around the umbilicus. Onset of neurologic symptomatology was heralded by the abrupt onset of fever, headache, and myalgia and by intense local reactions that appeared simultaneously at all the injection sites.[6–8]

Robert Koch discovered the tubercle bacillus in 1882. Shortly thereafter, he showed that guinea pigs injected subcutaneously with tubercle bacilli developed a nodule at the injection site approximately 2 weeks later. When a similar injection was made at another site in an already infected animal, the response was faster and more violent, with a dusky indurated lesion appearing within 2–3 days. Koch then showed that a similar response could be obtained with boiled culture filtrates of the organism. Old tuberculin (OT) and its successor, purified protein derivative (PPD), continue in use to this day as diagnostic tests for prior infection with tuberculosis.

Koch gave OT intravenously to patients with tuberculosis in the hope that it would be protective. Tuberculous recipients developed fever, headache, myalgia, lymphopenia, and sometimes collapse within a few hours of the injection and skin test anergy that lasted for a week or so. Looked at today, the systemic symptoms depended on pyrogenic cytokines released from sensitized lymphocytes activated by their exposure to OT. The transient anergy and lymphopenia reflected migration of antigen-activated T cells out of the blood into tissues throughout the body, so that they were no longer available to migrate into a cutaneous injection site. Cutaneous sensitivity rebounded 1 week after treatment was stopped, frequently with an intensity substantially greater than that observed before treatment. These features came to be known as the *systemic tuberculin reaction* (reviewed in reference 9).

Von Pirquet coined the term *allergy* shortly after the turn of the last century. The word derives from the Greek word "allos" for *altered* and "ergeia" for *reactivity*.[10] Von Pirquet studied vaccinia reactions.[11] He showed that when a patient who had never been vaccinated was given daily vaccinations, all the vaccination sites erupted simultaneously on the tenth day or thereabout. This reaction he called a *primary take*. If a patient had been vaccinated previously and was revaccinated, the reaction occurred much sooner with kinetics evocative of those of cutaneous tuberculin reactions in persons with a prior exposure to tuberculosis. This reaction he called a *secondary take*.

In my opinion, the constitutional symptoms that herald the onset of neuroparalytic accidents are those of a systemic tuberculin type or, in current parlance, a systemic delayed-type hypersensitivity (DTH) reaction. The abdominal skin reactions are a local DTH response and, based on the timing of their appearance, a primary take.

Rabies vaccination–induced encephalomyelitis is an acute process. The brunt of the insult may fall on the spinal cord in the form of an acute transverse myelitis; more often, cerebral symptoms predominate. An inflammatory neuritis can also complicate rabies vaccination. The illness is usually monophasic and of brief duration, but chronic and recrudescent cases have been described. In former times, the mortality was at least 20%. With the introduction of glucocorticoid therapy, mortality has declined to 5%, but survivors are often left with residual disabilities.

Most vaccinees were children, yet more than 90% of cases occurred in adults, in particular young adults,[6] an observation evocative of the age of onset of multiple sclerosis (MS). It was also suggested that the complication was more likely to occur in those of higher socioeconomic status,[6] a proposal advanced also by epidemiologists as a factor implicated in the propensity to develop MS. However, as a point of stark contrast with MS, the complication is seen throughout the world, including such countries as Thailand, where MS is exceedingly rare. Cases with the earliest onset during a course of vaccine injections tend to have the most severe disease. Here the parallel is with experimental autoimmune encephalomyelitis (EAE), in which the same pertains.

Pathologically, the cardinal features are multiple perivenous lymphocyte and macrophage infiltrates, all of like age, with demyelination at sites of cellular infiltration and relative but not absolute sparing of axons.[1,2,7,12] In a remarkable study of nine fatal cases from Japan, large confluent demyelinated lesions were noted in patients who had survived for 1–6 months after the onset of an acute monophasic illness that then stabilized. There was a predilection for the lesions to abut the lateral ventricles[13] in a pattern reminiscent of the lesions of MS. Extensive spinal cord involvement was noted as well.

One early brief report suggested that complement fixing antibrain antibodies might be elevated in rabies vaccination–induced encephalomyelitis,[14] but the first convincing direct evidence that rabies vaccine–induced encephalomyelitis is a hypersensitivity reaction was provided in 1987 by Hemachudha et al.,[8,15] 100 years after the first reports of the complication. Thirty-six patients were studied. The illness was monophasic in 33 patients and progressive in three, including one with a relapsing-remitting course. All had received a vaccine prepared from rabies virus–infected sheep brain that had been inactivated with 0.25% phenol. This vaccine was widely used in Thailand at the time. It was given to 15,000 persons each year; 1 in 400 developed neurologic complications.

A brisk proliferative response of patient lymphocytes to myelin was observed in three of four studied patients who were not receiving glucocorticoid treatment. Antibodies to brain white matter, to MBP, and to cerebroside were routinely found in patients with central nervous system (CNS) or peripheral nervous system disease and were not found in vaccinated patients without neurologic complications. Antibodies to MBP were also detected in the cerebrospinal fluid (CSF). Anti-myelin–associated glycoprotein antibodies were absent, indicating some specificity in the response observed. No antibody response to peripheral nerve was detected in any patient. It was concluded that MBP was likely to be the disease-relevant antigen in both the CNS and peripheral nervous system complications of rabies vaccination, the CNS complication was the human equivalent of EAE in laboratory animals, and the neuritis was akin to the Guillain-Barré syndrome.

Some years ago, a rabies vaccine prepared in suckling mouse brain was used widely in South America. The rationale was that newborn mouse brain would not provoke CNS neurologic complications, as it is unmyelinated; indeed, this proved to be the case. However, numerous cases of the Guillain-Barré syndrome were encountered.[16] The dissociation between CNS and peripheral nervous system complications observed with suckling mouse brain vaccine suggests to me that some antigen other than

MBP is likely to be responsible when the Guillain-Barré syndrome complicates rabies vaccination. Perhaps the South American vaccine was contaminated with cranial nerves. Myelination of cranial nerves precedes that of brain.

Only 1 vaccinee in 400 develops encephalomyelitis, so there must be some individually determined propensity to react to brain tissue. In MS, there is an inflammatory response directed against white matter and a genetically determined propensity to develop the disease. For these reasons, it is of interest to learn how MS patients fare when injected with brain material. Bauer[17] reported the results obtained by a Yugoslavian neurosurgeon who, for obscure reasons, transplanted porcine brain fragments to the subcutaneous abdominal fat of 24 MS patients. Neurologic complications occurred in at least five, leading in one instance to death. An additional patient developed a severe polyradiculoneuritis 11 days after swine brain implantation.[18] This patient was shown to have an immune response directed against gangliosides shared by the neural implant and his own tissues.[18]

Porcine MBP was administered to 11 MS patients by Salk et al.[19] Earlier work had established that administration of MBP could protect against development of EAE (see Treatment of Experimental Autoimmune Encephalomyelitis). The basic ideas were that MS and EAE are variant forms of the same disease, sensitivity to MBP exists in MS, and patients could be desensitized by antigen administration in the same way that subcutaneous allergen administration lessens symptoms of allergy.

There had been earlier trials of MBP treatment for MS,[20,21] but the doses given were relatively small. The authors noted neither a beneficial nor a deleterious effect, although it was remarked in one study that when questioned, patients blamed their deterioration on the treatment.[21] Salk et al. administered approximately 75 mg (sometimes more) of MBP subcutaneously daily for an indefinite period. High-titer immunoglobulin M (IgM) and IgG antibodies to MBP developed within weeks of starting treatment. Eosinophilia was universal. I point out later that an eosinophilic component to brain infiltrates has been noted in EAE in monkeys. DTH reactions developed at inoculation sites in the second and third weeks of treatment, sometimes associated with fever and, in several instances, with an accompanying CSF pleocytosis, not mentioned in the report.

Evidence of continuing disease activity to a greater or lesser degree was observed in all but two patients. One patient was admitted to the study with fulminant disease. She stabilized for a time on treatment (or despite it). Treatment was stopped when fulminant disease resumed. She promptly became quadriplegic and semicomatose and died 6 weeks later. Postmortem examination of the CNS was reported to have revealed lesions typical of severe MS.[19]

Because a brisk DTH response to MBP surfaced after 2–3 weeks of treatment, as evidenced by the development of injection site reactions after this interval, the possibility that the sensitivity observed was a primary take can be entertained (i.e., sensitivity to MBP may have developed de novo). A more prompt response might have been anticipated if MBP was the elusive antigen against which the immune response is directed in MS and if there was, for this reason, a preexisting sensitivity.

I reviewed the CNS tissue slides of the fatal case. There were multiple acute perivenular inflammatory lesions superimposed on a background of typical MS plaques (see also reference 22). The histology raised the nagging concern in my mind that EAE (or, if one will, a neuroparalytic accident) may have been superimposed onto MS in this case and perhaps to a lesser extent in others, given the CSF pleocytosis noted in several of them.

Acute Disseminated Encephalomyelitis

Acute disseminated encephalomyelitis (ADEM) is also known as *post-infectious encephalomyelitis* and *perivenous encephalomyelitis* (reviewed in references 1, 23, and 24). The illness presents as multifocal encephalitis or myelitis, or both. Onset is abrupt, with signs and symptoms pointing to damage of white matter. Headache and delirium may be followed by lethargy and coma. Focal signs include weakness or paralysis, loss of sphincter control, and sensory loss. The spinal fluid protein is usually increased, and lymphocytes, sometimes several hundred, are often (although not invariably) present. The pathologic picture is one of multiple small foci of perivenular mononuclear cell infiltration, all of like age, with demyelination that corresponds to the topography of the inflammatory infiltrates. Sometimes the inflammatory foci may be larger, even very large, and (but for their number) a not absolutely reliable criterion, indistinguishable by magnetic resonance imaging (MRI) scan from active MS lesions. The clinical and pathologic features are identical with those of rabies vaccination–induced encephalomyelitis, and I believe that the two are variants of the same basic process.

ADEM occurs throughout the world and at all ages, although children younger than 2 years are largely (and possibly totally) spared. The illness is monophasic in at least 95% of instances although the earliest recorded case (in 1790) reported two attacks, one in association with smallpox and the other in association with measles, and additional instances of recurrent ADEM have been documented over the years.[25] In former times, measles was by far the most common precipitant and, in countries with inadequate vaccination programs, this continues to be the case. ADEM usually follows the appearance of the measles rash by an interval of 5 days on average,[26] but onset may precede the rash and can be delayed for up to 2 weeks after the rash appears. The complication bears no relationship to the severity of the measles infection. Both genders are affected equally. Mortality is considerable, and 50% of survivors are left with residual deficits.

ADEM is also seen as a complication of varicella infection, rubella infection, and, in former times, smallpox.[1,27] At present, ADEM is an uncommon illness in developed countries, and most cases that do occur follow acute but nondescript upper respiratory infections.[28,29] ADEM is a recognized complication of *Mycoplasma pneumoniae* infection,[30–32] so the inciting organism need not be a virus. Once again, the severity of ADEM bears no relationship to the severity of the mycoplasmal infection. This can even be subclinical and detected only serologically. Prompt antibiotic treatment of the mycoplasmal illness does not in any way lessen the likelihood or severity of the complication. ADEM may also complicate infectious mononucleosis.[33,34]

A minority of cases occur without any evident antecedent infection. Some of these may be instances of clinically inapparent mycoplasmal infection or infectious mononucleosis. When there is no antecedent infection or if the infection is non-

descript, the distinction between ADEM and acute MS may be difficult (if not impossible) to make on clinical grounds, because MS attacks may follow respiratory infections. When CSF pleocytosis and fever are prominent, the distinction between ADEM and viral meningitis can also be difficult (if not impossible) to make on clinical grounds. MRI scan may clarify the issue.

Cell-mediated immunity and antibody to MBP can be detected in most ADEM patients studied at the onset of their disease.[35–37] ADEM is generally viewed as a human counterpart of EAE, and I share this opinion. The initial studies documenting abnormally elevated responses to MBP in ADEM were conducted in sporadic cases, one of whom had a brother with MS.[35] This left the concern that some of those who tested positive might have been experiencing a first attack of MS even though brisk T-cell responses to MBP are unusual in MS. It has long been appreciated that some cases of ADEM, perhaps as many as 20% of those with clinical diagnoses, will ultimately turn out to have MS (reviewed in reference 38). The concern with regard to the specificity of MBP sensitivity in ADEM was laid to rest when Johnson et al.[26] reported results of a study of a large series of ADEM cases that occurred during a measles outbreak in Peru. There, the diagnosis of ADEM was never in doubt. Eight of 17 cases evaluated for lymphocyte responsiveness to MBP had significant proliferative responses. Controls were uniformly negative. MBP is not the sole antigen that can cause EAE. Others include proteolipid protein (PLP) and myelin oligodendrocyte glycoprotein (MOG), as discussed later. To my knowledge, whether sensitivity to these encephalitogens is present in ADEM has never been studied.

Although the similarities in ADEM occurring on the background of different infectious illnesses outweigh the differences, there are differences nonetheless. ADEM complicating varicella is more likely to present clinically as a cerebellitis than ADEM complicating other infections, measles-induced ADEM is more likely to present as myelitis, and postvaccinial ADEM (see further on in this section) as encephalitis. Trismus was reported in 25% of cases of ADEM-complicating smallpox but has never, insofar as I am aware, ever been reported since as a feature of ADEM.[1] Curiously, ADEM-complicating smallpox most often presented as myelitis, according to the reports of the time, whereas ADEM-complicating vaccinia presented most often as encephalitis, despite the close structural similarities of the two viruses.

Given the differences in clinical presentation cited heretofore, it is possible that ADEM may occur as a response to discrete antigens in different infections, or, although reactivity to MBP may be universal, responses to additional antigens (antibodies?) may vary with the infection and determine topography of lesions and hence presentation. The notion has some attraction, given the fact that several different encephalitogens can cause EAE or contribute to demyelination in EAE, as discussed later.

Treatment of ADEM is with glucocorticoids, although their efficacy has never been subjected to formal study. Nonetheless, the mortality reported earlier by far exceeds that reported more recently, and I doubt that better nursing care accounts for it. The ability of glucocorticoids to favorably alter the natural history of ADEM, if true, may provide a point of contrast with MS. Glucocorticoids favorably affect acute symptomatology in MS but have no demonstrable beneficial effect on long-term outlook. Given the well-known ability of glucocorticoids to blunt DTH responses, their failure to alter long-term outlook in MS may argue for some process distinct from a DTH response or superimposed on it as a major operator in the pathogenesis of MS.

In the early 1920s, cases of smallpox resurfaced in western Europe, and extensive vaccination programs were undertaken. Postvaccinial encephalomyelitis had been first reported in 1860 as a curiosity, but an alarming number of cases were encountered in the United Kingdom and in Holland in the 1920s, and this became a matter of concern to public health authorities.[39,40] Postvaccinial ADEM was also reported from Germany, the Scandinavian countries, elsewhere in Europe, and the United States.[41] In France and Spain, very few cases were reported. This prompted use of Spanish vaccine in Holland, but there was no reduction in the frequency of ADEM. The finding indicated that the problem did not lie with the vaccine itself.

ADEM did not occur in children younger than age 2 years when vaccinated. A few developed an encephalopathy that would now be called *Reye's syndrome* but never a perivenous encephalomyelitis.[42,43] In the 1920s, vaccination in the first year of

life was mandatory in France and Spain but not in other countries. The complication was far more likely to be encountered on the background of a primary take than that of a secondary take. The explanation for its rarity in France and Spain related rather simply to the fact that the population had already had their primary take before the age when postvaccinial ADEM could develop. Most cases of postvaccinial ADEM occurred in children between the ages of 5–11 years, but this may be misleading in terms of relative risk, because children were far more likely than adults to be vaccinated and not to have been vaccinated previously, and numerous cases in adults are on record. The frequency varied but at times approached 1 in 1,000 vaccinees. Both genders were equally affected, including adult cases.

The clinical features were encephalitis or myelitis of brutally abrupt onset, encephalitis being by far the more common.[1,39–42] The illness began from 6 to 15 days after vaccination and most frequently on days 10–12. This time corresponded to the peak of the vaccinial reaction or more often fell just behind it. Some cases preceded the vaccination reaction peak by a few days, and others followed it by several days. There was no correlation between the intensity of the vaccinial response and either the occurrence of ADEM or its severity. Rare cases followed a secondary take that, as expected, showed precocious reactivity. Onset of ADEM was accelerated in these cases. Mortality in postvaccinial ADEM ranged from 20% to 50%, but recovery was remarkably complete in the vast majority of survivors despite the alarming nature with which their illness had presented—a point of contrast with ADEM-complicating measles. Virus could not be recovered from the CNS despite the fact that vaccinia is easy to propagate.

The pathologic features in patients dying within a few days of onset of their illness were indistinguishable from those of ADEM associated with other infectious processes. Multiple inflammatory perivenular infiltrates with substantial demyelination at sites of inflammation were noted.[44–48] Importantly, in patients dying within 24 hours of onset, inflammatory foci were duly noted, but demyelination was minimal or undetectable. This finding presaged the recognition many years later that an abrupt interruption of axonal function in demyelinating diseases can precede demyelination.

Of course, we now know that cytokines and nitric oxide (NO), released by invading inflammatory cells, can directly affect axonal function adversely and abruptly. Several patients with postvaccinial ADEM and clinically complete recovery died years later for sundry reasons and came to autopsy. Little was found and, in particular, there was no or, at best, minimal evidence of demyelination. Clearly, extensive remyelination had occurred.

Hurst[49] described acute necrotizing hemorrhagic leukoencephalitis (ANHL) in 1941, and several confirming reports appeared shortly thereafter.[50–52] The condition is rare but has unique features. Within a few days of a seemingly banal "influenza-like" infectious illness or a gastrointestinal upset, an encephalopathic process of apopleptic onset ensues with fever, neutrophilia, stiff neck, headache, and confusion that transitions quickly into stupor and then coma. Hemiplegia or quadriplegia quickly follows, and the condition is fatal within hours to a few days. The clinical picture resembles that of ADEM, save for the intensity of the process, its speed of progression, and its dismal outcome.

The spinal fluid shows neutrophils, often several hundred or even a few thousand; lymphocytes; red blood cells; and elevated protein with or without xanthochromia. Most cases have occurred in young adults; the genders are represented equally. Cases complicating varicella,[53] measles,[54] and smallpox vaccination[55] have been recorded, pointing to a tight link between ANHL and ADEM.

Pathologic examination reveals hemorrhagic areas, perivascular mononuclear and polymorphonuclear infiltrates, extensive exudation of fibrin, and frank necrosis of vessels. Extensive areas of white matter may be involved. Areas of demyelination surround small blood vessels or hemorrhagic areas, or both; massive necrosis and fibrinoid degeneration of blood vessels are prominent features.

The pathology mimics that of ADEM onto which a localized Shwartzman reaction has been superimposed. The situation can be duplicated experimentally by inducing a Shwartzman reaction in animals about to succumb to EAE[56] or by administering pertussis vaccine to rats during the induction phase of EAE so as to induce "hyperacute" EAE.[57–59] Adoptive transfer of EAE to virgin recipients given lymph node cells from rats with hyperacute EAE leads to ordinary EAE in the recipients.

Rarely, ANHL may be confined to the spinal cord,[60] and, extremely rarely, it may be superimposed onto MS on the background of a very recent respiratory illness.[61] In the only case that to my knowledge was studied in this way, a lymphocyte proliferative response after exposure to MBP, akin to that seen in ADEM, was demonstrated.[35] I draw attention to ANHL, despite its rarity, to signal that (1) a second process can be superimposed onto the initial one in demyelinating diseases, (2) demyelinating processes may have two or more distinct components contributing to their etiology, and (3) rare entities may represent a concurrence of two or more less rare entities.

Experimental Autoimmune Encephalomyelitis

In 1933, Rivers et al.[62] published the first convincing description of EAE. A more detailed follow-up study appeared 2 years later.[63] In essence, Rivers and his colleagues duplicated the Pasteur technique. As noted, the Pasteur technique consisted of a series of 14–20 daily subcutaneous injections of rabbit brain or spinal cord material containing killed rabies virus. Rivers and his colleagues administered a series of intramuscular injections of rabbit brain tissue to half-grown rhesus monkeys thrice weekly over a period of months. The monkeys were given intramuscular injections of aqueous emulsions of ground rabbit brain and alcohol-ether extracts of rabbit brain on an alternating schedule. After receiving 44–86 injections, the monkeys became sick with an inflammatory demyelinating disease.

As is often the case, this seminal study was met with indifference. Rivers lamented that what he viewed as his most important work was being ignored and, indeed, the first confirming paper did not appear until 1940.[64] With the passage of time, Rivers has been fully vindicated. EAE, the first described experimental autoimmune disease—thanks to Rivers—has become the most extensively studied of such diseases. Several thousand studies devoted to the unmasking of the mechanisms responsible for the genesis of EAE are currently extant.

The monkeys in the Rivers study showed extensive confluent areas of "moth-eaten" myelin loss in the cortex, brainstem, cerebellum, optic nerves, and, to a lesser extent, in the spinal cord. They were sacrificed shortly after the onset of clinical symptoms so that, given the considerable size of the demyelinated lesions observed, the process must have been ongoing for some time, and much damage must have accumulated before the illness declared itself clinically. Exactly the same sequence of events occurs in MS. This became evident only some 50 years later with the introduction of MRI scanning.

Perivascular infiltrates with a mononuclear predominance and loss of myelin sheaths with relative preservation of axons were noted on microscopic examination. Eosinophils were singled out as well, with the wisdom of retrospection an indication that the process was not purely and simply what would now be called a *Th1-type T-cell response*. Spinal fluid showed anywhere from 8 to 280 cells with a mononuclear cell predominance but with substantial numbers of polymorphonuclear cells as well. On a whimsical note, typical of the scientific writing of the era, we are informed that the monkeys ate bananas or oranges for breakfast and bread for lunch, were served heated milk for supper, and were given raw carrots and roasted peanuts periodically as a special treat.

Rivers hinted that his finding might provide a model for rabies vaccination–induced encephalomyelitis and for ADEM but chose not to take a stand. In his confirming reports, Ferraro and various colleagues[64–68] were bolder and argued that the process had to be an allergic reaction. Ferraro also drew attention to the fact that the process in monkeys could be acute, chronic, relapsing-remitting, or hemorrhagic.[66–68] It had been known since the 1920s that the brain contains organ-specific antigens that are not species specific, and there was a substantial earlier literature on anti-brain antibodies, although no disease was seen in animals with such antibodies nor did adoptive transfer of brain antibodies cause disease. Arthus-type reactions were known to be readily inducible in brain when animals, immunized systemically with a soluble protein antigen and with circulating antibodies to the immunogen, were given the immunogen intracisternally. The pathology of the Arthus reaction is that of a vasculitis and is totally different from that of EAE, but the principle that antibodies could cause brain disease had been established. It was natural, therefore, for Ferraro to assume that autoallergic encephalomyelitis was antibody mediated. As we shall see, he may not have been altogether wrong.

The next major advance came with the introduction of Freund's adjuvant. This development accelerated and simplified the induction of EAE and permitted its study in other species at reduced expense. Jules Freund was Hungarian. His compatriot, Louis Dienes, told me that he provided Freund with the basic idea for Freund's adjuvant. This was acknowledged by Freund. Dienes observed that injecting a protein such as egg white (i.e., egg albumin and conalbumin) into a tuberculous focus, even one containing killed tubercle bacilli, greatly augmented the magnitude of the antibody response generated in response to the egg white. More important, the injection led to the appearance of a tuberculin-type reaction to egg white in immunized animals when the egg white and tubercle bacilli were injected subcutaneously.[69] Onset of tuberculin-type hypersensitivity preceded that of antibody and, in animals with anti–egg white antibody, the magnitude of the tuberculin-type response and the antibody titer failed to correlate.

Dienes and Mallory[70] published an account of the histology of the tuberculin-type skin reaction to egg white and compared it to that seen in cutaneous anaphylaxis. They pointed out that large mononuclear phagocyte infiltration preceded the onset of inflammation and accordingly could not be a reaction to it; edema was absent or minimal, in contrast to antibody-mediated skin reactions; polymorphonuclear cells were present only if there was superimposed necrosis; and delayed skin reactivity could be seen before any circulating antibody could be detected. They stated, "It appears probable that we are dealing with an altered tissue reactivity as specific to the protein antigen arousing it as are the usual serum reactions" and went on to suggest that the "antibody" might be fixed to cells.[69] Remarkably, this occurred in 1932.

Freund's insight was to incorporate the tubercle bacilli in oil and to add an emulsifying agent so that water-soluble antigens could be incorporated into a water-in-oil emulsion.[71] How Freund's adjuvant worked was a mystery for many years. The muramyl peptides of *Mycobacterium tuberculosis* are now known to stimulate the prompt release of cytokines, such as interleukin-12 (IL-12), that drive immune responses along the Th1-type T-cell path. This polarization of the immune response toward a DTH response has obvious advantages for the rapid induction of acute EAE in a reproducible manner but may have an inadvertently polarized opinion as well.

In 1947, Kabat et al.[72] and Morgan,[73] working independently, reported the rapid induction of allergic encephalomyelitis in rhesus monkeys given monkey brain tissue in Freund's adjuvant 2–7 weeks earlier. In that same year, Kabat became the first recipient of a grant in the amount of $10,725 from the newly founded National Multiple Sclerosis Society. I believe he gave value for money: Perivenular infiltrates with mononuclear cells, demyelination, and axonal sparing were duly noted,[72–74] as were relapses and remissions. Notably, almost every monkey developed EAE. Interestingly, dorsal root ganglia are involved in monkeys with EAE,[67] a point of contrast with MS. Animals immunized with fetal (i.e., unmyelinated) brain did not develop disease.

Also in 1947, Freund et al.[75] reported EAE in guinea pigs after a single injection of brain and mycobacteria in water-in-oil emulsion. Although the guinea pigs became acutely ill, usually with a rapidly fatal paraplegia, and perivascular infiltrates with lymphoid cells were prominent, demyelination was reported as totally absent. Subsequent study has documented that a limited amount of demyelination does occur in guinea pigs with acute EAE.[76,77] The minimal (or absent) demyelination seen in guinea pigs with paralytic disease indicated that demyelination was not a sine qua non for EAE symptomatology. It reinforced the hint provided earlier by the finding that demyelination was lacking in children dying acutely from postvaccinial ADEM. The finding also suggested that the demyelinative component of EAE might involve something above and beyond the DTH that guinea pigs are known to develop to a marked degree but that nonetheless fails to protect them from tuberculosis.

EAE was induced in numerous other species in short order, including rats, mice, rabbits, dogs, chickens, and others (reviewed in reference 78). It was quickly established that white matter contained the encephalitogen; white matter from every mammalian and avian species tested was encephalitogenic, whereas myelin from amphibians and fish was not; fetal mammalian white matter lacking myelin was not encephalitogenic; and even a brain

biopsy sample from a monkey could be used to induce EAE in that same monkey.[79] It also soon became evident that the clinical features varied among species, as did the topography of lesions.[78,80]

In 1951, Waksman and Morrison[81] showed that rabbits immunized with whole spinal cord in adjuvant developed skin test positivity to proteolipid (see later) before the onset of clinical symptoms and that skin test intensity, unlike anti-brain antibody titers, correlated with the severity of subsequent clinical disease. The idea that cells might be the vectors of tissue damage was beginning to take hold. The proof of this notion required the successful adoptive transfer of disease with cells alone. However, initial attempts to do so failed.

Adoptive Transfer of Experimental Autoimmune Encephalomyelitis

The first successful transfer of tuberculin sensitivity was reported in 1910.[82] Transfer was achieved with whole blood but not with serum, suggesting a role for the formed elements of the blood rather than for antibody. The study was ignored. The next successful transfer of tuberculin sensitivity was reported by Chase[83] in 1945. Chase immunized guinea pigs with killed tubercle bacilli in mineral oil. Five weeks later, peritoneal exudate cells were harvested, and cells from 2 to 10 donors were given intraperitoneally or intravenously to individual recipients. Tuberculin was injected intradermally at the time of cell transfer, and positivity was observed 20–36 hours after intravenous transfer and 2–3 days after intraperitoneal transfer. Without providing details, Chase commented that lymph node and spleen cells would also transfer tuberculin sensitivity. Tellingly, he noted that the duration of transferability was extremely brief. The guinea pigs were outbred, and recipients promptly rejected the donated cells. Cellular transfer of EAE in outbred animals failed initially, because the transferred cells were eliminated before they could cause disease.

Lipton and Freund[84] reported the first successful transfer of EAE in 1953 using parabiont rat pairs. One of the pair had EAE, and these authors obtained histologic evidence for EAE in the other. Parabionts share blood supply through anastomotic vessels. This experiment could not distinguish between transfer via cells and transfer via antibody, but, given numerous failed prior attempts to transfer disease with antibodies, the study strongly suggested a role for cells.

Åström and Waksman[78,85] and Paterson[86] solved the adoptive transfer problem independently. Åström and Waksman gave recipient rabbits 400 rad of whole-body irradiation 1–8 days before cell transfer. This procedure retarded the rejection of injected cells. In addition, although the fact was not appreciated at the time, low-dose radiation kills host regulatory T cells selectively and for this reason facilitates adoptive transfer of disease.[87–90] Paterson chose to inject newborn rats with the spleen cells of future donor rats so as to induce immunologic tolerance. He immunized the spleen cell donors once the tolerized rats were grown and transferred donor cells into tolerized recipients. The cells were not rejected and caused disease in the recipients.

Adoptive transfer of disease was next accomplished in inbred strains that could not reject donor cells of their same strain. Inbred guinea pig strains were developed at the National Institutes of Health in Bethesda. One such strain, known as *strain 13*, proved to be susceptible to EAE, and Stone adoptively transferred EAE in this strain in 1961.[91] When inbred Lewis rats became available, they were found to be susceptible to a single episode of EAE, and Koprowski[92] reported adoptive transfer of EAE in them. As were the donors, recovered recipients were resistant to a second attack when immunized in the standard fashion. It subsequently was observed that recipients could be brought down with a second attack of adoptively transferred disease. This finding indicated that host restraint mechanisms worked better before cells became activated than once they had been activated.

In 1971, Werdelin and McCluskey[93] developed EAE and allergic adrenalitis in Lewis rats. They then adoptively transferred lymph node cells. Recipients had thermal injury lesions placed on the brain or on the adrenal surface, as this maneuver had been shown to facilitate cell homing.[94] Cells from EAE donors homed quickly to the area beneath the brain lesion; cells from adrenalitis donors homed to the adrenal. Donor cells were identifiable, because they had been labeled with thymidine or with adenosine in vitro. Cells that labeled with thymidine accumulated preferentially over adenosine-labeled cells, indicating that dividing cells homed best.

Mixed populations from adrenalitis and EAE donors were studied next. Cells from one or the other were labeled. Labeled cells from either donor accumulated to a comparable extent in either organ (i.e., recruitment was of activated proliferating cells but was far from antigen specific), a finding subsequently confirmed by Karin et al.,[95] who documented early specificity followed by extensive nonspecificity of CNS-invading T cells.

Recipients were then irradiated with 800 rad 5 days before transfer. Transferred cells did not accumulate in brain or adrenal, pointing to some host cell–derived facilitator of cell migration. When the bone marrow was shielded, lesions were once again seen, suggesting that a bone marrow–derived cell was the facilitator. That this was the case was established when irradiated recipients were injected immediately with bone marrow cells, and donor lymph node cells were transferred 5 days later. Typical lesions were observed. The finding pointed to a role for monocytes or for cytokines released by them in the initiation of adoptively transferred DTH responses.

Because the target organs had been heat treated, there remained the concern that the blood-brain barrier (BBB) beneath the heat lesions might have been compromised and that the findings might not be representative of what happened in the intact brain. This concern was set to rest by Wekerle et al.,[96] who extended the earlier results using animals with an intact BBB and also established that the CNS is constantly patrolled by low numbers of activated T cells. They also reported that intrathecally injected purified T cells would not transfer EAE. In earlier studies, intrathecal injections of cruder cell preparations did cause adoptively transferred disease,[85] indicating yet again a need for cooperation between cell types. The findings pointed to (1) a host cell contribution in the periphery under ordinary circumstances (or within the CNS under extraordinary circumstances) to the initiation of adoptively transferred disease and (2) a priming signal for T cells provided before entry into the CNS or perhaps provided by monocyte-primed CNS endothelial cells as the T cells traverse them.

CD4 and CD8 T cells home to the CNS.[97] B cells reportedly migrate poorly to the CNS in EAE,[97] yet some obviously find their way there in EAE, as in MS, as witnessed by the appearance of oligoclonal bands of IgG in the CSF in both diseases. Red blood cells and polymorphonuclear cells are not found in EAE lesions. It follows that migration cannot be passive, as would be expected if cell access to the CNS simply reflected a disruption of the tight junctions that join CNS endothelial cells one to the next, a point to which I will return.

Kosunen et al.[98] injected radiolabeled thymidine into rats before the onset of EAE so as to label dividing cells in the periphery. They documented that cells that had undergone multiple cycles of proliferation, as judged by dilution of label over time, accumulated preferentially in EAE lesions. Only large lymphocytes were labeled. In animals with disease ongoing for several days, cells in new lesions showed labeling less intense than that in cells in older lesions, indicating that infiltrating cells continued to proliferate in the periphery even after onset of disease, but they did so only transiently, if at all, once they had entered the CNS. The observation provides a possible point of contrast with DTH reactions at other sites. Kosunen et al.[99] showed brisk proliferative responses in situ by cells that had invaded the reaction site in DTH reactions in the skin. The issue is not trivial. T cells that enter the CNS do not remain there for long. If their specificity is for non-CNS antigens, they leave.[100] If their specificity is for CNS antigens, they remain, but their life span is limited, and they die by apoptosis. Some macrophages in the EAE lesions were labeled consistent with the derivation of precursor monocytes from a rapidly dividing bone marrow precursor pool.

Griscelli et al.[101] showed that when activated lymphocytes from gastrointestinal tract lymph nodes are injected systemically, they home selectively to gastrointestinal tract lymph nodes, whereas lymphocytes from lymph nodes draining the skin migrate preferentially to lymph nodes that drain the skin (see also references 102 and 103). EAE is induced by immunization protocols that activate lymphocytes in peripheral lymph nodes that drain the skin. It is obvious that T cells from such nodes can home to the CNS. Whether gastrointestinal tract–stimulated T cells can do so to the same extent remains an unresolved issue. The fact that orally administered MBP can protect in EAE suggests that they may well do so, but that does not prove the point.

Female animals are more susceptible to EAE than are males. Women are twice as likely to develop MS as men. It is sometimes argued that the gender difference in autoimmune processes reflects an increased T-cell responsiveness in females as compared to males. Adoptively transferred EAE requires activated donor T cells to be sure, but it also requires a contribution by host monocytes and macrophages. EAE does not develop in animals depleted of monocytes.[104] Adoptively transferred EAE is more severe in females than in males, given the same number of cells from the same donor. The finding argues that female host cells contribute to the adoptive transfer EAE process to a greater extent than do male host cells and that these contributions determine disease severity, at least in part. The finding suggests that monocyte functions, presumably including relative levels of cytokine secretion, differ between males and females, and they play a role in determining the severity of EAE. Might differences in monocyte function between the genders also bear on MS? I am unaware of studies that bear on this issue.

Adoptive transfer of EAE was shown to be facilitated by two maneuvers. Exposure of cells to the disease-inciting antigen in vitro led to their activation, even when cell proliferation was blocked, and, accordingly, it became evident that only activated cells could cause EAE.[105] It was also shown that simply driving host T cells through a cycle of proliferation with a T-cell mitogen and nonspecifically activating them in this manner[106] drastically reduced the number of cells required to transfer disease adoptively and even permitted transfer of disease with lymphocytes from animals that were recovered from EAE and were themselves refractory to a second attack of disease. This finding established that memory T cells with the potential to cause EAE are present in recovered animals and further indicated that the memory cells are somehow held in check in the milieu of the recovered animal. The finding bears on MS attacks triggered by viral infectious illnesses[107] wherein cytokines released by cells responding to the virus are thought to kindle memory T cells that then cause attacks. This kindling of effector T cells is likely to be accompanied by, or facilitated by, a compromise of restraint mechanisms as a second consequence of viral infection, and, indeed, CD8 "suppressor" cell function is defective at times of MS attacks. MS relapses run a finite course. Presumably, the ending of an attack bespeaks a reestablishment of check mechanisms. CD8 suppressor function rebounds as attacks end.

Next came the demonstration that CD4-type T cells were responsible for transfer.[88,100,108] Development of T-cell lines and clones with specificity for encephalitogenic peptides and documentation that they could adoptively transfer disease provided a further advance.[109] The recognition that CD4 T cells could be subdivided into Th1 and Th2 subsets was followed by the demonstration that cells of the Th1 subset could transfer disease, whereas cells of the Th2 subset could not (reviewed in reference 110). These aspects and subsequent developments are discussed elsewhere in this volume.

Genetics of Experimental Autoimmune Encephalomyelitis

As mentioned, strain 13 guinea pigs are susceptible to EAE. A second inbred strain, known as *strain 2*, proved resistant to EAE. These findings provided compelling evidence for a genetically determined propensity to develop disease and provided a possible explanation for why, as all had noticed, only a proportion of outbred rats, mice, or guinea pigs would develop EAE. The situation is to be contrasted with that observed in laboratory rhesus monkeys, almost all of whom are susceptible to EAE. Perhaps they are more inbred than is commonly thought. That there was a genetically determined component to susceptibility to develop EAE had actually been anticipated by seldom-cited earlier work.

Olitsky, Lee, and various colleagues[111–115] undertook studies of EAE in inbred mice in the late 1940s and early 1950s. They had access to mice bred by Webster for susceptibility or resistance to salmonella and for susceptibility or resistance to St. Louis encephalitis. The colony, established in 1929,[116] had been carried through brother-sister matings for well more than two decades. Four inbred strains were available, known as *BSVS* (for bacteria-sensitive and virus-sensitive), *BRVR* (bacteria-resistant and virus-resistant), *BSVR* (for bacteria-sensitive and virus-resistant), and *BRVS* (for bacteria-resistant and virus-sensitive). BSVS mice were largely (not always) susceptible to EAE. BRVR mice were largely (not always) resistant.[112,114] The other two strains showed intermediate sensitivity. This experiment documented the existence of a genetically

determined susceptibility to EAE within a given species. "Proteolipid" in complete Freund's adjuvant was given to induce disease. The mice were also injected with *Haemophilus pertussis* vaccine, a second adjuvant introduced by these workers to facilitate induction of EAE.[113]

Lee et al.[112] generated (BSVS × BRVR) F1 mice. The F1 mice were resistant to EAE, indicating that BRVR mice carried one or more EAE resistance factors. They did further backcrosses to BSVS mice and concluded that BRVR mice carried two distinct, independently segregating, dominant disease resistance factors and that either sufficed to protect from EAE. Susceptibility or resistance to EAE bore no relationship to ability to form antibodies, except that BSVS mice were sensitive to anaphylaxis, whereas BRVR mice were not.[114]

Along the same lines, Perlik and Zidek[117] conducted a limited study of genetic susceptibility to EAE in rats. These authors crossed EAE-susceptible Lewis rats with EAE-resistant AVN rats. The F1 rats were resistant to EAE but remained susceptible to adjuvant arthritis. Perlik and Zidek concluded that a dominant resistance factor, with some specificity for EAE, was present in AVN rats. These results are to be contrasted with those obtained by Williams and Moore,[12] who crossed EAE-sensitive Lewis rats with EAE-resistant Brown Norway rats. F1 rats were fully or almost fully susceptible, and a series of backcross experiments showed that susceptibility to EAE in the Lewis rat was linked to the major histocompatibility complex (MHC) locus, a finding amply confirmed by subsequent gene-mapping studies. That Brown Norway rats, unlike AVN rats, may lack a dominant protective allele seems distinctly possible, inasmuch as they can be brought down with EAE when a modified adjuvant and immunization route are used.[118]

Levine and Sowinski[119] documented that several strains of mice were susceptible to EAE but to varying degrees, suggesting hierarchical levels of susceptibility. In addition, by using strains that shared MHC identity, these authors found some strains that were susceptible to EAE and others that were resistant.[120] Similar results were obtained independently by Gasser et al.[121] It was concluded that inheritance of susceptibility to EAE is polygenic and that MHC endowment alone does not suffice.

Bernard[122] studied the genetics of EAE in mice and likewise concluded that susceptibility to EAE was determined only in part by the MHC. He found antibodies to MBP in all susceptible strains and in some (but not all) resistant strains. DTH responsiveness to MBP was found in all susceptible strains and not in resistant strains, although both susceptible and resistant strains developed brisk DTH responses to PPD. Earlier, Wilkie et al.[123] had shown that cutaneous DTH reactions to an acid-soluble protein extract of brain (the active ingredient of which was almost surely MBP) peaked before disease onset in susceptible guinea pigs and that EAE-resistant strain 2 guinea pigs did not develop skin sensitivity to acid-soluble brain protein extracts.[123] Yet, strain 2 guinea pigs developed brisk skin responses to PPD and to human serum albumin.[123]

From the foregoing findings, the basic principles of the immunogenetics of EAE emerged. These were that (1) the MHC has a major role but does not act alone; (2) inheritance of susceptibility is both hierarchical and antigen specific, and antigen specificity is probably tied to MHC endowment; (3) multiple genes are involved; and (4) there are protective and susceptibility alleles. In outbred populations, such as humans, protective alleles for MS would be difficult to detect.

Immune Mechanisms in Experimental Autoimmune Encephalomyelitis

Although it was evident from the outset that EAE was an inflammatory disease, it is perhaps difficult for the contemporary reader to fathom the ignorance that prevailed in the middle years of the last century concerning immune mechanisms. Which cells made antibody and how they did so were subjects of vituperative debate. The functions of lymphocytes were unknown. Phagocytosis by polymorphonuclear cells and by macrophages had been recognized from the time of Metchnikoff but was viewed, and totally so, as a means of defense and not as a means of attack. That antibodies could cause damage of free-floating blood cells had been established largely on the basis of Landsteiner's work with blood groups. The existence of tissue-specific antibodies directed against solid organs had been amply documented, but none had been shown to cause disease. The phenomenon of what is now called the *DTH phenomenon* had been recognized since the time of Robert Koch and exploited

diagnostically in the tuberculin reaction, but how tuberculin sensitivity developed, why it developed, and what its biological significance was were unanswered questions.

In the summer of 1959, I interrupted my neurology residency to begin work in the laboratory of Byron Waksman. The group there was studying antisera directed against lymphocytes, and I was plugged into this project. It soon became evident that animals treated with antilymphocyte antibodies were protected from EAE, and, for this reason, lymphocytes somehow had to be implicated in the disease.[124] Our antibody preparations were crude, but they established proof of principle. As improved methods for making and purifying antibodies developed over the years, and especially with the development of monoclonal antibody technology, it became possible to develop antibodies directed in a highly specific manner against lymphocytes (and, subsequently, against subsets of lymphocytes) and to use them for research purposes, for diagnostic purposes, and in human therapeutics. Their use continues to this day.

In 1956, Bruce Glick, a veterinarian, reported that chickens from which he had removed the bursa of Fabricius at birth were unable to mount antibody responses.[125] The *bursa of Fabricius* is an outpouching of the cloaca found in fowl but not in mammals. It became evident on the basis of this seminal work that the bursa was the site in which antibody-producing cells matured in birds. Hence came the B-cell name. In mammals, B cells mature in the bone marrow. By happenstance, bone marrow also begins with a *b* in the English language, and the name has stuck.

At that time, the thymus was widely viewed as a vestigial organ. Yet, given its large size at birth and the fact that it contained most of the lymphocytes in the body in the early weeks of life in rodents, it occurred to me, Byron Waksman, and Branislav Janković (a Yugoslavian immunologist who had joined the laboratory) that it might be interesting to remove the thymus at birth and see what happened to immune responses. I did the surgeries, and collectively we documented that rats thymectomized at birth were substantially protected against EAE.[126,127] Some years later, Gonatos and Howard[128] combined thymectomy with irradiation followed by reconstitution with bone marrow followed, in turn, by thoracic duct drainage. These authors succeeded in depleting what were by this time recognized as T cells to an extent beyond what we had been able to achieve. Protection from EAE was total.[128]

We showed in 1962 that some antibody responses were deficient in thymectomized rats, a finding that anticipated by some years the discovery of the role of helper T cells in the generation of what are now called *T-cell–dependent antibody responses*.[129] We also documented that there were regions in the lymph nodes and spleens of thymectomized rats from which lymphocytes were absent.[130] These regions subsequently came to be known as the *thymus-dependent areas*.

It turned out, although we did not know it at the time, that Miller[131] in London and Good et al.[132] in Minneapolis had also been studying immune function in thymectomized animals with results similar to ours. Their work and our own and the work on the bursa of Fabricius already mentioned brought to the fore the notion that there were discrete populations of lymphocytes with distinct functions, and a population that was present in the thymus at birth was responsible for EAE. The finding that agammaglobulinemic children totally lacking antibodies were capable of controlling viral infections and of developing DTH responses also had a considerable role in shaping opinion.

Birds have both a bursa of Fabricius and a thymus. Janković et al.[133] removed one or the other at birth and showed that chickens lacking a bursa developed EAE normally, perhaps even precociously, despite markedly reduced immunoglobulin levels, whereas those lacking a thymus had acute disease of reduced severity. The findings were not totally clear-cut, but they strongly suggested no obligatory role for antibody in the initial stages of EAE. In a subsequent study, bursectomy was combined with total body irradiation with 650 rad. Completely agammaglobulinemic birds were generated.[134] They developed EAE, thus confirming and extending the observations of Janković and his colleagues.

At this juncture, it seemed clear that EAE was mediated by lymphocytes of thymic origin. The issues then became as follows:

1. What was the antigen in nervous tissue against which the immune response was being generated?
2. What was the mechanism by which lymphocytes damaged the CNS?

3. How could the process be prevented or controlled?
4. What was the relevance of any of these factors for MS?

I deal with the search for the antigen first.

Encephalitogens. MBP constitutes some 30% of the protein of CNS myelin and was the first encephalitogen proven to be in cause in EAE. Nowadays, a high-school student working in the laboratory for the summer can purify MBP without difficulty, but, at the moment when several groups began to attack the problem of identifying and purifying the EAE encephalitogen, the challenges were daunting, to say the least. No one had ever succeeded in generating a DTH response to a sugar even though antibodies to sugars are easily obtained (reviewed in reference 135). The reason, so evident today given the structure of the MHC alleles and the T-cell receptor, was completely unknown at the time. Nonetheless, sugars as potential antigens were set aside early, and attention turned almost from the outset to the proteins of myelin, as it was clear that only proteins or haptens that bound to proteins induced DTH responses.[135] There was, however, the concern that the encephalitogen resisted boiling, a procedure that seriously damages most proteins. Antibody binding to heat-denatured proteins is usually seriously compromised (if not abolished), and the notion that DTH responses depended on something structurally akin to antibody was widely held.

The role of lipids was also unclear, and, in early reports, lipid preparations were reported to induce EAE, doubtless (in retrospect) because they contained contaminating protein. Similarly, proteins prepared from myelin were usually contaminated with lipid, leaving the issue in doubt as to just what, in this or that fraction, was responsible when a positive result was obtained.

Further complicating the issue, although not appreciated initially, was the fact that the lipid extraction procedures in use at the time seldom neutralized the proteases of myelin so that MBP was cleaved into various small peptides. Some peptides were encephalitogenic, and some were not. Confusion reigned for some years. Much credit for the identification of MBP as an encephalitogen in EAE must go to Kies and her team[136–139] working at the National Institutes of Health and to Alvord, who developed a technique for quantitating EAE severity and who used it to test the relative potencies of innumerable samples provided by the National Institutes of Health team.[136,138] Others who made major early contributions to the solving of this problem included Carnegie and Lumsden,[140–144] Kibler and Shapira,[145,146] and Nakao and Roboz-Einstein,[147–149] to name only some.

Kies recognized that when myelin lipids were extracted with chloroform-methanol, proteases were neutralized and intact MBP could be obtained. MBP is highly basic, and it developed that it could be solubilized by treatment with acid. These insights permitted recovery of intact MBP rather than protease-cleaved fractions thereof. MBP was then purified by column chromatography. With purified material at hand, it became possible to solve the sequence of MBP. Major contributors to the working out of the sequence of MBP were Eylar and colleagues[150–152] and many others (reviewed in reference 153).

It next developed that there were antigen-specific epitopes within MBP that could be synthesized. The epitopes were remarkably small, some not more than 10 amino acids in length. The nature of the T-cell receptor was completely unknown at the time, so it seemed surprising that a small linear array of amino acids would be antigenic, given that the putative T-cell receptor was viewed as similar, in all probability, to antibody, known to recognize three-dimensional configuration rather than linear sequence. Much was made of the open linear configuration of MBP as a way of explaining this seeming paradox.[153] Retrospectively, it is evident that the properties of the T-cell receptor and MHC-binding sites were being delineated by the systematic study of the amino acid sequences of peptides capable of binding to them. Beyond this, Hashim and Eylar[154–156] mutated the various amino acids in one of the encephalitogenic peptides and determined that only some residues were critical for encephalitogenicity, whereas others were not. These authors even showed that certain substitutions led to a peptide that was protective rather than encephalitogenic some 15 years before the degeneracy of the T-cell receptor became an established fact.

The second encephalitogen to be identified in EAE was PLP. PLP constitutes 50% of the total protein of myelin. Here, again, the history is checkered. The first reports that proteolipid-containing fractions were encephalitogenic were published in 1952 by Olitsky and Tal[157] and in 1954 by Waksman et al.[158] Interestingly and presciently, Waksman concluded that there had to be a second encephalitogen in addition to PLP.[159] With the discovery that MBP was *the* encephalitogen and presumably the *sole* encephalitogen, the prevailing view became that those proteolipid fractions that had been shown to induce EAE must have been contaminated with small amounts of MBP. The contention was impossible to refute at the time.

Working at the McLean Hospital in Boston, Folch-Pi and Lees developed a method to purify PLP, a remarkable achievement given its water insolubility and the methodologic problems involved in working with preparations that contain 70% lipid. (The interested reader may wish to consult Lees' delightful retrospective concerning the purification of PLP[160] and how it came to be recognized as one of the antigens capable of inducing EAE.)

Solomon and I briefly studied purified PLP provided to us by Lees. We satisfied ourselves that it was encephalitogenic and drew this to her attention.[160] On the basis of our findings, she and her collaborators returned to the PLP encephalitogenicity problem after a hiatus of 15 years. They were able to induce severe EAE in rabbits immunized with PLP.[160–163] Subsequently, Tabira and his collaborators[164–167] documented that PLP could induce EAE in guinea pigs,[164] rats,[165] and mice[166,167] and that PLP-responsive T-cell lines would transfer EAE.[167] Tuohy et al.[168] synthesized PLP peptides that caused disease. PLP-induced EAE shows diverse T-cell receptor Vβ gene usage, a point of contrast with MBP-induced disease in which T-cell receptor Vβ gene usage is restricted. Mouse strains resistant to MBP-induced EAE may be susceptible to PLP-induced EAE and vice versa. As with MBP, different epitopes may be responded to by different species and by different strains within the same species.[169]

The third major encephalitogenic protein is MOG. This protein was identified by Linington et al.[170] using a monoclonal antibody that Linington had generated.[170] The antibody was used in combination with MBP-sensitive T cells in adoptive transfer studies of EAE. T cells alone caused inflammation, and antibody alone caused nothing, but the combination produced extensive demyelination.[171] Demyelination was observed within 24 hours of antibody administration. The lesions evolved with remarkable rapidity, maximum size being achieved within 6 days. Antibody was detected within macrophages, providing evidence for intake of immune complexes. Later work documented T-cell responsiveness to a region of MOG. T-cell lines specific for MOG caused inflammation but no clinically evident disease.[172] Combination of T cells with antibody to MOG caused demyelination and clinical symptoms. Subsequently, successful induction of frank EAE in Lewis rats and in several mouse strains immunized with MOG was achieved.[173–176] The important point is that the DTH response to MOG is directed against a different part of the molecule than is the antibody response to MOG and that the two synergize to produce demyelination. It has been reported that response to MOG is common in MS, suggesting it as a candidate antigen in this disease.[173]

Mechanisms Involved in Delayed-Type Hypersensitivity Reactions. In 1928, Rich and Lewis[177] noted that cultured blood cells from tuberculous patients failed to migrate in tissue culture when exposed to OT, whereas cells from controls did so. These authors took the failure to migrate as evidence for cell death, and the observation lay fallow for many years. In 1962, George and Vaughan[178] had the wit to centrifuge peritoneal exudate cells from tuberculin-sensitive guinea pigs in microcapillary tubes, to seal the bottom of the tubes, to cut the tubes at the interface between the cells and the supernatant, and to lay the tubes in culture medium. Monocytes migrated out of the tubes in a fanlike configuration. Migration was drastically curtailed if cultured cells from sensitized donors were exposed to PPD. As a control, animals were immunized so as to generate high-titer antibody to egg albumin. Migration was not inhibited by exposure of cultured cells from egg albumin–sensitized guinea pigs to anti–egg albumin antibody, demonstrating that antibody was not responsible for migration inhibition and that the phenomenon depended on a DTH response. This was the origin of the migration inhibition assay for delayed hypersensitivity.

Shortly thereafter, David and Paterson[179] showed that migration out of capillary tubes of monocytes

from EAE rats was inhibited by exposure to MBP. David[180,181] then mixed purified lymphocytes from a sensitized donor with monocytes from an unsensitized donor and added antigen. Migration was inhibited, establishing that lymphocytes somehow signaled monocytes. Next, David added culture supernatants from antigen-exposed lymphocytes, and again migration was inhibited[180] (see also references 182–184). Clearly the lymphocytes were providing a signal by means of a soluble factor. The factor came to be known as the *migration inhibition factor*. Inhibitors of protein synthesis blocked expression of the factor, indicating that it was newly synthesized in response to exposure to antigen. Through use of fractionation techniques, migration inhibition factor was shown to have a molecular weight much lower than that of immunoglobulin. Purification proved difficult because of the minuscule amounts present. In fact, migration inhibition factor was not purified until its molecular cloning in 1989.[185]

Numerous other in vitro assays to assess lymphocyte function were developed in short order. These included assays for a soluble factor released by antigen-exposed lymphocytes that was mitogenic for other lymphocytes,[186] an assay in which culture supernatants injected intradermally induced DTH responses,[184] and assays that assessed killing of such selected targets as fibroblasts by means of a soluble factor in lymphocyte supernatants that came to be known as *lymphotoxin* (LT)[187–189] (among others). What quickly became apparent was that different factors were in play in the different assays, and the terms *lymphokines*[190] and, ultimately, *cytokines* came to be applied to these biologically active molecules as a class.

It was clear as early as 1969 that the factors, although still uncharacterized, could function not only as effectors of DTH responses but also as regulators,[190] and the amounts produced correlated with the intensity of DTH responses measured in the skin. Others will discuss the subsequent elucidation of the various cytokines and their myriad functions.

Pathology of Experimental Autoimmune Encephalomyelitis. Light microscopy had established that lymphocytes and macrophages were the two major populations of invading cells in EAE lesions, microglia were activated, oligodendrocytes were depleted in established lesions, and astrogliosis was sometimes seen. Further developments depended on electron microscopy and on immunohistochemistry.

Lampert and Carpenter[191] first reported on the electron microscopy of EAE lesions in 1965. Most of their conclusions have stood the test of time, but one, which profoundly influenced thinking of the time, I call into question. They reported that the tight junctions that join endothelial cells in the CNS were disrupted in EAE and that invading cells entered the CNS through these gaps. This conclusion was based on their finding that injected thorotrast passed between endothelial cells. The problem with this interpretation relates to the fact that thorotrast causes vascular injury. In addition, the animals had been given pertussis vaccine, and it too alters vascular permeability.[192] Others find tight junctions preserved[193,194] or at a minimum have been unable to prove that they are disrupted even while arguing that they should be.[195]

In 1969, Åström et al.[196] presented evidence that invading cells passed through endothelial cells rather than between them. The finding was not without precedent. Passage of lymphocytes through endothelial cells had already been documented for the high endothelial venular cells of lymph nodes and had even been given the name of *emperipolesis*, which translates from the Greek as "inside round about wandering." The 1969 study was conducted in animals with experimental allergic neuritis, rather than in EAE, but nerves have a blood-nerve barrier similar to that in the BBB. The study suggested that the same would pertain in EAE but, of course, did not prove that thesis. In the event, subsequent studies documented passage of invading cells through endothelial cells in EAE.[197] It was also established that endothelial cells became as plump as the high endothelial venule cells of lymph nodes at the onset of EAE. The initial observation was made in 1948.[66]

All are mindful that the BBB is disrupted in MS at times of attacks, evidenced by passage of gadolinium into the CNS, as revealed by MRI scanning. The same holds for acute EAE. If tight junctions remain intact, how then does gadolinium pass into the CNS? It transpires that fluid is actively transported across endothelial cells in vesicles and that, at least in experimental animals, injected gadolinium can be visualized within such vesicles.[198] The

process requires energy, and given that vesicles form by invagination and fusion on the luminal surface, any molecule present in the blood can be carried across into the CNS. Even IgM, with a molecular weight of 1 million, has been visualized in CNS endothelial cell vesicles in MS[199] and within MS lesions.[200] The findings cited here indicate that circulating antibodies have ready access to the CNS whenever there is an ongoing DTH response.

Working with Carpenter[191] and individually,[201,202] Lampert studied the demyelinative process in EAE. He noted that macrophages were the vectors of myelin destruction and that they attacked myelin from its outer surface, peeling off myelin lamellae or, when interdigitated at nodes of Ranvier, separated entire sheaths from axons. Presciently, he noted that invading inflammatory cells underwent degenerative changes, became "necrotic," and were phagocytosed. The concept of apoptosis was unknown at the time, but his pictures and his description of them render evident that apoptosis was being described. Thus, he noted a "spoke wheel appearance of the nucleus in some of these degenerating cells brought about by clumping of nuclear material."[201] Lampert also described remyelination, vesicular transformation of myelin in EAE lesions, and the focal nature of myelin dissolution.

Raine et al.,[203] Wisniewski et al.,[204] Epstein et al.,[205] and Prineas individually[206] and with Graham[207] showed that macrophages in EAE and in MS (see later) bound to myelin at sites of clathrin-coated pits. These are loci on the macrophage surface where receptors cluster, including receptors for the Fc portion of immunoglobulin and the third component of complement. Fc receptors are activated when immune complexes bind to them, and when complement is bound to the Fc molecules, engagement of the complement receptor further contributes to cell activation. Binding transduces signals that enhance release of proteases and reactive oxygen and nitrogen radicals from monocytes and potentiate their phagocytic capacity. Nyland et al.[208] demonstrated that macrophages in MS plaques would bind the Fc portion of IgG, but they failed to detect complement binding. Subsequently, others have documented the presence of C3 receptors on macrophages in MS[209,210] and of C3 itself in CNS endothelial vesicles, on the abluminal endothelial surface, and within MS plaques.[199,200] The implication from these findings is that antibodies directed against some component of myelin are likely to be involved in demyelination, and the DTH response that attracts monocytes into the lesions and activates them is potentiated by antigen-antibody complexes to which macrophages, having evolved from monocyte precursors under T-cell influence, respond by augmented myelinophagic activity.

Binding of immune complexes to the Fc receptors expressed on the surface of activated macrophages has additional consequences. One is a substantial upregulation of IL-10 and prostaglandin E_2 (PGE_2) production.[211,212] IL-10 and PGE_2 potently inhibit Th1 cells, DTH responses, and the activity of macrophages, including their ability to produce IL-12.[213,214] Immune complex binding activates macrophages initially but, by means of an induced negative feedback loop, subsequently restrains both macrophages and lymphocytes. As Newton put it, "For every action there is an equal and opposite reaction." It should also be noted that rapid clearance of compromised myelin by macrophages may facilitate remyelination. ·

EAE induced in adult strain 13 guinea pigs is an acute monophasic process but, in juvenile guinea pigs of the same strain, the onset of EAE is delayed.[203,215,216] Disease in juvenile animals is less severe at the outset than in adults, but it transitions into a relapsing and ultimately progressive process, provided the animals are immunized with whole spinal cord. Immunization of juvenile animals with MBP does not induce chronic disease.[217–219] Demyelination in spinal cord–induced chronic disease is extensive, and demyelination in MBP-induced acute disease is minimal. Pretreatment with MBP, usually with massive doses in incomplete Freund's adjuvant lacking tubercle bacilli, will protect against acute EAE when MBP in complete Freund's adjuvant is subsequently given (see Treatment of Experimental Autoimmune Encephalomyelitis). This maneuver fails to protect against chronic EAE induced by immunization with whole myelin once disease is underway. Raine et al.[218–219] and Moore[220] added galactocerebroside or total myelin lipids to MBP and immunized with the combinations. When this was done, extensive demyelination was seen. It was concluded that inflammation and demyelination in EAE represent discrete responses to discrete epitopes, and antibodies directed against lipids engrafted onto a DTH response directed against protein antigens are likely to be implicated in demyelination.[220]

As mentioned, MOG-induced EAE in rats is associated with widespread demyelination. When disease is adoptively transferred with MBP- or MOG-specific T cells, inflammation is extensive, but demyelination is minimal. When cells and anti-MOG antibody are transferred jointly, extensive demyelination ensues.[171,173,175] The findings point to a cooperation between a DTH and an antibody response in a progressive demyelinating process, with the two responses directed against the same protein (i.e., MOG-MOG) or against different proteins (i.e., MBP-MOG) in the instances cited.

The rabbit is unique in having two broad bands of myelinated nerves that extend horizontally from the nasal and temporal sides of the optic nerve head to a peripheral region just short of the equator in the retina. The vitreous contacts these myelinated fibers so that cells or serum injected into the posterior vitreous have direct access to myelin without having to traverse the BBB. Unpurified lymph node cells (i.e., T cells plus B cells) from immunized rabbits injected into the posterior vitreous infiltrate the myelinated retina and cause demyelination with swelling of the optic nerve head.[221] Brosnan and colleagues[222–224] showed that when culture supernatants of rabbit lymphocytes previously activated in vitro with PPD or a T-cell mitogen were injected into the posterior vitreous of rabbits immunized with spinal cord in complete Freund's adjuvant and already sick with EAE, demyelination in the retinal rays ensued. When cell culture supernatants were injected into normal rabbits, a mononuclear cell infiltrate was induced, but demyelination was minimal. When serum from EAE rabbits was injected into the vitreous of normal rabbits, no demyelination was seen, but when supernatants of activated lymphocytes and serum were both injected, there was extensive focal demyelination. The effect was shown to depend on IgG in the serum.[222,224] Several conclusions can be drawn:

1. Antibody has a role in demyelination in this system.
2. The T cells can be activated by PPD, an antigen that has nothing to do with myelin, or by a nonspecific mitogen and still attract monocytes and induce an inflammatory response.
3. In actively immunized rabbits, there is the strong implication that lymphocytes or more probably the monocytes that they attract "pull" antibody

into the lesion, possibly by activating endothelial cell vesicular transport of antibody, as discussed earlier.

Taken collectively, the foregoing data argue persuasively for a demyelination-promoting role for antibodies in EAE. By extension, they suggest a like role for antibodies in other autoimmune-demyelinating diseases including MS. The antibody must have access to its antigen on the surface of myelin. Thus, MOG is expressed on the outer face of myelin so that it is accessible to antibody. MBP is not expressed on the surface of myelin so that it is inaccessible to antibody, and, for this reason, antibodies to MBP do not enhance demyelination in adoptively transferred EAE. Note also that antibody in EAE may be directed against the same protein as the T-cell response, as in MOG-induced disease, or alternatively against something altogether different. If antibodies have a tissue-destructive role in MS (and they well may, because antibodies that can be detected in the serum of MS patients damage myelin in macrophage-containing CNS tissue culture preparations),[225–228] why has it proven so difficult to find the offending antigen against which the antibody response is directed?

In EAE and MS, anti-myelin antibody titers do not correlate with disease severity, or do so very imperfectly (reviewed in reference 229), although it is evident that antibodies can potentiate demyelination, at least in the case of EAE. The difficulty in reconciling a role for antibody in demyelinating processes with the seeming lack of correlation with antibody titer may be multifaceted. First, if antibodies do have a role, they do not act alone. Activated T cells, armed macrophages, and regulatory cells also come into play so that antibody is only one component of a multicomponent process. Second, the problem may be methodologic. Poor correlations have been observed for those antibodies that have been measurable to the present. Such antibodies are directed against antigens present in normal myelin. Antibodies directed against epitopes expressed only in compromised myelin within inflammatory MS foci have been measured only sparsely heretofore, and they might correlate with demyelination (see Genetics of Multiple Sclerosis).

Immunohistochemical studies of EAE using monoclonal antibodies specific for lymphocyte subsets and their products have been most informative.

The predominant invading T cell is CD4-positive, and these cells are prominent at lesion margins and just beyond them. CD8 cells are located mostly perivascularly, as are B cells.[216] Macrophages and activated microglia tend to outnumber T cells, dramatically so in chronic forms of EAE. The CD4 cells responsible for acute DTH responses in EAE are of the Th1 subclass. Th1 cells secrete interferon gamma (IFN-γ), IL-2, LT, and tumor necrosis factor (TNF). LT and TNF are toxic to oligodendrocytes.[230,231] The cells must be activated to enter the CNS. Initial antigen presentation within the CNS is generally held to be provided by MHC-expressing perivenular macrophages.[232] The Th1 cells attract monocytes from the blood that evolve into macrophages once within the CNS. The macrophages then actively engage in myelin stripping, as discussed earlier. The foregoing simplistic schema having been stated, the basis for tissue damage in EAE remains imperfectly understood. The current status of these matters is covered elsewhere in this volume.

Treatment of Experimental Autoimmune Encephalomyelitis. It has been known since 1947 that glucocorticoids exert a major beneficial effect on the course of EAE in monkeys, a species that, like humans, is relatively glucocorticoid resistant as compared to rats or mice.[68,233,234] Similarly, numerous immunosuppressive agents have been shown to favorably alter the course of EAE (reviewed in references 235 and 236). These findings have led to trials of glucocorticoids and immunosuppressive agents in MS, with disappointing results overall. Glucocorticoids profoundly inhibit DTH responses, but they have little effect on antibody titers.[237] Although they lessen the symptoms of acute MS attacks, they exert no long-term beneficial effect on progression of disability in MS. This failure suggests that some immune system component other than a T-cell–driven DTH response and one that is refractory to glucocorticoid influence has a major role in the causation of disability in MS. Similarly, T-cell–ablating immunosuppressive agents such as cladribine fail to slow disability progression in progressive MS.[238]

In general, it has proven much easier to prevent EAE from getting started using immunosuppressive agents than to favorably modify disease course once the disease is underway. The failure to improve MS using immunosuppressive drugs is sometimes explained away by the fact that the illness is invariably already established when treatment is commenced. This is not likely to be the explanation, however, as one of the immunosuppressive agents that suppresses EAE, including established and relapsing disease, is mitoxantrone,[239–242] and this drug also lessens progression of disability in progressive MS[243,244] and uniquely so to date. Mitoxantrone does not target T cells preferentially. The bulk of its effect is exerted on monocytes and on B cells.[239,245,246] Two points emerge: Drugs that favorably affect EAE may be effective in MS or they may not be. This raises questions as to the reliability of the EAE model as a predictor of response in MS.

A TNF-receptor fusion protein was tested in EAE. The basic idea was that TNF has a disease-promoting role in EAE and that its capture by a TNF receptor would favorably affect disease course. This proved to be the case in the EAE model systems studied,[247,248] although TNF can be protective in at least one EAE model system.[249] When the TNF-receptor fusion protein was tested in MS patients, attack frequency and attack severity rose, and the trial was abandoned.[250] From this finding, additional points emerge. Agents that favorably affect EAE may be contraindicated in MS, and one EAE model may not be predictive of another.

Administration of MBP, either systemically or in incomplete adjuvant (i.e., Freund's adjuvant without the tubercle bacilli), was shown long ago to attenuate the subsequent development of EAE induced by the standard administration of MBP in complete Freund's adjuvant and in some circumstances to prevent it (reviewed in reference 229). The same holds for MOG-induced EAE in mice.[251] Various explanations for this finding have been proposed over the years, including a blocking effect of antibody to MBP, induction of tolerance, and induction of regulatory or "suppressor" cells. MBP given in incomplete Freund's adjuvant may favor the production of anti-MBP antibodies at the expense of a DTH response to MBP. Antibody may capture and sequester MBP and, in this way, impede development of a DTH response to MBP. The Th2 cytokines thought to be generated in the course of the antibody response to MBP may exert a damping effect on DTH responses in keeping with the well-known yin-yang between Th1- and Th2-type T-cell responses. MBP–anti-MBP immune complexes may trigger disease-attenuating regulatory mechanisms as a consequence of their binding

to Fc receptors on NK cells and monocytes. That anti-MBP antibody is not likely to be the major factor responsible for protection from MBP-induced EAE emerges from studies showing that protection is abolished by treatment with antibody directed against T cells[252,253] and by the finding that anti-MBP antibody titers are no different in animals protected from EAE by prior administration of MBP in incomplete Freund's adjuvant than in unprotected animals after immunization with MBP in complete Freund's adjuvant.[254]

In 1976, Swierkosz and Swanborg[255] showed that lymph node cells from Lewis rats rendered unresponsive to EAE by a series of prior treatments with large doses of MBP in incomplete Freund's adjuvant transferred protection from clinical (although not from histologic) EAE. Swanborg[256] found that, in guinea pigs, the major encephalitogenic determinant resided in a part of the MBP molecule different from the determinant for unresponsiveness. The notion of harnessing protective cell-mediated regulatory mechanisms to control autoimmune processes remains attractive to this day.

There have been numerous attempts to vaccinate against EAE. The initial approach was to generate T-cell lines with specificity for MBP, neutralize them, and then to inject them so that the host would develop an anti-idiotypic regulatory response specific for the injected T cells. The approach worked[257] and subsequently came to be refined when it became evident that one could immunize with purified T-cell receptors and even with peptides derived from T-cell receptors, taking advantage of the restricted Vβ chain usage observed in some strains of rats and mice that are susceptible to MBP-induced EAE.[258–261] Clinical trials have been undertaken in MS using this approach but without much in the way of reported success. The approach presupposes that EAE is a valid model for MS and that MBP or PLP or MOG is the major antigenic determinant in MS. In my opinion, these contentions are far from proven.

With the advent of cytokines and the recognition of the complexity of their interactions, numerous trials were undertaken in which "good," or so-called anti-inflammatory, cytokines were given to EAE animals, with notable success reported for IL-10[262–266] and transforming growth factor β1 (TGF-β1).[267–269] In the same vein, studies in which "bad" or so-called proinflammatory cytokines were blocked, usually by monoclonal antibodies directed against them or by generating "knock outs," were conducted. TNF- and LT-deficient animals were shown to be protected from EAE by these methodologies,[270] as were IL-12–deficient animals.[271] Blocking of CD4 cells was also found to protect in EAE,[272] consistent with the dominant role of Th1-type CD4 cells in the initiation of acute EAE. Administration of antibodies to CD2 was also shown to protect. I return to CD2 in the section Genetics of Multiple Sclerosis.[273] Immunoglobulin was also shown to be protective in EAE.[274,275]

The approach has been productive in terms of understanding the roles of cytokines in the acute EAE process, but several caveats should be signaled if one plans to test such reagents in MS. Every cytokine has a built-in regulatory or feedback mechanism. Feedback comes into play as cytokine accumulates, serving to shut off output of the cytokine. Feedback may be either autocrine or paracrine. In the latter case, counter-regulatory cytokines are induced; these may have functions that may not be known or are at best ill understood, and some of them may be noxious. Because effects change as cytokine accumulates, dosage can make a difference. For example, small doses of anti–IL-10 protect against EAE, but large doses worsen it.[276,277] How does one decide what the dose should be in humans?

What a cytokine does in the periphery may be rather different from what it does within the CNS. TNF is toxic to oligodendrocytes in culture[230] and within the CNS when it is transgenically expressed there,[278] but TNF downregulates the MS process in the periphery.[250] Similarly, NO can damage oligodendrocytes[279] and is readily detectable within the CNS in EAE,[280–282] yet peripherally it favors apoptosis of T cells and for this reason attenuates disease, at least in the EAE model.[283–286] Further, IFN-γ, which is made by Th1 cells in acute EAE and apparently during MS attacks, has been reported to provoke attacks of MS,[287] yet the same cytokine protects in EAE,[288–296] and animals lacking IFN-γ develop progressive disease.[297,298] There may be unpleasant surprises as cytokine therapies that work in EAE come to be tested in MS.

The actions of cytokines are usually pleiotropic in the sense that they act on multiple cell types and mediate diverse biological effects. For this reason, the use of a cytokine for a desired clinical effect frequently leads to unwanted side effects. Mice do not complain of headaches when given cytokines but people may. Cytokines are also redundant. Blocking of one cytokine may come to be compensated for by the actions of others, a serious concern when long-term treatment is contemplated (as would almost surely be necessary in MS).

IFN-β preparations and glatiramer acetate are currently approved treatments for MS. Happily, both have been shown to exert a protective effect in EAE.[299–308] The findings indicate the potential usefulness of EAE for the screening of agents that might prove helpful in MS, despite the reservations mentioned earlier. Again, there is a caveat: Glatiramer acetate favorably alters the course of EAE within 1 or 2 days of its administration, whereas, in MS, the onset of the beneficial effect of glatiramer acetate is delayed 4–6 months, whether assessed by MRI scanning or in terms of attack frequency reduction. The difference in time of benefit onset raises the prospect that the mechanisms of action of glatiramer acetate in EAE and MS differ and that, although the effect of glatiramer acetate on EAE provided the rationale for its testing in MS, the basis for its efficacy in MS may be independent of the rationale that led to its testing. Glatiramer acetate is a highly basic molecule and is thought to compete with MBP for binding to MHC molecules (reviewed in reference 308). It may also lead to the generation of suppressor cells, at least in EAE.[303,306,307] However, are these actions relevant to MS, given the remarkably delayed onset of therapeutic efficacy of glatiramer acetate in MS? All patients receiving glatiramer acetate develop antibodies to it, with titers peaking between 4 months and 1 year after commencing treatment. The antibodies clearly do not interfere with efficacy, and it has even been reported that those patients with the highest antibody titers fare best.[309] Might glatiramer acetate–antiglatiramer acetate immune complexes actually contribute to efficacy?

Multiple Sclerosis

MS lesions were first illustrated by Carswell[310] in 1838 and by Cruveilhier[311] between 1835 and 1842. Charcot[312] described the major clinical features of MS in 1868. He was also the first to recognize that the cardinal pathologic feature of the process was demyelination with relative sparing of axons. Charcot believed that sclerosis in the lesions was primary, hence the name *sclerose en plaques*, although MS lesions viewed in three dimensions are spherical, ovoid, or tubular rather than plaque-like. Nevertheless, the name persists. The basis for the disease remained a mystery. Charcot postulated a major role for astrocytes in disease pathogenesis.

In his classic report of 1916, Dawson[313] studied nine autopsy cases of MS. He described lymphocytes and fat granule cells in early lesions and perivenous areas devoid of myelin. Inflammation is usually perivenular. This had been noted by Cohnheim[314] in his original description of the pathology of inflammation published in 1867. The outward flow of chemokines from the CNS to the blood is via venules, and the slow flow and low pressure in venules facilitates attachment of the chemokine-sniffing formed elements of the blood to venular endothelia and their subsequent passage into the CNS parenchyma. Because the venules course over the lateral ventricles to midline collecting veins, the topography of the periventricular and supraventricular "fingers" described by Dawson is for practical purposes pathognomonic of an inflammatory process.

Dawson noted hypercellularity at the borders of lesions and that this hypercellularity extended into surrounding, normal-appearing white matter. He viewed the small dark cells that he identified in the depth of plaques and on their margins as precursors of fat granule cells, distinguishing them from the small dark cells in perivascular cuffs. He viewed the latter as a secondary response to fat granule cell products and argued that inflammatory cuffs followed local fat granule cell formation. The formulation was in keeping with thinking of the time. Metchnikoff had described phagocytosis in 1882 but as a reaction to injury and not as a cause of injury. Antibodies had been recognized for 20 years. Round-cell infiltrates were viewed as a scavenger reaction to antibody- or otherwise-mediated pre-existing tissue damage. The notion that inflammatory cells might actually cause damage to self was not an accepted concept. Ehrlich's dictum of horror autotoxicus held sway.

Numerous additional light microscopic studies were published over the years, four of which are mentioned here. Adams and Kubik[315] compared the pathology of MS with that of ADEM. They pointed out that in acute MS, as in ADEM, there was a substantial perivenular lymphoid inflammatory infil-

trate and that the lesions in no way resembled those seen in viral infections. They also drew attention to the fact that the topography of lesions in MS differs from that in ADEM, an observation that suggests that the two processes differ in their etiologies. Finally, they drew attention to the presence of MS foci within the cortical mantle and commented that MS is not a disease of white matter alone. In a comprehensive study, Fog[316] stressed the perivenular nature of the MS process, going so far as to state that disease followed venules. Lumsden[317] pointed to what he viewed as major differences between the pathologies of MS and EAE. He considered shadow plaques to be areas of incomplete demyelination. The notion of myelin repair had not yet taken hold. Using immunohistochemistry, Boyle and McGeer[318] drew attention to the prominence of macrophages and to the fact that the macrophages were activated.

Further significant advances in understanding of MS pathology came with the development of electron microscopy. This technology revealed lymphocytes, subsequently recognized as T cells and, of course, revealed macrophages in MS lesions with the macrophages attacking myelin, attaching to it by coated pits, stripping it, ingesting it, and digesting it, exactly as in EAE.[206,207,319–321]

It became clear from the work of Prineas et al.[322,323] that remyelination was prominent within sites of a first MS attack. There was an initial depletion of oligodendrocytes in newly evolving demyelinated foci but, within 4 weeks or thereabout, new oligodendrocytes appeared at plaque margins, having migrated from the surround, and began to lay down new myelin that could be identified as such by the shortening of internodal distances and its thinness relative to the myelin it replaced. Current thinking is that oligodendrocyte precursors that are scattered throughout CNS white matter may have to undergo at least one cycle of mitosis before they can form myelin, they invade the plaque from its immediate perimeter, and they alone are responsible for remyelination. Sites of remyelination are now recognized as shadow plaques. As one attack follows another, the precursor pool comes to be depleted; remyelination becomes more and more problematic; ultimately, it ceases altogether; and oligodendrocytes vanish from established lesions.

Immunohistochemical studies of MS plaques have also been informative. Myelin proteins ingested by macrophages are degraded in days to weeks, whereas degradation of lipids in macrophages takes much longer. For this reason, it is possible by staining for myelin proteins and lipid to date plaques in terms of their acuteness or their chronicity. CD4-positive T cells are prominent in acute plaques[324,325] but, in at least some studies, CD8 cells far outnumber CD4 cells[326,327] in patients with more advanced disease, even though current thinking is that CD4 cells, arguing by analogy to the EAE model, provide the critical signals for macrophage activation. The finding of large numbers of CD8 cells perhaps points out the hazards of total reliance on the EAE model as a predictor of events in MS. MS is not simply a matter of attacks following one after the next. MS is a war, and there are offensive and defensive tactics in war. The immune system is tightly regulated so that the finding of large numbers of CD8 cells in established MS lesions could have three interpretations. CD8 cells have cytotoxic potential so that they may be engaged in attacks, a postulate for which there is scant evidence. They may be engaged in defense or they may be neutral. I favor the view that they are engaged in defense but would freely admit that finding a cell in a location may say little about why it is there. In favor of defense are the observations, admittedly in EAE and not in MS, that CD8-deficient mice are subject to relapses[328,329] and that CD8 cells become prominent in EAE lesions with recovery.[330,331]

Finding a cytokine in a location does not permit one to conclude that the functions of that cytokine, as observed in a dish, equate to functions occurring in situ. The issue is clouded by the presence at the same site within the CNS of numerous other cytokines that may synergize with the observed cytokine, act additively with it, antagonize it, or participate jointly with it in some ill-understood regulatory cascade.

In both primary and secondary-progressive MS, the predominant invading cell by far is the macrophage.[332] There may be a sea of macrophages throughout the parenchyma with (or even without) a cluster of T cells surrounding central veins. B cells are rare in acute early lesions. They tend to accumulate with chronicity, suggesting that intra-CNS immunoglobulin production is a consequence of the fundamental process or processes, rather than its cause. It has been argued that all the lesions in a given MS patient show like pathology,[333,334] but this begs the issue of whether the pathology at earlier times was the same as that encountered at time of autopsy or tissue sampling (see also the role of macrophages in progressive MS in Genetics of Multiple Sclerosis). The current status of the pathology or pathologies of MS is discussed elsewhere in this volume.

MS is more than a demyelinating disease; it is also an indolent meningoencephalitis. The cytokines, proteases, reactive oxygen and nitrogen radicals, and other factors released by CNS-invading cells are by no means confined within MS plaques. They readily diffuse beyond them and make their way into the CSF, where they can be detected in the lumbar spinal fluid, a sampling site far removed from their site of generation. If they diffuse down, they also diffuse up. Toxic products released by CNS-invading cells may adversely affect the function of neuronal cytons throughout the neuraxis, and, indeed, positron emission tomography scanning provides evidence that this is the case.[335,336] Global hypometabolism has been documented in MS by positron emission tomography scanning even early in the course of the disease and in areas where no MS lesions can be detected.

MS patients have cognitive difficulties, particularly so with short-term memory.[337,338] This problem can surface early on in patients with minimal disease burden. Without doubt, as the illness evolves, interruption of cortical pathways contributes to progressive cognitive decline in MS patients, and a correlation between overall disease burden and the magnitude of cognitive impairment can be demonstrated. However, the matter may not be so simple. In my opinion, not all the cognitive problems of MS patients depend on hard wiring. That component of cognitive decline that depends on metabolic derangement (and it may be substantial) will not be detected by pathologic studies of MS plaques or by quantitating disease burden by MRI scanning.

N-acetylaspartate (NAA) levels can be used to assess neuronal and axonal function. NAA can be measured by nuclear magnetic resonance spectroscopy. NAA levels are reduced in MS plaques.[339] The finding provides evidence for axonal damage. NAA levels are also significantly reduced in normal-appearing white matter in MS even when disease burden is minimal.[340] This finding has sometimes been interpreted as an indicator of axonal interruption in normal-appearing white matter, but this is unlikely to be the entire story. MS patients treated with IFN-β-1b show an increase in NAA levels in normal-appearing white matter 1 year into treatment, which is statistically meaningful as compared to control MS patients with a similarly modest disease burden who are not receiving treatment.[341] I interpret this positive change as evidence that viable axons and neuronal cytons are metabolically deranged in MS, and the derangement is at least partly reversible once the inflammatory response is quelled. The increase in NAA levels observed is delayed in normal-appearing white matter in MS patients treated with IFN-β-1b. Nothing is seen at 3 or 6 months into treatment, but a significant increase is noted at 1 year. These kinetics are totally different from those for gadolinium enhancement, which falls by 80% from pretreatment levels within the first 2–4 weeks of IFN-β-1b treatment[342,343] and for MS attacks, the frequency of which is meaningfully reduced by the second or third month into IFN-β-1b treatment (J. Wallenberg, personal communication). Different kinetics argue for different mechanisms. Perhaps recovery of neurons from a metabolic insult is a slow process. Cognition improves significantly in MS patients receiving IFN-β treatment.[338,344] In my experience, the improvement in cognition, as with the rise in NAA levels, is delayed.

Immunology of Multiple Sclerosis

The earliest studies of the immunology of MS were concerned with the colloidal gold reaction in the spinal fluid used formerly as a corroborating test for clinical diagnosis of the disease. In retrospect, the test was detecting immunoglobulin that, as is well known today, is synthesized within the CNS in MS, is present in increased amount in the CSF, and also exhibits oligoclonal banding on examination by electrophoresis or by isoelectric focusing. The initial documentation that CSF immunoglobulin was elevated in MS was provided by Kabat et al.,[345] whose contributions to EAE research have been mentioned. It was also appreciated early on that the spinal fluid lymphocyte count was often modestly elevated, and subsequent work established that the lymphocytes within the CSF were activated even in patients with seemingly quiescent disease.[346]

Oligoclonal bands within the CNS bespeak production of IgG by clones of B cells that have infil-trated the CNS. The significance of the finding in terms of MS pathogenesis remains enigmatic despite its diagnostic usefulness. Oligoclonal IgG bands are not unique to MS. They are also found in chronic CNS infections, such as subacute sclerosing panencephalitis (SSPE). This disease is a chronic measles virus infection of the CNS, and the oligoclonal bands detected in SSPE have been shown to be antimeasles antibodies. For this reason (and arguing by analogy that MS also must be an infectious process), much effort has been expended in a search for the MS-relevant antigen against which the oligoclonal IgG is directed in MS. Little has come of this effort. Elevated levels of antibodies to numerous viral infectious agents, of which measles will serve as the prototype, have been documented in MS, with elevated antibody levels to several viruses often noted in the same patient.[347] Although any given virus might be implicated in MS, it is highly unlikely that multiple viruses can be implicated. Even antibodies to diphtheria and tetanus toxoids have been shown to be synthesized intrathecally in MS,[348] and neither can be viewed as MS-relevant antigens.

As noted, elevated antimeasles antibody titers are found in the CSF in MS, indicating local synthesis within the CNS. CSF antimeasles antibodies in MS are oligoclonal, but they are not ordinarily appreciated as such because they are buried in the substantial multiclonal background IgG. In the end, all antibody responses are oligoclonal. *Polyclonality* simply bespeaks the presence of innumerable clones. Background "polyclonal" IgG is much lower in SSPE than in MS, indicating fewer nonspecific antibody-secreting B-cell clones in SSPE than in MS. Yet, both are chronic inflammatory processes. The finding argues for a difference between the two diseases in recruitment of random B-cell clones into the CNS and, by extension, some difference in the properties of the B-cell populations in the two diseases.

No antigen against which the oligoclonal IgG bands found in the CSF in MS are directed has been found. There is no consistent pattern to the isoelectric points of the IgG bands in MS, unlike the situation in SSPE in which the same clones may be reiterated among different patients. It is possible to raise monoclonal antibodies against IgG clones found in the CSF. When this is accomplished in SSPE, the same clone can be found in

20% of others with the disease.[349] This is not so in MS.[350] The lack of reiteration in MS suggests that the oligoclonal bands are directed against different antigens in different MS patients, presumably in a random manner. A recent study of CSF IgG using random peptide libraries displayed on phage supports this conclusion.[351] IgG bands eluted from different plaques of the same MS brain differ,[352] a finding in keeping with the formulation offered. All the foregoing findings suggest that B cells enter plaques randomly and that, once resident in plaques, they continue to produce antibody for years on end, presumably in the absence of antigen stimulation, just as they frequently do once they have made their way to the bone marrow.

Perhaps immortalized B cells are the cause. It is known that prior Epstein-Barr virus (EBV) infection can lead to persistent antibody production by B cells if they are in a milieu free of the normal short-range restraining influences ordinarily exerted on them by T cells. Bone marrow may qualify in this regard. Every adult MS patient is EBV-positive versus 85% of adult controls.[353-356] A history of frank serologically proven infectious mononucleosis is four times as common in MS as in age-matched controls. Anti-EBV antibody titers are higher in MS than in controls, but the significance of this finding is moot because titers of antibodies to other viruses are elevated as well. In my view, EBV is an attractive candidate for the elusive environmental factor that permits the MS process to get underway. Such a factor surely exists, as evidenced by the concordance frequency for MS in identical twins (see later). More often than not, the identical twin of an MS proband will not develop the disease, indicating that genetic endowment alone does not suffice.

MS is rare in developing countries, in which infection with EBV occurs at a much earlier age than it does in developed countries. Persons of Chinese extraction rarely contract MS, even when they live in the countries of the Western hemisphere. MS is rare in the Indian subcontinent, yet children of immigrants from the Indian subcontinent to Great Britain develop MS not infrequently.[357] Presumably, Chinese individuals seldom carry the genes that permit MS to surface, whereas disease susceptibility genes are present in a proportion of the East Indian population, but they rarely predispose to disease unless the environ-

ment changes. These geographic findings are consistent with the formulation advanced long ago by epidemiologists that a disease-predisposing infectious agent for MS is encountered at a later age in countries where MS is common than in countries where it is rare. In a small but provocative study, a cluster of MS patients in a Danish village was studied.[358] The MS patients were compared to others in the village. All the MS patients had been infected with the same subtype of EBV, whereas others in the village had not. If a virus or other infectious agent that sets MS in motion could be identified with certainty, the prospect of eradicating the disease by vaccination at an early age arises. (Recall that measles vaccination drastically reduced the incidence of ADEM.)

B cells are not invariably found in MS brains. They tend to accumulate as the disease evolves. B cells are rare in tissue samples obtained shortly after disease onset, and there are also autopsied MS patients with long-term established disease in whom no B cells were found in MS plaques, and oligoclonal IgG bands were not detectable in the CSF.[359] These findings make it improbable (in my opinion) that antibody produced within the CNS is a contributor to pathogenesis at the onset of MS, and it is unlikely to be a sine qua non for the perpetuation of the process. My view is that CSF antibodies in MS are likely to be "nonsense" antibodies in terms of disease pathogenesis. This is not to say that antibodies generated in the periphery, transported into MS plaques, and binding to myelin have no role in MS pathogenesis, as discussed farther on.

There have been innumerable studies of immunocyte function in MS (reviewed in references 360–362), but limited clarification has come from them, and reported results have often been outright contradictory, particularly so in the earlier literature (as reviewed in reference 360). One problem may relate to sampling of the blood in a disease in which the action occurs in the CNS. Those T cells that make their way into the CNS may be present in the blood in limited numbers for a brief period, and this can pose sampling problems. Also, the disease-promoting immune processes that operate during attacks surely differ from the disease-restraining immune processes that operate between attacks, and there are clearly substantial differences in immune function between patients experiencing an attack and those with progressive disease. In many early reports, the clinical status of the patients studied was not clearly indicated.

To my knowledge, the first clear-cut demonstration of an abnormality of T cells in MS was described by Oger et al.,[363] working in my laboratory. Oger showed that the rosetting properties of T cells exposed to sheep red blood cells was abnormal in MS, indicating something different about the T-cell surface. This finding was followed by numerous studies in which the numbers of T cells, B cells, monocytes, and their various subsets were counted and their surface properties were probed. Surprisingly, little came from this.

Antel,[364–366] also working with me, found that the regulatory capacity of CD8-type T cells was grossly deficient at times of disease activity in relapsing-remitting MS, with a rebound in activity as attacks ended. He also found that CD8-cell "suppressor" function was persistently subnormal in MS patients with progressive disease. The finding has been amply confirmed (reviewed in reference 360). Circulating CD8-cell numbers are normal in relapsing-remitting MS, whether the patient is in remission or experiencing an attack. This finding points to a dissociation between cell number and cell function (reviewed in reference 367). CD8 numbers are modestly reduced in progressive MS, yet function is compromised to a lesser extent than during relapses. CD8 density on the cell surface is reduced during attacks but is normal between attacks.[367] CD8 density is persistently reduced in progressive disease.[367] In contrast, β_2-adrenergic receptor density on the CD8-cell surface is elevated in progressive MS,[368] indicating that the cells are not simply sick (see also CD8 cells in Genetics of Multiple Sclerosis).

Much recent work has emphasized in vitro cytokine production by blood-derived T cells and monocytes from MS patients as compared to cells from controls. The literature is extensive and confusing (reviewed in references 361 and 362). A few points bear on the arguments to be elaborated in the final section (see Genetics of Multiple Sclerosis), as current understanding of these matters is considered elsewhere in this volume. It is established that T cells are activated before MS attacks with increased production of Th1-type cytokines, perhaps because of defective restraint. IL-10 inhibits DTH responses. IL-10 production has been reported to be deficient in

MS before relapses[369–372] and to rise with remission.[373–376] The findings are consistent with the prevailing view that IL-10, whether made by Th2 cells or by monocytes and macrophages, restrains Th1-type T-cell–initiated responses and does so by acting on T cells and on monocytes.

TGF-β1 is another cytokine that restrains T cells and monocytes. Production of TGF-β1 by peripheral blood lymphocytes from MS patients appears to be deficient, particularly at times of disease activity, and a decline in TGF-β1 production has been claimed to herald an impending attack.[376–380] TGF-β1 is made by many cell types and is thought to be a major product of CD8 suppressor cells,[381] the function of which (as mentioned) is defective at times of disease activity.

IL-12 is a marker for monocyte activation and a potent activator of NK cells, Th1-type CD4 T cells, and CD8 cells. IL-12 induces IFN-γ production by all three cell types. IL-12 production is markedly increased in secondary-progressive MS as compared to relapsing-remitting MS.[382–389] IFN-γ levels, presumably driven by IL-12, also tend to be elevated above control levels in secondary-progressive MS to an extent greater than that in relapsing-remitting MS.[390]

IL-12 is viewed as a major initiator of Th1-type T-cell responses, but I question whether the action of IL-12 in promoting disease depends simply on IFN-γ induction and Th1-type CD4 T-cell activation, in view of results obtained in EAE. IL-12 knockouts are utterly refractory to the development of EAE,[271] indicating an essential role for IL-12 in the initiation of the EAE process. Nevertheless, IFN-γ–deficient animals develop EAE after the customary incubation period postimmunization.[297] The finding indicates no critical role for IL-12–induced IFN-γ in the initiation of the EAE process. Further, IFN-γ–deficient animals do not recover from their attacks. This finding plus results of numerous studies in which either antibody to IFN-γ or IFN-γ itself was given to EAE animals indicate a restraining, attack-ending effect of IFN-γ on the established EAE process.[288–296] It follows that the reason why IL-12–deficient mice do not contract EAE must depend on some property of IL-12 other than its ability to induce IFN-γ production. For the reasons outlined, the elevated IL-12 found in monocytes of progressive MS patients does not provide prima facie evidence for an IL-12–induced augmentation of Th1-type T-cell responses as the basis for disability progression in secondary-progressive MS.

IFN-γ provokes production of inducible NO synthase (iNOS) by monocytes and macrophages. The consequence of this induction is release of NO. NO apoptoses T cells, and the restraining effect that IFN-γ exerts on the progression of EAE is thought to be mediated by iNOS-induced NO production, NO release, and NO-mediated apoptosis of T cells. Consistent with this formulation are the findings that T-cell apoptosis within lymph nodes is not observed in iNOS knockouts with EAE and that EAE induced in iNOS knockouts is inordinately severe and prolonged. Rodents appear to produce more NO and to be more sensitive to it than humans. For this reason, any extrapolation of the foregoing findings must be viewed as speculative. Perhaps IFN-γ–driven elevated iNOS, and, hence, elevated release of NO, favor apoptosis of T cells in the periphery in progressive MS, and perhaps this accounts for the reduced MS attack frequency observed in secondary-progressive MS as compared to relapsing-remitting MS, even though NO released by macrophages within the CNS contributes to axonal interruption.

My overall sense of the literature is that there are considerable differences in the cytokine profiles observed in relapsing-remitting MS as opposed to progressive MS. These differences are consistent with the postulate already advanced that there is a difference not simply in magnitude of response between the two forms of the disease but also one of kind, or, to adopt an intermediate position, there is a shift in dominance between two processes, both of which operate to a greater or lesser degree throughout the course of MS, with a DTH response dominating early and some other process dominating later.

Why Does Multiple Sclerosis Become Progressive?

MS usually begins as a relapsing-remitting illness, but, when patients are followed-up for a sufficient period, almost 90% of them eventually "switch" to an inexorably progressive course, a situation termed *secondary-progressive MS*.[391] Fifteen percent of MS cases are progressive from the outset. Such cases are known as *primary-progressive MS*. Many believe that there are mechanistic differences between primary-progressive and secondary-progressive MS.

The arguments for a mechanistic difference include (1) a later age of onset for primary-progressive MS; (2) absence of female preponderance in primary-progressive MS or, at a minimum, a less marked preponderance than in secondary-progressive MS; (3) far fewer lesions on brain MRI; and (4) some differences in the pathology (discussed elsewhere in this volume). The arguments against a difference include (1) identical human leukocyte antigen (HLA) endowment in the two groups[392]; (2) an identical tempo of evolution of disability, provided the clock starts in secondary-progressive patients when progression begins; and (3) a frequent history among primary-progressive MS cases of blood relatives with relapsing-remitting or secondary-progressive MS. Whether the two forms of MS are mechanistically similar or different is not resolvable at present, although, in my opinion, the similarities outweigh the differences.

If onset of progression in MS is determined by a "strategic hit" in descending neural pathways (see later), then the time of onset of progression will be determined by the moment at which the hit occurs. Once the strategic hit has occurred, gadolinium enhancement declines, the tempo at which newly appearing lesions accumulate falls, and attacks cease or become rare. When the strategic hit is delayed, which I postulate is the case in secondary-progressive MS, more cortical lesions will perforce have accumulated before onset of progression.

As noted, MS attack frequency declines coincident with the switch from relapsing-remitting to progressive disease and, in most patients, ultimately ceases altogether. Progression of gait disturbance is stressed in progressive MS, yet the decline in attack frequency is profound and will have to be taken into account in any coherent theory as to why MS becomes progressive. It is sometimes argued that attacks actually continue apace in progressive MS but are not perceived as such, because the extent of disability impedes the ability to detect their occurrence. I doubt this.

The distinction between relapsing-remitting and secondary-progressive MS is not absolute. The transition may be gradual, with attack frequency abating as progressive disability commences its advance. Thus, some patients may find themselves for a time on the cusp between the two forms.

Neurologists tend to view the segue from relapsing-remitting MS into secondary-progressive MS as in the nature of things, but the situation is surely far more common in MS than in other autoimmune processes and may even be quasi-unique to MS. Rheumatologists never speak of secondary-progressive rheumatoid arthritis, for example. The transition can be viewed in two ways:

1. The tissue-destructive process that operates in relapsing-remitting MS is fundamentally similar to that which operates in secondary-progressive MS, but the immune system oscillator comes, for obscure reasons, to be reset, so that instead of swinging widely between attack and remission, the oscillator settles at some intermediate point.
2. There are two distinct immunologic processes operating in MS; one predominates early, and the other predominates later.

As already indicated, I favor the second view.

Results of recent clinical trials perhaps offer a clue as to the basis for the "switch" from relapsing-remitting to secondary-progressive MS. There have been three trials of IFN-β in patients with secondary-progressive MS.[393–396] All three showed a 70–80% reduction in gadolinium-enhancing lesions and in accumulating burden of disease in MRI scans of treated patients as compared to MRI scans of those on placebo. The percentage reductions are almost identical to those seen earlier with IFN-β treatment of relapsing-remitting MS patients. Similarly, superimposed attacks on a background of progressive disease were reduced by approximately 30%. This percentage reduction was again similar to that reported earlier in relapsing-remitting MS. It should be noted that attack frequency is much reduced in secondary-progressive MS as compared to relapsing-remitting MS, as is the frequency with which gadolinium-enhancing lesions are observed. Nonetheless, in all three studies, IFN-β did favorably affect these measures in secondary-progressive MS in a highly statistically significant way.

In two of the three studies, there was no effect whatsoever on progression of disability as measured by the Kurtzke scale.[394,396] In the third study, there was a modest but nonetheless statistically significant beneficial effect on disability.[393] The patients in the third study were 6 years younger on average than were the patients in the other two trials, and more of them were on the cusp between relapsing-remitting and secondary-progressive MS.

The results of these trials were a disappointment but were also informative. It seems safe to conclude that there is no relation between gadolinium enhancement and disability progression in secondary-progressive MS, as gadolinium enhancement was reduced by 75% in those undergoing treatment as compared to those in the placebo group, whereas disability progression was unchanged. Disease burden as measured by MRI scanning accumulated four times as quickly in controls as in treated patients, yet disability progression was identical. These findings suggest that newly formed plaques and enlargement at the margins of existing plaques have little to do with disability progression. This leads me to conclude that the bulk of progression occurs within plaques that may have existed for years before the onset of the progressive phase of the disease. The implication that emerges from the foregoing data is that demyelinated axons that have survived earlier insults and have adapted to their demyelinated state for some reason come to be interrupted or otherwise functionally compromised by a process that is more prominent by far in progressive disease than in relapsing-remitting disease. The basis for the axonal loss is not clear, but I believe that it is immune system–mediated for several reasons.

Most believe that acute MS attacks are T-cell driven. This thinking has prompted trials in which T-cell ablation has been undertaken in MS. Cladribine potently kills T cells and is used to treat T-cell lymphomas for this reason. The agent was tested in progressive MS. Gadolinium enhancement was reduced by 80% by cladribine treatment, a finding that exactly duplicated the IFN-β results discussed earlier.[238] There was minimal effect on disability progression despite the fact that T cells had been drastically depleted and remained depleted over time. The finding suggests to me that T cells have little to do with progression of disability in MS.

Mitoxantrone is the sole immunosuppressive drug that has been reported to favorably affect disability progression in secondary-progressive MS in a statistically meaningful manner.[243,244] If one accepts that it truly does so, then immune mechanisms, rather than some ill-defined degenerative or axonal exhaustion process, are likely to be operative in secondary-progressive MS. Cladribine is T-cell specific, but it fails; mitoxantrone is not T-cell specific, yet it works at least partially. Mito-xantrone acts preferentially on monocytes and on B cells,[239,245,246] suggesting a major role for these cell types (acting largely independent of T-cell influence) in the progression of disability in MS. Mitoxantrone does not cross the BBB. This would additionally suggest, given its putative beneficial effect, that monocytes destined to become mac-rophages are continually recruited from the blood into the CNS in secondary-progressive MS.

Extensive apoptosis of macrophages is observed in plaques from progressive MS patients[397] and in EAE.[398–400] The authors of the MS report argued that the extent of apoptosis in progressive disease is such that there must be a continuous recruitment of monocytes from the blood to maintain the macro-phage pool in MS plaques. (Recall that macroph-ages are the predominant invading cell type by far in the plaques of secondary-progressive MS patients.)

There have been several trials of immune sys-tem ablation followed by bone marrow stem-cell transplantation in MS. The basic idea was to ablate the entire immune system and to reconstitute it with progenitor cells (i.e., to start over from scratch). The results of three bone marrow trans-plantation trials were reported at the North Ameri-can Council for Treatment and Research in Multiple Sclerosis meeting in the fall of 2000. The sense I took away from these presentations (although others may have seen it differently) was that the patients with progressive disease stabilized for a year or so after transplant, but once their immune system had been reconstituted, progression of dis-ability resumed pretty much as before. The failure to affect progression favorably in MS over the longer term by bone marrow transplantation is unlikely to be technical, as the same procedure pro-duces long-term benefit in systemic lupus erythe-matosus and in systemic sclerosis. Of note, when progression resumed, it did so without an evolu-tion of the disease from naïvety into sensitization of T cells to myelin antigens followed by T-cell–mediated attacks and only then on to progression (i.e., the sequence of events that earlier on had eventuated in progressive disease was not recapitu-lated). If I am correct in my interpretation of them, the findings indicate that the internal milieu of the progressive MS patient differs somehow from that found in other autoimmune diseases; secondary progression can resume in MS patients, despite the

introduction of a totally naïve immune system; and perhaps even that progression of disability can resume in the absence of de novo T-cell sensitiza-tion. The bone marrow transplantation results argue for a clear-cut distinction between attacks and inex-orable progression of disability in terms of the immune mechanisms involved.

If T cells are not necessary or only marginally so for progression of disability in MS, it follows that the role of the adaptive immune system is likely to be secondary or marginal to disability pro-gression, inasmuch as adaptive immunity depends totally on T cells. If the process is nonetheless immune system mediated, this leaves the innate immune system as the most likely major player. Based on the previous considerations, I postulate major roles for monocytes, B cells, and possibly for NK cells (see later) in the pathogenesis of dis-ability in progressive MS.

It is established that the immune system has two major arms: the innate and the adaptive immune systems. The innate immune system provides a first line of defense against infectious organisms. It acts more promptly and more crudely than does the adaptive immune system and buys time while more finely honed T-cell responses are being generated. The cells of the innate immune system include NK cells, monocytes, γδT cells, and B cells. In adap-tive immunity, T cells control the responses of B cells and monocytes so that B cells and monocytes must be viewed as components of the innate and adaptive arms of the immune response. The two systems are interactive. The innate system cooper-ates with the adaptive system to reinforce adaptive responses. Thus, bacteria induce monocytes to promptly make IL-12, which drives IFN-γ produc-tion by NK cells (innate) and subsequently by CD4 Th1-type T cells and by CD8 cells (adaptive). The initial IFN-γ production by NK cells contributes to T-cell activation. As will become apparent, the innate immune system also acts to restrain T-cell–mediated adaptive responses.

B cells respond to two distinct classes of anti-gens known as *T-cell–independent antigens* (innate) and *T-cell–dependent antigens* (adaptive). B cells make IgM-class antibody in response to T-cell–independent antigens, although they can also make small amounts of IgG in response to T-cell–independent antigens. B cells also make IgM as their initial response to T-cell–dependent antigens, but subsequently isotype switching occurs, immunoglobulin structure is modified in ways that increase antibody affinity, and the amount of immunoglobulin released is increased. All of this activity occurs under the guiding influence of T cells.

MS patients with primary-progressive or secondarily progressive disease are invariably spastic (in my experience). Spasticity bespeaks compromise of descending pyramidal tract pathways. Descending sympathetic pathways directly abut the pyramidal tract, and these too are usually, if not always, compromised in progressive MS. This can be easily documented by measuring something as simple as sympathetic nervous system (SNS)–mediated sweating responses in the feet.[401] Might a strategic hit of MS with interruption of descending sympathetic pathways have consequences for the immune system and preferentially so for the innate immune system? There is reason to think that it might, inasmuch as the SNS exerts a rather substantial restraining influence on immune responses, including innate immune responses.

Some years ago, Chelmicka-Schorr and I examined the consequences of sympathetic ablation for immune responses in rats and mice (reviewed in references 402 and 403). Mice or rats were given 6-hydroxydopamine at birth. The agent is taken up by SNS nerve endings, oxidizes within them, and destroys them. In rodents, there are 15,000 neurons in the superior cervical ganglion at birth. Three weeks later, there are 5,000. Two-thirds of the neurons die, because only those neurons that succeed in making contact with target tissues and receive target cell–derived nerve growth factor survive. All others undergo programmed cell death. If all SNS nerve endings are blown in the newborn period, then no axons contact target tissues, all SNS neurons undergo programmed cell death, and a total sympathectomy is achieved.

The consequences of sympathetic ablation for the immune system are numerous and far from trivial. EAE induced in SNS-ablated animals is of significantly increased severity and frequently becomes progressive rather than monophasic and self-limited.[404,405] Adoptively transferred EAE is much more severe in sympathectomized recipients than in controls, given the same number of T cells from the same donor, pointing to an increased activity of host monocytes as one consequence of inter-

rupted sympathetic outflow. Peritoneal exudate mononuclear cells from adult mice sympathectomized as pups were exposed to lipopolysaccharide and compared to controls for in vitro production of TNF and IL-1. Cytokine production by macrophages from sympathectomized donors was increased threefold over that by macrophages from controls.[406] This finding indicates a "spontaneous" overactivity of monocytes in the milieu of the sympathectomized animal and perhaps duplicates the cytokine shift seen in progressive MS.

Antibody responses were also studied. IgM responses to T-cell–independent antigens were increased three- to fivefold in sympathectomized mice as compared to controls, whereas IgG responses to T-cell–dependent antigens did not differ between sympathectomized animals and controls.[407] The finding suggests a preferential activation of the innate activity of B cells over their adaptive responsiveness as a major consequence of interrupted sympathetic outflow.

Chelmicka-Schorr and I also studied the effects of sympathetic agonists on immune responses. β_2-Adrenergic agonists protected against EAE, including chronic disease.[408,409] SNS-ablated mice showed upregulated β_2-adrenergic receptors on their lymphocytes, possibly reflecting denervation hypersensitivity.[410] This finding prompted my colleagues and me to measure β_2-adrenergic receptors on lymphocytes from MS patients. Receptors are upregulated threefold on CD8 cells from progressive MS patients as compared to controls but are not upregulated on CD8 cells from relapsing-remitting MS patients even during attacks,[401,411,412] although others find them to be elevated during MRI-confirmed MS attacks.[413] The receptors are fully functional.[412] In a short-term trial of the β_2-adrenergic agonist terbutaline in MS patients, we noted a reduction in adrenergic receptor number on T cells and an increase in CD8-cell–mediated suppressor function that promptly declined significantly when treatment was stopped (E. Chemicka-Schorr, A. Reder, and B.G. Arnason, unpublished observations).

Activated monocytes and macrophages synthesize and release NO. NO has many actions. Its ability to apoptose T cells has been mentioned. An additional short-range action of NO is to nitrosylate cysteines on proteins expressed on the surface of cells in the immediate vicinity of activated monocytes and macrophages. Boullerne et al.[414]

postulated that natural (i.e., innate immune system) IgM antibodies directed against nitrosylated cysteine might exist and showed that IgM antibody to nitrosylated cysteine is in fact present in the normal population. They reported that titers of IgM anti-nitrosylated cysteine antibody were elevated in a significant proportion of MS patients as compared to healthy controls, but the clinical status of many of the patients was uncertain.[414] In a more recent study,[415] clinical status was carefully documented in a group of MS patients evaluated for their titers of anti-nitrosylated cysteine antibodies. Patients experiencing overt MS attacks invariably showed elevated IgM anti-NO cysteine antibody titers. In every instance, titers were higher than were titers observed in any of 20 healthy controls. Clinically assessed titers in MS patients in remission exceeded the highest control value some 30% of the time. In relapsing-remitting MS patients receiving IFN-β, the frequency of elevated titers was 15%. Three-fourths of patients with progressive MS showed persistently elevated titers when studied serially, regardless of whether they were being treated with IFN-β. Thus, titers of this "natural" T-cell–independent antibody appear to correlate reasonably well with disease activity.

Anti-nitrosylated cysteine antibody titers were also measured in Lewis rats immunized with MBP.[415] Titers increased promptly after immunization, with peak values observed at 1 week. The antibodies were mostly of the IgM class, although elevated IgG titers were also found. At 1 week, the increment over baseline averaged some 10-fold for the IgM response and threefold for the IgG response. Titers varied substantially from one animal to the next. Peak antibody titers did not correlate with the severity of clinical EAE but did correlate significantly with the extent of demyelination measured at autopsy on day 35, some 2 weeks after the animals had recovered clinically.

How relevant these observations may be to demyelination in MS is uncertain, but it is fair to remark that IgM anti-NO cysteine antibody titers are persistently elevated several times in the majority of progressive MS cases as compared to controls and are invariably elevated during attacks in patients with relapsing-remitting disease. IgM does have access to the CNS in MS[199] and can be readily detected in MS plaques[200] (as noted). IgM has also been observed within macrophages in MS plaques, indicating the presumed prior ingestion of immune complexes.[200]

Invading macrophages within the CNS in MS have been documented to release NO.[416,417] Released NO might be expected to nitrosylate cysteines on myelin proteins, so that antibody directed against myelin proteins modified in this way would be expected to bind to the modified myelin and thence via the Fc portion of the immunoglobulin molecule to the clathrin-coated pits by which macrophages make contact with myelin.

Natural IgM antibodies are generally of low affinity,[418] as are anti-nitrosylated cysteine antibodies.[414] For this reason, nitrosylated cysteines must reach a certain threshold density on the cell surface before IgM (valence 10) can bind. Such antibodies are of course neither organ nor MS specific. For example, elevated titers are seen after immunization of rats with complete Freund's adjuvant alone, although at a substantially lower titer than that observed when the adjuvant contains MBP.[415]

As has been pointed out, there is firm evidence for persistent monocyte activation in secondary-progressive MS. This is evidenced by increased production of the proinflammatory cytokine IL-12 and by decreased production of the anti-inflammatory cytokine IL-10 and of PGE$_2$, a second inhibitory molecule. If monocytes are prime movers in the disability of secondary-progressive MS, as I propose, one goal of therapy might be to lower IL-12 production by finding ways to increase IL-10 and PGE$_2$ production. This may be feasible, as engagement of CD16 (the FcγRIIIa receptor) on monocytes and macrophages is followed by markedly increased IL-10 and PGE$_2$ production and the release of both molecules.[419–422] If T cells are irrelevant, what then lures the activated monocytes to the CNS? No answer can be given. Release of chemokines from angry astrocytes comes to mind as one possibility (shades of Charcot?). Astrocyte hypertrophy and gliosis are prominent features of established demyelinated EAE lesions, a phenomenon first noted in 1948.[66]

NK cells comprise another component of the innate immune system. Their role in MS is unclear. In the EAE model, however, depletion of NK cells is followed by disease of increased severity and duration, pointing to a restraining role for NK cells in EAE.[423] Arguing by analogy, failed NK-cell function, for whatever reason, could be a contributor to MS disease progression. NK-cell properties are known to be altered by SNS ablation.[424]

NK-cell function has traditionally been assessed by the ability of NK cells to lyse selected target cell lines. The literature is not in agreement as to NK-cell killing of target cells in MS, but many find it to be normal, and those who find it abnormal find it to be so in only a minority of patients (reviewed in reference 360). The overall sense I carry is that if killing by NK cells is compromised in MS, it is compromised to an extremely limited extent. The problem is that activated NK cells are not simply killers. They also abundantly secrete cytokines, notably IFN-γ, TNF, and to some extent TGF-β1, and it transpires that their cytokine-secreting capacity is far more relevant to their ability to control the initial events in viral infections than is their cytolytic capacity.[425] Importantly, NK-cell–mediated killing and NK-cell–mediated cytokine secretion are regulated independently[426] so that normal target-cell killing in MS does not preclude abnormal cytokine secretion.

NK cells can be triggered to proliferate and secrete cytokines via engagement of CD16 (the FcγRIIIa receptor) expressed on the surface of these cells and on macrophages, as mentioned earlier. CD16 binds IgG immune complexes, and CD16 ligation by immune complexes activates proliferation of NK cells and their cytokine production. Proliferative responses of NK cells from MS patients are only 50% of those of controls after CD16 ligation (M. Jensen, D. White, and B.G. Arnason, unpublished observations), hinting at a defect in NK function in MS. NK cells can also be driven to secrete cytokines by ligation of CD2. CD2 and CD16 use the same downstream signaling path in NK cells. As pointed out earlier, CD2 ligation exerts a protective effect in EAE.

NK cells activated by ligation of CD16 or CD2 provide a priming signal to CD8 regulatory cells via secretion of nanogram amounts of TGF-β1.[427–430] The CD8 cells, once primed by TGF-β1 and provided they have received additional priming signals from CD4 cells via IL-2[431] and monocytes via PGE$_2$,[432,433] secrete TGF-β1 in large amount. TGF-β1 exerts potent downregulating effects on Th1-type T-cell responses.[434–436] TGF-β1 also restrains monocytes[437,438] so that the well-documented failure of CD8-cell–mediated sup-

pressor function in progressive MS would be expected to promote monocyte activation. Perhaps defective NK cell function contributes to the deficiency of CD8 suppressor cell function in progressive MS. Deficient PGE$_2$ production by monocytes may also contribute.

Female individuals are more likely than male individuals to develop MS, indicating a difference in immune function between the genders. The usual thinking is that this occurs because immunocyte function and cytokine secretion are greater in female than in male individuals. Possibly augmented immune function facilitates becoming pregnant, just as the Th1-to-Th2 shift that occurs during pregnancy (thought to be responsible for the reduction in attack frequency observed during pregnancy in relapsing-remitting MS patients) facilitates maintaining pregnancy. However, there may be another side to the equation. Perhaps activity of the male immune system is set lower than that of the female system for some equally biologically relevant reason. The obvious reason would be that a downregulation of the male immune system somehow favors successful impregnation. Semen contains substantial amounts of cytokines, notably TGF-β1 and prostaglandins, plus a lesser amount of TNF. In paraplegics, semen levels of TGF-β1 are significantly lower than those in controls, whereas levels of TNF are significantly higher.[439] Fertility is seriously compromised in paraplegics. These observations are interesting inasmuch as they mimic the cytokine shift seen in progressive MS in a circumstance that has nothing to do with autoimmunity. The commonality with MS, of course, is the interruption of descending spinal cord pathways.

Genetics of Multiple Sclerosis

It has been recognized since 1972 that HLA endowment is a major factor in determining propensity to develop MS.[440–443] As is well-known, the HLA A7-B3-DR2-DQW1 haplotype is significantly overrepresented in white MS populations. Because HLA alleles present antigens and HLA allelic preponderances have been observed in innumerable other autoimmune processes, the finding of an increased representation of the HLA A7-B3-DR2-DQW1 haplotype provides strong supporting evidence for an autoimmune pathogenesis for MS.

As in EAE, it is also evident that HLA endowment alone does not suffice to cause MS.

Inheritance of susceptibility to MS is surely polygenic. Concordance for MS in siblings is of the order of 3% but, for identical twins, it is 25% on clinical grounds and rises to 40% if MRI or CSF findings consistent with MS in a seemingly unaffected twin are taken as paraclinical evidence for disease.[444] Siblings share one-half of their genes, and identical twins share all of their genes. The eightfold difference in MS concordance between the two groups is incompatible with the idea that a single gene or gene cluster determines whether MS will develop.

Much effort has gone into a search for additional genes that predispose to MS with numerous candidate gene regions identified, but no actual gene identified has been proven to be related to susceptibility to develop disease. Ongoing efforts to find additional MS-relevant genes will, I predict, bear fruit in the not-too-distant future.

Some autoimmune diseases tend to cluster. Accordingly, there has been an intense search for associations between MS and other autoimmune processes. Cases of MS occurring concurrently with demyelinating inflammatory neuropathies, inflammatory bowel disease, myasthenia gravis, and possibly with diabetes mellitus have all been recorded, and it is possible that these joint occurrences exceed background expectation. Even so, such putative associations, even should they prove to be valid, are rare.

One unusual complication of IFN-β treatment for MS is the development of rheumatoid arthritis or a systemic lupus erythematosus–rheumatoid arthritis overlap syndrome. I have encountered several such cases and carry the sense that their occurrence is far higher in IFN-β–treated patients than in MS patients not so treated. The complication was earlier documented in persons receiving IFN-α preparations (reviewed in reference 445). IFN-α exerts a beneficial effect in MS[446] and binds to the same receptor as IFN-β.

Lenercept is a fusion protein that contains the p55 TNF receptor. The agent, as mentioned earlier, was given to MS patients and was associated with an increase in attack frequency. The agent did exert a beneficial effect on rheumatoid arthritis,[447] although it was not brought to market for this indication. Another fusion protein containing the other TNF receptor, known as *p75*, is approved for treatment of rheumatoid arthritis. Several cases of MS, transverse myelitis, and optic neuritis have occurred in rheumatoid arthritis patients receiving this agent. If, as seems likely, successful treatment of MS can permit rheumatoid arthritis to surface, whereas successful treatment of rheumatoid arthritis can permit inflammatory demyelinating processes to surface, the issue of disease propensity–promoting genes shared by the two diseases can be entertained. There is precedent for this. The nonobese diabetic mouse spontaneously develops diabetes mellitus. Inheritance of susceptibility is polygenic. Some 15 disease-predisposing genes have been identified in the nonobese diabetic mouse, including some that carry relative risks as low as 1.2.[448] Inheritance of susceptibility to EAE is also polygenic. Some disease susceptibility genes are shared by nonobese diabetic mice and mice of EAE susceptible strains.[448] It follows that gene mapping for susceptibility-associated genes in MS may benefit from successful identification of susceptibility genes in other autoimmune processes. If there are shared genes that predispose to disease, the not-infrequent reporting by MS patients that they have relatives with systemic lupus erythematosus may find a ready explanation.

Depression is extremely common in MS. More than 50% of MS patients will experience one or more bouts of depression over the course of their illness. The situation is to be contrasted with that in rheumatoid arthritis, another crippling disease but one with only a 15% incidence of depression. MS patients often ascribe their depression to their disease. A commonly voiced sentiment is, "If you had this illness, you would be depressed too." However, depression in MS does not correlate with disease burden, attacks of disease, activity as measured by MRI scanning, or extent of disability.[449] Because depression appears to be independent of the other features of MS, one wonders what the basis for it may be. MS attacks occur most often in the spring and the fall in Chicago and are commonly ascribed to "the flu." Depression occurs most often in the spring and the fall and is often ascribed to the light. Might a gene that predisposes to MS and a gene that predisposes to depression overlap? A seasonal clock gene comes to mind as a candidate. If depression in MS is genetically based, one might anticipate a substantial frequency of depression in other family members. In my experience, the incidence of depression in other family members is very high, much higher than I would have anticipated on the basis of the literature. Before I ask MS patients about depression in family members, I tell them why I am asking. Perhaps MS patients are more candid about depression in the family when they believe it is in their interest to be so.

Acknowledgments

Original work cited in this communication was supported by a grant from the National Multiple Sclerosis Society, a grant from Berlex Inc., the Alan Friend MS Research Fund, and a gift from the Butz Foundation.

References

1. Lhermitte F. Les Leuco-Encéphalites. Paris: Éditions Médicales Flammarion, 1950.
2. Jellinger K, Seitelberger F. Akute tödliche Entmarkungsencephalitis nach wiederholten Hirntrockenzelleninjektionen. Klin Wschr 1958;36:437–441.
3. Prussin G, Katabi G. Dorsolumbar myelitis following anti-rabies vaccination with duck embryo vaccine. Ann Intern Med 1964;60:114–116.
4. Harrington RB, Olin R. Incomplete transverse myelitis following rabies duck embryo vaccination. JAMA 1971;216:2137–2138.
5. Label LS, Batts DH. Transverse myelitis caused by duck embryo rabies vaccine. Arch Neurol 1982;39:426–430.
6. Stuart G, Krikorian KS. The neuroparalytic accidents of anti-rabies treatment. Ann Trop Med Parasit 1928;22:327–377.
7. Bassoe P, Grinker RR. Human rabies and rabies vaccine encephalomyelitis. A clinicopathologic study. Arch Neurol Psychiatry 1930;23:1138–1160.
8. Hemachudha T, Phanaphak R, Johnson RT, et al. Neurologic complications of Semple-type rabies vaccine: clinical and immunologic studies. Neurology 1987;37:550–556.
9. Arnason BGW, Waksman BH. Tuberculin Sensitivity. In Advances in Tuberculosis Research. Basel: Karger, 1964;13:1–97.
10. Von Pirquet CE. Allergy. Arch Intern Med 1911;7:259–288,383–436.
11. Von Pirquet CF. Klinische Studien über Vakzination und vakzinale Allergie. Leipzig F: Deuticke, 1907.
12. Williams RM, Moore MJ. Linkage of susceptibility to experimental allergic encephalomyelitis to the major histocompatibility locus in the rat. J Exp Med 1973;138:775–783.
13. Uchimuri I, Shiraki H. A contribution to the classification and the pathogenesis of demyelinating encephalomyelitis: with special reference to the central nervous system lesion caused by preventive inoculation against rabies. J Neuropathol Exp Neurol 1957;16:139–203.
14. Kirk RC, Ecker EE. Time of appearance of antibodies to brain in the human receiving antirabies vaccine. Proc Soc Exp Biol Med 1949;70:734–737.
15. Hemachudha T, Griffin DE, Giffels JJ, et al. Myelin basic protein as an encephalitogen in encephalomyelitis and polyneuritis following rabies vaccination. N Engl J Med 1987;316:369–374.
16. Held JR, Lopez Adaros H. Guillain-Barré syndrome associated with immunization against rabies: epidemiologic aspects. Res Publ Assoc Res Nerv Ment Dis 1971;49:178–186.
17. Bauer HJ. Umschrittene MS therapie. Nervenarzt 1983;54:400–405.
18. Knorr-Held S, Brendel W, Kiefer H, et al. Sensitization against brain gangliosides after therapeutic swine brain implantation in a multiple sclerosis patient. J Neurol 1986;233:54–56.
19. Salk J, Romine JS, Westall FC, Wiederholt WC. Myelin Basic Protein Studies in Experimental Allergic Encephalomyelitis and Multiple Sclerosis: A Summary with Theoretical Considerations of Multiple Sclerosis Etiology. In Davison AN, Cuzner ML (eds), The Suppression of Experimental Allergic Encephalomyelitis and Multiple Sclerosis. London: Academic Press, 1980;141–156.
20. Campbell B, Vogel PJ, Fisher E, Lorenz R. Myelin basic protein administration in multiple sclerosis. Arch Neurol 1973;29:10–15.
21. Gonsette RE, Delmotte P, Demonty L. Failure of basic protein therapy for multiple sclerosis. J Neurol 1977;216:27–31.
22. Juba A. Die maligne exacerbation der multiplen sklerose. Arch Psychiatry 1939;145;275–289.
23. Miller HG, Stanton JB, Gibbons JL. Para-infectious encephalomyelitis and related syndromes, a critical review of the neurological complications of certain specific fevers. QJM 1956;25:427–505.
24. Miller HG, Stanton JB, Gibbons JL. Acute disseminated encephalomyelitis and related syndromes. BMJ 1957;1:668–672.
25. Alcock NS, Hoffman HL. Recurrent encephalomyelitis in childhood. Arch Dis Child 1962;37:40–44.
26. Johnson RT, Griffin DE, Hirsch RL, et al. Measles encephalomyelitis—clinical and immunological studies. N Engl J Med 1984;310:137–141.
27. Finley KH. Perivenous changes in acute encephalitis associated with vaccination, variola, and measles. Arch Neurol Psychiatry 1937;37:505–513.
28. Greenfield JG. Acute disseminated encephalomyelitis as sequel to influenza. J Pathol Bacteriol 1930;33:453–462.
29. Grinker RR, Bassoe P. Disseminated encephalomyelitis—its relation to other infections of nervous system. Arch Neurol Psychiatry 1931;25:723–747.
30. Klimek JJ, Russman BS, Quintiliani R. *Mycoplasma pneumoniae* meningoencephalitis and transverse myelitis in association with low cerebrospinal fluid glucose. Pediatrics 1976;58:133–135.

31. Nicholson G. Transverse myelitis complicating *Mycoplasma pneumoniae* infection. Postgrad Med J 1977;53: 86–87.

32. Westenfelder GO, Akey DT, Corwin SJ, Vick NA. Acute transverse myelitis due to *Mycoplasma pneumoniae* infection. Arch Neurol 1981;38:317–318.

33. Cotton PB, Webb-Peploe MM. Acute transverse myelitis as a complication of glandular fever. BMJ 1966;1:654–655.

34. Helgason CM, Arnason BGW. Demyelinating Diseases Affecting the Spinal Cord. In Davidoff RA (ed), Spinal Cord Handbook. New York: Marcel Dekker 1987;559–606.

35. Behan PO, Geschwind N, Lamarche JB, et al. Delayed hypersensitivity to encephalitogenic protein in disseminated encephalomyelitis. Lancet 1968;2:1009–1012.

36. Lisak RP, Behan PO, Zweiman B, Shetty T. Cell-mediated immunity to myelin basic protein in acute disseminated encephalomyelitis. Neurology 1974;24:560–564.

37. Lisak RP, Zweiman B. In vitro cell-mediated immunity of cerebrospinal fluid lymphocytes to myelin basic protein in primary demyelinating diseases. N Engl J Med 1977;297: 850–853.

38. Van Bogaert L. Post-infectious encephalomyelitis and multiple sclerosis. The significance of perivenous encephalomyelitis. J Neuropathol Exp Neurol 1950;9:219–249.

39. Turnbull HM, Mac Intosh J. Encephalomyelitis following vaccination. Br J Exp Pathol 1926;7:181–222.

40. Bouwdijk-Bastiannse FS. Encéphalite consécutive à la vaccination antivariolique. Bull Acad Nat Med 1925;94: 815–821.

41. Greenberg M, Appelbaum E. Post vaccinal encephalitis. A report of 45 cases in New York City. Am J Med Sci 1948;216:565–570.

42. De Vries E. Postvaccinial Perivenous Encephalitis. Amsterdam: Elsevier, 1960.

43. Reye RDK, Morgan G, Baral J. Encephalopathy and fatty degeneration of the viscera. Lancet 1963;2:749–752.

44. Perdrau JR. The histology of post-vaccinal encephalitis. J Path Bact 1928;31:17–32.

45. Mulligan RM, Neubuerger KT. Post vaccinal encephalitis in adults. J Neuropathol Exp Neurol 1942;1:416–421.

46. Marsden JP, Hurst EW. Acute perivascular myelinoclasis (acute disseminated encephalitis) in small pox. Brain 1900;55:181.

47. Grose C, Henle W, Henle G, Feorino PM. Primary Epstein-Barr virus infections in acute neurologic diseases. N Engl J Med 1975;292:392–396.

48. Rousseau JJ, Franck G. Les complications neurologiques de la mononucléose infectieuse. Acta Neurol Belg 1977; 77:25–40.

49. Hurst EW. Acute haemorrhagic leucoencephalitis, a previously undefined entity. Med J Aust 1941;2:1–6.

50. Adams RD, Cammermeyer J, Denny-Brown D. Acute necrotizing hemorrhagic encephalopathy. J Neuropathol Exp Neurol 1949;8:1–29.

51. Crawford T. Acute haemorrhagic leucoencephalitis. J Clin Pathol 1954;7:1–9.

52. Gosztonyi G. Acute Hemorrhagic Leucoencephalitis (Hurst's Disease). In PJ Vinken, GW Bruyn (eds), Handbook of Clinical Neurology. Amsterdam: North Holland, 1978;587–604.

53. Lander H. A case of acute haemorrhagic leucoencephalitis (Hurst) complicating varicella. J Pathol Bacteriol 1955; 70:157–165.

54. Shallard B, Latham O. A case of acute haemorrhagic leucoencephalitis. Med J Aust 1945;32:145–148.

55. Giedion A. Die hamorrhagische encephalomyelitis postvaccinalis. Schweiz Z Allg Pathol 1952;15:234–253.

56. Waksman BH, Adams RD. Studies of the effect of the generalized Shwartzman reaction on the lesions of experimental allergic encephalomyelitis. Am J Pathol 1957; 23:131–153.

57. Levine S. Hyperacute, neutrophilic, and localized forms of experimental allergic encephalomyelitis: a review. Acta Neuropathol (Berl) 1974;28:179–189.

58. Levine S, Wenk EJ. Allergic encephalomyelitis: a hyperacute form. Science 1964;146:1681–1682.

59. Levine S, Hirano A, Zimmerman HM. Hyperacute allergic encephalomyelitis: electron microscopic observations. Am J Pathol 1965a;47:209–221.

60. Russell DS. The nosological unity of acute haemorrhagic leucoencephalitis and acute disseminated encephalomyelitis. Brain 1955;78:369–374.

61. Foncin JF, Breton J, Chodkiewicz JP. Leucoéncephalite aiguë hemorrhagique de Hurst et plaque de sclerose. Rev Neurol 1969;121:491–494.

62. Rivers TM, Sprunt DH, Berry GP. Observations on attempts to produce acute disseminated encephalomyelitis in monkeys. J Exp Med 1933;58:39–53.

63. Rivers TM, Schwentker FF. Encephalomyelitis accompanied by myelin destruction experimentally produced in monkeys. J Exp Med 1935;61:689–702.

64. Ferraro A, Jervis GA. Experimental disseminated encephalopathy in monkey. Arch Neurol Psychiatry 1940;43: 195–290.

65. Ferraro A. Pathology of demyelinating diseases as an allergic reaction of the brain. Arch Neurol Psychiatry 1944;52:443.

66. Ferraro A, Cazzullo CL. Chronic experimental allergic encephalomyelitis in monkeys. J Neuropathol Exp Neurol 1948;7:235–260.

67. Ferraro A, Roizin L. Neuropathologic variations in experimental allergic encephalomyelitis. Hemorrhagic encephalomyelitis, perivenous encephalomyelitis, diffuse encephalomyelitis, patchy gliosis. J Neuropathol Exp Neurol 1954;13:60–89.

68. Ferraro A, Roizin L. Experimental allergic encephalomyelitis during and following cortone acetate treatment. J Neuropathol Exp Neurol 1953;12:373–386.

69. Dienes L, Schoenheit EW. Certain characteristics of the infectious processes in connection with the influence exerted on the immunity response. J Immunol 1930;19: 41–61.

70. Dienes L, Mallory TB. Histological studies of hypersensitive reactions. Part 1. The contrast between the histological responses in the tuberculin (allergic) type and the anaphylactic type of skin reactions. Am J Pathol 1932;8:689–709.

71. Freund J, McDermott K. Sensitization to horse serum by means of adjuvants. Proc Soc Exp Biol Med 1942;49:548–553.

72. Kabat EA, Wolf A, Bezer AE. The rapid production of acute disseminated encephalomyelitis in rhesus monkeys by injection of heterologous and homologous brain tissue with adjuvants. J Exp Med 1947;85:117–129.

73. Morgan IM. Allergic encephalomyelitis in monkeys in response to injection of normal monkey nervous tissue. J Exp Med 1947;85:131–140.

74. Wolf A, Kabat EA, Bezer AE. The pathology of acute disseminated encephalomyelitis produced experimentally in the rhesus monkey and its resemblance to human demyelinating disease. J Neuropathol Exp Neurol 1947;6:333–357.

75. Freund J, Stern ER, Pisani TM. Isoallergic encephalomyelitis and radiculitis in guinea pigs after one injection of brain and mycobacteria in water-in-oil emulsion. J Immunol 1947;57:179.

76. Jervis GA, Koprowski H. Experimental allergic encephalomyelitis. J Neuropathol Exp Neurol 1948;7:309–320.

77. Koprowski H, Jervis GA. Further studies in experimental allergic encephalitis in the Guinea pig. Proc Soc Exp Biol Med 1948;69:472–476.

78. Waksman BH. Experimental allergic encephalomyelitis and the "auto-allergic" diseases. Int Arch Allergy Appl Immunol 1959;14(Suppl):1–87.

79. Kabat EA, Wolf A, Bezer AE. Studies of acute disseminated encephalomyelitis in rhesus monkeys. IV. Disseminated encephalomyelitis produced in monkeys with their own brain tissue. J Exp Med 1949;89:395–398.

80. Waksman BH, Adams RD. An histologic study of the early lesion in experimental allergic encephalomyelitis in the guinea pig and rabbit. Am J Pathol 1962;41:135–150.

81. Waksman BH, Morrison LR. Tuberculin type hypersensitivity to spinal cord antigen in rabbits with isoallergic encephalomyelitis. J Immunol 1951;66:421–444.

82. Bail O. Uebertragung der Tuberkulinempfindlichkeit. Z Immunitaetsforsch 1910;4:470–485.

83. Chase MW. Cellular transfer of cutaneous hypersensitivity to tuberculin. Proc Soc Exp Biol Med 1945;59:134–135.

84. Lipton MM, Freund J. The transfer of experimental allergic encephalomyelitis in the rat by means of parabiosis. J Immunol 1953;71:380–384.

85. Åström K-E, Waksman BH. The passive transfer of experimental allergic encephalomyelitis and neuritis with living lymphoid cells. J Pathol Bacteriol 1962;83:89–106.

86. Paterson PY. Transfer of allergic encephalomyelitis in rats by means of lymph node cells. J Exp Med 1960;111:119–135.

87. Bernard CCA, Leydon J, MacKay IR. T cell necessity in the pathogenesis of experimental autoimmune encephalomyelitis in mice. Eur J Immunol 1976;6:655.

88. Bernard CCA, McKay IR. Transfer of murine experimental autoimmune encephalomyelitis and cell-mediated immunity to myelin protein is effected by Lyt-1 cells. J Neuroimmunol 1983;4:61–65.

89. Kuchroo VK, Martin CA, Greer JM, et al. Cytokines and adhesion molecules contribute to the ability of myelin proteolipid protein-specific T cell clones to mediate experimental allergic encephalomyelitis. J Immunol 1993;151:4371–4382.

90. Paterson PY, Harvey JM. Irradiation potentiation of cellular transfer of EAE: time course and locus of effect in irradiated recipient Lewis rats. Cell Immunol 1978;41:256–263.

91. Stone SH. Transfer of allergic encephalomyelitis by lymph node cells in inbred guinea pigs. Science 1961;134:619–620.

92. Koprowski H. The role of hyperergy in measles encephalitis. Am J Dis Child 1962;103:273–178.

93. Werdelin O, McCluskey RT. The nature and the specificity of mononuclear cells in experimental autoimmune inflammations and the mechanisms leading to their accumulation. J Exp Med 1971;133:1242–1263.

94. Levine S, Hoenig EM. Induced localization of allergic adrenalitis and encephalomyelitis at sites of thermal injury. J Immunol 1968;100:1310–1318.

95. Karin N, Szafer F, Mitchell D, Gold DP, et al. Selective and nonselective stages in homing of T lymphocytes to the central nervous system during experimental allergic encephalomyelitis. J Immunol 1993;150:4116–4124.

96. Wekerle H, Linington C, Lassmann H, Meyermann R. Cellular immune reactivity within the CNS. Trends Neurosci 1986;9:271–277.

97. Trotter J, Steinman L. Homing of Lyt-2$^+$ and Lyt-2$^-$ T cell subsets and B lymphocytes to the central nervous system of mice with acute experimental allergic encephalomyelitis. J Immunol 1984;132:2919–2923.

98. Kosunen TU, Waksman BH, Samuelsson IK. Radioautographic study of cellular mechanisms in delayed hypersensitivity. II. Experimental allergic encephalomyelitis in the rat. J Neuropathol Exp Neurol 1963;22:367–380.

99. Kosunen TU, Waksman BH, Samuelsson IK. Radioautographic study of cellular mechanisms in delayed hypersensitivity. J Neuropathol Exp Med 1963;22:367–380.

100. Hickey WF. Migration of hematogenous cells through the blood-brain barrier and the initiation of CNS inflammation. Brain Pathol 1991;1:97–105.

101. Griscelli C, Vassalli P, McCluskey RT. The distribution of large dividing lymph node cells in syngeneic recipient rats after intravenous injection. J Exp Med 1969;130:1427–1442.

102. Butcher EC, Scollay RG, Weissman IL. Organ specificity of lymphocyte migration: mediation by highly selective lymphocyte interaction with organ-specific determinants on high endothelial venules. Eur J Immunol 1980;10:556–561.

103. Kraal G, Weissman IL, Butcher EC. Differences in in vivo distribution and homing of T cell subsets to mucosal vs. nonmucosal lymphoid organs. J Immunol 1983;130:1097–1102.

104. Brosnan CF, Bornstein MB, Bloom BR. The effects of macrophage depletion on the clinical and pathologic expression of experimental allergic encephalomyelitis. J Immunol 1981;126:614–620.

105. Richert JR, Driscoll BF, Kies MW, Alvord EC Jr. Adoptive transfer of experimental allergic encephalomyelitis: incubation of rat spleen cells with specific antigen. J Immunol 1979;122:494–496.

106. Panitch HS, McFarlin DE. Experimental allergic encephalomyelitis: enhancement of cell-mediated transfer by concanavalin A. J Immunol 1977;119:1134–1137.

107. Sibley WA, Bamford CR, Clark K. Clinical viral infections and multiple sclerosis. Lancet 1985;1:1313.

108. Pettinelli CB, McFarlin DE. Adoptive transfer of experimental allergic encephalomyelitis in SJL/J mice after in vitro activation of lymph node cells by myelin basic protein: requirement for Lyt $1^+ 2^-$ T lymphocytes. J Immunol 1981;127:1420–1423.

109. Ben-Nun A, Wekerle H, Cohen IR. The rapid isolation of clonable antigen-specific T lymphocyte lines capable of mediating autoimmune encephalomyelitis. Eur J Immunol 1981;11:195–199.

110. Wekerle H. CD4 Effector Cells in Autoimmune Diseases of the Central Nervous System. In RE Keane, WF Hickey (eds), Immunology of the Nervous System. New York: Oxford University Press, 1997;460–492.

111. Olitsky PK, Yager RH. Experimental disseminated encephalomyelitis in white mice. J Exp Med 1949;90:213–224.

112. Lee JM, Olitsky PK, Schneider HA, Zinder ND. Role of heredity in experimental disseminated encephalomyelitis in mice. Proc Exp Biol Med 1954;85:430–432.

113. Lee JM, Olitsky PK. Simple method for enhancing development of acute disseminated encephalomyelitis in mice. Proc Soc Exper Biol Med 1955;89:263–266.

114. Olitsky PK, Lee JM. The immunologic response of mice from stocks resistant and susceptible to acute disseminated encephalomyelitis. J Lab Clin Med 1955;45:81–86.

115. Lee JM, Schneider HA. Critical relationships between constituents of the antigen-adjuvant emulsion affecting experimental allergic encephalomyelitis in a completely susceptible mouse genotype. J Exp Med 1962; 115:157–168.

116. Webster LT. Inheritance of resistance of mice to enteric bacterial and neurotropic virus infections. J Exp Med 1937;65:261–286.

117. Perlik F, Zidek Z. The susceptibility of several inbred strains of rats to adjuvant-induced arthritis and experimental allergic encephalomyelitis. Z Immunitaetsforsch 1974;147:191–193.

118. Levine S, Sowinski R. Allergic encephalomyelitis in the reputedly resistant Brown Norway strain of rats. J Immunol 1975;114:597–601.

119. Levine S, Sowinski R. Experimental allergic encephalomyelitis in inbred and outbred mice. J Immunol 1973; 110:139.

120. Levine S, Sowinski R. Experimental allergic encephalomyelitis in congenic strains of mice. Immunogenetics 1974;1:352–356.

121. Gasser DL, Newlin CM, Palm J, Gonatos NK. Genetic control of susceptibility to experimental allergic encephalomyelitis in rats. Science 1973;181:872.

122. Bernard CCA. Experimental autoimmune encephalomyelitis in mice: genetic control of susceptibility. J Immunogenetics 1976;3:263–274.

123. Wilkie MH, Kies MW, Alvord EC, Shaw CM. Homologous delayed-type skin responses and experimental allergic encephalomyelitis (EAE) in guinea pigs. Fed Proc 1963;22:671(abst).

124. Waksman BH, Arbouys S, Arnason BG. The use of specific "lymphocyte" antisera to inhibit hypersensitive reactions of the "delayed" type. J Exp Med 1961;114:997–1022.

125. Glick B, Chang TS, Jaap RG. The bursa of Fabricius and antibody production. Poultry Sci 1956;35:224.

126. Arnason BG, Janković BD, Waksman BH. Effect of thymectomy on 'delayed' hypersensitive reactions. Nature (Lond) 1962;194:99–100.

127. Arnason BG, Janković BD, Waksman BH, Wennersten C. Role of the thymus in immune reactions in rats. II. Suppressive effect of thymectomy at birth on reactions of delayed (cellular) hypersensitivity and the circulating small lymphocyte. J Exp Med 1962;116:177–186.

128. Gonatos NK, Howard JC. Inhibition of experimental allergic encephalomyelitis in rats severely depleted of T cells. Science 1974;186:839–841.

129. Janković BD, Waksman BH, Arnason BG. Role of the thymus in immune reactions in rats. I. The immunologic response to bovine serum albumin (antibody formation, Arthus reactivity, and delayed hypersensitivity) in rats thymectomized or splenectomized at various times after birth. J Exp Med 1962;116:159.

130. Waksman BH, Arnason BG, Janković BD. Role of the thymus in immune reactions in rats. III. Changes in the lymphoid organs of thymectomized rats. J Exp Med 1962; 116:187.

131. Miller JFAP. Immunological function of the thymus. Lancet 1961;2:748.

132. Good RA, Dalmasso AP, Martinez C, et al. The role of the thymus in development of immunologic capacity in rabbits and mice. J Exp Med 1962;116:773.

133. Janković BD, Išvaneski M. Experimental allergic encephalomyelitis in thymectomized, bursectomized and normal chickens. Int Arch Allergy 1963;23:188.

134. Blaw ME, Cooper MD, Good RA. Experimental allergic encephalomyelitis in agammaglobulinemic chickens. Science 1967;158:1198–1200.

135. Raffel S. Delayed hypersensitivities. Progr Allergy 1954; 4:173–198.

136. Kies MW, Murphy JB, Alvord EC Jr. Fractionation of guinea pig brain proteins with encephalitogenic activity. Fed Proc 1960;19:207(abst).

137. Kies MW. Chemical studies on an encephalitogenic protein from guinea pig brain. Ann N Y Acad Sci 1965;122:161–170.

138. Kies MW, Alvord EC Jr., Martenson RE, LeBaron FN. Encephalitogenic activity of bovine basic proteins. Science 1966;151:821–822.

139. Martenson RE, Deibler GE, Kies MW. Myelin basic proteins of the rat central nervous system. Purification, encephalitogenic properties, and amino acid compositions. Biochim Biophys Acta 1970;200:353–362.

140. Carnegie PR, Lumsden CE. Encephalitogenic peptides from spinal cord. Nature 1966;209:1354–1355.

141. Carnegie PR. N-terminal sequence of an encephalitogenic protein from human myelin. Biochem J 1969;111:240–242.

142. Carnegie PR, Lumsden CE. Fractionation of encephalitogenic polypeptides from bovine spinal cord by gel filtration in phenol-acetic acid-water. Immunology 1967;12: 133–145.

143. Carnegie PR. Proposed technique for classifying and identifying encephalitogens. Nature 1967;214:407–408.

144. Carnegie PR, Bencina B, Lamoureux G. Experimental allergic encephalomyelitis. Isolation of basic proteins and polypeptides from central nervous tissue. Biochem J 1967;105:559–568.

145. Kibler RF, Fox RH, Shapira R. Isolation of a highly purified encephalitogenic protein from bovine cord. Nature 1964;204:1273–1275.

146. Kibler RF, Shapira R, McKneally S, et al. Encephalitogenic protein: structure. Science 1969;164:577–580.

147. Nakao A, Davis WJ, Roboz-Einstein E. Basic proteins from the acidic extract of bovine spinal cord. I. Isolation and characterization. Biochim Biophys Acta 1966;130:163–170.

148. Nakao A, Davis WJ, Roboz-Einstein E. Basic proteins from the acidic extract of bovine spinal cord. II. Encephalitogenic, immunologic and structural interrelationships. Biochim Biophys Acta 1966;130:171–179.

149. Chao L-P, Roboz-Einstein E. Isolation and characterization of an active fragment from enzymatic degradation of encephalitogenic protein. J Biol Chem 1968;243:6050–6055.

150. Eylar EH, Hashim GA. Allergic encephalomyelitis: the structure of the encephalitogenic determinant. Proc Natl Acad Sci U S A 1968;61:644–650.

151. Eylar EH, Salk J, Beveridge GC, Brown LV. Experimental allergic encephalomyelitis: an encephalitogenic basic protein from bovine myelin. Arch Biochem 1969;132:34–48.

152. Eylar EH, Thompson M. Allergic encephalomyelitis: the physical–chemical properties of the basic protein encephalitogen from bovine spinal cord. Arch Biochem Biophys 1969;129:468–479.

153. Eylar EH. The Induction and Suppression of EAE. In AN Davison, ML Cuzner (eds), The Suppression of Experimental Allergic Encephalomyelitis and Multiple Sclerosis. London: Academic Press, 1980;59–78.

154. Hashim GA, Eylar EH. Allergic encephalomyelitis: enzymatic degradation of the encephalitogenic basic protein from bovine spinal cord. Arch Biochem 1969a;129:635–644.

155. Hashim GA, Eylar EH. Allergic encephalomyelitis: isolation and characterization of encephalitogenic peptides form the basic protein of bovine spinal cord. Arch Biochem 1969b;129:645–654.

156. Hashim GA. T-Cell Activation and Suppression in Experimental Allergic Encephalomyelitis and Multiple Sclerosis. In AN Davison, ML Cuzner (eds), The Suppression of Experimental Allergic Encephalomyelitis and Multiple Sclerosis. London: Academic Press, 1980;79–104.

157. Olitsky PK, Tal C. Acute disseminated encephalomyelitis produced in mice by brain proteolipid (Folch-Lees). Proc Soc Exp Biol Med 1952;79:50–53.

158. Waksman BH, Porter H, Lees MD, et al. A study of the chemical nature of components of bovine white matter effective in producing allergic encephalomyelitis in the rabbit. J Exp Med 1954;100:451–471.

159. Waksman BH. Activity of Proteolipid-Containing Fractions of Nervous Tissue in Producing Experimental "Allergic" Encephalomyelitis. In MW Kies, EC Alvord (eds), "Allergic" Encephalomyelitis. Springfield, Illinois: CC Thomas, 1959; 263–272.

160. Lees MB. A history of proteolipids: a personal memoir. Neurochem Res 1998;23:261–271.

161. Williams RM, Lees MB, Cambi F, Macklin WB. Chronic experimental allergic encephalomyelitis induced in rabbits with bovine white matter proteolipid apoprotein. J Neuropathol Exp Neurol 1982;41:508–521.

162. Cambi F, Lees MB, Williams RM, Macklin WB. Chronic experimental allergic encephalomyelitis produced by bovine proteolipid apoprotein: immunological studies in rabbits. Ann Neurol 1983;13:303–308.

163. Sobel RA, van der Veen R, Lees MB. The immunopathology of chronic experimental allergic encephalomyelitis induced in rabbits with bovine proteolipid protein. J Immunol 1986;136:157–163.

164. Yoshimura T, Kunishita T, Sakai K, et al. Chronic experimental allergic encephalomyelitis in guinea pigs induced by proteolipid protein. J Neurol Sci 1985;69:47–58.

165. Yamamura T, Namikawa T, Endoh M, et al. Experimental allergic encephalomyelitis induced by proteolipid protein in Lewis rats. J Neuroimmunol 1986;12:143–153.

166. Endoh M, Tabira T, Kunishita T. Antibodies to proteolipid apoprotein in chronic relapsing experimental allergic encephalomyelitis. J Neurol Sci 1986;73:31–38.

167. Satoh J, Sakai K, Endoh M, et al. Experimental allergic encephalomyelitis mediated by murine encephalitogenic T cell lines specific for myelin proteolipid apoprotein. J Immunol 1987;138:179–184.

168. Tuohy VK, Lu Z, Sobel RA, et al. A synthetic peptide from myelin proteolipid protein induces experimental allergic encephalomyelitis. J Immunol 1988;141:1126–1130.

169. Tuohy VK, Sobel RA, Lees MB. Myelin proteolipid protein-induced experimental allergic encephalomyelitis: Variations in disease expression in different strains of mice. J Immunol 1988;140:1868–1873.

170. Linington C, Webb M, Woodhams PL. A novel myelin-associated glycoprotein defined by a mouse monoclonal antibody. J Neuroimmunol 1984;6:387–396.

171. Linington C, Bradl M, Lassmann H, et al. Augmentation of demyelination in rat acute allergic encephalomyelitis by circulating mouse monoclonal antibodies directed against a myelin/oligodendrocyte glycoprotein. Am J Pathol 1988;130:443–454.

172. Linington C, Berger T, Perry L, et al. T cells specific for the myelin oligodendrocyte glycoprotein mediate an unusual autoimmune inflammatory response in the central nervous system. Eur J Immunol 1993;23:1364–1372.

173. Kerleo de Rosbo N, Mendel I, Ben-Nun A. Chronic relapsing experimental autoimmune encephalomyelitis with a delayed onset and an atypical clinical course, induced in PL/J mice by myelin oligodendrocyte glycoprotein (MOG)–derived peptide: preliminary analysis of MOG T cell epitopes. Eur J Immunol 1995;25:985–993.

174. Mendel I, Kerlero de Rosbo N, Ben-Nun A. A myelin oligodendrocyte glycoprotein peptide induces typical chronic experimental autoimmune encephalomyelitis in H-2^b mice: fine specificity and T cell receptor Vβ expression of encephalitogenic T cells. Eur J Immunol 1995;25:1951–1959.

175. Johns TG, Kerleo de Rosbo N, Menon KK, et al. Myelin oligodendrocyte glycoprotein induces a demyelinating encephalomyelitis resembling multiple sclerosis. J Immunol 1995;154:5536–5541.

176. Amor S, Groome N, Linington C, et al. Identification of epitopes of myelin oligodendrocyte glycoprotein for the induction of experimental allergic encephalomyelitis in SJL and Biozzi AB/H mice. J Immunol 1994;153:4349–4356.

177. Rich AR, Lewis MR. Mechanism of allergy in tuberculosis. Proc Soc Exp Biol Med 1928;25:596–598.

178. George M, Vaughan JH. In vitro cell migration as a model for delayed hypersensitivity. Proc Soc Exp Biol Med 1962;111:514–521.

179. David JR, Paterson PY. In vitro demonstration of cellular sensitivity in allergic encephalomyelitis. J Exp Med 1965;122:1161–1171.

180. David JR. Delayed hypersensitivity in vitro: its mediation by cell free substances formed by lymphoid cell-antigen interaction. Proc Natl Acad Sci U S A 1966;56:72–76.

181. David JR. Lymphocyte mediators and cellular hypersensitivity. N Engl J Med 1973;288:143–149.

182. Bloom BR, Bennett B. Mechanism of a reaction in vitro associated with delayed-type hypersensitivity. Science 1966;153:80–82.

183. Bennett B, Bloom BR. Studies on the migration inhibition factor associated with delayed-type hypersensitivity: cytodynamics and specificity. Transplantation 1967;5:996–1000.

184. Bennett B, Bloom BR. Biological activity of a partially purified migration inhibitory factor (MIF) associated with delayed-type hypersensitivity. Fed Proc 1968;27:263.

185. Weiser WY, Temple PA, Witek-Giannotti JS, et al. Molecular cloning of a cDNA encoding a human macrophage inhibitory factor. Proc Natl Acad Sci 1989;86:7522–7527.

186. Maini RN, Bryceson ADM, Wolstencroft RA, Dumonde DC. Lymphocyte mitogenic factor in man. Nature 1969; 224:43–44.

187. Ruddle NH, Waksman BH. Cytotoxicity mediated by soluble antigen and lymphocytes in delayed hypersensitivity. I. Characterization of the phenomenon. J Exp Med 1968;128:1237–1254.

188. Ruddle NH, Waksman BH. Cytotoxicity mediated by soluble antigen and lymphocytes in delayed hypersensitivity. II. Correlation of the in vitro response with skin reactivity. J Exp Med 1968;128:1255–1265.

189. Ruddle NH, Waksman BH. Cytotoxicity mediated by soluble antigen and lymphocytes in delayed hypersensitivity. III. Analysis of mechanism. J Exp Med 1968;128:1267–1278.

190. Dumonde DC, Wolstencroft RA, Panayi GS, et al. 'Lymphokines': non antibody mediators of cellular immunity generated by lymphocyte activation. Nature (Lond) 1969; 224:38–42.

191. Lampert PW, Carpenter S. Electron microscopic studies on the vascular permeability and the mechanism of demyelination in experimental allergic encephalomyelitis. J Neuropathol Exp Neurol 1965;24:11–24.

192. Levine S, Wenk EJ. Exacerbation and transformation of allergic encephalomyelitis by pertussis vaccine. Proc Soc Exp Biol (NY) 1966;122:115–118.

193. Brown WJ. The capillaries in acute and subacute multiple sclerosis plaques: a morphometric analysis. Neurology 1978;28:84–92.

194. Claudio L, Raine CS, Brosnan CF. Evidence of persistent blood-brain barrier abnormalities in chronic-progressive multiple sclerosis. Acta Neuropathol 1995;90:228–238.

195. Hirano A, Dembitzer HM, Becker NH, et al. Fine structural alterations of the blood-brain barrier in experimental allergic encephalomyelitis. J Neuropath Exp Neurol 1970;29:432–440.

196. Åström KE. Webster HD, Arnason BG. The initial lesion in experimental allergic neuritis. A phase and electron microscopic study. J Exp Med 1968;128:469–496.

197. Lossinsky AS, Vorbrodt AW, Wisniewski HM. Ultracytochemical studies of vesicular and canalicular transport structures in the injured mammalian blood brain barrier. Acta Neuropathol (Berl) 1983;61:239–245.

198. Hawkins CP, Munro PMG, Mackenzie F, et al. Duration and selectivity of blood-brain-barrier breakdown in chronic relapsing experimental allergic encephalomyelitis studied by gadolinium-DTPA and protein markers. Brain 1990;113:365–378.

199. Gay D, Esiri M. Blood-brain barrier damage in acute multiple sclerosis plaques: An immunocytological study. Brain 1991;114:557–572.

200. Kwon EE, Prineas JW. Blood-brain barrier abnormality in long-standing multiple sclerosis lesions. J Neuropathol Exp Neurol 1994;53:625–636.

201. Lampert PW. Demyelination and remyelination in experimental allergic encephalomyelitis: further electron microscopic observations. J Neuropathol Exp Neurol 1965;24: 371–385.

202. Lampert PW. Electron microscopic studies on ordinary and hyperacute experimental allergic encephalomyelitis. Acta Neuropathol (Berl) 1967;9:99–126.

203. Raine CS, Snyder DH, Valsamis MP, Stone SH. Chronic experimental allergic encephalomyelitis in inbred guinea pigs. An ultrastructural study. Lab Invest 1974;31:369–380.

204. Wisniewski H, Prineas J, Raine CS. An ultrastructural study of experimental demyelination and remyelination I. acute experimental allergic encephalomyelitis in the peripheral nervous system. Lab Invest 1969;21:105.

205. Epstein LG, Prineas JW, Raine CS. Attachment of myelin to coated pits on macrophages in experimental allergic encephalomyelitis. J Neurol Sci 1983;61:341–348.

206. Prineas JW. The Neuropathology of Multiple Sclerosis. In PJ Vinken, GW Bruyn, HL Klawans (eds), Handbook of Clinical Neurology. Amsterdam: North Holland Publishing, 1985;213–257.

207. Prineas JW, Graham JS. Multiple sclerosis: capping of surface immunoglobulin G on macrophages engaged in myelin breakdown. Ann Neurol 1981;10:149–158.

208. Nyland HR, Matre R, Mork S. Fc receptors on microglial lipophages in multiple sclerosis. N Engl J Med 1980;302: 120–121.

209. Piddleson SJ, Lassmann H, Zimprich F, et al. The demyelinating potential of antibodies to myelin oligodendrocyte glycoprotein is related to their ability to fix complement. Am J Pathol 1993;143:555–564.

210. Genain CP, Cannella B, Hauser SL, Raine CS. Identification of auto antibodies with myelin damage in multiple sclerosis. Nat Med 1999;5:170–175.

211. Moore KW, O'Garra A, de Waal Malefyt R, et al. Interleukin-10. Annu Rev Immunol 1993;11:165–190.

212. Tripp CS, Wolf SF, Unanue ER. Interleukin 12 and tumor necrosis factor α are costimulators of interferon γ production by natural killer cells in severe combined immunodeficiency mice with listeriosis, and interleukin 10 is a

physiologic antagonist. Proc Natl Acad Sci U S A 1993;90:3725–3729.

213. van der Pouw Kraan TCTM, Boeije LCM, Smeenk RJT, et al. Prostaglanding-E2 is a potent inhibitor of human interleukin-12 production. J Exp Med 1995; 181:775–779.

214. D'Andra A, Aste-Amezaga M, Valiante NM, et al. Interleukin-10 (IL-10) inhibits human lymphocytes interferon gamma production by suppressing natural killer cell stimulatory factor/IL-12 synthesis in accessory cells. J Exp Med 1993;178:1041–1048.

215. Stone SH, Lerner EM. Chronic disseminated allergic encephalomyelitis in guinea pigs. Ann N Y Acad Sci 1965;122:227–241.

216. Traugott V, Shevach E, Chiba J, et al. Chronic relapsing experimental allergic encephalomyelitis: identification and dynamics of T and B cells within the central nervous system. Cell Immunol 1982;68:261–265.

217. Raine CS, Stone SH. Suppression of chronic Allergic Encephalomyelitis: relevance to multiple sclerosis. Science 1978;201:445–447.

218. Raine CS, Traugott V, Farooq M, et al. Augmentation of immune-mediated demyelination by lipid haptens. Lab Invest 1981;45:174–182.

219. Raine CS, Traugott V, Farooq M, et al. Helper antigens are needed for demyelination. J Neuropath Exp Neurol 1980;39:385(abst).

220. Moore GRW, Traugott V, Farooq M, et al. Experimental autoimmune encephalomyelitis. Augmentation of demyelination by different myelin lipids. Lab Invest 1984;51:416–424.

221. Wray SH, Cogen GG, Arnason BGW. Experimental allergic encephalomyelitis. Passive transfer by the intraocular injection of sensitized cells. Arch Neurol 1976;33:183.

222. Brosnan CF, Stoner GL, Bloom BR, Wisniewski HM. Studies on demyelination by activated lymphocytes in the rabbit eye. II. Antibody-dependent cell-mediated demyelination. J Immunol 1977;118:2103–2110.

223. Stoner GL, Brosnan CF, Wisniewski HM, Bloom BR. Studies on demyelination by activated lymphocytes in the rabbit eye. I. Effects of a mononuclear cell infiltrate induced by products of activated lymphocytes. J Immunol 1977;118:2094–2102.

224. Wisniewski HM, Brosnan CF, Bloom BR. Bystander and Antibody-Dependent Cell-Mediated Demyelination. In AN Davison, ML Cuzner (eds), The Suppression of Experimental Allergic Encephalomyelitis and Multiple Sclerosis. New York: Academic Press, 1980;45–48.

225. Lebar R, Boutry J-M, Vincent C, et al. Studies on autoimmune encephalomyelitis in the guinea pig. II. An in vitro investigation on the nature, properties and specificity of the serum-demyelinating factor. J Immunol 1976;116: 1439.

226. Lebar E, Lubetzki C, Vincent C, et al. The M2 autoantigen of central nervous system myelin, a glycoprotein present in oligodendrocyte membrane. Clin Exp Immunol 1986;66:423–443.

227. Bornstein MB, Crain SM. Functional studies of cultured brain tissue as related to 'demyelinative disorders.' Science 1965;148:1242–1244.

228. Berg O, Källen B. An in vitro gliotoxic effect of serum from animals with experimental allergic encephalomyelitis. Acta Path Microbiol Scand 1962;54:425–433.

229. Alvord Jr. EC. Acute Disseminated Encephalomyelitis and "Allergic" Neuroencephalopathies. In PJ Vinken, GW Bruyn (eds), Handbook of Clinical Neurology. Amsterdam: North Holland, 1970;9:500–571.

230. Selmaj KW, Raine CS. Tumor necrosis factor mediates myelin and oligodendrocyte damage in vitro. Ann Neurol 1988;23:339.

231. Selmaj KM, Raine CS, Farooq M, et al. Cytokine toxicity against oligodendrocytes: apoptosis induced by lymphotoxin. J Immunol 1991;147:1522–1529.

232. Hickey WF, Kimura H. Perivascular microglial cells of the CNS are bone marrow-derived and present antigen in vivo. Science 1988;239:290–292.

233. Kabat EA, Wolf A, Bezer AE. Studies on acute disseminated encephalomyelitis produced experimentally in rhesus monkeys. VII. The effect of cortisone. J Immunol 1952;68:265.

234. Gammon GA, Dilworth MJ. Effect of corticotropin on paralysis of experimental allergic encephalomyelitis. Arch Neurol Psychiatry 1953;69:649.

235. Brandriss MW, Smith JW, Friedman RM. Suppression of experimental allergic encephalomyelitis by antimetabolites. Ann N Y Acad Sci 1965;122:356–368.

236. Bolton C, Cuzner ML. Modification of EAE by Nonsteroidal Anti-Inflammatory Drugs. In AN Davison, ML Cuzner (eds), The Suppression of Experimental Allergic Encephalomyelitis and Multiple Sclerosis. New York: Academic Press, 1980;189–197.

237. Claman HN. How corticosteroids work. J Allergy Clin Immunol 1975;55:145–151.

238. Rice GPA, Cladribine Study Group. Cladribine and chronic progressive multiple sclerosis: the results of a multicenter trial. Neurology 1997;48:1730.

239. Watson CM, Davison AN, Baker D, et al. Suppression of demyelination by mitoxantrone. Int J Immunopharmacol 1991;13:923–930.

240. Levine S, Saltzman A. Regional suppression, therapy after onset and prevention of relapses in experimental allergic encephalomyelitis by mitoxantrone. J Neuroimmunol 1986;13:175–181.

241. Lublin FD, Lavasa M, Viti C, Knobler RL. Suppression of acute and relapsing allergic encephalomyelitis with mitoxantrone. Clin Immunol Immunopathol 1987;45:122–128.

242. Ridge SC, Sloboda AE, McReynolds RA, et al. Suppression of experimental allergic encephalomyelitis by mitoxantrone. Clin Immunol Immunopathol 1985;35:35–42.

243. Hartung HP, Gonsette R, and the MIMS-Study Group. Mitoxantrone in progressive multiple sclerosis (MS): clinical results and three year follow-up of the MIMS Trial. Mult Scler 1999;5(Suppl 1):515.

244. Hartung HP, Gonsette R, and the MIMS-Study Group. Mitoxantrone in progressive multiple sclerosis: a placebo-controlled, randomized, observer-blind phase III trial: clinical results and three-year follow-up. Neurology 1999;52(Suppl 2):A290.

245. Fidler JM, De Joy SQ, Smith FR III, Gibbons JJ Jr. Selective immunomodulation by the antineoplastic agent mitoxantrone. II. Nonspecific adherent suppressor cells

derived from mitoxantrone-treated mice. J Immunol 1986;136:2747–2754.

246. Fidler JM, De Joy SQ, Gibbons JJ Jr. Selective immuno-modulation by the antineoplastic agent mitoxantrone. I. Suppression of B lymphocyte function. J Immunol 1986;137:727–732.

247. Klinkert WE, Kojima K, Lesslauer W, et al. TNF-alpha receptor fusion protein prevents experimental autoimmune encephalomyelitis and demyelination in Lewis rats: an overview. J Neuroimmunol 1997;72:163–168.

248. Baker D, Butler D, Scallon BJ, O'Neill JK, et al. Control of established experimental allergic encephalomyelitis by inhibition of tumor necrosis factor (TNF) activity within the central nervous system using monoclonal antibodies and TNF receptor-immunoglobulin fusion proteins. Eur J Immunol 1994;24:2040–2048.

249. Liu J, Marino MW, Wong G, et al. TNF is a potent anti-inflammatory cytokine in autoimmune-mediated demyeli-nation. Nat Med 1998;4:78–83.

250. The Lenercept Multiple Sclerosis Study Group and the University of British Columbia MS/MRI Analysis Group. TNF neutralization in MS: results of a randomized, pla-cebo-controlled multicenter study. Neurology 1999;53: 457–465.

251. Devaux B, Enderlin F, Wallner B, Smilek DE. Induction of EAE in mice with recombinant human MOG, and treat-ment of EAE with a MOG peptide. J Neuroimmunol 1997;75:169–173.

252. Swanborg RH. Immunological response to altered encephali-togenic protein in guinea pigs. J Immunol 1969;102:381–388.

253. Swanborg RH. Antigen-induced inhibition of experimen-tal allergic encephalomyelitis. I. Inhibition in guinea pigs injected with non-encephalitogenic modified myelin basic protein. J Immunol 1972;109:540–546.

254. Ortiz-Ortiz L, Weigle WO. Cellular events in the induc-tion of experimental allergic encephalomyelitis in rats. J Exp Med 1976;144:604–616.

255. Swierkosz JE, Swanborg RH. Suppressor cell control of unresponsiveness to experimental allergic encephalomy-elitis. J Immunol 1975;115:631–633.

256. Swanborg RH. Antigen-induced inhibition of experimen-tal allergic encephalomyelitis. III. Localization of an inhibitory site distinct from the major encephalitogenic determinant of myelin basic protein. J Immunol 1975;114:191–194.

257. Ben-Nun A, Wekerle H, Cohen IR. Vaccination against autoimmune encephalomyelitis with T-lymphocyte cell lines reactive against myelin basic protein. Nature 1981; 293:60–61.

258. Howell MD, Winters ST, Olee T, et al. Vaccination against experimental allergic encephalomyelitis with T cell recep-tor peptides. Science 1989;246:668–670.

259. Acha-Orbea H, Mitchell DJ, Timmermann L, et al. Limited heterogeneity of T cell receptors from lymphocytes mediat-ing autoimmune encephalomyelitis allows specific immune intervention. Cell 1988;54:263–273.

260. Urban JL, Kumar V, Kono DH, et al. Restricted use of T cell receptor V genes in murine autoimmune encephalomy-elitis raises possibilities for antibody therapy. Cell 1988;54:577–592.

261. Vandenbark AA, Hashim G, Offner H. Immunization with a synthetic T cell receptor V-region peptide protects against experimental autoimmune encephalomyelitis. Nature 1989;341:541–544.

262. Rott O, Fleischer B, Cash E. Interleukin-10 prevents experimental allergic encephalomyelitis in rats. Eur J Immunol 1994;24:1434–1440.

263. Nagelkerken L, Blauw B, Tielemans M. IL-4 abrogates the inhibitory effect of IL-10 on the development of experimental allergic encephalomyelitis in SJL mice. Int Immunol 1997;9:1243–1251.

264. Samoilova EB, Horton JL, Chen Y. Acceleration of exper-imental autoimmune encephalomyelitis in interleukin-10-deficient mice: roles of interleukin-10 in disease progres-sion and recovery. Cell Immunol 1998;188:118–124.

265. Cua DJ, Groux H, Hinton DR, et al. Transgenic interleu-kin 10 prevents induction of experimental autoimmune encephalomyelitis. J Exp Med 1999;189:1005–1010.

266. Legge KL, Min B, Bell JJ, et al. Coupling of peripheral tolerance to endogenous interleukin 10 promotes effective modulation of myelin-activated T cells and ameliorates experimental allergic encephalomyelitis. J Exp Med 2000;191:2039–2051.

267. Racke MK, Jalbut SD, Cannella B, et al. Prevention and treatment of chronic relapsing experimental allergic encephalomyelitis by transforming growth factor β1. J Immunol 1991;146:3012–3017.

268. Johns LD, Flanders KC, Ranges GE, Sriram S. Successful treatment of experimental allergic encephalomyelitis with transforming growth factor-β1. J Immunol 1991;147: 1792–1796.

269. Kurvvilla AP, Shah R, Hochwald GM, et al. Protective effect of transforming growth factor β1 in experimental autoimmune diseases in mice. Proc Natl Acad Sci U S A 1991;88:2918–2921.

270. Ruddle NH, Bergman CM, McGrath KM, et al. An anti-body to lymphotoxin and tumor necrosis factor prevents transfer of experimental allergic encephalomyelitis. J Exp Med 1990;172:1193–1200.

271. Segal BM, Dwyer BK, Shevach EM. An interleukin (IL-10/IL-12) immunoregulatory circuit controls susceptibil-ity to autoimmune disease. J Exp Med 1998;187:537–546.

272. Sedgwick JD, Mason DW. The mechanism of inhibition of experimental allergic encephalomyelitis in the rat by monoclonal antibody against CD4. J Neuroimmunol 1986;13:217–232.

273. Jung S, Toyka K, Hartung HP. Suppression of experimen-tal autoimmune encephalomyelitis in Lewis rats by anti-bodies against CD2. Eur J Immunol 1995;25:1391–1398.

274. Pashov A, Dubey C, Kaveri SV, et al. Normal immunoglo-bulin G protects against experimental allergic encephalo-myelitis by inducing transferable T cell unresponsiveness to myelin basic protein. Eur J Immunol 1998;28:1823–1831.

275. Ahiron A, Margalit R, Hershkoviz R, et al. Intravenous immunoglobulin treatment of experimental T cell-medi-ated autoimmune disease. J Clin Invest 1994;93:600–605.

276. Skias DD, Reder AT. IL-10 inhibits EAE. Neurology 1995;45(Suppl 4):A349.

277. Cannella B, Gao YL, Brosnan C, Raine CS. IL-10 fails to abrogate experimental autoimmune encephalomyelitis. J Neurosci Res 1996;45:735–746.

278. Taupin V, Renno T, Bourbonniere L, et al. Increased severity of experimental autoimmune encephalomyelitis, chronic macrophage/microglial reactivity, and demyelination in transgenic mice producing tumor necrosis factor-alpha in the central nervous system. Eur J Immunol 1997;27:905–913.

279. Merrill JE, Ignarro LJ, Sherman RP, Melinek J, et al. Microglial cell cytotoxicity of oligodendrocytes is mediated through nitric oxide. J Immunol 1993;151:2132.

280. Mac Micking JD, Willenborg DO, Weidemann MJ, et al. Elevated secretion of reactive nitrogen and oxygen intermediates by inflammatory leukocytes in hyperacute experimental autoimmune encephalomyelitis: enhancement by the soluble products of encephalitogenic T cells. J Exp Med 1992;176:303–307.

281. Cross AH, Keeling RM, Goorha S, et al. Inducible nitric oxide synthase gene expression and enzyme activity correlate with disease activity in murine experimental autoimmune encephalomyelitis. J Neuroimmunol 1996; 71:145–153.

282. Okuda Y, Sakoda S, Fujimura H, Yanagihara T. Expression of the inducible isoform of nitric oxide synthase in the central nervous system of mice correlates with the severity of actively induced experimental allergic encephalomyelitis. J Neuroimmunol 1995;62:103–112.

283. Willenborg DO, Fordham SA, Staykova MS, et al. IFN-γ is critical to the control of murine autoimmune encephalomyelitis and regulates both in the periphery and in the target tissue: a possible role for nitric oxide. J Immunol 1999;163:5278–5286.

284. Zettl UK, Mix E, Zielasek J, Stangel M, et al. Apoptosis of myelin-reactive T cells induced by reactive oxygen and nitrogen intermediates in vitro. Cell Immunol 1997;178:1–8.

285. Van der Veen RC, Dietlin TA, Dixon Gary J, Gilmore W. Macrophage-derived nitric oxide inhibits the proliferation of activated T helper cells and is induced during antigenic stimulation of resting T cells. Cell Immunol 2000;199;43–49.

286. Ruuls SR, Van der Linden S, Sontrop K, et al. Aggravation of experimental allergic encephalomyelitis (EAE) by administration of nitric oxide (NO) synthase inhibitors. Clin Exp Immunol 1996;103:467–474.

287. Panitch HS, Hirsch AL, Haley AS, Johnson KP. Exacerbation of multiple sclerosis in patients treated with gamma interferon. Lancet 1987;1:893–895.

288. Chu C-Q, Wittmer S, Dalton DK. Failure to suppress the expansion of the activated CD4 T cell population in interferon γ-deficient mice leads to exacerbation of experimental autoimmune encephalomyelitis. J Exp Med 2000;192:123–128.

289. Willenborg DO, Fordham S, Bernard CA, et al. IFN-gamma plays a critical down-regulatory role in the induction and effector phase of myelin oligodendrocyte glycoprotein-induced autoimmune encephalomyelitis. J Immunol 1996;157:3223–3227.

290. Billiau AH, Heremans F, Van de Kerckove R, et al. Enhancement of experimental allergic encephalomyelitis in mice by antibodies against IFN. J Immunol 1988;140:1506–1510.

291. Heremans H, Dillen C, Groenen M, et al. Chronic relapsing experimental autoimmune encephalomyelitis (CREAE) in mice: enhancement by monoclonal antibodies against interferon-gamma. Eur J Immunol 1996;26:2393–2398.

292. Duong TT, Finkelman FD, Singh B, Strejan GH. Effect of anti-interferon-gamma monoclonal antibody treatment on the development of experimental allergic encephalomyelitis in resistant mouse strains. J Neuroimmunol 1994;53:101–107.

293. Duong TT, St. Louis J, Gilbert JJ, et al. Effect of anti-interferon-gamma and anti-interleukin-2 monoclonal antibody treatment on the development of actively and passively induced experimental allergic encephalomyelitis in the SJL/J mouse. J Neuroimmunol 1992;36:105–115.

294. Lublin FD, Knobler RL, Kalman B, et al. Monoclonal anti-gamma interferon antibodies enhance experimental allergic encephalomyelitis. Autoimmunity 1993;16:267–274.

295. Voorthuis J, VitdeHaag B, De Groot C, et al. Suppression of experimental allergic encephalomyelitis by intraventricular administration of interferon-gamma in Lewis rats. Clin Exp Immunol 1990;81:183–188.

296. Heremans H, Dillen C, Dijkmans A, et al. The role of cytokines in various animal models of inflammation. Lymphokine Res 1989;8:329–333.

297. Ferber IA, Brocke S, Taylor-Edwards C, et al. Mice with a disrupted IFN-gamma gene are susceptible to the induction of experimental autoimmune encephalomyelitis (EAE). J Immunol 1996;156:5–7.

298. Krakowski M, Owens T. Interferon-gamma confers resistance to experimental autoimmune encephalomyelitis. Eur J Immunol 1996;26:1641–1646.

299. Abreu SL. Interferon in experimental autoimmune encephalomyelitis (EAE): effects of exogenous interferon on the antigen-enhanced adoptive transfer of EAE. Int Arch Allergy Appl Immunol 1982;11:1–7.

300. Abreu SL, Tondreau J, Levine S, Sowinski R. Inhibition of passive localized experimental allergic encephalomyelitis by interferon. Int Arch Allergy Appl Immunol 1983;72:30–33.

301. Hertz F, Deghenghi R. Effect of rat and β-human interferons on hyperacute experimental allergic encephalomyelitis in rats. Agents Actions 1985;16:397–403.

302. Abreu SL, Thampoe I, Kaplan P. Interferon in experimental autoimmune encephalomyelitis: intraventricular administration. J Interferon Res 1986;6:627–632.

303. Arnon R, Sela M, Teitelbaum D. New insights into the mechanism of action of copolymer 1 in experimental allergic encephalomyelitis and multiple sclerosis. J Neurol 1996;243(Suppl 1):S8–S13.

304. Teitelbaum D, Fridkis-Hareli M, Arnon R, Sela M. Copolymer 1 inhibits chronic relapsing experimental allergic encephalomyelitis induced by proteolipid protein (PLP) peptides in mice and interferes with PLP-specific T cell responses. J Neuroimmunol 1996;64:209–217.

305. Gran B, Tranquill L, Zhou W, et al. Copolymer-1 modulates autoreactive, myelin basic protein reactive T cells and induces specific T-helper 2 T cell clones. Neurology 1999;52(Suppl 1):abstract.

306. Aharoni R, Teitelbaum D, Sela M, Arnon R. Copolymer 1 induces T cells of the T helper Type 2 that crossreact with

myelin basic protein and suppress experimental autoimmune encephalomyelitis. Proc Natl Acad Sci U S A 1997; 94:10821–10826.

307. Aharoni R, Teitelbaum D, Sela M, Arnon R. Bystander suppression of experimental autoimmune encephalomyelitis by T cell lines and clones of the Th2 type induced by copolymer 1. J Neuroimmunol 1998;91:135–146.

308. Bran B, Tranquill LR, Chen M, et al. Mechanisms of immunomodulation by glatiramer acetate. Neurology 2000; 55:1704–1714.

309. Brenner T, Meiner Z, Abramsky O, et al. Humoral responses to copolymer 1 in multiple sclerosis patients: preferential production of IgG1 over IgG2. Ann Neurol 1996;40:518(abst).

310. Carswell R. Pathological Anatomy: Illustrations on the Elementary Forms of Disease. London: Longman, Orme, Brown, Green and Longman, 1838.

311. Cruveilhier J. Anatomie pathologique du corps humain. Paris: J.B. Bailliere, 1829–1842.

312. Charcot J-M. Histologie de la sclerose en plaques. Gaz Hop de Paris 1868;41:554–555, 557–558, 566.

313. Dawson JW. The histology of disseminated sclerosis. Trans roy soc Edinb 1916;50:517–740.

314. Cohnheim J. Über Entzündung und Eiterung. Virch Arch f path Anat 1867;40:1–79.

315. Adams RD, Kubik CS. The morbid anatomy of the demyelinative diseases. Am J Med 1952;12:510–546.

316. Fog T. The topography of plaques in multiple sclerosis. Acta Neurol Scand 1965;41(Suppl 15):1–162.

317. Lumsden CE. The Neuropathology of Multiple Sclerosis. In PJ Vinken, GW Bruyn (eds), Handbook of Clinical Neurology, vol. 9, Multiple Sclerosis and other Demyelinating Diseases. New York: Elsevier, 1970:217–309.

318. Boyle EA, McGeer PL. Cellular immune-response in multiple sclerosis plaques. Am J Pathol 1990;137:575–584.

319. Suzuki K, Andrews JM, Waltz JM, Terry RD. Ultrastructural studies of multiple sclerosis. Lab Invest 1969;20:444–454.

320. Prineas J. Pathology of the early lesion in multiple sclerosis. Hum Pathol 1975;6:531–554.

321. Prineas JW, Raine CS. Electron microscopy and immunoperoxidase studies of early multiple sclerosis lesions. Neurology 1976;26:29–32.

322. Prineas JW, Barnard RO, Kwon EE, et al. Multiple sclerosis: remyelination of nascent lesions. Ann Neurol 1993;33: 137–151.

323. Prineas JW, Kwon EE, Cho E-S, Sharer LR. Continual breakdown and regeneration of myelin in progressive multiple sclerosis plaques. Ann N Y Acad Sci 1984;436:11–32.

324. Traugott U, Reinherz EL, Raine CS. Multiple sclerosis distribution of T cells, T cell subsets and Ia-positive macrophages in lesions of different ages. J Neuroimmunol 1983;4:201–221.

325. Traugott U, Reinherz EL, Raine CS. Multiple sclerosis: distribution of T cell subsets within chronic active lesions. Science 1983;219:308–310.

326. Weiner HL, Bhan AK, Burks J, et al. Immunohistochemical analysis of the cellular infiltrates in multiple sclerosis lesions. Neurology 1984;34(Suppl 1):112.

327. Boos J, Esiri MM, Tourtellotte WW, Mason DY. Immunohistological analysis of T lymphocyte subsets in the central nervous system in chronic progressive multiple sclerosis. J Neurol Sci 1983;62:219–232.

328. Jiang HJ, Zhang SI, Pernis B. Role of CD8+ T cells in murine experimental allergic encephalomyelitis. Science 1992;256:1213–1215.

329. Koh DR, Fung-Leung WP, Ho A, et al. Less mortality but more relapses in experimental allergic encephalomyelitis in CD8-1-mice. Science 1992;256:1210–1213.

330. Lassmann H, Vass K, Brunner C, Seitelberger F. Characterization of inflammatory infiltrates in experimental allergic encephalomyelitis. Prog Neuropathol 1986;6:33–62.

331. Hickey W, Gonatas NK. Suppressor T-lymphocytes in the spinal cord of Lewis rats recovered from acute experimental allergic encephalomyelitis. Cell Immunol 1984;85:284–288.

332. Bruck W, Sommermeier N, Bergmann M, et al. Macrophages in multiple sclerosis. Immunobiology 1996;195:588–600.

333. Lucchinetti CF, Brück W, Rodriguez M, Lassmann H. Distinct patterns of multiple sclerosis pathology indicates heterogeneity of pathogenesis. Brain Pathol 1996;6:259–274.

334. Lucchinetti C, Brück W, Parisi J, et al. Heterogeneity of multiple sclerosis lesions: implications for the pathogenesis of demyelination. Ann Neurol 2000;47:707–717.

335. Bakshi R, Miletich RS, Kinkel PR, et al. High-resolution fluorodeoxyglucose positron emission tomography shows both global and regional cerebral hypometabolism in multiple sclerosis. J Neuroimaging 1998;8:228–234.

336. Roelcke U, Kappos L, Lechner-Scott J, et al. Reduced glucose metabolism in the frontal cortex and basal ganglia of multiple sclerosis patients with fatigue: a 18F-fluorodeoxyglucose positron emission tomography study. Neurology 1997;48:1566–1571.

337. Rao SM, Leo GJ, Bernardin L, Unverzagt F. Cognitive dysfunction in multiple sclerosis: I. Frequency, patterns, and prediction. Neurology 1991;41:685–691.

338. Pliskin NH, Hamer DP, Goldstein DS, et al. Improved neuropsychological function in multiple sclerosis patients receiving interferon beta-1b. Neurology 1996;47:1463–1468.

339. Miller DH, Austin SJ, Connelly A, et al. Proton magnetic resonance spectroscopy of an acute and chronic lesion in multiple sclerosis (letter). Lancet 1991;337:58–59.

340. Arnold DL, Matthews PM. Measures for Quantification of Axonal Damage In Vivo Based on Magnetic Resonance Spectroscopic Imaging. In RA Rudick, DE Goodkin (eds), Multiple Sclerosis Therapeutics. London: Martin Dunitz, 1999;119–128.

341. Narayanan S, De Stefano N, Francis GS, et al. Restoration of cerebral axonal function in multiple sclerosis patients treated with interferon β-1b. Neurology 2000;54(Suppl 3): A232.

342. Stone LA, Frank JA, Albert PS, et al. The effect of interferon beta on blood-brain barrier disruptions demonstrated by contrast-enhanced magnetic resonance imaging in relapsing/remitting multiple sclerosis. Ann Neurol 1995; 37:611–619.

343. Calabresi PA, Stone LA, Bash CN, et al. Interferon beta results in immediate reduction of contrast-enhanced MRI lesions in multiple sclerosis patients followed by weekly MRI. Neurology 1997;48:1446–1448.

344. Broderick CF, Hsu LM, Massoth NA. Neuropsychological performance of MS patients with and without the use of Avonex (interferon-β-1a). Neurology 1999;52(Suppl 2): A499–500(abst).

345. Kabat EA, Moore DH, Landow H. An electrophoretic study of the protein components in the cerebrospinal fluid and their relationship to serum proteins. J Clin Invest 1942;21:571–577.

346. Noronha ABC, Richman DP, Arnason BGW. Detection of vivo stimulated cerebrospinal fluid lymphocytes by flow cytometry in patients with multiple sclerosis. N Engl J Med 1980;303:713–717.

347. Norrby E. Viral antibodies in multiple sclerosis. Prog Med Virol 1978;24:1–39.

348. Salmi A, Viljanen M, Reunanen M. Intrathecal synthesis of antibodies to diphtheria and tetanus toxoids in multiple sclerosis patients. J Neuroimmunol 1981;1:333–341.

349. Ebers GC, Zabriskie JB, Kunkel HG. Oligoclonal immunoglobulins in subacute sclerosing panencephalitis and multiple sclerosis—a study of idiotypic determinants. Clin Exp Immunol 1979;35:67–75.

350. Ebers GC. A study of CSF idiotypes in multiple sclerosis. Scand J Immunol 1982;16:151–161.

351. Cortese I, Capone S, Luchetti S, et al. CSF-enriched antibodies do not share specificities among MS patients. Mult Scler 1998;4:118–123.

352. Mattson DH, Roos RP, Arnason BGW. Isoelectric focusing of IgG eluted from multiple sclerosis and subacute sclerosing panencephalitis brains. Nature 1980;287:335–337.

353. Larsen PD, Bloomer LC, Bray PF. Epstein-Barr nuclear antigen and viral capsid antigen antibody titers in multiple sclerosis. Neurology 1985;35:435–438.

354. Sumaya CV, Myers LW, Ellison GW, Ench Y. Increased prevalence and titer of Epstein-Barr virus antibodies in patients with multiple sclerosis. Ann Neurol 1985;7:371–377.

355. Lindberg C, Andersen O, Vahlne A, et al. Epidemiological investigation of the association between infectious mononucleosis and multiple sclerosis. Neuroepidemiology 1991;10:62–65.

356. Wandinger K-P, Jabs W, Siekhaus A, et al. Association between clinical disease activity and Epstein-Barr virus reactivation in MS. Neurology 2000;55:178–184.

357. Elian M, Nightingale S, Dean G. Multiple sclerosis among United Kingdom-born children of immigrants from the Indian subcontinent, Africa and the West Indies. J Neurol Neurosurg Psychiatry 1990;53:906–911.

358. Munch MHJ, Christensen T, Møller-Larsen A, Haahr S. A single subtype of Epstein-Barr virus in members of multiple sclerosis clusters. Acta Neurol Scand 1998;98:395–399.

359. Farrell MA, Kaufmann JCE, Gilbert JJ, et al. Oligoclonal bands in multiple sclerosis: clinical-pathologic correlation. Neurology 1985;35:212–218.

360. Reder AT, Arnason BGW. Immunology of Multiple Sclerosis. In PJ Vinken, CW Bruyn (eds), Handbook of Clinical Neurology, vol. 3. New York: Elsevier, 1985:337–395.

361. Martin R, McFarland HF, McFarlin DE. Immunological aspects of demyelinating diseases. Annu Rev Immunol 1992;10:153–187.

362. Martin R, McFarland HF. Immunological aspects of experimental allergic encephalomyelitis and multiple sclerosis. Crit Rev Clin Lab Sci 1995;32:121–182.

363. Oger JJ-F, Arnason BGW, Wray SH, Kistler J. A study of B and T cells in multiple sclerosis. Neurology 1975;25: 444–447.

364. Arnason BGW, Antel JP. Suppressor cell function in multiple sclerosis. Ann Immunol (Inst Pasteur) 1978;129C: 159–170.

365. Antel JP, Arnason BGW, Medof ME. Suppressor cell function in multiple sclerosis: correlation with clinical disease activity. Ann Neurol 1979;5:338–342.

366. Antel JP, Bania MB, Reder A, Cashman N. Activated suppressor cell dysfunction in progressive multiple sclerosis. J Immunol 1985;137:137.

367. Reder AT, Antel JP, Oger JJ-F, et al. Low T8 antigen density on lymphocytes in active multiple sclerosis. Ann Neurol 1984;16:242–249.

368. Karaszewksi JW, Reder AT, Anlar B, et al. Increased lymphocyte beta-adrenergic receptor density in progressive multiple sclerosis is specific for the CD8+, CD28-suppressor cell. Ann Neurol 1991;30:42–47.

369. van Boxel-Dezaire AHH, Hoff SCJ, van Oosten BW, et al. Decreased interleukin-10 and increased interleukin-12p40 mRNA are associated with disease activity and characterize different disease stages in multiple sclerosis. Ann Neurol 1999;45:695–703.

370. Rieckmann P, Albrecht M, Kitze B, et al. Cytokine mRNA levels in mononuclear blood cells from patients with multiple sclerosis. Neurology 1994;44:1523–1526.

371. Musette P, Benveniste O, Lim A, et al. The pattern of production of cytokine mRNAs is markedly altered at the onset of multiple sclerosis. Res Immunol 1996;147:435–441.

372. Özenci V, Kouwenhoven M, Huang Y-M, et al. Multiple sclerosis: levels of interleukin-10 secreting blood mononuclear cells are low in untreated patients but augmented during interferon-β-1b treatment. Scand J Immunol 1999;49:554–561.

373. Navikas V, Link J, Palasik W, et al. Increased mRNA expression of IL-10 in mononuclear cells in multiple sclerosis and optic neuritis. Scand J Immunol 1995;41:171–178.

374. Crucian B, Dunne P, Friedman H, et al. Alterations in peripheral blood mononuclear cell cytokine production in response to phytohemagglutinin in multiple sclerosis patients. Clin Diagn Lab Immunol 1995;2:766–769.

375. Brod SA, Nelson LD, Khan M, Wolinsky JS. Increased in vitro induced CD4+ and CD8+ cell IFN-γ and CD4+ T cell IL-10 production in stable relapsing multiple sclerosis. Int J Neurosci 1997;90:187–202.

376. Monteyne P, Van Laere V, Marichal R, et al. Cytokine mRNA expression in CSF and peripheral blood mononuclear cells in multiple sclerosis: detection by RT-PCR without in vitro stimulation. J Neuroimmunol 1997;80: 137–142.

377. Mokhtarian F, Shi Y, Shirazian D, et al. Defective production of anti-inflammatory cytokine, TGF-β by T cell lines of patients with active multiple sclerosis. J Immunol 1994;152:6003–6010.

378. Bertolotto A, Capobianco M, Malucchi S, et al. Transforming growth factor β1 (TGFβ1) mRNA level correlates

with magnetic resonance imaging disease activity in multiple sclerosis patients. Neurosci Lett 1999;263:21–24.

379. Beck J, Rondot P, Jullien P, et al. TGF-β-like activity produced during regression of exacerbations in multiple sclerosis. Acta Neurol Scand 1991;84:452–455.

380. Nicoletti F, Di Marco R, Patti F, et al. Blood levels of transforming growth factor-beta 1 (TGF-β1) are elevated in both relapsing remitting and chronic progressive multiple sclerosis (MS) patients and are further augmented by treatment with interferon-beta 1b (IFN-β1b). Clin Exp Immunol 1998;113:96–99.

381. Miller A, Lider O, Roberts AB, et al. Suppressor T cells generated by oral tolerization to myelin basic protein suppress both in vitro and in vivo immune responses by the release of transforming growth factor beta after antigen specific triggering. Proc Natl Acad Sci U S A 1992;89:421–425.

382. Nicoletti F, Patti F, Cocuzza C, et al. Elevated serum levels of interleukin-12 in chronic progressive multiple sclerosis. J Neuroimmunol 1996;70:87–90.

383. Balashov KE, Comabella M, Ohashi T, et al. Defective regulation of IFNgamma and IL-12 by endogenous IL-10 in progressive MS. Neurology 2000;55:192–198.

384. Comabella M, Balashov K, Issazadeh S, et al. Elevated interleukin-12 in progressive multiple sclerosis correlates with disease activity and is normalized by pulse cyclophosphamide therapy. J Clin Invest 1998;102:671–678.

385. Fassbender K, Ragoschke A, Rossol S, et al. Increased release of interleukin-12p40 in MS: association with intracerebral inflammation. Neurology 1998;51:753–758.

386. Ferrante P, Fusi ML, Saresella M, et al. Cytokine production and surface marker expression in acute and stable multiple sclerosis: altered IL-12 production and augmented signaling lymphocytic activation molecule (SLAM)-expressing lymphocytes in acute multiple sclerosis. J Immunol 1998;160:1514–1521.

387. Reder AT, Genç K, Byskosh PV, et al. Monocyte activation in multiple sclerosis. Mult Scler 1998;4:162–168.

388. Matusevicius D, Kivisäkk P, Navikas V, et al. Interleukin-12 and perforin mRNA expression is augmented in blood mononuclear cells in multiple sclerosis. Scand J Immunol 1998;47:582–590.

389. Balashov KE, Smith DR, Khoury SJ, et al. Increased interleukin-12 production in progressive multiple sclerosis: induction by activated CD4+ T cells via CD40 ligand. Proc Natl Acad Sci U S A 1997;94:599–603.

390. Becher B, Giacomini PS, Pelletier D, et al. Interferon-γ secretion by peripheral blood T cell subsets in multiple sclerosis: correlation with disease phase and interferon-β therapy. Ann Neurol 1999;45:247–250.

391. Cottrell DA, Kremenchutzky M, Rice GPA, et al. The natural history of multiple sclerosis: a geographically based study. 6. Applications to planning and interpretation of clinical therapeutic trials in primary progressive multiple sclerosis. Brain 1999;122:641–647.

392. McDonnell GV, Middleton D, Graham CA, et al. Primary progressive multiple sclerosis (MS) is associated with HLA-DR2 in Northern Ireland. Neurology 1998;(Suppl 1):A209–A210(abst).

393. European Study Group on interferon beta-1b in secondary progressive MS. Placebo-controlled multicentre randomised trial of interferon beta-1b in treatment of secondary progressive multiple sclerosis. Lancet 1998;352:1491–1497.

394. Goodkin DE, North American Study Group on interferon beta-1b in secondary prevention MS. Interferon beta-1b in secondary progressive MS: clinical and MRI results of a 3-year randomized controlled trial. Neurology 2000;54 (Suppl):2352.

395. Miller DH, Molyneux PD, Barker GJ, et al. Effect of interferon β-1b on magnetic resonance imaging outcomes in secondary progressive multiple sclerosis: results of a European multicenter, randomized, double-blind, placebo-controlled trial. Ann Neurol 1999;46:850–859.

396. Blumhardt LD. Interferon beta-1a (Rebif) in the treatment of secondary progressive multiple sclerosis. I. Clinical results. Presented at the 9th European Neurological Society Meeting: June 7, 1999: Milan Italy. Abstract #37.

397. Dowling P, Husar W, Mennona J, et al. Cell death and birth in multiple sclerosis brain. J Neurol Sci 1997;149:1–11.

398. Tabi Z, McCombe PA, Pender MP. Apoptotic elimination of Vβ8.2+ cells from the central nervous system during recovery from experimental autoimmune encephalomyelitis induced by the passive transfer of Vβ8.2+ encephalitogenic T cells. Eur J Immunol 1994;24:2609–2617.

399. Smith T, Schmied M, Hewson AK, et al. Apoptosis of T cells and macrophages in the central nervous system of intact and adrenalectomized lewis rats during experimental allergic encephalomyelitis. J Autoimmun 1996;9:167–174.

400. Nguyen KB, McCombe PA, Pender MP. Increased apoptosis of T lymphocytes and macrophages in the central and peripheral nervous system of lewis rats with experimental autoimmune encephalomyelitis treated with dexamethasone. J Neuropath Exp Neurol 1997;56:58–69.

401. Karaszewski JW, Reder AT, Maselli R, et al. Sympathetic skin responses are decreased and lymphocyte beta-adrenergic receptors are increased in progressive multiple sclerosis. Ann Neurol 1990;27:366–372.

402. Chelmicka-Schorr E, Arnason BGW. Interactions between the sympathetic nervous system and the immune system. Brain Behav Immun 1999;12:271–278.

403. Arnason BGW. Immunology and the Autonomic Nervous System. In O Appenzeller (ed), Handbook of Clinical Neurology, vol. 75, The Autonomic Nervous System. Amsterdam: Elsevier, 2000:551–566.

404. Chelmicka-Schorr E, Checinski M, Arnason BGW. Chemical sympathectomy augments the severity of experimental allergic encephalomyelitis in rats. Ann N Y Acad Sci 1988;540:707–708.

405. Muthyala S, Wiegmann K, Kim DH, et al. Experimental allergic encephalomyelitis, β-adrenergic receptors and interferon gamma-secreting cells in β-adrenergic agonist-treated rats. Int J Immunopharmac 1995;17:895–901.

406. Chelmicka-Schorr E, Kwasniewski MN, Czlonkowska A. Sympathetic nervous system modulates macrophage function. Int J Immunopharmacol 1992;14:841–846.

407. Miles K, Quintans J, Chelmicka-Schorr E, Arnason BGW. The sympathetic nervous system modulates antibody response to thymus-dependent antigens. J Neuroimmunol 1981;1:101–106.

408. Chelmicka-Schorr E, Kwasniewski MN, Thomas BE, Arnason BGW. The β-adrenergic agonist isoproterenol suppresses experimental allergic encephalomyelitis in Lewis rats. J Neuroimmunol 1989;25:203–207.

409. Wiegmann K, Muthyla S, Kim D, et al. Beta-adrenergic agonists suppress chronic-relapsing experimental allergic encephalomyelitis (CREAE) in Lewis rats. J Neuroimmunol 1995;56:201–206.

410. Miles K, Atweh S, Otten G, et al. β-Adrenergic receptors on splenic lymphocytes from axotomized mice. Int J Immunopharmacol 1984;6:171–177.

411. Karaszewski JW, Reder AT, Anlar B, et al. Increased lymphocyte beta-adrenergic receptor density in progressive multiple sclerosis is specific for the CD8+,CD28-suppressor cell. Ann Neurol 1991;30:42–47.

412. Karaszewski JW, Reder A, Anlar B, Arnason BGW. Increased high affinity beta-adrenergic receptor densities and cyclic AMP responses of CD8 cells in multiple sclerosis. J Neuroimmunol 1993;43:1–8.

413. Zoukos Y, Kidd D, Woodroofe MN, et al. Increased expression of high affinity IL-2 receptors and β-adrenoreceptors in peripheral blood mononuclear cells is associated with clinical and MRI activity in multiple sclerosis. Brain 1994;117:307–315.

414. Boullerne AI, Petry KG, Meynard M, Geffard M. Indirect evidence for nitric oxide involvement in multiple sclerosis by characterization of circulating antibodies directed against conjugated S-nitrosocysteine. J Neuroimmunol 1995;60:117–124.

415. Boullerne AI, Rodríguez JJ, Touil T, et al. Anti-SNO-cysteine antibodies are a predictive marker for demyelination in experimental autoimmune encephalomyelitis: implications for multiple sclerosis. J Neurosci 2002;22:123–132.

416. Bö L, Dawson TM, Wesselingh S, et al. Induction of nitric oxide synthase in demyelinating regions of multiple sclerosis brain. Ann Neurol 1994;36:778–786.

417. Bagasra O, Michaels FH, Zheng YM, et al. Activation of the inducible form of nitric oxide synthase in the brains of patients with multiple sclerosis. Proc Natl Acad Sci U S A 1995;92:12041–12045.

418. Avrameas S, Ternynck T. The natural autoantibodies system: between hypothesis and facts. Molecular Immunol 1993;30:1133–1142.

419. Berger S, Chandra R, Balló H, et al. Immune complexes are potent inhibitors of interleukin-12 secretion by human monocytes. Eur J Immunol 1997;27:2994–3000.

420. Passwell JH, Dayer J-M, Merler E. Increased prostaglandin production by human monocytes after membrane receptor activation. J Immunol 1979;123:115–120.

421. Bonney RJ, Naruns P, Davies P, Humes JL. Antigen-antibody complexes stimulate the synthesis and release of prostaglandins by mouse peritoneal macrophages. Prostaglandins 1979;18:605–616.

422. Berger S, Balló H, Stutte HJ. Immune complex-induced interleukin-6, interleukin-10 and prostaglandin secretion by human monocytes: a network of pro-and anti-inflammatory cytokines dependent on the antigen: antibody ratio. Eur J Immunol 1996;26:1297–1301.

423. Zhang B, Yamamura T, Kondo T, et al. Regulation of experimental autoimmune encephalomyelitis by natural killer (NK) cells. J Exp Med 1997;186:1677–1687.

424. Reder AT, Checinski M, Chelmicka-Schorr E. The effect of chemical sympathectomy on natural killer cells in mice. Brain Behav Immun 1989;3:110–118.

425. Orange JS, Biron CA. An absolute and restricted requirement for IL-12 in natural killer cell IFN-γ production and antiviral defense. J Immunol 1996;156:1138–1142.

426. Orange JS, Biron CA. Characterization of early IL-12, IFN-αβ, and TNF effects on antiviral state and NK cell response during murine cytomegalovirus infection. J Immunol 1996;156:4746–4756.

427. Gray JD, Hirokawa M, Ohtsuka K, Horwitz DA. Generation of an inhibitory circuit involving CD8+ T cells, IL-2, and NK cells-derived TGF-β: contrasting effects of anti-CD2 and anti-CD3. J Immunol 1998;160:2248–2254.

428. Gray JD, Hirokawa M, Horwitz DA. The role of transforming growth factor β in the generation of suppression: an interaction between CD8+ T and NK cells. J Exp Med 1994;180:1937–1942.

429. Lee H-M, Rich S. Differential activation of CD8+ T cells by transforming growth factor-β1. J Immunol 1993;151:668–677.

430. Chavin KD, Qin L, Yon R, et al. Anti-CD2 mAbs suppress cytotoxic lymphocyte activity by the generation of Th2 suppressor cells and receptor blockade. J Immunol 1994;152:3729–3739.

431. Fox EJ, Cook RG, Lewis DE, Rich RR. Proliferative signals for suppressor T cells. Helper cells stimulated with pokeweed mitogen in vitro produce a suppressor cell growth factor. J Clin Invest 1986;78:214–220.

432. Fischer A, Durandy A, Griscelli C. Role of prostaglandin E₂ in the induction of nonspecific T lymphocyte suppressor activity. J Immunol 1981;126:1452–1455.

433. El Masry MN, Fox EJ, Rich RR. Sequential effects of prostaglandins and interferon-γ on differentiation of CD8+ suppressor cells. J Immunol 1987;139:688–694.

434. Marth T, Strober W, Kelsall BL. High dose oral tolerance in ovalbumin TCR-transgenic mice. Systemic neutralization of IL-12 augments TGF-β secretion and T cell apoptosis. J Immunol 1996;157:2348–2357.

435. Marth T, Strober W, Seder RA, Kelsall BL. Regulation of transforming growth factor-β production by interleukin-12. Eur J Immunol 1997;27:1213–1220.

436. Karp CL, Birm CA, Irani DN. Interferon-β in multiple sclerosis: is IL-12 suppression the key? Immunol Today 2000;21:24–28.

437. Vodovotz Y, Bogdan C. Control of nitric oxide synthase expression by transforming growth factor-beta: implications for homeostasis. Prog Growth Factor Res 1994;5:341–351.

438. Vodovotz Y, Geiser AG, Chesler L, et al. Spontaneously increased production of nitric oxide and aberrant expression of the inducible nitric oxide synthase in vivo in the transforming growth factor β1 null mouse. J Exp Med 1996;183:2337–2342.

439. Brackett NK, Basu S, Aballa TC, et al. Inflammatory cytokines—a possible role for infertility in men with spinal cord injury. Soc Neurosci 1992;14:841–846.

440. Bertrams J, Kuwert E. HL-A antigen frequencies in multiple sclerosis. Significant increase of HL-A3, HA-A10 and W5, and decrease of HL-A12. Eur Neurol 1972;7:74.

441. Jersild CA, Svejgaard A, Fog T. HL-A antigens and multiple sclerosis. Lancet 1972;1:1240–1241.

442. Naito S, Namerow N, Mickey MR, Terasaki P. Multiple Sclerosis: association with HL-A3. Tissue Antigens 1972;2:1–4.

443. Arnason BGW, Fuller TC, Lehrich JR, Wray SH. Histocompatibility antigens in multiple sclerosis and optic neuritis. J Neurosci Sci 1974;22:419.

444. Sadovnick AD, Armstrong H, Rice GP, et al. A population-based study of multiple sclerosis in twins: update. Ann Neurol 1993;33:281–285.

445. Arnason BGW, Reder AT. Interferons and multiple sclerosis. Clin Neuropharmacol 1994;17:495–574.

446. Durelli L, Bongioanni MR, Cavallo R, et al. Chronic systemic high-dose recombinant interferon alpha-2a reduces relapse rate, MRI signs of disease activity, and lymphocyte interferon gamma production in relapsing remitting multiple sclerosis. Neurology 1994;44:406–413.

447. Sanders O, Ran R, van Riel P, et al. Neutralization of TNF by lenercept (TNFR55-IgG, Ro 45-2081) in patients with rheumatoid arthritis treated for 3 months: results of a European phase II trial. Arthritis Rheum 1996;39(Suppl 9):242.

448. Vyse TJ, Todd JA, Kotzin BL. Non-MHC Genetic Contributions to Autoimmune Disease. In NR Rose, IR Mackay (eds), The Autoimmune Diseases. San Diego: Academic Press, 1998;85–118.

449. Cella DF, Dineen K, Arnason B, et al. Validation of the functional assessment of multiple sclerosis quality of life instrument. Neurology 1996;47:129–139.

Chapter 2

Molecular Basis of Myelination

Sharon Lefebvre and Timothy Vartanian

Myelination of axons involves the extension and biochemical modification of the plasma membranes of oligodendrocytes and Schwann's cells.[1] In the adult, myelin acts as an electrical insulator, a high-resistance, low-capacitance membrane allowing faster signal transmission along the axon. The essential role of myelin in the normal function of the nervous system is demonstrated by the profound effects of myelin loss in the peripheral nervous system (PNS), as in Guillain-Barré syndrome and Charcot-Marie-Tooth disease, and the central nervous system (CNS), as seen in multiple sclerosis.

Myelin Physiology and Function

Action potentials are generated in the axon in response to the opening of voltage-gated Na^+ channels localized at nodes of Ranvier. The local depolarization at the node of Ranvier spreads passively along the axon segment within the internode until arriving at the subsequent node of Ranvier where it is regenerated actively. Conduction velocity is increased through myelination due both to an increase in axonal diameter of myelinated axons and to the process of saltatory conduction. The amount of current flowing along the axon from the trigger zone is not enough to discharge the capacitance along the entire length of the axon; therefore, the action potential gradually diminishes as it travels along the axon. This effect is counteracted by high densities of Na^+ channels clustered at the nodes of Ranvier.[1] These sodium channels are acti-

vated by the depolarization of the axonal membrane induced by an influx of positively charged sodium ions. Additional depolarization is passively transmitted along the axon by the sodium gradient to the next node, where a new action potential is generated. This process, by which the action potential appears to jump from node to node, is known as *saltatory conduction*.

Structure of Myelin

Myelin is a lipid-protein membrane primarily found in the white matter of the CNS and in peripheral nerves containing large motor axons. Myelin is similar in composition to other plasma membranes, consisting of 70% lipid and 30% protein. The composition of myelin sheath lipids is approximately 25% cholesterol, 29% galactolipid, and 46% phospholipid.[2] The major galactolipid in myelin is galactocerebroside. The lipid molecules are arranged such that the hydrophilic portions provide the interface between the aqueous spaces, both intra- and extracellular, and the hydrophobic core produced by the acyl chains. The bilayer dimensions remain fairly constant throughout myelin, whereas the aqueous spaces differ in their degree of compaction.

The myelin sheath is arranged in concentric layers. Myelinated segments of nerve are separated by regularly spaced nodes of Ranvier.[1] The voltage-gated sodium channels that are responsible for the action potential are clustered at the nodes, in contrast to the arrangement in unmyelinated nerves where the channels are spread throughout the axolemma.[3] It is in the paranodal region—the region adjacent to the node—where the axon and the myelinating cell come into close contact, forming a tight interaction.[4]

Myelin Proteins

The major protein of mature PNS myelin is P0. P0 has a molecular weight of 28 kDa, having a single transmembrane domain and being found in compact myelin. P0 is a member of the immunoglobulin (Ig) superfamily. The Ig domains located on the glycosylated extracellular portion of the protein may play a role in the compaction of myelin. Loss of the P0 locus is associated with Charcot-Marie-Tooth disease type 1b.[5] In mice lacking P0, properties of the early stages of myelination, such as the ability of Schwann's cells to segregate axon bundles and to assume a 1 to 1 relationship with large-diameter axons, are not affected. However, these Schwann's cells are unable to form compact myelin.[6] P0 is thought to be involved in intraperiod line compaction.

Peripheral myelin protein 22 (PMP22) is a 22-kDa glycoprotein present in compact PNS myelin. PMP22 has a single site for N-linked glycosylation. The protein has four putative transmembrane domains. Carbohydrate residues in the protein may be involved in cell adhesion.[7] PMP22 mutations are associated with Charcot-Marie-Tooth disease type 1a, the most common inherited peripheral neuropathy in humans, and with hereditary neuropathy with liability to pressure palsies. *Trembler* mice, which lack a functional PMP22, exhibit peripheral nerve hypomyelination and continuous Schwann's cell proliferation into adulthood.[8]

The major protein of CNS myelin is proteolipid protein (PLP). Although PLP messenger RNA is expressed by Schwann's cells, the PLP protein is not found in PNS myelin.[9] The PLP gene encodes two alternatively spliced transcripts. The full-length PLP transcript encodes a 30-kDa protein, whereas the shorter transcript encodes the 26-kDa protein DM-20. PLP plays an important role in oligodendrocyte development. Absence of PLP results in premature cell death and hypomyelination.[10] The importance of PLP has largely been elucidated through the study of mice containing PLP

point mutations. The *jimpy* mouse exhibits axial body tremors followed by tonic seizures and subsequent death. Myelin in *jimpy* mice is diminished and abnormal.[11] Oligodendrocytes in *jimpy* mice die prematurely during CNS development, before the onset of myelination.

Myelin basic protein (MBP) exists in multiple isoforms that are derived from exon splicing and post-translational modifications such as phosphorylation and methylation. MBP is present in PNS and CNS compact myelin. Unlike other myelin proteins, MBP is not a transmembrane protein. MBP is located at the major dense line where it is involved in compaction of the myelin sheath. *Shiverer* mice, which lack functional MBP, show intention tremor, convulsions, and premature death. Although myelin at the intraperiod line appears normal, no major dense line is present. When injected into mice, MBP causes a T-cell–mediated inflammatory response known as *experimental autoimmune encephalomyelitis*, which has been used as a model for multiple sclerosis.

Myelin-associated glycoprotein (MAG) is a member of the Ig superfamily and contains five extracellular Ig-like domains and an intracellular domain that can be modified via phosphorylation and alternative messenger RNA splicing.[12] There are two MAG isoforms: 64 kDa and 60 kDa. MAG has been shown to interact with Fyn tyrosine kinase, focal adhesion kinase, and phospholipase Cγ, suggesting a role in transducing signals between axons and glia.[13,14] Indeed, MAG-deficient mice have been found to have axonal abnormalities, indicating a role in transmitting signals from myelinating glia to neurons.[15] Interestingly, MAG is phosphorylated by protein kinase C in cultured oligodendrocytes,[16] and protein kinase C has been found to be involved in oligodendrocyte differentiation and process formation.[17] MAG also contains an RGD (Arg-Gly-Asp) sequence that is known to play an important part in attachment to the integrin family.[18]

Myelin oligodendrocyte glycoprotein is a 26- to 28-kDa transmembrane glycoprotein that is also a member of the Ig superfamily. It has one Ig-like domain and two hydrophobic domains[19] and has a single site for N-linked glycosylation. Myelin oligodendrocyte glycoprotein is concentrated on the outside surfaces of oligodendrocytes and myelin sheaths but is absent from compact myelin.[20]

The oligodendrocyte-myelin glycoprotein is a 120-kDa glycoprotein. It is linked to the extracellular surface of oligodendrocytes by a glycosylphos-phatidylinositol anchor. The oligodendrocyte-myelin glycoprotein contains a cysteine-rich motif at its N-terminus and a series of leucine-rich repeats similar to those found in other proteins involved in cell adhesion.[21]

Transcriptional Control in Myelinating Glia

Regulation of the genes encoding myelin proteins is largely controlled at the transcriptional level. Several families of transcription factors that are expressed in myelinating glia have been recently identified.

The first glia-specific transcription factors were identified in invertebrates. The *Drosophila pointed* gene is expressed exclusively in glia of the embryonic CNS and is required for differentiation.[22] *Pointed* is a member of the ETS family of DNA-binding proteins that function as transcriptional activators.[23] *Engrailed* is another glia-specific transcription factor found in Drosophila. The *engrailed* gene encodes a homeodomain protein involved in determining segment polarity. There are two *engrailed* genes in vertebrates: en-1 and en-2.[24] En-2 knockout mice display structural defects in their cerebellum.[25]

Another homeodomain protein involved in glial development is paired-box homeotic gene (Pax3), which is expressed during early development in the dorsal part of the spinal cord and in cells of the neural crest.[26] Pax3-deficient mice exhibit neural tube defects, such as spina bifida and exencephaly and a dramatic loss of Schwann's cells.[27] Pax3 may be involved in determining the myelinating phenotype of Schwann's cells, as microinjection of Pax3 causes increased expression of markers characteristic of nonmyelinating Schwann's cells and causes a decrease in expression of MBP.[28] Mutations in *Pax3* have been seen in cases of Waardenburg's syndrome, suggesting a role in neural crest development, which is characterized by defects in the development of melanocytes and of the enteric nervous system.[29]

Tst-1/Oct6/SCIP is another homeodomain protein found in myelinating glia. This protein is a member of the POU group of homeodomain proteins and is expressed in Schwann's cells and oligodendrocytes. Expression of Tst-1/Oct6/SCIP is first detected in promyelinating cells,[30] and mice null for this gene exhibit Schwann's cells developmentally arrested at the promyelinating phase.[31,32] Tst-1/Oct6/SCIP is expressed in oligodendrocyte precursors but not in mature oligodendrocytes. However, loss of function has no effect on CNS myelination.[31,33] This may be due to overlapping functions by the oligodendrocyte-expressed Brn-1 and Brn-2.

Krox-20/Egr2 is a member of the zinc finger family of transcription factors, which is expressed in Schwann's cells but not in oligodendrocytes. *Krox-20/Egr2* is expressed at the onset of Schwann's cell development, and disruption of this gene leads to defects in PNS myelination.[34] Mutations in *Krox-20/Egr2* have been found in patients with congenital hypomyelinating neuropathy and Charcot-Marie-Tooth disease.[35]

MyTI (*myelin transcription factor I*) is a zinc finger protein expressed in the early stages of oligodendrocyte development. MyTI was isolated on the basis of its ability to bind to the *PLP* promoter. *Gtx* (*glia-* and *testis-specific homeobox gene*) is expressed in astrocytes and oligodendrocytes of adult mice.

The Sox proteins belong to the high-mobility-group family of DNA-binding proteins. Sox4 and Sox11 are expressed in oligodendrocyte precursors,[36] whereas Sox10 is first expressed in the neural crest and later is confined to mature oligodendrocytes and Schwann's cells.[37] Sox10-deficient mice show defects in the cranial ganglia and enteric nervous system and a dramatic loss of Schwann's cells.[38–40] Inoue et al.[40] recently described a *Sox10* mutation believed to exert a dominant negative effect in a patient with Waardenburg's syndrome. This individual exhibits myelin defects in both the PNS and CNS.

Last, a group of ubiquitously expressed transcription factors may play a role in myelination. These include Sp1, nuclear factor 1, cyclic AMP-responsive element-binding protien, and c-jun, among others. These proteins may function in concert with glia-specific factors to effect myelination.

Schwann's Cell Development

Schwann's cells originate from a region of ectoderm known as the *neural crest*, which develops adjacent to the dorsal neural ectoderm destined to form the neural tube. Schwann's cells migrate to populate the peripheral nerve. This migration is dependent on the extracellular matrix produced by mesenchymal cells.[41,42] This extracellular matrix contains fibronectin, laminin, collagen, proteoglycans, and tenascin.[43] Cell-surface adhesion molecules such as neural cell adhesion molecule and neuronal cadherin are also involved in neural crest cell migration.[44]

Mature Schwann's cells are elongated, extending longitudinally along the axons of peripheral nerve, with a centrally located nucleus. Mature Schwann's cells can be of two types: myelinating and nonmyelinating. Differentiation of Schwann's cells into either type is affected by axon diameter.[45] Nonmyelinating Schwann's cells do not produce myelin and are associated with small-diameter axons (less than 1 μM). Myelinating Schwann's cells are associated with large-diameter (more than 1 μM) axons. Myelinating Schwann's cells require constant contact with the axon to maintain the myelinating phenotype. Transection of peripheral nerve results in dedifferentiation of the myelinating Schwann's cell into a premyelinating Schwann's cell.

During development in the PNS, Schwann's cells line up along the peripheral nerve with intervals between them that will eventually become the nodes. The external cell membrane of the Schwann's cell, known as the *plasmalemma*, then surrounds a single axon, forming a double-membrane structure known as the *mesaxon*, which then elongates and wraps around the axon in concentric layers. During this process, the processes of the Schwann's cell are condensed into the compact lamellae of mature myelin.

Oligodendrocyte Development

Oligodendrocytes are derived from neural stem cells in the subventricular zone dorsal to the floor plate in the developing spinal cord. Oligodendrocyte precursors mature through a series of stages characterized by the expression of different cell-surface antigens and morphologic and motility changes as well as responsiveness to specific growth factors.[46] Oligodendrocytes develop from glial progenitor cells known as *O-2A cells*, which derive their name from their ability to develop into either oligodendrocytes or type 2 astrocytes in vitro. O-2A cells have a bipolar morphology, are highly motile, and can be labeled with the mono-

clonal antibody A2B5.[47] O-2A cells proliferate in response to platelet-derived growth factor and, to a lesser extent, to basic fibroblast growth factor-2 (FGF-2)[48–50] As they mature, O-2A cells become multipolar and less motile and are labeled by the monoclonal antibody O4.[51] O4+ cells lose their responsiveness to platelet-derived growth factor but still respond to FGF-2. Mature, differentiated oligodendrocytes have a complex multiprocessed morphology and can be labeled by galactocerebroside, the major glycolipid in myelin.[52]

Unlike Schwann's cells, oligodendrocytes can extend multiple processes, ensheathing multiple nerves. Myelination begins with contact between the oligodendrocyte and axonal membranes, followed within the cytoplasmic space by a compaction process that results in the apposition of the two opposing bilayers. The intracellular apposition is known as the *major dense line*, which derives its name from its appearance in electron micrographs. The extracellular apposition is known as the *intraperiod line*.

Axonal Signals of Myelination

In the PNS, the proliferation, differentiation, and survival of Schwann's cell precursors is dependent on the presence of axons.[53] It has been determined that the signal for engulfment and ensheathment of the nerve by Schwann's cells originates in the axons that are in contact with the mature Schwann's cells.[54–56]

In contrast, myelin formation in the CNS does not appear to be as dependent on axonal signals. In vitro oligodendrocytes are capable of proliferation and differentiation in the absence of neurons.[46] In addition, these mature oligodendrocytes are capable of producing myelin proteins.[57–59] Mature oligodendrocytes maintained in culture are able to extend at the tip of their processes large unfolded membranes that are able to form myelin-like structures.[60,61] However, myelin formed in the absence of neurons is not as well compacted as myelin associated with neurons.[62,63]

Studies have shown that oligodendrocyte precursors in culture can be stimulated to divide in vitro by soluble- and contact-mediated signals derived from nerves.[64–67] Additionally, oligodendrocytes fail to develop normally in transected optic nerve, suggesting the necessity of neuronally derived survival factors.[68–71] In the rodent ventral spinal cord, motoneurons arise approximately 2 days before the appearance of oligodendrocytes, suggesting a possible axonal signal.[72] This factor may be neuregulin (NRG), as E10 spinal cords explants from NRG[–/–] mice show neurite outgrowth but do not generate O-2As.[73]

Neuregulin and Neuregulin Receptors

The NRGs are a group of growth factors derived from alternative splicing of a single gene. These proteins have been independently identified as glial growth factor, acetylcholine receptor inducing activity, neu differentiation factor, and heregulin. NRGs belong to the epidermal growth factor superfamily of proteins. Alternative splicing of the NRG gene produces multiple isoforms, both membrane-bound and soluble. In addition to the 50- to 60-amino acid epidermal growth factor domain, NRG isoforms may contain an Ig-like domain or a cysteine-rich domain, also called the *sensory and motor neuron–derived factor*.[74] Production of NRGs in mice begins at embryonic day 9.

NRG signals are transduced through the ErbB family of receptor protein tyrosine kinases expressed in glial cells and postsynaptic cells. NRG binds to and phosphorylates both ErbB-3 and ErbB-4 but only interacts with ErbB-2 through receptor dimerization.[75,76] The ErbB receptors are 170- to 185-kDa proteins with a single transmembrane domain, two cysteine-rich regions in the extracellular region, and a relatively large cytoplasmic tail that contains numerous tyrosine residues that can be phosphorylated on stimulation with NRG.

NRG has been shown to be a survival factor for Schwann's cells in culture.[77] NRG also plays a role in the induction of proliferation of Schwann's cells by axons. NRG bound to the axonal membrane interacts with ErbB2 on the Schwann's cell.[78] In addition to promoting survival and proliferation, NRG appears to regulate programmed cell death in the developing nerve. Schwann's cells in vivo normally undergo developmentally regulated programmed cell death in neonatal sciatic nerve. This cell death can be prevented by the addition of NRG.[79] ErbB3 is also essential for Schwann's cell development, as mice lacking ErbB3 lack Schwann's cell precursors and mature Schwann's cells.[80]

NRG plays an important role in oligodendrocyte development. Its expression is seen at E14 in the ventral ventricular zone, where oligodendrocytes are believed to originate.[81] In spinal cord explants prepared from NRG knockout mice, oligodendrocytes are not produced unless they are cultured in the presence of added NRG.[73] In vitro, NRG promotes proliferation of both O-2As and mature oligodendrocytes.[82]

Myelin Damage and Remyelination

Damage to myelin can result from exposure to toxins, infection, injury, degeneration, or autoimmune disease. Myelin damage is accompanied by a decrease in conduction velocity and a loss of cell-cell interactions between the axon and myelinating glia, which can result in destabilizing changes in the axonal cytoskeleton.[83] Active lesions found in the brains of patients with multiple sclerosis contain both damaged myelin and transected axons.[84] Areas of demyelination are populated by macrophages, neutrophils, lymphocytes, and microglia. It is the phagocytic macrophages that are mainly responsible for the destruction of myelin by the immune system in patients with multiple sclerosis. The major goals of multiple sclerosis treatment are the suppression of the inflammatory immune response and restoration of glial and neuronal function.[85]

Remyelination in the CNS can be divided into two phases: a recruitment phase during which oligodendrocytes proliferate and migrate to the site of injury and a differentiation phase during which oligodendrocytes contact the axon and form a myelin sheath.[86] Each of these steps is driven by growth factors expressed in the CNS. Growth factor expression varies at each step of remyelination. Platelet-derived growth factor and FGF-2, which have been shown to enhance oligodendrocyte motility, are expressed at highest levels during the recruitment phase. During the differentiation phase, FGF-2 levels decrease, whereas insulin-like and transforming growth factor-β1 levels increase.[87]

Conclusions

Knowledge of the composition, organization, structure, and regulation of myelin proteins and lipids is necessary for an understanding of diseases of CNS white matter. Examining the myelination process suggests potential therapeutic targets, and studying oligodendrocyte development may lead to new remyelination strategies.

References

1. Morell P, Quarles R, Norton W. Myelin Formation, Structure, and Biochemistry. New York: Raven Press Ltd, 1994;117–144.
2. Brante G. Studies on lipids in the nervous system with special reference to quantitative chemical determinations and topical distribution. Acta Physiol Scand 1949;18:1–24.
3. Black J, Kocsis J, Waxman S. Ion channel organization of the myelinated fiber. Trends Neurosci 1990;13:48–54.
4. Rosenbluth J. Glial Membranes and Axonal Junctions. New York: Oxford University Press, 1995.
5. Oakey R, Watson M, Seldin M. Construction of a physical map on mouse and human chromosome 1: comparison of 13 Mb of human DNA. Hum Mol Genet 1992; 1:613–620.
6. Giese K, Martini R, Lemke G, et al. Disruption of the P0 gene in mice leads to hypomyelination, abnormal expression of recognition molecules, and degeneration of myelin and axons. Cell 1992;71(4):565–576.
7. Snipes G, Suter U, Shooter E. Human peripheral myelin protein-22 carries the L2/HNK-1 carbohydrate epitope. J Neurochem 1993;61:1961–1964.
8. Aguayo A, Atiwell M, Trecarte J, et al. Abnormal myelination in transplanted Trembler mouse Schwann cells. Nature 1977;265:73–75.
9. Puckett C, Hudson L, Ono K, et al. Myelin specific proteolipid protein is expressed in myelinating Schwann cells but not incorporated into myelin sheaths. J Neurosci Res 1987;18:511–518.
10. Nave K, Milner R. Proteolipid proteins: structure and genetic expression in normal and myelin-deficient mice. Crit Rev Neurobiol 1989;5:65–91.
11. Duncan I. Dissection of the phenotype and genotype of X-linked myelin mutants. Ann N Y Acad Sci 1990;605:110–121.
12. Quarles R, Coleman D, Salzer J, Trapp B. Myelin-associated glycoprotein: structure-function relationships and involvement in neurological diseases. Boca Raton: CRC Press, 1992.
13. Jaramillo M, Afar D, Almazan G, Bell J. Identification of tyrosine 620 as the major phosphorylation site of myelin-associated glycoprotein and its implications in interacting with signaling molecules. J Biol Chem 1994;269:27240–27245.
14. Umemori H, Sato S, Yagi T, et al. Initial events of myelination involve Fyn tyrosine kinase signaling. Nature 1994;367:572–576.
15. Fruttiger M, Montag D, Schachner M, Martini R. Crucial role for myelin-associated glycoprotein in the mainte-

nance of axon-myelin integrity. Eur J Neurosci 1995;7:511–515.
16. Bambrick L, Braun P. Phosphorylation of myelin-associated glycoprotein in cultured oligodendrocytes. Dev Neurosci 1991;13:412–416.
17. Vartanian T, Szuchet S, Dawson G, Campagnoni A. Oligodendrocyte adhesion activates protein kinase C-mediated phosphorylation of myelin basic protein. Science 1986; 234:1395–1398.
18. Rouslahti E, Piersbacher M. New perspectives in cell adhesion and integrins. Science 1987;238:491–497.
19. Gardinier M, Amiguet P, Linington C, Mettieu J. Myelin/oligodendrocyte glycoprotein is a unique member of the immunoglobulin superfamily. J Neurosci Res 1992;33: 177–187
20. Brunner C, Lassmann H, Waehneldt T, et al. Differential ultrastructural localization of myelin basic protein, myelin/oligodendroglial glycoprotein, and 2',3'-cyclic nucleotide 3'-phosphodiesterase in the CNS of adult rats. J Neurochem 1989;52:296–304.
21. Quarles R. Glycoproteins of myelin sheaths. J Mol Neurosci 1997;8:1–12.
22. Klaes A, Menne T, Stollewerk A, et al. The Ets transcription factors encoded by the Drosophila gene pointed direct glial cell differentiation in the embryonic CNS. Cell 1994;78:149–160.
23. Wasylyk B, Hahn S. The Ets family of transcription factors. Eur J Biochem 1993;211:7–18.
24. Joyner A, Hanks M. The engrailed genes: evolution of fuction. Semin Dev Biol 1991;2:435–445.
25. Millen K, Wurst W, Herrup K, Joyner A. Abnormal cerebellar development and patterning of postnatal foliation in two mouse Engrailed-2 mutants. Development 1994;120:695–706.
26. Read A, Newton V. Waardenburg Syndrome. J Med Genet 1997;34:656–665.
27. Goulding M, Chalepakis G, Deutsch U, et al. Pax-3, a novel murine DNA binding protein expressed during early neurogenesis. EMBO J 1991;10:135–147.
28. Kioussi C, Gross M, Gruss P. Pax3: a paired domain gene as a regulator in PNS myelination. Neuron 1995;15:553–562.
29. Tassabehji M, Newton V, Leverton K, et al. PAX3 gene structure and mutations: close analogies between Waardenburg syndrome and the Splotch mouse. Hum Mol Genet 1994;3:1069–1074.
30. Arroyo E, Bermingham J, Rosenfeld M, Scherer S. Promyelinating Schwann cells express Tst-1/Oct-6/SCIP. J Neurosci 1998;18:7891–7902.
31. Bermingham J, Scherer S, O'Connell S, et al. Tst-1/Oct-6/SCIP regulates a unique step in peripheral myelination and is required for normal respiration. Genes Dev 1996;10:1751–1762.
32. Jaegle M, Mandemakers W, Broos L, et al. The POU factor Oct-6 and Schwann cell differentiation. Science 1996;41:372–378.
33. Jaegle M, Meijer D. Role of Oct-6 in Schwann cell differentiation. Microsc Res Tech 1998;41(5):372–378.
34. Topilko P, Schneider M, Levi G, et al. Krox-20 controls myelination in the peripheral nervous system. Nature 1994;371:796–799.

35. Warner L, Mancias P, Butler I, et al. Mutations in the early growth response 2 (EGR2) gene are associated with hereditary myelinopathies. Nat Genet 1998;18:383–384.

36. Kuhlbrodt K, Herbarth B, Sock E, et al. Cooperative function of POU proteins and Sox proteins in glial cells. J Biol Chem 1998a;273(26):16050–16057.

37. Kuhlbrodt K, Herbarth B, Sock E, et al. Sox10, a novel transcription modulator in glial cells. J Neurosci 1998b; 18:237–250.

38. Herbarth B, Pingault V, Bondurand N, et al. Mutation in the Sry-related Sox10 gene in Dominant megacolon, a mouse model for human Hirschsprung disease. Proc Natl Acad Sci U S A 1998;95:5161–5165.

39. Southard-Smith E, Kos L, Pavan W. Sox10 mutation disrupts neural crest development in Dom Hirschsprung mouse model. Nat Genet 1998;18:60–64.

40. Inoue K, Tanabe Y, Lupski J. Myelin deficiencies in both the central and peripheral nervous system associated with a Sox10 mutation. Ann Neurol 1999;46:313–318.

41. Bronner-Fraser M. Analysis of the early stages of trunk neural crest migration in avian embryos using monoclonal antibody HNK-1. Dev Biol 1986;115:44–55.

42. Le Douarin N, Teillet M. Experimental analysis of the migration and differentiation of neuroblasts of the autonomic nervous system and of neuroectodermal mesenchymal derivatives, using a biological cell marking technique. Dev Biol 1974;41(1):162–184.

43. Lallier T, Bronner-Fraser M. Avian neural crest cell attachment to laminin: involvement of divalent cation dependent and independent integrins. Development 1991; 113:1069–1084.

44. Akitaya, T, Bonner-Fraser M. Expression of cell adhesion molecules during initiation and cessation of neural crest cell migration. Dev Dyn 1992;194:12–20.

45. Voyvodic J. Target size regulates calibre and myelination of sympathetic nerves. Nature 1989;342:430–433.

46. Pfeiffer S, Warrington A, Bansal R. The oligodendrocyte and its many cellular processes. Trends Cell Biol 1993;3: 191–197.

47. Eisenbarth G, Walsh F, Nirenburg M. Monoclonal antibody to a plasma membrane antigen of neurons. Proc Natl Acad Sci U S A 1979;76:4913–4917.

48. Gard A, Pfeiffer S. Glial cell mitogens bFGF and PDGF differentially regulate development of O4+ GalC-oligodendrocyte progenitors. Dev Biol 1993;159:618–630.

49. Nobel M, Murray K, Strooband P, et al. Platelet-derived growth factor promotes division and motility and inhibits premature differentiation of the oligodendrocyte/type-2 astrocyte progenitor cell. Nature 1988;333:560–562.

50. Richardson W, Pringle N, Mosley M, et al. A role for platelet-derived growth factor in normal gliogenesis in the central nervous system. Cell 1988;53:309–319.

51. Sommer I, Schachner M. Monoclonal antibodies (O1 to O4) to oligodendrocyte cell surfaces: an immunocytological study in the central nervous system. Dev Biol 1981;83:311–327.

52. Raff M, Mirsky R, Fields K, et al. Galactocerebroside: a specific cell surface antigenic marker for oligodendrocytes in culture. Nature 1978;274:813–816.

53. Jessen M, Mirsky R. Schwann cell precursors and their development. Glia 1991;4:185–194.

54. Owens G, Bunge R. Evidence for an early role for myelin-associated glycoprotein in the process of myelination. Glia 1989;2:119–128.

55. Scherer S, Vogelbacker H, Kamholtz J. Axons modulate the expression of proteolipid protein in the CNS. J Neurosci Res 1992;32:138–148.

56. Scherer S, Wang D, Kuhn R, et al. Axons regulate Schwann cell expression of the POU transcription factor SCIP. J Neurosci 1994;14:1930–1942.

57. Dubois-Dalq M, Behar T, Hudson L, Lazzarini R. Emergence of three myelin proteins in oligodendrocytes cultured without neurons. J Cell Biol 1986;102:384–392.

58. Hudson L, Friedrich V, Behar T, et al. The initial events in myelin synthesis: orientation of proteolipid protein in the plasmid membrane of cultured oligodendrocytes. J Cell Biol 1989;109:717–727.

59. Mirsky R, Winter J, Abney E, et al. Myelin-specific proteins and glycolipids in rat Schwann cells and oligodendrocytes in culture. J Cell Biol 1980;84(3):483–494.

60. Sarlieve L, Rao G, Campbell G, Pieringer R. Investigations on myelination in vitro: biochemical and morphological changes in cultures of dissociated brain cells from embryonic mice. Brain Res 1980;189:79–90.

61. Szuchet S, Polak P, Yim S. Mature oligodendrocytes cultured in the absence of neurons recapitulate the ontogenic development of myelin membranes. Dev Neurosci 1986;8:208–221.

62. Althaus H, Montz H, Neuroff V. Isolation and cultivation of mature oligodendroglial cells. Naturwissench 1984;71: 309–315.

63. Lubetzki C, Demerens C, Anglade P. Even in culture, oligodendrocytes myelinate solely axons. Proc Natl Acad Sci U S A 1993;90:6820–6824.

64. Edgar A, Pfeiffer S. Extracts from Neuron-enriched cultures of chick telencephalon stimulate the proliferation of rat oligodendrocytes. Dev Neurosci 1985;7:206–215.

65. Giuilian D, Young D. Brain peptides and glial growth. II. Identification of cells that secrete glia-promoting factors. J Cell Biol 1986;102:812–820.

66. Levine J. Neuronal influences on glial progenitor cell development. Neuron 1989;3:103–113.

67. Wood P, Bunge R. Evidence that axons are mitogenic for oligodendrocytes isolated from adult animal. Nature 1986;320:756–758.

68. David S, Miller R, Patel R, Raff M. Effects of neonatal transection in the rat optic nerve: evidence that the oligodendrocyte-type-2 astrocyte cell lineage depends on axons for its survival. J Neurocytol 1984;13:961–974.

69. Fulcrand J, Privat A. Neuroglia reactions secondary to Wallerian degeneration in the optic nerve of the postnatal rat: ultrastructural and quantitative study. J Comp Neurol 1997;176:189–224.

70. Privat A, Valat J, Fulcrand J. Proliferation of neuroglial cells in the degenerating optic nerve of a young rat: an autoradiographic study. J Neuropath Exp Neurol 1981;40: 46–60.

71. Valat J, Privat A, Fulcrand J. Multiplication and differentiation of glial cells in the optic nerve of the postnatal rat. Anat Embryol (Berl) 1983;167:335–346.

72. Miller R. Oligodendrocyte origins. Trends Neurosci 1996;19:92–96.

73. Vartanian T, Fischbach G, Miller R. Failure of spinal cord oligodendrocyte development in mice lacking neuregulin. Proc Natl Acad Sci U S A 1999;96:731–735.

74. Ho W, Armanini M, Nuijens A, et al. Sensory and motor neuron-derived factor. A novel heregulin variant highly expressed in sensory and motor neurons. J Biol Chem 1995;270:14523–14532.

75. Sliwkowski M, Schaefer G, Akita R, et al. Coexpression of ErbB-2 and ErbB-3 protein reconstitutes a high affinity receptor for heregulin. J Biol Chem 1994;269(20):14661–14665.

76. Tzahar E, Levlowitz G, Karunagaran D, et al. ErbB-3 and ErbB-4 function as the respective low and high affinity receptors of all Neu differentiation factor/heregulin isoforms. J Biol Chem 1994;269:25226–25233.

77. Dong Z, Brennan A, Liu N, et al. Neu differentiation factor is a neuron-glial signal and regulates survival, proliferation, and maturation of rat Schwann cell precursors. Neuron 1995;15:585–596.

78. Morrissey T, Levi A, Nuijens A, et al. Axon-induced mitogenesis of human Schwann cells involves heregulin and p185erbB2. Proc Natl Acad Sci U S A 1995;92(5):1431–1435.

79. Syroid D, Maycox P, Burrola P, et al. Cell death in the Schwann cell lineage and its regulation by neuregulin. Proc Natl Acad Sci U S A 1995;93:9229–9234.

80. Riethmacher D, Sonnenberg-Riethmacher E, Brinkmann V, et al. Severe neuropathies in mice with targeted mutations in the ErbB3 receptor. Nature 1997;389:725–730.

81. Vartanian T, Corfas G, Li Y, et al. A role for the acetylcholine receptor-inducing protein ARIA in oligodendrocyte development. Proc Natl Acad Sci U S A 1994;91:11626–11630.

82. Canoll P, Musacchio J, Hardy R, et al. GGF/neuregulin is a neuronal signal that promotes the proliferation and survival and inhibits the differentiation of oligodendrocyte progenitors. Neuron 1996;17:229–243.

83. Kirkpatrick L, Brady S. Modulation of the axonal microtubule cytoskeleton by myelinating Schwann cells. J Neurosci 1994;14:7440–7450.

84. Trapp B, Peterson J, Ransohoff R, et al. Axonal transection in the lesions of multiple sclerosis. N Engl J Med 1998;338:278–285.

85. Compston A. Future prospects for the management of multiple sclerosis. Ann Neurol 1994;36:S146–S150.

86. Franklin R, Hinks G. Understanding CNS remyelination: clues from developmental and regeneration biology. J Neurosci Res 1999;58:207–213.

87. Hinks G, Franklin R. Distinctive patterns of PDGF-A, FGF-2, IGF-I, and TGF-1 gene expression during remyelination of experimentally-induced spinal cord demyelination. Mol Cell Neurosci 1999;14:153–168.

Chapter 3

Role of Neural Stem and Oligodendrocyte Progenitor Cells in Demyelinating Diseases: Insights into Disease Mechanisms and Therapeutic Potential

Jaime Imitola, Karim Makhlouf, and Samia J. Khoury

Multiple sclerosis (MS) is the most commonly diagnosed neurologic disease in young adults,[1] and this chronic debilitating disorder represents a high cost to society in terms of productivity and health care.[2] The current treatment of MS relies on immunologic manipulations; however, it is becoming clear that remyelination should be considered as a goal for treatment. Although demyelination is a key feature in MS pathology, current evidence suggests that remyelination also occurs.[3,4] As these mechanisms become better understood, neural repair may emerge as a target for new therapies. The objective of this chapter is to review what is known about the role of neural stem cells (NSCs) and progenitor cells in demyelinating diseases. We first discuss basic concepts of NSC and progenitor biology, especially oligodendrocyte progenitor cells (OPCs) in the developing and the mature central nervous system (CNS). We next review the cytokines and other molecules involved in NSC and OPC proliferation, differentiation, and apoptosis; then we discuss the role of NSC and progenitor cells during demyelination and remyelination in animal models and MS. Finally, we analyze the therapeutic potential of NSCs.

Neurobiology of Neural Stem Cells and Oligodendrocyte Progenitor Cells

Definitions and Anatomy

In this chapter, we use the term *precursors* to define multipotent cells that include both stem cells and progenitor cells. The current definition of NSC relies on "operational" criteria rather than on a set of molecular markers alone; NSCs are cells from the CNS and peripheral nervous system that are multipotent and self-renewing.[5] Multipotency is the ability of a single cell clone to give rise to the three major types of cells in the CNS: neurons, oligodendrocytes, and astrocytes. The term *self-renewal* is used to define the capacity of a clone to generate progeny of new stem cells, preserving their properties from generation to generation. Moreover, NSCs have a specific proliferative response to the cytokines epidermal growth factor (EGF) and basic fibroblast growth factor-2 (FGF-2) and are able to replace endogenous cells when damaged (Figure 3-1).[5]

Progenitor cells are a step farther than NSCs in the differentiation process, as they have committed to a route of differentiation and begin to express

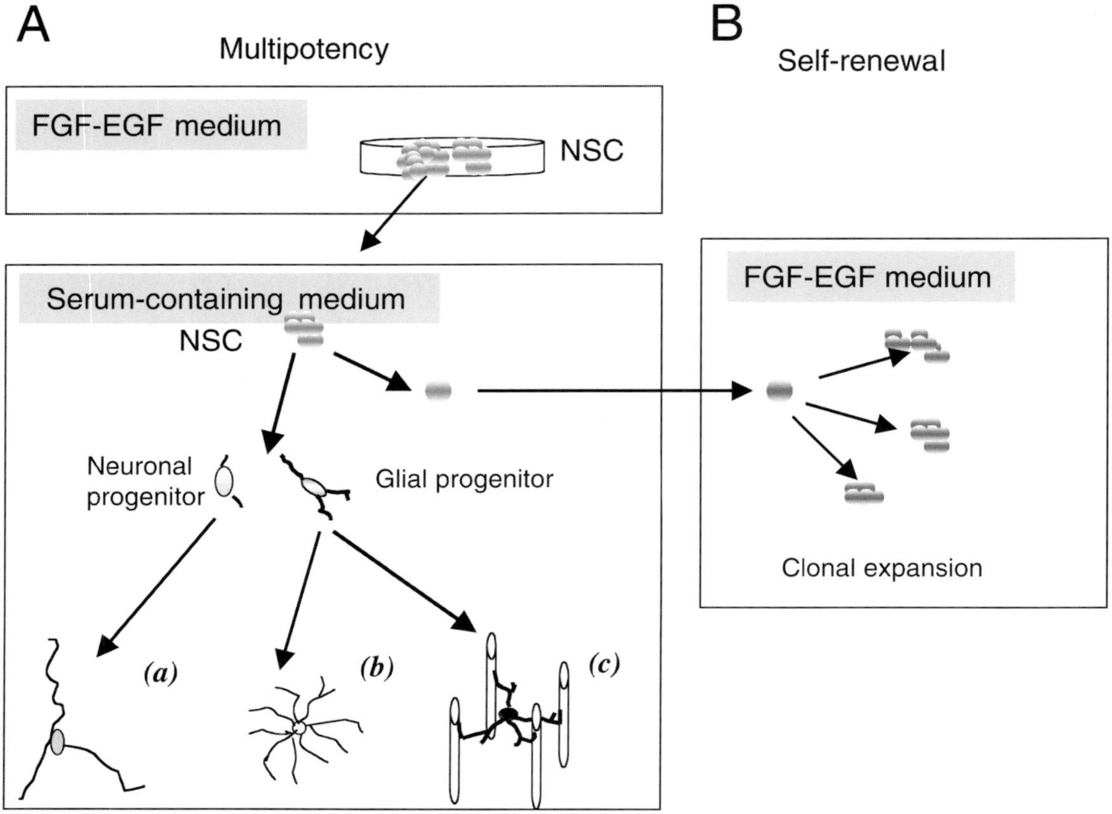

Figure 3-1. Operational definition of neural stem cells (NSCs). **A.** NSCs exhibit multipotency when cultured in medium containing serum. NSCs give rise to neuronal and glial progenitors and subsequently more mature and terminally differentiated cells: neurons (a), astrocytes (b), and oligodendrocytes (c). **B.** These multipotent cells can give rise to secondary neurospheres, demonstrating self-renewing capacity. (EGF = epidermal growth factor; FGF = fibroblast growth factor.)

lineage-specific markers. However, already committed progenitor cells such as OPCs can exhibit "stemness" and thus are able to generate neurons, astrocytes, and oligodendrocytes in vitro (Figure 3-2).[6–8] Even fully differentiated cells have been demonstrated to possess this property as well: Adult ependymal cells have been shown to exhibit properties of stem cells when cultured in vitro and in vivo. In vivo, these cells generate neurons that migrate to the olfactory bulb and astrocytes that respond to injury,[9] although controversy exists about the real stemness of ependymal cells.[10,11] Finally, others have found NSCs in a glial population from postnatal and adult cortex as well as adult optic nerve, which give rise to neurons and glia.[11,12] These provocative results are likely to

reflect the existence of a heterogenous population of NSCs in the adult CNS (Table 3-1).

NSCs reside in a relative dormant status throughout the CNS after completion of embryonic brain development. In the adult mammalian CNS, they can be isolated from the subventricular zone (SVZ), striatum, hippocampus, and cortex.[12,13] There are specific germinative zones in the embryonic and adult mammalian CNS[14] that can be considered as sources of NSCs. These zones include the SVZ, the external germinal layer of the cerebellum, the subgranular zone of the dentate gyrus, and the ependymal layer of the spinal cord.[15]

The SVZ is a heterogenous three-dimensional complex of several layers of cells adjacent to the ependyma, surrounding the lateral ventricles.

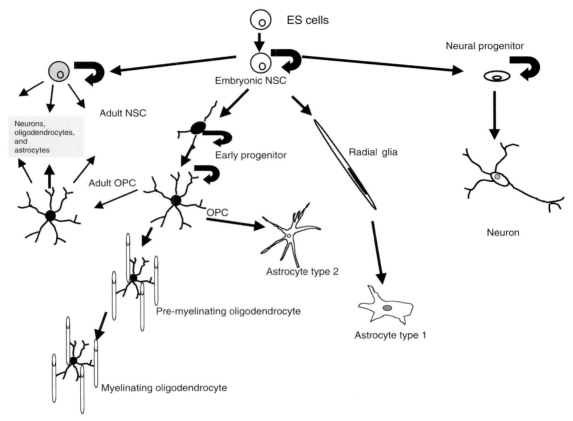

Figure 3-2. Neural stem cell (NSC) development. The developmental cascade from the embryonic stem (ES) cells to the mature neural cells is presented. NSCs and some progenitor cells are self-renewing (*curved arrows*) and differentiate into mature neural cells (*straight arrows*). Some progenitor cells previously thought to have a more restricted lineage commitment may exhibit multipotency (e.g., adult oligodendrocyte progenitor cells [OPCs] and NSCs).

There are so far four different types of cells in the SVZ: migrating neuronal precursors that migrate to the olfactory bulb; nestin-positive, glial fibrillary acidic protein (GFAP)–positive astrocytes that exhibit NSC properties; nestin-positive multipotent stem cells; and the ependymal cells that line the ventricle and are NSCs as well (see Color Plate 1).[9,16,17]

The SVZ is a source of NSCs and progenitor cells in vivo.[18] During development, neuronal and glial cells are born in the SVZ from NSCs that become progenitors, as these cells migrate out using the radial glia as a scaffold to reach the cortex.[19–22] NSCs in adults participate in the neurogenesis that is responsible for the seasonal changes of songs in the songbird,[23] the adult neurogenesis in humans,[24] and the response to injury in models of mammalian brain injury.[25]

The relative dormancy of NSCs is represented by a slow cell cycle in the adult CNS; in vivo NSCs of the SVZ divide symmetrically with the production of two NSCs, one of which dies by apoptosis while the other maintains the number of cells during the life span of the individual. During development or when external triggering occurs (such as injury), NSCs proliferate either by symmetric division, in which each cell divides into two new NSCs, or by asymmetric division, in which the NSC gives rise to one new NSC and a progenitor cell (see Color Plate 2). When asymmetric division predominates, a great number of rapidly proliferating progenitors that are generated migrate out.

Table 3-1. Neural Stem Cells Isolated to Date*

Cell Source	Species	Growth Factor and Dose	Developmental Stage
Astrocytic stem cell	Mouse	EGF + FGF at 10 ng/ml	Adult SVZ
			E18-P2 astrocyte monolayers
Astrocytic stem cell	Mouse	EGF + FGF at 20 ng/ml	Adult SVZ
Cortical glial cell	Rat	FGF at 20 ng/ml	Adult
Periventricular region	Human	FGF + EGF at 20 ng/ml	15-wk gestation
SVZ cell	Human	FGF + EGF at 20 ng/ml	Fetal
Oligodendrocyte progenitor cell	Rat	FGF at 20 ng/ml	P6
External germinal layer of cerebellum	Mouse	EGF at 20 ng/ml	E17
Striatum	Mouse	EGF at 20 ng/ml	Adult
Hippocampus	Rat	FGF at 20 ng/ml	Adult
Neural crest cell	Mouse	FGF at 20 ng/ml	E14.5
Cortical cells	Mouse	EGF + FGF at 10 ng/ml	E10-P2

EGF = epidermal growth factor; FGF = fibroblast growth factor; SVZ = subventricular zone.
*Work from research groups that have isolated these neural stem cells is cited throughout the text.

Characterization and Isolation of Neural Stem Cells

NSCs require EGF and FGF-2 to proliferate, and this is used as a strategy to isolate them from the CNS by using the neurosphere assay: A cell suspension from the adult SVZ or embryonic forebrain is generally plated without substrate in culture media with FGF-2 or EGF, or both. Most of the time, a cluster of undifferentiated cells will appear, and some cells can attach to the culture dish, but the great majority will proliferate and tend to grow into cell clusters called *neurospheres.* These neurospheres represent the clonal expansion of a single NSC. Depending on the time in culture, as these neurospheres grow, asymmetric as well as symmetric division occurs, and, after several rounds of cellular division, progenitors appear in the neurospheres.[9,19,26–31] Once these cells are plated in substrate with serum-containing medium, astrocytes, neurons, and oligodendrocytes appear, demonstrating multipotency of the plated NSC. These cultures also contain undifferentiated cells. When cells from these cultures are plated at clonal density (single cell per well), the growth of multipotent neurospheres from these single undifferentiated cells demonstrates the self-renewal ability. It was recently suggested that cultures of NSC in reduced O_2 levels (5%), which more closely approximates physiologic oxygen levels, lead to a purer population of stem cells (see Color Plate 3).[32]

To distinguish NSCs from others neural cells, biological markers have been investigated. Nestin, an intermediate filament protein, has been useful to study NSC.[27,33] Nestin is expressed by a variety of cells that includes reactive astrocytes, endothelial cells, SVZ neuronal progenitor cells, and ependymal cells.[34,35] However, it can also be expressed by others type of cells, in particular by non-NSCs such as embryonic stem (ES) cells.[36] Furthermore, nestin-positive pancreatic stem cells have also been isolated.[37] Taken together, these findings suggest that nestin is a true stem-cell marker. Multipotent neural progenitor cells from the SVZ also can express vimentin and the polysialic form of neural cell adhesion molecule.[38,39]

Some studies have identified and isolated populations of NSCs on the basis of flow cytometric characteristics in response to staining with the DNA dye Hoechst, as has been conducted in other stem cells.[40,41] The isolation is based on the differential efflux of the dye by a multidrug transporter, and the population isolated in this way is called *side population fraction* and is demonstrated to be NSCs.[42] Furthermore, the novel hematopoietic stem-cell marker CD133 has been used to define a population of human neural precursor cells that exhibit a $CD133^+CD34^-CD45^-$ phenotype and fulfill all the criteria for human NSCs. However, it is not clear whether these cells are a distinct population of NSCs or just express distinct markers.[43] Other NSCs, such as neural crest stem cells, have been isolated from

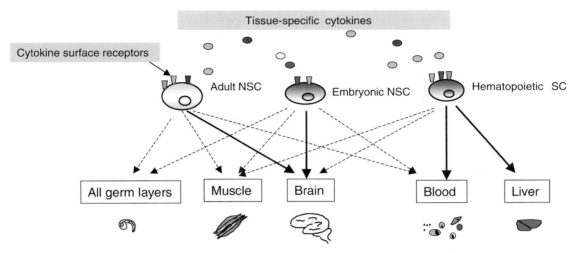

Figure 3-3. Pluripotency of neural stem cells (NSCs): developmental plasticity of NSCs. Adult and embryonic NSCs primarily give rise to neural cells (*solid arrow*). However, in low-density cultures, they can give rise to muscle or, in vivo, can contribute to all embryonic germ layers and become mature hematopoietic cells (*dashed arrows*). Hematopoietic stem cells (SCs) give rise primarily to blood derivates (*solid arrows*); however, in vivo they can become liver cells (*solid arrow*) or travel to the adult central nervous system and express neural markers (*dashed arrows*). This differentiation potential appears to be determined by the temporal and spatial encounter of SC surface receptors with tissue-specific cytokines and growth factors.

fetal mouse sciatic nerve using cell-surface antigens, such as p75, the low-affinity neurotrophin receptor, and P_0, a peripheral myelin protein: These cells exhibit phenotype $p75^+P_0^-$, are capable of self-renewal, and generate neurons and glia.[44]

Although it is likely that nestin is a stem-cell marker, it is possible that not all NSCs express it. Likewise, not all nestin-positive cells can be considered as NSCs, which is why practitioners have relied on the operational criterion of the neurosphere assay for the initial characterization of NSCs. Probably a heterogeneous population of NSCs exists in the CNS.

Differentiation Potential of Neural Stem Cells

The term *totipotency* refers to the capacity of ES cells to give rise to different types of cells and tissues in an organism. This most extensive differentiation potential was thought to be a specific property of ES cells; however, several key observations since 1999 have demonstrated that other stem cells, especially NSCs, can have such a differentiation potential, albeit to a smaller degree. Thus, NSCs can give rise to mature nonneural cells.[45] Adult mouse NSCs

can become mature hematopoietic cells after injection in an irradiated host, and express markers of mature T cells such as CD3.[46] Others have shown that, when injected into early-stage mice and chick embryos, adult NSCs differentiate into fully mature cells from gastrointestinal tract, heart, and kidney tissues, expressing markers typically found in these tissues in a nontumorigenic manner (see Color Plate 4).[30] NSCs can also produce skeletal myotubes in vitro and in vivo.[47] This behavior is also observed in other stem cells, such as hematopoietic stem cells that after intravenous injection in mice travel to the CNS, express neuronal markers, and generate an astroglial phenotype (Figure 3-3).[48,49]

The extraordinary differentiation potential of stem cells, in particular NSCs, and their ability to differentiate according to a specific environment suggest a critical role for cytokines and cell-to-cell contact signals. Thus, terminal differentiation of these cells will depend on the spatiotemporal expression and interactions of multiple cytokines with their receptors on the NSC surface.[50] This complexity has been suggested from work on ES cells, in which just a single cytokine can induce ES differentiation into various cell types.[51] This biological behavior is important to consider during pathologic conditions in which cytokines are predominant and stem cells are likely to be involved.

Oligodendrocyte Progenitor Cells

In the mature CNS, oligodendrocytes are terminally differentiated cells, and new oligodendrocytes must originate from OPCs and NSCs,[52] because there is production of new oligodendrocytes in the adult forebrain[53] and spinal cord.[54] OPCs can be identified by several markers: the ganglioside GD3, A2B5, O4 antigen, 14F7, the glycoprotein AN2,[55] the spliced form of 2',3'-cyclic nucleotide 3'-phosphohydrolase (CNPase) gene,[56] and the integral membrane proteoglycan NG2.[57–59] Through the use of these markers, OPCs have been detected in adult CNS.[60]

Around embryonic day 15, oligodendrocytes arise from a subpopulation of precursor cells within the ventral ventricular zone of the spinal cord and the SVZ.[22,61] Reynolds et al.[60] characterized the time course of oligodendrocyte marker expression and differentiation using the anti–ganglioside GD3 antibody: These cells arise from subependymal layers, migrate out, and subsequently express galactocerebrosidase-C (GalC) and at the same time express the myelin-associated protein CNPase. Myelin basic protein (MBP) is expressed 2–3 days later, before myelin formation.[52,62]

During oligodendrocyte development, OPCs undergo several maturation stages determined by specific antigenic expression and developmental potential. The OPCs isolated from neonatal optic nerve were initially termed *O-2A progenitor cells*[63] and are characterized as proliferative, self-renewing, bipotent glial precursor cells that stain with anti-GD3, vimentin, A2B5, and NG2 antibodies. In serum-free medium, they differentiate into oligodendrocytes, whereas, in serum-containing medium, they become astrocytes.[64] Adult optic nerves also contain a similar type of cell that conserved some properties of the perinatal counterpart.[65]

In the initial stages of development, OPCs exhibit the NG2[+] platelet-derived growth factor (PDGF) receptor-α[+] O4[−] phenotype. These cells give rise to more advanced progenitors expressing O4, and these, in turn, generate premyelinating oligodendrocytes that lose the expression of NG2 and gain the expression of proteolipid protein, to later mature as oligodendrocytes expressing MBP and CNPase.[64] Expression of O4 is a first step in terminal oligodendrocyte differentiation[66] and indicates a more committed stage with less proliferative potential.[67] GalC expression is associated with terminal differentiation and is followed by MBP, proteolipid protein, and myelin oligodendrocyte glycoprotein expression (see Color Plate 5).[68]

Some of the foregoing precursors persist as adult OPCs that differ from their perinatal counterparts in several respects, including motility, cell cycle, and differentiation stage but maintain self-renewing capacity. Adult OPCs can be identified by NG2, PDGF-α, O4, and FGF receptor expression and can differentiate into mature oligodendrocytes in the adult brain.[69] OPCs have been isolated from brains of healthy humans and of MS patients and express the p75[NTR] (neurotrophin receptor) that is implicated in oligodendrocyte survival and apoptosis (see Color Plate 6).[70]

Adult OPCs persist in the CNS and are maintained in a quiescent state by a mechanism that involves both AMPA receptors[71] and the cell-cycle inhibitor p27Kip1[72] and by a mechanism involving Notch. OPCs express Notch receptor, the activation of which blocks OPC differentiation in the developing optic nerve.[73] Owing to their abundance in the CNS and the fact that their processes contact the nodes of Ranvier,[74] OPCs have been suggested to fulfill the plasticity, synaptic remodeling function, and stem-cell function in the adult CNS.[75,76] Recent data point to a broader differentiation potential of OPCs in which, depending on the cytokine milieu, they exhibit NSC characteristics.[6,12]

OPCs express several functional cytokine receptors such as FGF-2R[77] and PDGF-α receptor,[78] which have been used as a marker for OPCs.[79] OPCs express c-kit, a marker for hematopoietic stem cells, which is lost when they differentiate into postmitotic oligodendrocytes.[80]

In vitro oligodendroglial development can be recapitulated from NSCs: Zhang et al.[81] demonstrated that human oligodendrocytes appear from neurospheres and express PDGF-α receptor. The proliferation of these human OPCs was augmented by coculture with neurons and astrocytes. Furthermore, human neurospheres increase their yield of oligodendrocyte production when cultured with triiodothyronine (T3).[82] Finally, control of OPC differentiation timing requires extracellular signals such as PDGF-α and T3.[83]

Growth Factors and Cytokines for Neural Stem and Oligodendrocyte Progenitor Cells

The signals responsible for controlling proliferation and differentiation of precursor cells in the CNS are starting to be elucidated. Among these molecules, the cytokines EGF and FGF-2 and their receptors are critical for the proliferation of NSCs.[27,84,85] However, many other molecules are involved.

EGF and FGF-2 signal through extracellular signal-regulated kinases and induce the proliferation of NSCs and progenitors.[38] NSCs express both receptors with varying levels of expression in individual cells. Furthermore, there are specific FGF- or EGF-responsive NSCs. FGF-responsive NSCs are present early, and EGF-responsive NSCs emerge later in development. Both FGF- and EGF-responsive NSCs retain their self-renewal and multipotency.[86,87] The activity of FGF is mediated by FGF receptor-1. The acquisition of NSC identity from ES cells is mediated by leukemia inhibitory factor (LIF)[88] and is enhanced by FGF-2.

Transforming growth factor α (TGF-α) is also critical for SVZ precursor cells. TGF-α knockout mice exhibit decreased proliferation of the SVZ cells, owing to decreased progenitor numbers in the SVZ and reduced numbers of neuronal progenitors that migrate to the olfactory bulb. However, the stem-cell number does not change.[89] More important, intraventricular infusion of TGF-α increases cell proliferation in the SVZ (Figure 3-4).[90]

FGF regulates the differentiation of NSCs. At low dosage, FGF-2 induces neurogenic differentiation, but it induces oligodendroglial differentiation at high dosage.[91] FGF-2 requires a novel autocrine cofactor—a glycosylated form of cystatin C that synergizes with FGF-2 to stimulate neurogenesis differentiation of NSC in vivo.[92] In vivo, EGF and FGF exhibit a differential effect on the SVZ NSCs; FGF-2 increases the rate of newborn cells, especially neurons, whereas EGF increases the numbers of glia in the hippocampus.[93] FGF is also mitogenic for oligodendrocytes and OPCs.[78] The importance of FGF-2 is revealed by the observation that introduction of a dominant-negative version of FGF receptor-1 into OPCs results in cells that are not responsive to FGF-2 and that fail to migrate in vivo.[94]

Some members of the Eph family of tyrosine kinase receptors are expressed by cells of the SVZ and have been shown to be involved in the migration of neuronal progenitors in the adult SVZ. The infu-

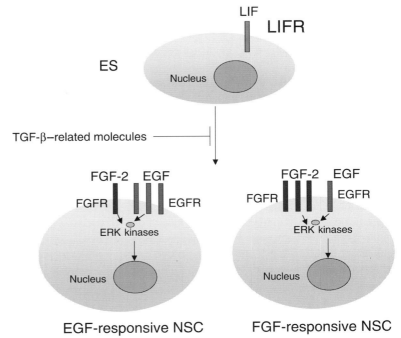

Figure 3-4. Cytokines for neural stem cell (NSC) proliferation. Several cytokines control the emergence and proliferation of NSCs; these cytokines include leukemia inhibitory factor (LIF), which induces embryonic stem (ES) cells to become NSCs in a process that can be blocked by transforming growth factor β (TGF-β)–related molecules. Epidermal growth factor (EGF) and fibroblast growth factor (FGF) are growth factors for NSCs and signal through extracellular signal-regulated kinases (ERKs). NSCs can express both EGF and FGF; however, there are specific subpopulations of EGF- and FGF-responsive NSCs. (EGFR = epidermal growth factor receptor; FGFR = fibroblast growth factor receptor; LIF = leukemia inhibitory factor receptor.)

sion of a truncated version of EphB2 or ephrin-B2 into the lateral ventricle disrupted migration of neuronal progenitors and increased proliferation of NSCs.[95] Other molecules such as basic helix loop helix (bHLH) transcription factors are related to the differentiation of NSC to glia and to neurons, and the bHLH transcription factor neurogenin inhibits the differentiation of NSC into astrocytes. Neurogenin promotes neurogenesis by functioning as a transcriptional activator and inhibits the signal transducers and activators of transcription (STAT) associated with astrocytic differentiation.[96]

Other cytokines are involved in the lineage commitment of NSCs. Brain-derived neurotrophic factor increases the morphologic and antigenic differentiation of neuronal progenitors derived from NSCs.[97] Hematopoietic cytokines also regulate NSC differentiation: Using immortalized hippocampal stem cells, Mehler et al.[98] showed that cytokines that participate in T-cell maturation, immunoglobulin synthesis, and hematopoiesis induce progressive neuronal differentiation. The cytokine interleukin-11 (IL-11) induces the differentiation of NSCs to immature neurons. However, IL-5, IL-7, and IL-9 induce differentiation of NSCs into more mature neurons when combined with TGF-α after pretreatment with FGF-2. These findings may be relevant in the context of the potential interaction between T-cell–derived cytokines and precursor cells during immune-mediated demyelination and injury (Figure 3-5).

O-2A cells express receptors for bone morphogenetic protein and require this cytokine for astroglial development.[99] Bone morphogenetic protein induces selective expression of astrocytic progenitor cells and mature astrocytes and induces an inhibition of oligodendrocytes.[100] Insulin-like growth factor 1 (IGF-1), neurotrophin 3 (NT-3), and gp130 receptor subunit–related ligands induce the proliferation of OPCs and postmitotic oligodendrocytes.[101] In addition, different gp130-associated neuropoietic cytokines—ciliary neurotrophic factor, LIF, oncostatin-M, and hematopoietic cytokines (IL-6, IL-11, IL-12, and granulocyte colony stimulating factor)—have differential trophic effects on oligodendroglial lineage.[102]

The terminal maturation of OPCs derived from multipotent stem cells is dependent on factors that activate gp130–LIF-β receptors, such as ciliary neurotrophic factor.[103] Ciliary neurotrophic factor enhances the proliferation of OPC as well as the generation of oligodendrocytes in vivo.[104] The

downstream signaling pathways responsible for differentiation after gp130 engagement involve the STAT family of transcription factors.[105] IL-6 and LIF (both of which signal through gp130) modulate the growth of NSCs and progenitors in vitro via a STAT-3–dependent mechanism that requires the transcriptional coactivator p300.[106] STAT-5 also plays a role in proliferation of progenitor cells after cytokine receptor stimulation.[107] Although neurogenin promotes neurogenesis by functioning as a transcriptional activator, it inhibits astrocyte differentiation by inhibiting the activation of STAT factors that are necessary for gliogenesis.[96]

The Notch family of proteins is critical for neural precursor biology. Notch1 has been used to isolate ependymal stem cells.[9] Notch receptor activation inhibits OPC maturation and myelination in the CNS.[73] It also inhibits neural crest stem-cell differentiation into neurons. Even a transient exposure to Notch ligands causes an irreversible change from neurogenesis to gliogenesis.[108] Chambers et al.[109] studied the effects of Notch in vivo and found that an excess of activated Notch markedly inhibited the generation of neurons from precursors and increased the generation of astroglial progeny. Notch can also inhibit OPC differentiation during development.[73] Others have found that activated Notch can induce the generation of radial glia that then become periventricular astrocytes.[110] Presenilin-1 is involved in neuronal progenitors' fate. Presenilin-1 cleaves Notch and induces an activated form that maintains the neuronal progenitors pool. Presenilin-1[−/−] mice exhibit premature neuronal differentiation associated with aberrant neuronal migration and disorganization of architecture of the cerebral hemisphere via alteration of the notch pathway (see Figure 3-5).[111]

Neuregulins are cytokines present in motor neurons and the ventral ventricular zone, where they exert their influence on early OPCs. The neuregulin glial growth factor-2 (GGF-2) is mitogenic for OPCs and is able to maintain OPC plasticity by reverting their phenotype to nestin-expressing precursor cells.[112,113] Vartanian et al.[114] demonstrated that neuregulin is necessary to obtain mature oligodendrocytes from OPCs in the spinal cord. PDGF-α is the main mitogen for OPCs[115] and is involved in generating OPCs.[78] PDGF-α can also induce chemotaxis of NSCs[116] and inhibit further terminal differentiation into oligodendrocytes.[115]

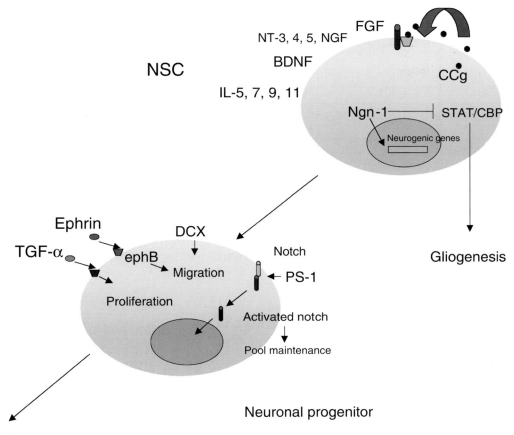

Figure 3-5. Cytokines and transcription factors that influence neuronal differentiation, migration, and survival. Multiple cytokines affect the generation of new neurons from neural stem cells (NSCs), with some cytokines having overlapping effects on other lineages; some of these effects depend on synergism with other molecules and effective levels. These molecules include fibroblast growth factor (FGF), brain-derived neurotrophic factor (BDNF), and interleukins (ILs). These molecules activate neural-specific transcription factors that control the expression of neurogenic genes. Neural transcription factors can block the signaling pathways of astrocytic differentiation. During neuronal differentiation, restricted neuronal progenitors appear. These cells express the doublecortin gene (DCX) related to the migratory capacity of these cells. The proliferation of these cells is modulated by Notch, Ephrin, or transforming growth factor α (TGF-α). (CCg = cystatin C; CBP = cAMP response element-binding [CREB] protein; NGF = nerve growth factor; Ngn-1 = neurogenin-1; NT-3 = neurotrophin 3; PS-1 = presenilin-1; STAT = signal transducer activators of transcription.)

During development, bHLH proteins regulate formation of neurons from multipotent progenitor cells. The HLH protein Id4 stimulates cell proliferation and blocks OPC differentiation. Downregulation of this molecule is required for OPCs to exit the cell cycle and differentiate.[117] The genes Olg-1 and Olg-2 that also encode for bHLH proteins are associated with development of OPCs.[118] Hormones such as T3 are important in oligodendroglial development: Treatment of human neural

spheres with T3 increases the number of oligodendrocytes (Figure 3-6).[82]

Thus, several cytokines, including ILs, play a role in proliferation and apoptosis of NSCs and progenitors cells, not only during development but also in the adult CNS. These immune molecules have an unexpected functional role in the CNS, as demonstrated by the critical role of major histocompatibility complex (MHC)-I and CD3-zeta, on the plasticity of connections between neurons dur-

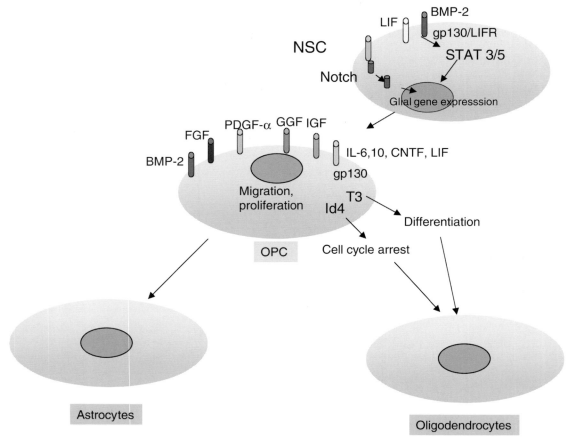

Figure 3-6. Cytokines and transcription factors that influence glial differentiation and migration. Multiple cytokines affect the generation of new glial cells from neural stem cells (NSCs). These molecules include cytokines acting through surface receptors that activate astroglial transcription. Several cytokines have differential effects on astrocytic versus oligodendrocyte differentiation (see text for details). Other molecules include hormones (e.g., T3), and lineage-restricted transcription factors are involved in the timing of generation of oligodendroglial cells. (BMP = bone morphogenetic protein; CNTF = ciliary neurotrophic factor; FGF = fibroblast growth factor; GGF = glial growth factor; IGF = insulin-like growth factor; IL = interleukin; LIFR = leukemia inhibitory factor receptor; OPC = oligodendrocyte progenitor cell; PDGF = platelet derived growth factor; STAT = signal transducers and activators of transcription.)

ing development and adulthood.[119] Consequently, these same molecules may be involved in CNS pathologic states that are characterized by an inflammatory component such as brain and spinal cord injury and MS.[120] Therefore, the study of molecules such as cytokine and chemokine receptors, costimulatory and adhesion molecules in NSCs, and progenitor cells will help us to better understand the biology during development and adult CNS and the vulnerability of these cells during neurodegenerative diseases and also provide us with possible therapeutic options.

Experimental and Clinical Evidence of Involvement of Endogenous Precursors in Demyelinating Diseases

Experimental Models of Multiple Sclerosis

The role of NSCs and progenitor cells in CNS injury in general is demonstrated by an incremental response in the form of proliferation and migration of these cells from the SVZ toward the lesions in injury models. It has been shown that nestin immunoreactivity in the SVZ is increased after injury. These nestin-positive cells can differentiate into astrocytes in response to traumatic brain injury[121] and into neurons in an experimental model of dopaminergic neurodegeneration.[122] Ependymal stem cells also migrate out of the central canal and differentiate into astrocytes in response to longitudinal fasciculus injury.[123] Experimental cortical lesions increase the cellular proliferation and induce expression of the polysialic form of neural cell adhesion molecule in the SVZ.[124] Magavi et al.[25] found de novo neurogenesis from SVZ precursor cells of adult mouse CNS in an experimental model of targeted neuronal apoptosis.

Experimental autoimmune encephalomyelitis (EAE), an animal model of MS, is characterized by an infiltration in the CNS of autoreactive T cells and macrophages, accompanied by the production of proinflammatory Th1 cytokines[125] and oxidative injury mediators.[126] During EAE, there is increased proliferation of cells in the SVZ, suggesting that stem or progenitor cells in this area proliferate in response to demyelination damage.[127] Furthermore, using a model of EAE combined with either injection of myelin oligodendrocyte glycoprotein antibodies to induce inflammatory demyelination or nonspecific mouse immunoglobulins to induce an inflammatory response without demyelination, Di Bello et al.[128] suggested that remyelination by OPCs in this model appears to be associated more with demyelination than with inflammation. However, the greater increase in OPCs in inflammatory demyelinated lesions as compared with that in lesions induced by anti-GalC antibodies suggests a mitogenic role of cytokines and growth factors released during inflammation.[129]

Several models of experimental demyelination have shown that spontaneous remyelination by precursor cells occurs.[130] In a lysolecithin-induced demyelination model, it has been demonstrated that progenitor cells of the adult mouse SVZ proliferate, migrate, and differentiate into oligodendrocytes.[131,132] Other research groups have confirmed these results with retrovirus labeling of proliferating cells, demonstrating that endogenous progenitors in the subcortical white matter migrate and engage in repair of the lesion (see Color Plate 7).[133–135] IGF-1 is a mitogen for OPCs, and several reports have suggested involvement of IGF-1 and PDGF-α during remyelination in lysolecithin-[136] and cuprizone-mediated demyelination models.[137] In EAE,

some groups have reported clinical amelioration after IGF-1 treatment,[138,139] but others have reported less encouraging results.[140]

Previous studies suggest that during demyelinating insults induced by gliotoxic agents and during EAE, there is hypertrophy and proliferation of OPCs, reaching maximum numbers at the peak of remyelination and suggesting a response to the local environment, although direct evidence for the formation of remyelinating oligodendrocytes from OPCs in EAE is lacking.[128,141] These results indicate that the environment during demyelination may be permissive to OPCs. Furthermore, studies of demyelination induced by injection of anti-GalC antibodies and serum complement in the rat spinal cord suggest that remyelination is carried out by OPCs rather than by surviving oligodendrocytes but that repeated insults lead to chronic depletion of the OPC pool in the CNS.[142] Similarly, repeated episodes of myelin destruction eventually result in the formation of chronic demyelinated lesions that fail to remyelinate, as observed in MS brain tissues.[143,144] There are several hypotheses to explain this lack of remyelination in chronic MS lesions: (1) the destruction of OPCs and exhaustion of the OPC or NSC pools by apoptosis; (2) the inability of adult OPCs to differentiate fully into myelinating oligodendrocytes, owing to an ongoing humoral immune reaction; (3) the lack of appropriate signals or the existence of negative signals for OPC differentiation because of destroyed axons and neurons; and (4) the inhibitory effect of astrogliosis. The following sections outline the experimental data that support these hypotheses.

Evidence for Precursor Cell Death by Molecular Mediators of Immune Demyelination

There is evidence that precursor cells might be susceptible to cytokine-induced apoptosis.[145,146] Therefore, the fate of stem and progenitor cell pools in MS and EAE may depend on the balance between apoptosis-inducing cytokines and proliferation and differentiation-inducing factors such as T-cell and neuropoietic cytokines that are dynamically regulated during inflammatory neurodegeneration.[120,125,147]

For example, proinflammatory cytokines can induce cell death of precursor cells via Fas-FasL interactions.[148,149] Oligodendrocytes and OPCs are vulnerable to apoptosis by a Fas-mediated mecha-

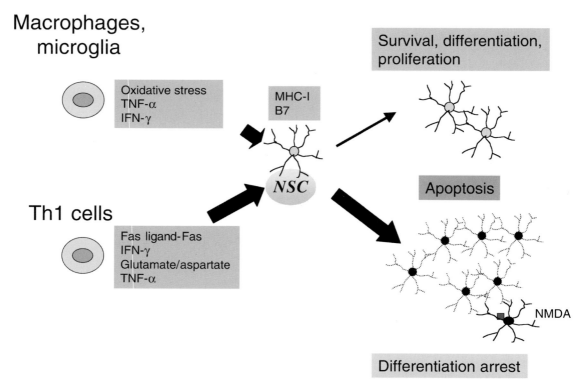

Figure 3-7. Role of cytokines in precursor cell apoptosis during demyelination. Cytokines and other inflammatory media-tors induce cell death of oligodendrocyte progenitor cells and other precursors by multiple pathways that involve Th1 cyto-kines, oxidative stress, and glutamate. The fate of these cells may be worsened by the expression of immunogenic molecules such as class I major histocompatibility complex (MHC-I) and costimulatory molecules. Surviving precursors can arrest their differentiation through *N*-methyl-D-aspartate (NMDA)–mediated signaling. These events would induce a shift in the balance toward apoptosis of the endogenous pool (*thick arrows*). (IFN-γ = interferon gamma; NSC = neural stem cell; TNF-α = tumor necrosis factor-α.)

nism.[150,151] Tumor necrosis factor alpha is upregu-lated during EAE and MS[152] and can mediate OPC apoptosis in vitro.[145] Tumor necrosis factor alpha also potentiates the apoptotic effects of interferon gamma (IFN-γ) on OPC cells, and this effect is par-tially reversible by caspase inhibitors.[151] IFN-γ and LPS induce apoptosis of mature oligodendrocytes and OPCs via endogenous nitric oxide production.[146]

Infiltrating immune cells are a source of glutamate and can induce damage by excitotoxic-ity.[153,154] Glutamate receptor AMPA-mediated exci-totoxicity is an independent and additional source of oligodendrocytes and axonal damage in EAE[155] and has been shown to induce apoptosis of mature differentiating oligodendrocytes.[155,156] Excitotoxic-ity may cause damage to other progenitor and stem cells as well, because both multipotent uncommit-

ted and committed progenitors express functional AMPA receptors.[157] Furthermore, glutamate ago-nists induce growth arrest and inhibit oligodendro-cyte progenitors differentiation (Figure 3-7).[158]

Oligodendrocytes and adult O-2A progenitors of adult rats are specifically susceptible to lytic effects of complement.[159] However, there are other potential damaging mechanisms for NSCs and pro-genitors during demyelinating injury, such as the expression of molecules that may render these cells immunogenic to the attack of T or B cells; IFN-γ induces the expression of MHC-I on neural pro-genitors, thus rendering these cells potential targets during an immune response.[31,160] Cytokine-stimu-lated human immature neuroepithelial cell precur-sors express intercellular adhesion molecule-1 and interact with neutrophils by intercellular adhesion

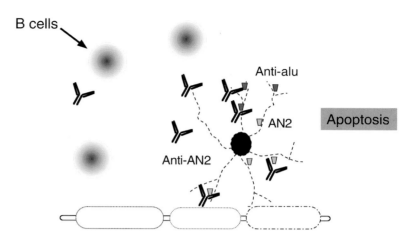

Figure 3-8. Ongoing immune responses against human oligodendrocyte progenitors in multiple sclerosis. Some patients with multiple sclerosis demonstrate an ongoing immune response against progenitor-specific molecules. These molecules can be critical for progenitor cell function and include AN2—a glycoprotein expressed by oligodendrocyte progenitor cells and important for myelination in vivo. These events would increase the rate of cell death of the endogenous progenitors pool, limiting the innate ability of these cells to engage in repair. Anti-alu peptide responses have been detected in the serum and cerebrospinal fluid of multiple sclerosis patients.

molecule-1–lymphocyte function–associated antigen-1 ligation.[161] We have demonstrated that murine NSCs in vitro express MHC-I and functional CD80 and CD86 costimulatory molecules, which are upregulated after IFN-γ stimulation and during stress-induced apoptosis.[162]

Inability of Adult Oligodendrocyte Progenitor Cells to Differentiate Fully into Myelinating Oligodendrocytes

Data from MS pathology support a role for NSCs and progenitor cells in the pathogenesis of MS.[163] The analysis of demyelinating lesions in MS during the chronic phase shows that a limited amount of remyelination occurs[164] and appears to be provided by migrating OPCs or NSCs that reside near the lesions. Some authors have shown that MS lesions contain a significant number of quiescent OPCs.[165,166] Using PDGF-α receptor as a marker, Scolding et al.[4] identified OPCs in the CNS of healthy adults and of MS patients. Others have identified a relatively quiescent population of OPCs expressing NG2. These OPCs have been observed in lesions of patients with all the clinical subtypes of MS.[143] In the chronic stages of the disease, most immature oligodendrocytes did not appear to be engaged in myelination,[143] suggesting that oligodendrocyte differentiation of precursor cells is impaired in chronic MS, which is consistent with the general failure of myelin repair observed during the later stages of this disease.[144]

The lack of remyelination in MS may be owing to factors that induce OPC cell death before the cells can fully mature into myelinating oligodendrocytes, leading to the exhaustion of the progenitors' pool. Archelos et al.[167] demonstrated that serum and CSF from 44% of patients with relapsing-remitting MS react with a protein-bearing Alu peptide sequence that is found only in OPCs, suggesting that there is an ongoing immune response to OPCs in MS. Similarly, cerebrospinal fluid from patients with relapsing-remitting active MS but not from stable MS contains antibodies against AN2, a glycoprotein critical for myelination and expressed only by OPCs.[168] In vitro experiments confirmed the importance of AN2[55] in myelination: In myelinating cultures, anti-AN2 antibody suppressed the synthesis of myelin protein, supporting the hypothesis that an immunologic attack on AN2-positive OPCs may be responsible for the impaired remyelination capacity (Figure 3-8).[168]

Lack of Appropriate Signal from Destroyed Axons and Neurons

Normal axons and neurons produce signals that induce oligodendroglial differentiation.[169,170] Neurons, oligodendrocytes, and astrocytes not only form an anatomic unit that maintains nerve transmission but also perpetuate a reciprocal paracrine loop between axons, myelin, and oligodendrocytes.[171] However, immunologic attacks severely affect the

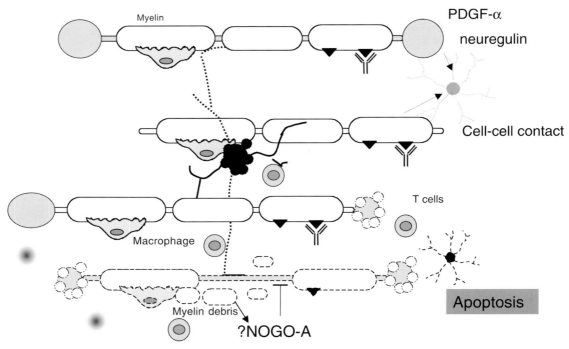

Figure 3-9. Effect of the disturbance of the axon-myelin unit on oligodendrocyte progenitor cells (OPCs) and diagram of alterations of the axon-myelin unit that may alter proliferation and differentiation of OPCs during multiple sclerosis. OPCs generate adult myelinating cells, requiring soluble and cell-cell contact signals from neurons and axons. During autoimmune demyelination, the destruction of oligodendrocytes and the ensuing neuronal degeneration may cause a lack of necessary signals for OPC generation, and this process may be worsened by the release of molecules that inhibit axonal regeneration, such as myelin-associated neurite outgrowth inhibitor (NOGO). (PDGF-α = platelet-derived growth factor alpha.)

integrity of this unit.[171] OPCs are influenced by the axonal and neuronal environment through diffusible and contact-mediated signals such as neuregulin, PDGF-α and -β, and FGF.[172-174] OPCs are influenced to undergo proliferation by the axonal signals. During the course of MS, there is evidence of neuronal abnormalities[175] and of early axonal damage that can jeopardize the ability of neurons to maintain oligodendrocyte homeostasis and may be responsible for the absence of OPC differentiation and generation.[112,176,177] Even myelin can inhibit the maturation of OPCs in a concentration-dependent manner, suggesting an effect of membrane-associated proteins.[178] Furthermore, axonal regeneration can be inhibited by molecules from the injured oligodendrocytes and myelin that exert negative signals. Thus, the potential repair signals from neurons and axons may be worsened by the presence of negative signals for axonal regeneration that are released during myelin destruction. It has been shown that a molecule with negative effects on axonal regenera-

tion, such as myelin-associated neurite outgrowth inhibitor (NOGO-A), is released after myelin and oligodendrocyte injury.[179-181] However, it is not known whether these molecules are released during MS injury or whether they are responsible for the remyelination failure in MS (Figure 3-9).

Inhibitory Effects of Astrogliosis

The lack of remyelination in MS may result in part from the suppressive effects of gliotic astrocytes on myelin formation. EAE and MS lesions are characterized by an increase in astrocyte reactivity demonstrated by hypertrophy and enhanced expression of GFAP but no proliferation, although in vitro MBP peptides are mitogenic for astrocytes.[182] In vivo and in vitro experiments have shown that an astrocytic environment is not permissive for migration of OPCs or for axonal regrowth.[183] Reactive astrocytes limit the remyelination capacity of Schwann's cells injected into the CNS.[184,185] Furthermore, in MS patients, Schwann's cell remyelination is seen in spinal cord lesions in areas devoid of astroglial scars.[186]

In vitro data support these in vivo observations: Astrocyte explants were shown to inhibit axonal myelination.[187] Although astrocytes may induce a nonpermissive environment by diffusible factors, data from the GFAP[-/-] mice suggest that GFAP, the intermediate filament gene expressed by astrocytes, is required for long-term maintenance of CNS myelination. When EAE is induced in GFAP[-/-] mice, they exhibit a worsened disease despite remyelination, indicating a distinct functional role of intermediate filament protein GFAP expressed in astrocytes in the control of the disease.[188]

Astrocytes can modify the migratory properties of oligodendrocyte progenitors. Fok-Seang et al.[189] studied the ability of cytokine-stimulated astrocytes on OPC migration and neurite outgrowth and found that IFN-γ exerts an inhibitory effect on migration of OPCs, whereas IL-1α plus bFGF greatly increased axon outgrowth, and this effect could be blocked by TGF-β and IFN-γ. Interestingly, others have found permissive signals from astrocytes as well.[190] Taken together, these data suggest that cytokine activation of astrocytes may influence the degree of axonal growth and migration of OPCs. In the case of immune-mediated demyelination, it is likely that the cytokine production results in blockade of axonal regeneration that, together with other molecular mediators released during demyelinating injury (tenascin, brevican, neurocan, N-cadherin[183,191]), may result in a nonpermissive environment for remyelination and axonal regeneration (see Color Plate 8).

Evidence of Neuroprotection and Trophic Effects of Cytokines for Precursors during Demyelination

Some anti-inflammatory cytokines and neurotrophins released during injury appear to be protective in experimental models of MS and able to induce the differentiation of OPCs and NSCs in vitro. Certain models of EAE mimic the relapsing-remitting form of MS and are characterized by remission periods that correlate with a shift toward Th2 cytokine production in the CNS such as TGF-β and IL-10.[125] Experimental treatments used in EAE may induce a change toward Th2. For example, CD28-B7 costimulatory blockade inhibits Th1 but spares Th2 cytokines in the CNS.[192] In addition to producing cytokines, T cells are able to produce neurotrophins such as NT-3, nerve growth factor (NGF), and brain-derived neurotrophic factor.[147,193] In EAE, there is an increase in NGF immunoreactivity in the SVZ.[127] It is well-known that human NGF protects the common marmoset against EAE by inducing a Th2 cytokine switch within the CNS by IL-10 upregulation on astrocytes.[194] More interestingly, neurotrophins such as NGF are mitogenic for NSCs.[195] NT-3 promotes survival, clonal expansion, and proliferation of OPCs,[196] and Th2 cytokines favor oligodendroglial development from NSCs.[102] The cytokine GGF-2 promotes the proliferation, survival, and expansion of oligodendrocytes and enhances remyelination in animals with EAE,[197] which show reduced relapses and increased remyelination, as well as IL-10 expression in the CNS and upregulation of exon-2 of MBP, indicative of remyelination.[198] Furthermore, OPCs have been found to express receptors for GGF-2.[199] There is more evidence suggesting that Th2 cytokines may function in support of progenitors cells: IL-10 and IL-4 receptors are expressed in OPCs, and these cytokines protect OPCs from oxidative stress and apoptosis.[146]

Although some of these data come from in vitro work, these results suggest a protective role of Th2 and neuropoietic cytokines in the survival and differentiation of OPCs in the CNS during demyelinating injury such as in EAE and MS (Figure 3-10) and suggest that the combination of neurotrophin and Th2 cytokine secretion may lessen disease not only by downregulation of autoreactive T cells but also by improving NSC oligodendroglial survival and replenishing the oligodendrocyte population.

A Model of the Role of Precursor Cells in Demyelinating Diseases

The heterogenous pathology of MS suggests a diversity in the disease mechanisms.[200] The failure of oligodendrocytes to repair demyelinated axons contributes to the cumulative neurologic disability in MS.[201] However, it is clear from the experimental and clinical evidence that in the diverse pathologic types, OPCs and NSCs are likely to be implicated. A model consistent with alterations of the endogenous potential and sur-

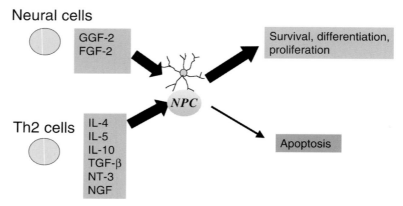

Figure 3-10. Role of neuropoietic cytokines and Th2 cytokines in survival and differentiation of precursors. Th2 and neuropoietic cytokines influence proliferation and differentiation of oligodendrocyte progenitor cells. Several interleukins (ILs) (especially Th2-derived cytokines), growth factors, and neurotrophins appear to be protective and induce proliferation or differentiation of precursor cells. These molecules have been associated with remyelination and neuroprotection and include glial growth factor-2 (GGF-2), IL-10, and nerve growth factor (NGF). (FGF-2 = fibroblast growth factor-2; NPC = neural progenitor cell; NT-3 = neurotrophin 3; TGF-β = transforming growth factor β.)

vival of stem cells and OPCs is presented in Figure 3-10.

The acute lesion of MS may be initiated by an attack from autoreactive T cells and activated macrophages and the production of Th1 cytokines that induce demyelination. OPCs and stem cells may undergo apoptosis through excitotoxicity, oxidative stress, proapoptotic cytokines, and antibody-mediated cytotoxicity. Some surviving OPCs may increase their numbers, accounting for the initial increase in NG2 cells (see Color Plate 9A). Inactive lesions during the remission phase may show an increase in OPCs with some remyelination (see Color Plate 9B). However, during the chronic phase of demyelination, the fate and the viability of endogenous progenitors would be determined by the balance between neuroprotective versus neurotoxic cytokines and the alteration of the neuron-OPC signals. The initial increase in OPC numbers may be lost during the chronic phase. Relapses may induce OPC apoptosis directly or indirectly via alterations of axons and neurons, resulting in a lack of positive signals or the induction of negative signals that arrest the differentiation of surviving OPCs. Finally, repeated attacks over a prolonged period would induce the exhaustion of the pool of cells with repair ability, resulting in a complete failure of remyelination (see Color Plate 9C).

Therapeutic Potential of Precursor Cells in Demyelinating Diseases

Endogenous Precursor Cells

Various observations have shown that promotion of endogenous precursors may be a potential strategy in CNS neurodegenerative diseases.[5,135,166,202] However, to exploit the biological properties of precursors and to promote specifically their differentiation into remyelinating oligodendrocytes, it is necessary to learn more about the molecular pathways governing the NSC and OPC pools. It has been demonstrated that the intraventricular injection of TGF-α in an animal model of Parkinson's disease induces a massive proliferation of forebrain NSCs and migration to the striatum of neural and glial progenitors, accompanied by significant clinical improvement.[90]

Cannella et al.[198,199] showed that neuregulin and GGF-2 induced clinical improvement and remyelination in EAE. One of the potential mechanisms of recovery could be mediated by the effects of GGF-2 on OPCs. OPCs survive and proliferate when exposed to neuregulin.[112,113,174] IGF-1 is also important for OPC proliferation, and several reports have shown positive effects in gliotoxic models of demyelination and EAE[139]; however, there are also reports showing lack of efficacy.[140] The continuous infusion of exogenous cytokines could induce SVZ hyperplasia, raising questions about the tumorigenic potential of such manipulations.[93]

Transplantation of Progenitors and Stem Cells in Models of Demyelination

The rationale for neural transplant is twofold: to replace a protein or to replace a cell that is missing. NSCs are able to differentiate into the three major cell types in the mammalian CNS, thus offering promising strategies for neural cell transplants and for gene therapy protocols.[203]

NSCs and progenitor cells have been successfully isolated,[204,205] genetically manipulated, and transplanted to replace cells and introduce genes in models of neurodegenerative disease in mice.[203,206–209] Several authors have shown that NSCs survive and differentiate in diverse disease models; Brustle et al.[210] have shown chimerism after injecting human NSC in fetal recipients. Results obtained so far demonstrate the feasibility of NSC transplants with prolonged survival, integration, and differentiation in the adult brain.[211]

Injection of murine NSCs in the neonatal SVZ of *shiverer* mice results in widespread engraftment[212] and myelination of 40% of the host neuronal process with evident clinical improvement. However, these findings may not be applicable to adult animals because of the limited migration of transplants in adults as compared with that in the neonatal SVZ. EGF-responsive neural progenitors differentiate into oligodendrocytes when injected into *shaking* pup canine myelin mutants.[213,214] Transplanted OPCs were able to repair focal demyelinated areas in the neonatal and adult canine mutants.[215] In the *md* rat, which carries a myelin proteolipid protein mutation, injected OPCs result in myelin formation and wide distribution in the host parenchyma.[216]

These results indicate that transplanted cells receive environmental cues that drive their differentiation and migration toward oligodendrocytes.[217] However, porcine progenitors isolated from the SVZ required in vitro induction to oligodendroglial lineage to achieve myelination in vivo.[218] Nestin-positive human neural precursor cells removed from surgical specimens have been used to induce repair in rat spinal cord with extensive remyelination.[219] OPCs can be isolated from the rat SVZ as well and produce robust myelin after transplantation.[220]

ES cells also differentiate into oligodendrocytes and myelinate in culture and after spinal cord transplantation in *shiverer* mice[36] and *md* rats.[221] EGF-responsive NSCs have also shown efficacy when transplanted into the thoracolumbar region of *md* rats.[214] Others using denervation models have shown that pig-rat xenotransplants with olfactory glial progenitors induce axonal regeneration and remyelination.[222]

Several reports have demonstrated the clinical efficacy of NSCs and progenitor cells in experimental models of CNS neurodegenerative diseases.[203,206,208,209] However, it is not known whether a particular CNS disease in humans may benefit from NSC transplantation.[223] The chances for success would be better in those diseases in which clinical efficacy is determined by a single defined biological mechanism, such as Parkinson's or Huntington's disease. The challenge in MS is the widespread pathology affecting multiple sites in the CNS. In this case, targeting localized lesions that cause a great disability, such as a lesion in the spinal cord, can be envisioned. The survival of the transplanted cells in a potentially toxic environment is an important consideration. One report showed encouraging data on migration and proliferation of transplanted OPCs in the EAE model[224]: Fifty days after transplantation, the cells had migrated 6 cm from the site of the injection.

Nonetheless, research in relevant models of immune demyelinating disease is needed, because the myelin mutant models do not reflect all clinicopathologic features of MS such as relapses and remissions, axonal damage, sustained oxidative injury, and immune cell infiltrates.

NSCs may be a better source of myelinating transplants than OPCs,[202] as they can be obtained in greater numbers with no need to predifferentiate them in vitro, because environmental cues at the transplantation site can drive their differentiation.[225] NSCs also possess the ability of wide migration toward the pathologic site.[28,212] Finally, these cells may provide additional neurotrophic factors to repair axonal and neuronal abnormalities present in MS and EAE.

Conclusions

The goal for MS therapy is the induction and maintenance of immunologic tolerance toward self-antigens, promotion of remyelination, and prevention of the axonal degeneration as soon as the diagnosis is made. To address the entire spectrum of this disease, a comprehensive and interdisciplinary analysis of MS biology is needed. The complex dynamics between the cellular mechanisms responsible for symptoms and for neurodegenerative damage pose important questions that must be addressed. Regardless of the initial mechanism, disability is cumulative. That is why considering MS as an inflammatory neurodegenerative disorder is likely to reflect the true nature of this disease and should prompt us to develop a more comprehensive therapy.

Although there are now therapies that can prevent exacerbations, we still lack knowledge about how to promote remyelination. Adult brain contains adult stem cells and progenitors scattered throughout the CNS in regional pools, and these cells are able to engage in some endogenous repair. However, the size of the lesion may overcome the capacity for endogenous precursor cells to repair the damage.[5,24] Conversely, precursor cells could be targets of pathology as well, with great repercussions on the CNS's innate ability to repair.

Boosting the endogenous pool can be achieved by manipulation of specific molecular signals to induce a preferential differentiation of endogenous NSCs and their derived progenitors toward cells with remyelinating capability. More research is needed to understand the signaling pathways so as to obtain highly specific molecular targets without inducing aberrant neurogenesis or perhaps tumorogenic proliferation.

An alternative would be to transplant exogenous stem cells, possibly genetically modified, to promote remyelination and support axonal repair. The future clinical application of transplantation for MS will require a greater amount of experimental research on the extent of remyelination, cell migration, and the repercussion of the MS tissue environment on NSCs. These are the challenges that must be addressed by researchers to render NSC-based therapies a new option for MS.

References

1. Noseworthy JH, Lucchinetti C, Rodriguez M, Weinshenker BG. Multiple sclerosis. N Engl J Med 2000;343(13): 938–952.

2. Catanzaro M, Weinert C. Economic status of families living with multiple sclerosis. Int J Rehabil Res 1992;15(3): 209–218.

3. Scolding NJ, Rayner PJ, Compston DA. Identification of A2B5-positive putative oligodendrocyte progenitor cells and A2B5-positive astrocytes in adult human white matter. Neuroscience 1999;89:1–4.

4. Scolding N, Franklin R, Stevens S, et al. Oligodendrocyte progenitors are present in the normal adult human CNS and in the lesions of multiple sclerosis. Brain 1998;121: 2221–2228.

5. Gage FH. Mammalian neural stem cells. Science 2000;287:1433–1438.

6. Kondo T, Raff M. Oligodendrocyte precursor cells reprogrammed to become multipotential CNS stem cells. Science 2000;289:1754–1757.

7. Marmur R, Mabie PC, Gokhan S, et al. Isolation and developmental characterization of cerebral cortical multipotent progenitors. Dev Biol 1998;204:577–591.

8. Ben-Hur T, Rogister B, Murray K, et al. Growth and fate of PSA-NCAM+ precursors of the postnatal brain. J Neurosci 1998;18:5777–5788.

9. Johansson CB, Momma S, Clarke DL, et al. Identification of a neural stem cell in the adult mammalian central nervous system. Cell 1999;96:25–34.

10. Doetsch F, Caille I, Lim DA, et al. Subventricular zone astrocytes are neural stem cells in the adult mammalian brain. Cell 1999;97:703–716.

11. Laywell ED, Rakic P, Kukekov VG, et al. Identification of a multipotent astrocytic stem cell in the immature and adult mouse brain. Proc Natl Acad Sci U S A 2000;97: 13883–13888.

12. Palmer TD, Markakis EA, Willhoite AR, et al. Fibroblast growth factor-2 activates a latent neurogenic program in neural stem cells from diverse regions of the adult CNS. J Neurosci 1999;19:8487–8497.

13. Reynolds BA, Weiss S. Generation of neurons and astrocytes from isolated cells of the adult mammalian central nervous system. Science 1992;255:1707–1710.

14. Alvarez-Buylla A, Temple S. Stem cells in the developing and adult nervous system. J Neurobiol 1998;36:105–110.

15. Gage FH, Kempermann G, Palmer TD, et al. Multipotent progenitor cells in the adult dentate gyrus. J Neurobiol 1998;36:249–266.

16. Doetsch F, Garcia-Verdugo JM, Alvarez-Buylla A. Cellular composition and three-dimensional organization of the subventricular germinal zone in the adult mammalian brain. J Neurosci 1997;17:5046–5061.

17. Levison SW, Goldman JE. Multipotential and lineage restricted precursors coexist in the mammalian perinatal subventricular zone. J Neurosci Res 1997;48:83–94.

18. Lois C, Alvarez-Buylla A. Proliferating subventricular zone cells in the adult mammalian forebrain can differentiate into neurons and glia. Proc Natl Acad Sci U S A 1993;90:2074–2077.

19. Hunter-Schaedle KE. Radial glial cell development and transformation are disturbed in reeler forebrain. J Neurobiol 1997;33:459–472.

20. Morshead CM, Craig CG, van der Kooy D. In vivo clonal analyses reveal the properties of endogenous neural stem

cell proliferation in the adult mammalian forebrain. Development 1998;125:2251–2261.

21. Goldman JE, Zerlin M, Newman S, et al. Fate determination and migration of progenitors in the postnatal mammalian CNS. Dev Neurosci 1997;19:42–48.

22. Levison SW, Goldman JE. Both oligodendrocytes and astrocytes develop from progenitors in the subventricular zone of postnatal rat forebrain. Neuron 1993;10:201–212.

23. Kirn JR, Fishman Y, Sasportas K, et al. Fate of new neurons in adult canary high vocal center during the first 30 days after their formation. J Comp Neurol 1999;411:487–494.

24. Eriksson PS, Perfilieva E, Bjork-Eriksson T, et al. Neurogenesis in the adult human hippocampus. Nat Med 1998;4:1313–1317.

25. Magavi SS, Leavitt BR, Macklis JD. Induction of neurogenesis in the neocortex of adult mice. Nature 2000;405:951–955.

26. Morshead CM, Reynolds BA, Craig CG, et al. Neural stem cells in the adult mammalian forebrain: a relatively quiescent subpopulation of subependymal cells. Neuron 1994;13:1071–1082.

27. Villa A, Snyder EY, Vescovi A, Martinez-Serrano A. Establishment and properties of a growth factor-dependent, perpetual neural stem cell line from the human CNS. Exp Neurol 2000;161:67–84.

28. Aboody KS, Brown A, Rainov NG, et al. From the cover: neural stem cells display extensive tropism for pathology in adult brain: evidence from intracranial gliomas. Proc Natl Acad Sci U S A 2000;97:12846–12851.

29. Chiasson BJ, Tropepe V, Morshead CM, van der Kooy D. Adult mammalian forebrain ependymal and subependymal cells demonstrate proliferative potential, but only subependymal cells have neural stem cell characteristics. J Neurosci 1999;19:4462–4471.

30. Clarke DL, Johansson CB, Wilbertz J, et al. Generalized potential of adult neural stem cells. Science 2000;288:1660–1663.

31. McLaren FH, Svendsen CN, Van der Meide P, Joly E. Analysis of neural stem cells by flow cytometry: cellular differentiation modifies patterns of MHC expression. J Neuroimmunol 2001;112:35–46.

32. Morrison SJ, Csete M, Groves AK, et al. Culture in reduced levels of oxygen promotes clonogenic sympathoadrenal differentiation by isolated neural crest stem cells. J Neurosci 2000;20:7370–7376.

33. Lendahl U, Zimmerman LB, McKay RD. CNS stem cells express a new class of intermediate filament protein. Cell 1990;60:585–595.

34. Lin RC, Matesic DF, Marvin M, et al. Re-expression of the intermediate filament nestin in reactive astrocytes. Neurobiol Dis 1995;2:79–85.

35. Messam CA, Hou J, Major EO. Coexpression of nestin in neural and glial cells in the developing human CNS defined by a human-specific anti-nestin antibody. Exp Neurol 2000;161:585–596.

36. Liu S, Qu Y, Stewart TJ, et al. Embryonic stem cells differentiate into oligodendrocytes and myelinate in culture and after spinal cord transplantation. Proc Natl Acad Sci U S A 2000;97:6126–6131.

37. Zulewski H, Abraham EJ, Gerlach MJ, et al. Multipotential nestin-positive stem cells isolated from adult pancreatic islets differentiate ex vivo into pancreatic endocrine, exocrine, and hepatic phenotypes. Diabetes 2001;50:521–533.

38. Shihabuddin LS, Ray J, Gage FH. FGF-2 is sufficient to isolate progenitors found in the adult mammalian spinal cord. Exp Neurol 1997;148:577–586.

39. Zerlin M, Levison SW, Goldman JE. Early patterns of migration, morphogenesis, and intermediate filament expression of subventricular zone cells in the postnatal rat forebrain. J Neurosci 1995;15:7238–7249.

40. Goodell MA, Brose K, Paradis G, et al. Isolation and functional properties of murine hematopoietic stem cells that are replicating in vivo. J Exp Med 1996;183:1797–1806.

41. Goodell MA, et al. Dye efflux studies suggest that hematopoietic stem cells expressing low or undetectable levels of CD34 antigen exist in multiple species. Nat Med 1997;3:1337–1345.

42. Hulspas R, Quesenberry PJ. Characterization of neurosphere cell phenotypes by flow cytometry. Cytometry 2000;40:245–250.

43. Uchida N, Buck DW, He D, et al. Direct isolation of human central nervous system stem cells. Proc Natl Acad Sci U S A 2000;97:14720–14725.

44. Morrison SJ, White PM, Zock C, Anderson DJ. Prospective identification, isolation by flow cytometry, and in vivo self-renewal of multipotent mammalian neural crest stem cells. Cell 1999;96:737–749.

45. Snyder EY, Vescovi AL. The possibilities/perplexities of stem cells [news]. Nat Biotechnol 2000;18:827–828.

46. Bjornson CR, Rietze RL, Reynolds BA, et al. Turning brain into blood: a hematopoietic fate adopted by adult neural stem cells in vivo. Science 1999;283:534–537.

47. Galli R, Borello U, Gritti A, et al. Skeletal myogenic potential of human and mouse neural stem cells. Nat Neurosci 2000;3:986–991.

48. Brazelton TR, Rossi FM, Keshet GI, Blau HM. From marrow to brain: expression of neuronal phenotypes in adult mice. Science 2000;290:1775–1779.

49. Mezey E, Chandross KJ, Harta G, et al. Turning blood into brain: cells bearing neuronal antigens generated in vivo from bone marrow. Science 2000;290:1779–1782.

50. Tsai RY, McKay RD. Cell contact regulates fate choice by cortical stem cells. J Neurosci 2000;20:3725–3735.

51. Schuldiner M, Yanuka O, Itskovitz-Eldor J, et al. From the cover: effects of eight growth factors on the differentiation of cells derived from human embryonic stem cells. Proc Natl Acad Sci U S A 2000;97:11307–11312.

52. Hardy R, Reynolds R. Proliferation and differentiation potential of rat forebrain oligodendroglial progenitors both in vitro and in vivo. Development 1991;111:1061–1080.

53. Wu HY, Dawson MR, Reynolds R, Hardy RJ. Expression of QKI proteins and MAP1B identifies actively myelinating oligodendrocytes in adult rat brain. Mol Cell Neurosci 2001;17:292–302.

54. Horner PJ, Power AE, Kempermann G, et al. Proliferation and differentiation of progenitor cells throughout the

intact adult rat spinal cord. J Neurosci 2000;20:2218–2228.

55. Niehaus A, Stegmuller J, Diers-Fenger M, Trotter J. Cell-surface glycoprotein of oligodendrocyte progenitors involved in migration. J Neurosci 1999;19:4948–4961.

56. Yu WP, Collarini EJ, Pringle NP, Richardson WD. Embryonic expression of myelin genes: evidence for a focal source of oligodendrocyte precursors in the ventricular zone of the neural tube. Neuron 1994;12:1353–1362.

57. Nishiyama A, Chang A, Trapp BD. NG2+ glial cells: a novel glial cell population in the adult brain. J Neuropathol Exp Neurol 1999;58:1113–1124.

58. Yoshimura K, Sakurai Y, Nishimura D, et al. Monoclonal antibody 14F7, which recognizes a stage-specific immature oligodendrocyte surface molecule, inhibits oligodendrocyte differentiation mediated in co-culture with astrocytes. J Neurosci Res 1998;54:79–96.

59. Levine JM, Stincone F, Lee YS. Development and differentiation of glial precursor cells in the rat cerebellum. Glia 1993;7:307–321.

60. Reynolds R, Hardy R. Oligodendroglial progenitors labeled with the O4 antibody persist in the adult rat cerebral cortex in vivo. J Neurosci Res 1997;47:455–470.

61. Noll E, Miller RH. Oligodendrocyte precursors originate at the ventral ventricular zone dorsal to the ventral midline region in the embryonic rat spinal cord. Development 1993;118:563–573.

62. Reynolds R, Wilkin GP. Development of macroglial cells in rat cerebellum. II. An in situ immunohistochemical study of oligodendroglial lineage from precursor to mature myelinating cell. Development 1988;102:409–425.

63. Raff MC, Miller RH, Noble M. A glial progenitor cell that develops in vitro into an astrocyte or an oligodendrocyte depending on culture medium. Nature 1983;303:390–396.

64. Espinosa de los Monteros A, Zhang M, De Vellis J. O2A progenitor cells transplanted into the neonatal rat brain develop into oligodendrocytes but not astrocytes. Proc Natl Acad Sci U S A 1993;90:50–54.

65. Wolswijk G, Riddle PN, Noble M. Coexistence of perinatal and adult forms of a glial progenitor cell during development of the rat optic nerve. Development 1990;109:691–698.

66. Gard AL, Pfeiffer SE. Two proliferative stages of the oligodendrocyte lineage (A2B5+O4– and O4+GalC–) under different mitogenic control. Neuron 1990;5:615–625.

67. Warrington AE, Barbarese E, Pfeiffer SE. Differential myelinogenic capacity of specific developmental stages of the oligodendrocyte lineage upon transplantation into hypomyelinating hosts. J Neurosci Res 1993;34:1–13.

68. Scolding NJ, Frith S, Linington C, et al. Myelin-oligodendrocyte glycoprotein (MOG) is a surface marker of oligodendrocyte maturation. J Neuroimmunol 1989;22:169–176.

69. Levison SW, Young GM, Goldman JE. Cycling cells in the adult rat neocortex preferentially generate oligodendroglia. J Neurosci Res 1999;57:435–446.

70. Yoon SO, Casaccia-Bonnefil P, Carter B, Chao MV. Competitive signaling between TrkA and p75 nerve growth factor receptors determines cell survival. J Neurosci 1998;18:3273–3281.

71. Patneau DK, Wright PW, Winters C, et al. Glial cells of the oligodendrocyte lineage express both kainate- and AMPA-preferring subtypes of glutamate receptor. Neuron 1994;12:357–371.

72. Casaccia-Bonnefil P, Hardy RJ, Teng KK, et al. Loss of p27Kip1 function results in increased proliferative capacity of oligodendrocyte progenitors but unaltered timing of differentiation. Development 1999;126:4027–4037.

73. Wang S, Sdrulla AD, diSibio G, et al. Notch receptor activation inhibits oligodendrocyte differentiation. Neuron 1998;21:63–75.

74. Bergles DE, Roberts JD, Somogyi P, Jahr CE. Glutamatergic synapses on oligodendrocyte precursor cells in the hippocampus. Nature 2000;405:187–191.

75. Wren D, Wolswijk G, Noble M. In vitro analysis of the origin and maintenance of O-2Aadult progenitor cells. J Cell Biol 1992;116:167–176.

76. Noble M, Wren D, Wolswijk G. The O-2A (adult) progenitor cell: a glial stem cell of the adult central nervous system. Semin Cell Biol 1992;3:413–422.

77. Messersmith DJ, Murtie JC, Le TQ, et al. Fibroblast growth factor 2 (FGF2) and FGF receptor expression in an experimental demyelinating disease with extensive remyelination. J Neurosci Res 2000;62:241–256.

78. Redwine JM, Blinder KL, Armstrong RC. In situ expression of fibroblast growth factor receptors by oligodendrocyte progenitors and oligodendrocytes in adult mouse central nervous system. J Neurosci Res 1997;50:229–237.

79. Pringle NP, Richardson WD. A singularity of PDGF alpha-receptor expression in the dorsoventral axis of the neural tube may define the origin of the oligodendrocyte lineage. Development 1993;117:525–533.

80. Ida JA, Jr., Dubois-Dalcq M, McKinnon RD. Expression of the receptor tyrosine kinase c-kit in oligodendrocyte progenitor cells. J Neurosci Res 1993;36:596–606.

81. Zhang SC, Ge B, Duncan ID. Tracing human oligodendroglial development in vitro. J Neurosci Res 2000;59:421–429.

82. Murray K, Dubois-Dalcq M. Emergence of oligodendrocytes from human neural spheres. J Neurosci Res 1997;50:146–156.

83. Durand B, Raff M. A cell-intrinsic timer that operates during oligodendrocyte development. Bioessays 2000;22:64–71.

84. Kitchens DL, Snyder EY, Gottlieb DI. FGF and EGF are mitogens for immortalized neural progenitors. J Neurobiol 1994;25:797–807.

85. Gritti A, Frolichsthal-Schoeller P, Galli R, et al. Epidermal and fibroblast growth factors behave as mitogenic regulators for a single multipotent stem cell-like population from the subventricular region of the adult mouse forebrain. J Neurosci 1999;19:3287–3297.

86. Tropepe V, Sibilia M, Ciruna BG, et al. Distinct neural stem cells proliferate in response to EGF and FGF in the developing mouse telencephalon. Dev Biol 1999;208:166–188.

87. Martens DJ, Tropepe V, van Der Kooy D. Separate proliferation kinetics of fibroblast growth factor-responsive and epidermal growth factor-responsive neural stem cells within the embryonic forebrain germinal zone. J Neurosci 2000;20:1085–1095.

88. Tropepe V, Hitoshi S, Sirard C, et al. Direct Neural Fate Specification from Embryonic Stem Cells. A Primitive Mammalian Neural Stem Cell Stage Acquired through a Default Mechanism. Neuron 2001;30:65–78.

89. Tropepe V, Craig, CG, Morshead CM, van der Kooy D. Transforming growth factor-alpha null and senescent mice show decreased neural progenitor cell proliferation in the forebrain subependyma. J Neurosci 1997;17:7850–7859.

90. Fallon J, Reid S, Kinyamu R, et al. In vivo induction of massive proliferation, directed migration, and differentiation of neural cells in the adult mammalian brain. Proc Natl Acad Sci U S A 2000:97:14686–14691.

91. Qian X, Davis AA, Goderie SK, Temple S. FGF2 concentration regulates the generation of neurons and glia from multipotent cortical stem cells. Neuron 1997;18:81–93.

92. Taupin P, Ray J, Fischer WH, et al. FGF-2-Responsive neural stem cell proliferation requires CCg, a novel Autocrine/Paracrine cofactor. Neuron 2000;28:385–397.

93. Kuhn HG, Winkler J, Kempermann G, et al. Epidermal growth factor and fibroblast growth factor-2 have different effects on neural progenitors in the adult rat brain. J Neurosci 1997:17:5820–5829.

94. Osterhout DJ, Ebner S, Xu J, et al. Transplanted oligodendrocyte progenitor cells expressing a dominant-negative FGF receptor transgene fail to migrate in vivo. J Neurosci 1997;17:9122–9132.

95. Conover JC, Doetsch F, Garcia-Verdugo JM, et al. Disruption of Eph/ephrin signaling affects migration and proliferation in the adult subventricular zone. Nat Neurosci 2000;3:1091–1097.

96. Sun Y, Nadal-Vicens M, Misono S, et al. Neurogenin Promotes Neurogenesis and Inhibits Glial Differentiation by Independent Mechanisms. Cell 2001;104:365–376.

97. Ahmed S, Reynolds BA, Weiss S. BDNF enhances the differentiation but not the survival of CNS stem cell-derived neuronal precursors. J Neurosci 1995;15:5765–5778.

98. Mehler MF, Rozental R, Dougherty M, et al. Cytokine regulation of neuronal differentiation of hippocampal progenitor cells. Nature 1993;362:62–65.

99. Gross RE, Mehler MF, Mabie PC, et al. Bone morphogenetic proteins promote astroglial lineage commitment by mammalian subventricular zone progenitor cells. Neuron 1996;17:595–606.

100. Mabie PC, Mehler MF, Marmur R, et al. Bone morphogenetic proteins induce astroglial differentiation of oligodendroglial-astroglial progenitor cells. J Neurosci 1997; 17:4112–4120.

101. Barres BA, Schmid R, Sendtner M, Raff MC. Multiple extracellular signals are required for long-term oligodendrocyte survival. Development 1993;118:283–295.

102. Mehler MF, Marmur R, Gross R, et al. Cytokines regulate the cellular phenotype of developing neural lineage species. Int J Dev Neurosci 1995;13:213–240.

103. Marmur R, Kessler JA, Zhu G, et al. Differentiation of oligodendroglial progenitors derived from cortical multipotent cells requires extrinsic signals including activation of gp130/LIFbeta receptors. J Neurosci 1998;18:9800–9811.

104. Barres BA, Burne JF, Holtmann B, et al. Ciliary neurotrophic factor enhances the rate of oligodendrocyte generation. Mol Cell Neurosci 1996;8:146–156.

105. Molne M, Studer L, Tabar V, et al. Early cortical precursors do not undergo LIF-mediated astrocytic differentiation. J Neurosci Res 2000;59:301–311.

106. Nakashima K, Yanagisawa M, Arakawa H, et al. Synergistic signaling in fetal brain by STAT3-Smad1 complex bridged by p300. Science 1999;284:479–482.

107. Cattaneo E, et al. Activation of the JAK/STAT pathway leads to proliferation of ST14A central nervous system progenitor cells. J Biol Chem 1996;271:23374–23379.

108. Morrison SJ, Perez SE, Qiao Z, et al. Transient Notch activation initiates an irreversible switch from neurogenesis to gliogenesis by neural crest stem cells. Cell 2000;101:499–510.

109. Chambers CB, Peng Y, Nguyen H, et al. Spatiotemporal selectivity of response to Notch1 signals in mammalian forebrain precursors. Development 2001;128:689–702.

110. Gaiano N, Nye JS, Fishell G. Radial glial identity is promoted by Notch1 signaling in the murine forebrain. Neuron 2000;26:395–404.

111. Handler M, Yang X, Shen J. Presenilin-1 regulates neuronal differentiation during neurogenesis. Development 2000;127:2593–2606.

112. Canoll PD, Musacchio JM, Hardy R, et al. GGF/neuregulin is a neuronal signal that promotes the proliferation and survival and inhibits the differentiation of oligodendrocyte progenitors. Neuron 1996;17:229–243.

113. Canoll PD, Kraemer R, Teng KK, et al. GGF/neuregulin induces a phenotypic reversion of oligodendrocytes. Mol Cell Neurosci 1999;13:79–94.

114. Vartanian T, Fischbach G, Miller R. Failure of spinal cord oligodendrocyte development in mice lacking neuregulin. Proc Natl Acad Sci U S A 1999;96:731–735.

115. Tang DG, Tokumoto YM, Raff MC. Long-term culture of purified postnatal oligodendrocyte precursor cells. Evidence for an intrinsic maturation program that plays out over months. J Cell Biol 2000;148:971–984.

116. Forsberg-Nilsson K, Behar TN, Afrakhte M, et al. Platelet-derived growth factor induces chemotaxis of neuroepithelial stem cells. J Neurosci Res 1998;53:521–530.

117. Kondo T, Raff M. The Id4 HLH protein and the timing of oligodendrocyte differentiation. EMBO J 2000;19:1998–2007.

118. Lu QR, Yuk D, Alberta JA, et al. Sonic hedgehog—regulated oligodendrocyte lineage genes encoding bHLH proteins in the mammalian central nervous system. Neuron 2000;25:317–329.

119. Huh GS, Riquelme PA, Brotz TM, et al. Functional requirement for class I MHC in CNS development and plasticity. Science 2000;290:2155–2159.

120. Begolka WS, Vanderlugt CL, Rahbe SM, Miller SD. Differential expression of inflammatory cytokines parallels progression of central nervous system pathology in two clinically distinct models of multiple sclerosis. J Immunol 1998;161:4437–4446.

121. Holmin S, Almqvist P, Lendahl U, Mathiesen T. Adult nestin-expressing subependymal cells differentiate to astrocytes in response to brain injury. Eur J Neurosci 1997;9:65–75.

122. Kay JN, Blum M. Differential response of ventral midbrain and striatal progenitor cells to lesions of the nigros-

triatal dopaminergic projection. Dev Neurosci 2000;22: 56–67.

123. Frisen J, Johansson CB, Torok C, et al. Rapid, widespread, and longlasting induction of nestin contributes to the generation of glial scar tissue after CNS injury. J Cell Biol 1995;131:453–464.

124. Szele FG, Chesselet MF. Cortical lesions induce an increase in cell number and PSA-NCAM expression in the subventricular zone of adult rats. J Comp Neurol 1996; 368:439–454.

125. Issazadeh S, Navikas V, Schaub M, et al. Kinetics of expression of costimulatory molecules and their ligands in murine relapsing experimental autoimmune encephalomyelitis in vivo. J Immunol 1998;161:1104–1112.

126. Hooper DC, Bagasra O, Marini JC, et al. Prevention of experimental allergic encephalomyelitis by targeting nitric oxide and peroxynitrite: implications for the treatment of multiple sclerosis. Proc Natl Acad Sci U S A 1997;94:2528–2533.

127. Calza L, Giardino L, Pozza M, et al. Proliferation and phenotype regulation in the subventricular zone during experimental allergic encephalomyelitis: in vivo evidence of a role for nerve growth factor. Proc Natl Acad Sci U S A 1998;95:3209–3214.

128. Di Bello IC, Dawson MR, Levine JM, Reynolds R. Generation of oligodendroglial progenitors in acute inflammatory demyelinating lesions of the rat brain stem is associated with demyelination rather than inflammation. J Neurocytol 1999;28:365–381.

129. Keirstead HS, Levine JM, Blakemore WF. Response of the oligodendrocyte progenitor cell population (defined by NG2 labelling) to demyelination of the adult spinal cord. Glia 1998;22:161–170.

130. Blakemore WF. Remyelination of the superior cerebellar peduncle in the mouse following demyelination induced by feeding cuprizone. J Neurol Sci 1973;20:73–83.

131. Oumesmar BN, Vignais L, Duhamel-Clerin E, et al. Expression of the highly polysialylated neural cell adhesion molecule during postnatal myelination and following chemically induced demyelination of the adult mouse spinal cord. Eur J Neurosci 1995;7:480–491.

132. Nait-Oumesmar B, Decker L, Lachapelle F, et al. Progenitor cells of the adult mouse subventricular zone proliferate, migrate and differentiate into oligodendrocytes after demyelination. Eur J Neurosci 1999;11:4357–4366.

133. Carroll WM, Jennings AR, Ironside LJ. Identification of the adult resting progenitor cell by autoradiographic tracking of oligodendrocyte precursors in experimental CNS demyelination. Brain 1998;121:293–302.

134. Carroll WM, Jennings AR. Early recruitment of oligodendrocyte precursors in CNS demyelination. Brain 1994; 117:563–578.

135. Gensert JM, Goldman JE. Endogenous progenitors remyelinate demyelinated axons in the adult CNS. Neuron 1997;19:197–203.

136. Hinks GL, Franklin RJ. Delayed changes in growth factor gene expression during slow remyelination in the CNS of aged rats. Mol Cell Neurosci 2000;16:542–556.

137. Mason JL, Jones JJ, Taniike M, et al. Mature oligodendrocyte apoptosis precedes IGF-1 production and oligodendrocyte progenitor accumulation and differentiation during demyelination/remyelination. J Neurosci Res 2000;61:251–262.

138. Liu X, Yao DL, Webster H. Insulin-like growth factor I treatment reduces clinical deficits and lesion severity in acute demyelinating experimental autoimmune encephalomyelitis. Mult Scler 1995;1:2–9.

139. Yao DL, Liu X, Hudson LD, Webster HD. Insulin-like growth factor I treatment reduces demyelination and upregulates gene expression of myelin-related proteins in experimental autoimmune encephalomyelitis. Proc Natl Acad Sci U S A 1995;92:6190–6194.

140. Cannella B, Pitt D, Capello E, Raine CS. Insulin-like growth factor-1 fails to enhance central nervous system myelin repair during autoimmune demyelination. Am J Pathol 2000;157:933–943.

141. Redwine JM, Armstrong RC. In vivo proliferation of oligodendrocyte progenitors expressing PDGFalphaR during early remyelination. J Neurobiol 1998;37:413–428.

142. Blakemore WF, Keirstead HS. The origin of remyelinating cells in the central nervous system. J Neuroimmunol 1999;98:69–76.

143. Chang A, Nishiyama A, Peterson J, et al. NG2-positive oligodendrocyte progenitor cells in adult human brain and multiple sclerosis lesions. J Neurosci 2000;20:6404–6412.

144. Wolswijk G. Oligodendrocyte survival, loss and birth in lesions of chronic-stage multiple sclerosis. Brain 2000; 123:105–115.

145. Cammer W. Effects of TNFalpha on immature and mature oligodendrocytes and their progenitors in vitro. Brain Res 2000;864:213–219.

146. Molina-Holgado E, Vela JM, Arevalo-Martin A, Guaza C. LPS/IFN-gamma cytotoxicity in oligodendroglial cells: role of nitric oxide and protection by the anti-inflammatory cytokine IL-10. Eur J Neurosci 2001;13:493–502.

147. Hammarberg H, Lidman O, Lundberg C et al. Neuroprotection by encephalomyelitis: rescue of mechanically injured neurons and neurotrophin production by CNS-infiltrating T and natural killer cells. J Neurosci 2000;20:5283–5291.

148. D'Souza SD, Bonetti B, Balasingam V, et al. Multiple sclerosis: Fas signaling in oligodendrocyte cell death. J Exp Med 1996;184:2361–2370.

149. Sabelko-Downes KA, Russell JH, Cross AH. Role of Fas—FasL interactions in the pathogenesis and regulation of autoimmune demyelinating disease. J Neuroimmunol 1999;100:42–52.

150. Pouly S, Becher B, Blain M, Antel JP. Interferon-gamma modulates human oligodendrocyte susceptibility to Fas-mediated apoptosis. J Neuropathol Exp Neurol 2000;59: 280–286.

151. Andrews T, Zhang P, Bhat NR. TNFalpha potentiates IFN-gamma-induced cell death in oligodendrocyte progenitors. J Neurosci Res 1998;54:574–583.

152. Probert L, Eugster HP, Akassoglou K, et al. TNFR1 signalling is critical for the development of demyelination and the limitation of T-cell responses during immune-mediated CNS disease. Brain 2000;123:2005–2019.

153. Piani D, Frei K, Do KQ, et al. Murine brain macrophages induced NMDA receptor mediated neurotoxicity in vitro by secreting glutamate. Neurosci Lett 1991;133:159–162.

154. Piani D, Spranger M, Frei K, et al. Macrophage-induced cytotoxicity of *N*-methyl-D-aspartate receptor positive neurons involves excitatory amino acids rather than reactive oxygen intermediates and cytokines. Eur J Immunol 1992;22:2429–2436.

155. Pitt D, Werner P, Raine CS. Glutamate excitotoxicity in a model of multiple sclerosis. Nat Med 2000;6:67–70.

156. McDonald JW, Althomsons SP, Hyrc KL, et al. Oligodendrocytes from forebrain are highly vulnerable to AMPA/kainate receptor-mediated excitotoxicity. Nat Med 1998; 4:291–297.

157. Gallo V, Pende M, Scherer S, et al. Expression and regulation of kainate and AMPA receptors in uncommitted and committed neural progenitors. Neurochem Res 1995; 20:549–560.

158. Gallo V, Zhou JM, McBain CJ, et al. Oligodendrocyte progenitor cell proliferation and lineage progression are regulated by glutamate receptor-mediated K+ channel block. J Neurosci 1996;16:2659–2670.

159. Wren DR, Noble M. Oligodendrocytes and oligodendrocyte/type-2 astrocyte progenitor cells of adult rats are specifically susceptible to the lytic effects of complement in absence of antibody. Proc Natl Acad Sci U S A 1989; 86:9025–9029.

160. Bailey KA, Drago J, Bartlett PF. Neuronal progenitors identified by their inability to express class I histocompatibility antigens in response to interferon-gamma. J Neurosci Res 1994;39:166–177.

161. Birdsall HH. Induction of ICAM-1 on human neural cells and mechanisms of neutrophil-mediated injury. Am J Pathol 1991;139:1341–1350.

162. Imitola J, Snyder EY, Sayegh MH, Khoury SJ. Differential upregulation of B7-1 costimulatory molecule during stress induced-apoptosis in neural stem cells. Neurology 1999;52:A336.

163. Prineas JW, Barnard RO, Kwon EE, et al. Multiple sclerosis: remyelination of nascent lesions. Ann Neurol 1993; 33:137–151.

164. Rodriguez M, Scheithauer B. Ultrastructure of multiple sclerosis. Ultrastruct Pathol 1994;18:3–13.

165. Wolswijk G. Oligodendrocyte precursor cells in chronic multiple sclerosis lesions. Mult Scler 1997;3:168–169.

166. Wolswijk G. Chronic stage multiple sclerosis lesions contain a relatively quiescent population of oligodendrocyte precursor cells. J Neurosci 1998;18:601–609.

167. Archelos JJ, Trotter J, Previtali S, et al. Isolation and characterization of an oligodendrocyte precursor-derived B-cell epitope in multiple sclerosis. Ann Neurol 1998; 43(1):15–24.

168. Niehaus A, Shi J, Grzenkowski M, et al. Patients with active relapsing-remitting multiple sclerosis synthesize antibodies recognizing oligodendrocyte progenitor cell surface protein: implications for remyelination. Ann Neurol 2000;48:362–371.

169. Butt AM, Berry M. Oligodendrocytes and the control of myelination in vivo: new insights from the rat anterior medullary velum. J Neurosci Res 2000;59:477–488.

170. Lubetzki C, Stankoff B. [Role of axonal signals in myelination of the central nervous system.] Pathol Biol (Paris) 2000;48:63–69.

171. Merrill JE, Scolding NJ. Mechanisms of damage to myelin and oligodendrocytes and their relevance to disease. Neuropathol Appl Neurobiol 1999;25:435–458.

172. Hardy R, Reynolds R. Rat cerebral cortical neurons in primary culture release a mitogen specific for early (GD3+/04–) oligodendroglial progenitors. J Neurosci Res 1993; 34:589–600.

173. Zajicek J, Compston A. Myelination in vitro of rodent dorsal root ganglia by glial progenitor cells. Brain 1994;117:1333–1350.

174. Fernandez PA, Tang DG, Cheng L, et al. Evidence that axon-derived neuregulin promotes oligodendrocyte survival in the developing rat optic nerve. Neuron 2000;28: 81–90.

175. Black JA, Dib-Hajj S, Baker D, et al. Sensory neuron-specific sodium channel SNS is abnormally expressed in the brains of mice with experimental allergic encephalomyelitis and humans with multiple sclerosis. Proc Natl Acad Sci U S A 2000;97:11598–11602.

176. Kornek B, Storch MK, Weissert R, et al. Multiple sclerosis and chronic autoimmune encephalomyelitis: a comparative quantitative study of axonal injury in active, inactive, and remyelinated lesions. Am J Pathol 2000;157:267–276.

177. De Stefano N, Narayanan S, Francis GS, et al. Evidence of Axonal Damage in the Early Stages of Multiple Sclerosis and Its Relevance to Disability. Arch Neurol 2001;58:65–70.

178. Miller RH. Contact with central nervous system myelin inhibits oligodendrocyte progenitor maturation. Dev Biol 1999;216:359–368.

179. Chen MS, Huber AB, van der Haar ME, et al. Nogo-A is a myelin-associated neurite outgrowth inhibitor and an antigen for monoclonal antibody IN-1. Nature 2000;403:434–439.

180. GrandPre T, Nakamura F, Vartanian T, Strittmatter SM. Identification of the Nogo inhibitor of axon regeneration as a Reticulon protein. Nature 2000;403:439–444.

181. Hunter SF, Leavitt JA, Rodriguez M. Direct observation of myelination in vivo in the mature human central nervous system. A model for the behaviour of oligodendrocyte progenitors and their progeny. Brain 1997;120:2071–2082.

182. South SA, Deibler GE, Tzeng SF, et al. Myelin basic protein (MBP) and MBP peptides are mitogens for cultured astrocytes. Glia 2000;29:81–90.

183. Fawcett JW, Asher RA. The glial scar and central nervous system repair. Brain Res Bull 1999;49:377–391.

184. Blakemore WF, Crang AJ, Franklin RJ, et al. Glial cell transplants that are subsequently rejected can be used to influence regeneration of glial cell environments in the CNS. Glia 1995;13:79–91.

185. Shields SA, Blakemore WF, Franklin RJ. Schwann cell remyelination is restricted to astrocyte-deficient areas after transplantation into demyelinated adult rat brain. J Neurosci Res 2000;60:571–578.

186. Itoyama Y, Ohnishi A, Tateishi J, et al. Spinal cord multiple sclerosis lesions in Japanese patients: Schwann cell remyelination occurs in areas that lack glial fibrillary acidic protein (GFAP). Acta Neuropathol 1985;65:217–223.

187. Ishikawa M, Tsukamoto T, Yamamoto T. Long-term cultured astrocytes inhibit myelin formation, but not axonal growth in the co-cultured nerve tissue. Mult Scler 1996;2:91–95.

188. Liedtke W, Edelmann W, Chiu FC, et al. Experimental autoimmune encephalomyelitis in mice lacking glial fibrillary acidic protein is characterized by a more severe clinical course and an infiltrative central nervous system lesion. Am J Pathol 1998;152:251–259.

189. Fok-Seang J, DiProspero NA, Meiners S, et al. Cytokine-induced changes in the ability of astrocytes to support migration of oligodendrocyte precursors and axon growth. Eur J Neurosci 1998;10:2400–2415.

190. Fok-Seang J, Smith-Thomas LC, Meiners S, et al. An analysis of astrocytic cell lines with different abilities to promote axon growth. Brain Res 1995;689:207–223.

191. Wilby MJ, Muir EM, Fok-Seang J, et al. N-Cadherin inhibits Schwann cell migration on astrocytes. Mol Cell Neurosci 1999;14:66–84.

192. Khoury SJ, Akalin E, Chandraker A, et al. CD28-B7 costimulatory blockade by CTLA4Ig prevents actively induced experimental autoimmune encephalomyelitis and inhibits Th1 but spares Th2 cytokines in the central nervous system. J Immunol 1995;155:4521–4524.

193. Moalem G, Gdalyahu A, Shani Y, et al. Production of neurotrophins by activated T cells: implications for neuroprotective autoimmunity. J Autoimmun 2000;15:331–345.

194. Villoslada P, Hauser SL, Bartke I, et al. Human nerve growth factor protects common marmosets against autoimmune encephalomyelitis by switching the balance of T helper cell type 1 and 2 cytokines within the central nervous system. J Exp Med 2000;191:1799–1806.

195. Cattaneo E, McKay R. Proliferation and differentiation of neuronal stem cells regulated by nerve growth factor. Nature 1990;347:762–765.

196. Barres BA, Raff MC, Gaese F, et al. A crucial role for neurotrophin-3 in oligodendrocyte development. Nature 1994;367:371–375.

197. Marchionni MA, Cannella B, Hoban C, et al. Neuregulin in neuron/glial interactions in the central nervous system. GGF2 diminishes autoimmune demyelination, promotes oligodendrocyte progenitor expansion, and enhances remyelination. Adv Exp Med Biol 1999;468:283–295.

198. Cannella B, Hoban CJ, Gao YL, et al. The neuregulin, glial growth factor 2, diminishes autoimmune demyelination and enhances remyelination in a chronic relapsing model for multiple sclerosis. Proc Natl Acad Sci U S A 1998;95:10100–10105.

199. Cannella B, Pitt D, Marchionni M, Raine CS. Neuregulin and erbB receptor expression in normal and diseased human white matter. J Neuroimmunol 1999;100:233–242.

200. Lucchinetti C, Bruck W, Parisi J, et al. Heterogeneity of multiple sclerosis lesions: implications for the pathogenesis of demyelination. Ann Neurol 2000;47:707–717.

201. Lovas G, Szilagyi N, Majtenyi K, et al. Axonal changes in chronic demyelinated cervical spinal cord plaques. Brain 2000;123:308–317.

202. Rogister B, Ben-Hur T, Dubois-Dalcq M. From neural stem cells to myelinating oligodendrocytes. Mol Cell Neurosci 1999;14:287–300.

203. Lacorazza HD, Flax JD, Snyder EY, Jendoubi M. Expression of human beta-hexosaminidase alpha-subunit gene (the gene defect of Tay-Sachs disease) in mouse brains upon engraftment of transduced progenitor cells. Nat Med 1996;2:424–429.

204. Nakafuku M, Nakamura S. Establishment and characterization of a multipotential neural cell line that can conditionally generate neurons, astrocytes, and oligodendrocytes in vitro. J Neurosci Res 1995;41:153–168.

205. Hulspas R, Tiarks C, Reilly J, et al. In vitro cell density-dependent clonal growth of EGF-responsive murine neural progenitor cells under serum-free conditions. Exp Neurol 1997;148:147–156.

206. Flax JD, Aurora S, Yang C, et al. Engraftable human neural stem cells respond to developmental cues, replace neurons, and express foreign genes. Nat Biotechnol 1998;16:1033–1039.

207. Ryder EF, Snyder EY, Cepko CL. Establishment and characterization of multipotent neural cell lines using retrovirus vector-mediated oncogene transfer. J Neurobiol 1990;21:356–375.

208. Snyder EY, Taylor RM, Wolfe JH. Neural progenitor cell engraftment corrects lysosomal storage throughout the MPS VII mouse brain. Nature 1995;374:367–370.

209. Rosario CM, Yandava BD, Kosaras B, et al. Differentiation of engrafted multipotent neural progenitors towards replacement of missing granule neurons in meander tail cerebellum may help determine the locus of mutant gene action. Development 1997;124:4213–4224.

210. Brustle O, Choudhary K, Karram K, et al. Chimeric brains generated by intraventricular transplantation of fetal human brain cells into embryonic rats. Nat Biotechnol 1998;16:1040–1044.

211. Gage FH, Coates PW, Palmer TD, et al. Survival and differentiation of adult neuronal progenitor cells transplanted to the adult brain. Proc Natl Acad Sci U S A 1995;92:11879–11883.

212. Yandava BD, Billinghurst LL, Snyder EY. "Global" cell replacement is feasible via neural stem cell transplantation: evidence from the dysmyelinated shiverer mouse brain. Proc Natl Acad Sci U S A 1999;96:7029–7034.

213. Milward EA, Lundberg CG, Ge B, et al. Isolation and transplantation of multipotential populations of epidermal growth factor-responsive, neural progenitor cells from the canine brain. J Neurosci Res 1997;50:862–871.

214. Hammang JP, Archer DR, Duncan ID. Myelination following transplantation of EGF-responsive neural stem cells into a myelin-deficient environment. Exp Neurol 1997;147:84–95.

215. Archer DR, Cuddon PA, Lipsitz D, Duncan LD. Myelination of the canine central nervous system by glial cell transplantation: a model for repair of human myelin disease. Nat Med 1997;3:54–59.

216. Espinosa de los Monteros A, Zhao P, Huang C, et al. Transplantation of CG4 oligodendrocyte progenitor cells in the myelin-deficient rat brain results in myelination of axons and enhanced oligodendroglial markers. J Neurosci Res 1997;50:872–887.

217. Franklin RJ, Blakemore WF. Transplanting oligodendrocyte progenitors into the adult CNS. J Anat 1997;190:23–33.

218. Smith PM, Blakemore WF. Porcine neural progenitors require commitment to the oligodendrocyte lineage prior to transplantation in order to achieve significant remyelination of demyelinated lesions in the adult CNS. Eur J Neurosci 2000;12:2414–2424.

219. Akiyama Y, Honmou O, Kato T, et al. Transplantation of clonal neural precursor cells derived from adult human brain establishes functional peripheral myelin in the rat spinal cord. Exp Neurol 2001;167:27–39.

220. Zhang SC, Ge B, Duncan ID. Adult brain retains the potential to generate oligodendroglial progenitors with extensive myelination capacity. Proc Natl Acad Sci U S A 1999;96:4089–4094.

221. Brustle O, Jones KN, Learish RD, et al. Embryonic stem cell-derived glial precursors: a source of myelinating transplants. Science 1999;285:754–756.

222. Imaizumi T, Lankford KL, Burton WV, et al. Xenotransplantation of transgenic pig olfactory ensheathing cells promotes axonal regeneration in rat spinal cord. Nat Biotechnol 2000;18:949–953.

223. Bjorklund A, Lindvall O. Cell replacement therapies for central nervous system disorders. Nat Neurosci 2000;3:537–544.

224. Tourbah A, Linnington C, Bachelin C, et al. Inflammation promotes survival and migration of the CG4 oligodendrocyte progenitors transplanted in the spinal cord of both inflammatory and demyelinated EAE rats. J Neurosci Res 1997;50:853–861.

225. Snyder EY, Yoon C, Flax JD, Macklis JD. Multipotent neural precursors can differentiate toward replacement of neurons undergoing targeted apoptotic degeneration in adult mouse neocortex. Proc Natl Acad Sci U S A 1997;94:11663–11668.

Chapter 4

Genetic and Metabolic Aspects of Leukodystrophies

Edwin H. Kolodny

Leukodystrophies

The term *leukodystrophy* is generally understood to mean inherited diseases primarily affecting brain white matter that are progressive and for which a specific biochemical or molecular cause has been identified. Some definitions emphasize histologic characteristics such as demyelination[1,2] or affection primarily of oligodendroglial cells or myelin.[3] Other definitions focus on the abnormal metabolism of myelin constituents.[4] The common elements are (1) a genetic basis, (2) a progressive clinical course, (3) primary involvement of brain white matter, and (4) a demonstrable biochemical or molecular defect.

Rapid advances in techniques for imaging the brain now challenge the meaning of the term leukodystrophy. Although cranial magnetic resonance imaging (MRI) findings of a low-density signal in cerebral white matter on T_1-weighted images and a high-intensity signal on T_2-weighted images are characteristic for the inherited demyelinating diseases, these particular neuroradiologic signs are not specific for the genetic leukodystrophies. A similar pattern is observed in MRI studies in (1) infants with nonprogressive diseases due to prenatal or perinatal insults, (2) disorders primarily affecting neurons and their axons, (3) diseases involving metabolic pathways not directly concerned with the synthesis or maintenance of myelin, and (4) toxic neurometabolic conditions. It is useful, therefore, to separate out from this larger collection of leukoencephalopathies those diseases that primarily affect myelin syn-

thesis and catabolism from those due to secondary causes resulting in delayed myelination, glial cell loss, or damage to neurons and axons and those due to a toxic metabolite or deficiency of a substrate.

The question of a possible leukodystrophy arises often in the practice of pediatric neurology. At one children's hospital, 215 of 7,784 MRI scans performed in a 1-year period revealed some type of white-matter abnormality.[5] Nevertheless, a detailed analysis might reveal a precise neurologic diagnosis in less than one-half of such cases. In a study of 26 children with cerebral white-matter abnormalities, a Swedish group found that the clinical course was progressive in 11 and nonprogressive in 15.[6] Those with a nonprogressive course tended to have prenatal stigmata and asymmetrical white-matter lesions.

Some authors maintain the distinction between primary leukodystrophic and secondary nonleukodystrophic white-matter changes.[7] However, this chapter includes within the leukodystrophies all genetically determined degenerative diseases affecting brain white matter whether the primary pathology is demyelinating or is some other process. It is assumed that the clinician has ruled out other causes of leukoencephalopathy, including inflammatory and infectious diseases, tumors, vascular diseases, and exogenous neurotoxins.[8]

Clinical Features

A period of normal development usually precedes the onset of neurologic signs and symptoms. Spasticity develops that is usually bilateral and symmetrical. Other long-tract signs include motor weakness and ataxia. Optic atrophy occurs late. If peripheral myelin is affected, then neuropathy with loss of ankle reflexes is seen. Seizures are uncommon but can be encountered in Krabbe's disease, metachromatic leukodystrophy (MLD),[9] and adrenoleukodystrophy (ALD).

Behavioral and cognitive changes can occur at any stage. The degree and type of impairment will depend on the distribution of white-matter lesions. Diffuse dysfunction is more common than focal impairment.[10] We encounter more severe behavioral changes such as blunted affect and lack of spontaneity in which frontal lobe white matter is involved. In the case of parieto-occipital lesions, intellectual functioning may remain intact. However, even in asymptomatic patients, neuropsychological testing can reveal deficits. In the study of Riva et al.[11] that examined asymptomatic and symptomatic boys with X-linked ALD, performance on neuropsychological testing directly correlated with the extent of white-matter lesions as visualized by MRI.

Neuroimaging

The development of MRI has provided enormous impetus to the study of the leukodystrophies. In contrast to computed tomography and ultrasonography, MRI has greater sensitivity in revealing small changes in the water content of brain tissue, changes in the binding of free water (revealed by magnetization transfer), and the extent and anisotropy of water diffusion (revealed by diffusion imaging). Thus, it can provide a noninvasive means for demonstrating anatomic and physiologic changes in brain white matter. MRI has been used to assess the pattern of myelination in developing infants,[12] map white-matter pathways, and detect metabolic abnormalities.

As myelination progresses, the intensity of the white-matter signal on the T_1-weighted image increases.[13] The loss of water that accompanies myelination reduces the proton density and, hence, the signal on T_2-weighted images. Conversely, the loss of myelin that accompanies a leukodystrophy results in an increase in water and high-signal intensity on T_2-weighted images.

In primary leukodystrophies, the abnormal signal is usually bilateral and symmetrical but can first appear in the periventricular region, especially at the atria and then spread toward the subcortical region. A characteristic feature of the genetic leukodystrophies is the preservation of the subcortical arcuate fibers. A notable exception is Canavan's disease.

Specific patterns of myelin loss are seen in particular disorders. For example, frontal lobe white matter is preferentially affected in late-onset MLD and parieto-occipital white matter is primarily involved in late-onset globoid cell leukodystrophy (GLD). Pontomedullary corticospinal tract involvement appears to be specific for X-linked ALD.[14]

Delayed myelination is a common feature of many inherited metabolic diseases, including disorders of amino acid and organic acid metabolism, the lysosomal storage diseases,[15] the mitochondrial encephalopathies, and some chromosomal disorders. This can be demonstrated by failure to meet the milestones for high-signal intensity on T_1-weighted images. A severe failure of myelin to form occurs in Pelizaeus-Merzbacher disease (PMD).

Additional information, including the extent of gliosis, can be obtained in certain cases with the use of the fluid-attenuated inversion recovery sequence, which minimizes the cerebrospinal fluid (CSF) signal and improves the signal from the periventricular, subcortical, and cortical regions. MR spectroscopy is a noninvasive means for studying cerebral metabolites, brain pH, and some neurotransmitters. It is useful for quantitating such chemical species in brain as (1) N-acetylaspartate, a putative neuronal marker, which can be elevated in brain white matter of Canavan's disease; (2) choline, which is increased in demyelination; and (3) lactate, which is raised in diseases of energy metabolism (i.e., mitochondrial defects).

Pathology of the Leukodystrophies

One can rarely make a correct diagnosis on the basis of imaging studies alone. However, tissue pathology can be very helpful, because histologic criteria differ among the various forms of leukodystrophy. Table 4-1 lists a few of the inherited leukodystrophies with their characteristic histologic features. Certain aspects, however, are common to the leukodystrophies. Extracellular fluid, reactive astrocytes, and inflammatory cells are increased. Myelin-specific components decrease and the amount of glial fibrillary acidic protein (GFAP) increases. The cholesterol becomes esterified and fills phagocytes producing sudanophilia. Extensive demyelination can secondarily lead to axonal degeneration and loss of neurons, with diffuse dysfunction of axonal conduction in such long-myelinated tracts as the pyramidal and spinocerebellar pathways. In cases of delayed myelination, the central white matter appears irregular and patchy. Status spongiosus is characteristic of Canavan's disease, vanishing white-matter disease, and megalencephalic leukodystrophy.

Further Testing

An electroencephalogram (EEG) is obtained to rule out static encephalopathy due to a seizure disorder such as West's syndrome, Lennox-Gastaut syndrome, or Landau-Kleffner syndrome. The usual finding in the leukodystrophies is progressive slowing of background rhythms. Visual-, auditory-, and somatosensory-evoked potentials are abnormal in shape and show increased latency owing to their passage through diseased white-matter tracts. Nerve conduction velocities will be reduced in MLD and its variants, GLD and Cockayne syndrome (CS), because peripheral as well as central myelin is affected in these diseases.

A skin biopsy may be obtained for studying Schwann's cells or other elements of dermal nerves by electron microscopy for MLD or GLD and for documenting tissue storage in the lysosomal enzyme–deficiency states. The skin specimen may also be used to grow fibroblasts in tissue culture for use in metabolic studies and DNA analyses. However, for most biochemical and molecular studies, a specimen of peripheral blood will suffice, from which leukocytes can be isolated for enzyme analyses, and DNA can be extracted for polymerase chain reaction amplification and sequencing.

Urine is obtained for quantitating mucopolysaccharides (in the mucopolysaccharidoses), oligosaccharides (in mannosidosis, fucosidosis, aspartylglucosuria, and sialyluria), sulfatide (in MLD and its variants), and amino acids and organic acids (including *N*-acetylaspartate in Canavan's disease).

Table 4-1. Examples of Neuropathologic Features Characteristic of Specific Leukodystrophies

Disease	Histopathology
Adrenoleukodystrophy	Perivascular lymphocytic cuffing
Alexander's disease	Rosenthal fibers
Canavan's disease	Vacuolization and enlarged protoplasmic astrocytes
Fucosidosis	Clear vacuoles, plus vacuoles with multilamellar membrane-bound inclusions
Krabbe's disease	Globoid cells
Leigh syndrome	Bilateral striatal necrosis
Metachromatic leukodystrophy	Metachromatic granules

Classification

The leukodystrophies are listed in Table 4-2. Disorders of *hypomyelination* are due to failure of the synthesis of a particular myelin protein. *Delayed myelination* is the result of an inadequate supply of myelin precursors or the accumulation of metabolites toxic to oligodendroglia and myelin formation. In disorders of *primary demyelination*, the accumulating storage material causes normally formed myelin to break down. These include the *vacuolating myelinopathies* in which the degenerating white matter is replaced by fluid and vacuolization. *Secondary demyelination* occurs when myelin is lost after a wallerian degeneration process, in which neurons and axons are destroyed.

Disorders of Hypomyelination (Myelin Protein Disorders)

Central nervous system (CNS) myelin is composed of 30% protein and 70% lipid. The two major myelin proteins are (1) proteolipid protein (PLP) and the structurally related protein DM20 and (2) myelin basic protein (MBP). Together, they represent 80–90% of total myelin protein.[16]

PLP is composed of 276 amino acids (of which 35 are absent from the alternatively spliced variant DM20). It accounts for one-half of the protein mass of CNS myelin but less than 1% of peripheral myelin protein (in Schwann's cells). It is localized in the

Table 4-2.   Genetic Bases of the Leukodystrophies

Disorder	Metabolite	Gene Location	Mode of Inheritance
Hypomyelination			
Pelizaeus-Merzbacher	Proteolipid protein	Xq22	X-linked recessive disease
18q– syndrome	Myelin basic protein	18q	Sporadic
Delayed myelination			
Amino acidopathies	Example: phenylketonuria	—	Autosomal recessive
Organic acidopathies	Example: maple syrup urine disease	—	Autosomal recessive
Fatty acid disorders	Example: multiple coenzyme A dehydrogenase deficiency	—	Autosomal recessive
Mitochondrial disorders	Example: complex I–IV deficiency, Kearns-Sayre syndrome, MELAS, Leber's hereditary optic neuropathy, MNGIE	—	Autosomal recessive, mitochondrial DNA mutations, and sporadic
Primary demyelination			
Globoid cell leukodystrophy	Galactosylceramide	14q21-q31	Autosomal recessive
Metachromatic leukodystrophy	Sulfatide	22q13	Autosomal recessive
Multiple sulfatase deficiency	Sulfatide, mucopolysaccharides	—	Autosomal recessive
Adrenoleukodystrophy	Very-long-chain fatty acids	Xq28	X-linked
Alexander's disease	GFAP	17q21	Sporadic dominant
Vacuolating myelinopathies			
Canavan's disease	N-acetylaspartate	17p13-ter	Autosomal recessive
Leukodystrophy with vanishing white matter	?	3q27	Unknown
Vacuolating megalencephalic leukoencephalopathy	?	22qtel	Autosomal recessive
Secondary demyelination			
Lysosomal storage diseases	Example: G_{M1}- and G_{M2}-gangliosidoses, fucosidosis, Niemann-Pick disease, sialic acid storage disease	Multiple	Autosomal recessive
Merosin-deficient congenital muscular dystrophy	Merosin (laminin-α2)	6q2	Autosomal recessive
Sjögren-Larsson syndrome	—	17p11.2	Autosomal recessive
Cockayne syndrome	Defective nucleotide excision repair	10q11-q21 (for the *ERCC6* gene)	Autosomal recessive
Cerebrotendinous xanthomatosis	Cholestanol	2q33-qter	Autosomal recessive
CADASIL	Granular osmophilic bodies	19p13.2-p12	Autosomal dominant
Proximal myotonic myopathy	—	7q35	Autosomal dominant
SOX10 deficiency	—	—	Autosomal recessive
Leukodystrophies of unknown etiology			
Leukodystrophy with ovarian dysgenesis	—	—	—
Aicardi-Goutières syndrome	—	—	—
Hereditary leukoencephalopathy and palmoplantar keratoderma	—	(?18q12.1)	—

CADASIL = cerebral autosomal dominant arteriopathy with subcortical infarcts and leukoencephalopathy; GFAP =glial fibrillary acidic protein; MELAS = mitochondrial encephalomyopathy, lactic acidosis, and stroke-like episodes; MNGIE = mitochondrial neurogastrointestinal encephalomyopathy.

outer portion of the cell membrane and extends into the extracellular space. PLP interacts homophilically with similar PLP chains on the surface of the myelin membrane. The lipophilic amino acid tryptophan is present on the outer surface edge of the PLP and may interact with galactocerebrosides in the outer lipid membrane of the adjacent myelin spiral.

PLP and DM20 are not necessary for normal myelin assembly but are essential for the maintenance of normal axonal integrity. *Jimpy* mice that are genetically deficient in PLP develop widespread wallerian degeneration. In individuals with a null mutation producing no functional PLP, there is also a demyelinating peripheral neuropathy. *MBP* forms dimers within the cytoplasm of the myelin sheath and likely stabilizes the myelin spiral at the major dense line by interacting with negatively charged lipids at the cytoplasmic surface of the lipid membrane. Other CNS myelin proteins are (1) 2',3'-cyclicnucleotide 3'-phosphodiesterase, (2) myelin-associated glycoprotein, (3) oligodendrocyte-specific protein, and (4) myelin oligodendrocyte glycoprotein.

Myelin-associated glycoprotein is the major mediator of the axonal-glial contacts that are essential for the initiation of myelination. It also serves as scaffolding, keeping the oligodendroglial cell process at a regular distance apart while the major structural proteins are being formed and plays a role in axonal guidance, because it is the component of myelin that represses growth of neurites (axons and dendrites). However, myelin-associated glycoprotein is ultimately excluded as a major structural component of the mature, compact myelin sheath.

Various mouse models have been described that are characterized by deficiencies in specific myelin proteins.[16] Among humans, two disorders are linked to a failure of synthesis of a particular CNS myelin protein: PLP in the case of PMD and MBP in the 18q– syndrome.

Pelizaeus-Merzbacher disease

Pelizaeus in 1885[17] and Merzbacher in 1910[18] reported one family in which several members had nystagmus, spastic quadriparesis, ataxia, and cognitive impairment. Both recognized that the disorder was X-linked, although two of the affected were female. Postmortem study of one patient revealed a severe lack of myelin staining with occasional small

areas of preserved myelin especially surrounding blood vessels, creating a patchy or tigroid appearance. A connatal form of this condition was subsequently recognized by Seitelberger.[19] These patients present in the neonatal period with nystagmus, pharyngeal weakness and stridor, hypotonia, severe spasticity, and seizures. There is a complete absence of myelin, and death occurs in childhood. The clinical spectrum of this rare disease now includes a milder form known as *SPG2*, which presents as a spastic paraplegia with or without nystagmus and ataxia.[20]

Characteristics of the classic variant are a history of reduced intrauterine movements, nystagmus that is often rotatory and may decrease with age, dysarthric or absent speech, diffuse muscle weakness and atrophy, head titubation, pyramidal and extrapyramidal signs, choreoathetosis, and mental deficiency. Many cannot sit upright and never learn to walk. Kyphoscoliosis and pes cavus develop, and the head size is small. Death occurs in the second to forth decades.

The brain stem auditory–evoked potentials show prolonged latencies in waves II–V.[21] The visual-evoked responses are also abnormal.[22] Electromyography and nerve conduction studies are normal. On MRI, the corpus callosum is thin and high-signal intensity is present in T_2-weighted images throughout the cerebral white matter, including the arcuate fibers, brain stem, and cerebellar peduncles. The cerebellum and brain stem in the connatal form are small.[23]

Neuropathologic studies disclose atrophy with poor demarcation between the gray and white matter, hypomyelination, reduced numbers of oligodendroglial cells, and a dense fibrillary astrocytosis. The axonal processes are tightly packed and there are microislands of a few irregular myelin sheaths. Electron microscopic images disclose abnormal layering and compaction of myelin.[24]

In 1964, Zeman et al. hypothesized a defect in PLP or other myelin proteins as the cause of PMD.[25] This was confirmed by Koeppen et al. in 1987 who showed an absence of PLP by immunostaining brain from a case of PMD.[26] Further support for PLP deficiency is the finding that the *PLP* gene localized to the X chromosome (Xq22).[27,28]

PLP accounts for one-half of the protein mass of CNS myelin but less than 1% of peripheral myelin protein. It is an extremely hydrophilic membrane protein comprising 276 amino acid residues within four transmembrane-spanning domains and highly charged extra cytosolic loops. As mentioned, an alternatively spliced isoform, DM20 lacks 35 amino acid residues from a portion of the second intracellular membrane loop. DM20 is expressed in newborn oligodendrocyte progenitor cells,[29] whereas PLP has adhesive properties and is responsible for compaction of myelin and maintenance of axonal integrity.[30] In the absence of PLP, the double-spaced intraperiod dense line is missing, and *N*-acetylaspartic acid is reduced owing to progressive axonal loss.[31] *Jimpy* mice that are genetically deficient in PLP develop widespread wallerian degeneration, and in those individuals with the null mutation producing nonfunctional PLP, there is also a demyelinating peripheral neuropathy.

The most common mutation present in 50–70% of patients is a duplication of the *PLP* gene that is detectable by fluorescence in situ hybridization analysis.[32,33] The clinical phenotype tends to be severe and of the connatal or classic form.

In approximately 15–20% of cases of PMD, point mutations occur in the PLP-coding region causing, in most cases, an amino acid substitution. These cause abnormal folding of PLP (gain-of-function mutation) and prevent it from exiting the endoplasmic reticulum and integrating into the cell surface.[34] Single amino acid changes in highly conserved regions of the DM20 protein cause the most severe forms of PMD.[35] Milder forms of PMD and SPG2 result from substitutions of less conserved amino acids, truncations, and absence of PLP. The *His139Tyr* mutation in exon 3B of males with SPG2 lies outside the coding region of DM20, the alternatively spliced transcript of the *PLP* gene. Although the mutation results in a mutant PLP, its DM20 isoform is normal, hence the less severe manifestations. Curiously, this mutation was present not only in the first-described X-linked SPG family [36] but also is also found in the *rumpshaker* mouse, a less severely affected model of PMD than the *jimpy* mouse, which has a point mutation in intron 4 that disrupts splicing.[37] A small percentage of human cases have also been described with mutations in introns of the PLP gene.[38]

Female heterozygotes with the less severe mutations are more likely to be clinically affected than those with a more severe mutation. This is because those oligodendrocytes expressing the severe mutation undergo cell death and are eliminated during myelination, whereas, with the less severe mutation, the abnormal oligodendrocytes are more apt to remain and produce defective myelin. This probably accounts for the inclusion of affected females in Merzbacher's 1910 report on the original family of Pelizaeus.[39]

The pattern of X-chromosome inactivation could also influence the phenotypic expression in carriers. Carriers of a PLP duplication have been shown to preferentially inactivate the X-chromosome bearing the duplication. In contrast, the pattern of X inactivation in point mutation carriers is random.[40]

18q– Syndrome

First described by de Grouchy et al. in 1964,[41] the 18q– syndrome is one of the most common chromosomal deletion syndromes. Clinical manifestations include short stature, microcephaly, midface hypoplasia, malformed ears, stenotic ear canals, flat philtrum, carp-shaped mouth, prognathism, tapered fingers, proximal thumbs, prominent fingerprint whirls, hypotonia, hearing loss, nystagmus, and mental retardation.[42,43] Nearly all patients also show delayed or incomplete myelination by MR imaging.[43–45] Autopsy studies have confirmed the presence of reduced cerebral white matter.[46,47]

The deletion most often involves the distal portion of the long arm of chromosome 18 from q21 to qter. The gene for *MBP* maps in this region at 18q22.3. All of the patients with abnormal white matter on their MRIs have been found to be missing one copy of the *MBP* gene.[43] One patient with a large interstitial deletion in the distal portion of 18q that did not include the *MBP* locus had a normal brain MRI. Also, patients with 18q23 deletions do not manifest white-matter abnormalities.[48] These exceptions suggest that the critical deleted region specific for abnormal myelination includes the site of the *MBP* gene. Interestingly, mice that are heterozygous for the *shiverer* mutation, which involves the *MBP* gene, are phenotypically normal,[49] whereas CNS myelination is defective in the s*hiverer* mouse with homozygous loss of the *MBP* gene.[50] Kline et al[51] have noted that the degree to which myelination is affected appears to correlate with the severity of other features of the 18q– syndrome. Therefore, they conclude that other deleted genes more proximal to the MBP locus may also contribute to the defect in myelination in these patients.

Delayed Myelination

Delay in myelination is a common finding in many of the inherited metabolic diseases. In these cases, the supply of certain endogenous substances that are needed for myelin synthesis is inadequate or metabolites that accumulate are toxic to oligodendroglia.

MRI at the mild end of the spectrum reveals poor gray-white differentiation and an immature pattern of myelination. In more severe cases, there is a diffuse symmetric white-matter signal abnormality involving both the deep and subcortical regions and also an alteration in cerebellar white matter. There have been few neuropathologic studies to correlate these images with the histology of white matter. In certain of these disorders, the brain MRI findings are reversible so that the leukodystrophic changes are probably not demyelinating.

Delay in myelination occurs in phenylketonuria and other aminoacidopathies. In one study of patients with phenylketonuria, improvement was noted in the brain scans of 5 of 21 patients on dietary therapy and 4 of 15 patients who made no dietary change. There was a significant association between the MRI findings and the blood phenylalanine concentration.[52]

A leukodystrophy has been found as well in many of the disorders of organic acid metabolism. An example is maple syrup urine disease.[53] Acquired leukodystrophy is also observed in certain of the inherited fatty acid disorders. Two examples are 2-methyl-3-hydroxybutyryl-coenzyme A dehydrogenase deficiency[54] and multiple acylcoenzyme A dehydrogenase deficiency.[55] The brain MRI of one 2-year-old boy with the latter condition improved on treatment with a course of ketones.[55]

Mitochondrial disorders represent yet another class of metabolic conditions causing delayed myelination.[56,57] These disturbances in respiratory chain energy production have an estimated incidence of 1 in 10,000 live births. Lactate may be increased in the serum and CSF, and a substantial lactate peak is frequently found in MR spectroscopy of the brain white matter.

Complex I defects causing cytochrome c oxidase deficiency are the most common. Although the usual presentation is Leigh syndrome, a diffuse white-matter abnormality may occur instead, producing cyst-like changes.[58,59] Among the more than 35 complex I subunits encoded by nuclear genes,

mutations in the *SURF1* gene[60] and the *NDUFV1* gene[61] of complex I have been implicated.

Similar MRI changes have been described in a 10-month-old boy with complex II (succinate dehydrogenase) deficiency. His neurologic impairment improved with riboflavin administration.[62]

This author has seen two teenage brothers with complex III deficiency and MRI evidence of leukodystrophy. Examination of the brain of one brother who died at age 21 years failed to demonstrate any change in the central white matter. Leukodystrophy has also been reported in cases of complex IV[56] and of pyruvate dehydrogenase complex deficiency.[56]

Abnormal brain white-matter signals are also a feature of defects in mitochondrial DNA. Kearns-Sayre syndrome; mitochondrial encephalomyopathy, lactic acidosis, and stroke-like episodes; Leber's hereditary optic neuropathy; progressive external ophthalmoplegia; and mitochondrial neurogastrointestinal encephalomyopathy syndrome fall into this category. The white-matter lesions in mitochondrial encephalomyopathy, lactic acidosis, and stroke-like episodes tend to be posterior and overlap with cortex. They do not follow a vascular distribution and over time may partially resolve. The mitochondrial neurogastrointestinal encephalomyopathy syndrome has been mapped to chromosome 22q13.32-qter, and mutations described in the gene for thymidine phosphorylase are located in this chromosomal region.[63]

An inborn error of polyol metabolism was suspected in the case of a 14-year-old boy with seizures, bilateral optic atrophy, nystagmus, dysarthria, cerebellar ataxia, pyramidal tract signs, and polyneuropathy. His MRI revealed extensive involvement of the cerebral white matter, including the arcuate fibers, relative sparing of the periventricular white matter, and complete sparing of the corpus callosum and internal capsule. His urine, plasma, and CSF contained marked elevations of arabitol and ribitol.[64]

Leukodystrophies due to Primary Demyelination

Inherited leukodystrophies with myelin destruction occurring as the primary event include two lysosomal storage diseases (i.e., GLD and MLD) and a peroxisomal disorder (i.e., ALD). Each is clinically heterogeneous. Early recognition is important, because these conditions can be ameliorated by bone marrow transplantation.

Globoid Cell Leukodystrophy

The classic form of this autosomal recessive disease, known as *Krabbe's disease*, is characterized by marked irritability and tonic spasms beginning at 3–6 months of age. Generalized rigidity and opisthotonic posturing also occur early and are soon followed by psychomotor regression and feeding difficulties. The child develops a flaccid polyneuropathy and optic atrophy and becomes microcephalic, blind, and cachectic, usually before the age of 15–18 months. Late infantile, juvenile, and adult variants are also encountered. In some of these later onset forms of GLD, the intellect is preserved, peripheral nerves are not involved, and disease progression may be very slow.

Laboratory testing reveals a marked elevation of total protein in the CSF, decrease in nerve conduction velocities, and central white matter demyelination initially in the periventricular regions of the posterior part of the cerebral hemispheres. The molecular basis of the disease is a deficiency in galactocerebroside β-galactosidase, the enzyme that normally hydrolyzes galactocerebroside to ceramide and galactose. The gene for this protein is located on chromosome 14q21-q31. Approximately one-half of all disease-causing alleles contain a large deletion at the 3' end of the gene in association with a $C^{502} \rightarrow T$ polymorphism. Pathologic examination discloses widespread demyelination, reactive astrocytosis, marked reduction in the number of oligodendrocytes, and sparing of the subcortical arcuate fibers and gray matter. Scattered throughout the demyelinated areas are large periodic acid-Schiff–positive multinucleated globoid cells containing numerous inclusions by electron microscopy.[65]

Metachromatic Leukodystrophy

MLD, the late infantile form of this autosomal recessive sphingolipidosis, is the most common variant. It begins insidiously in the second year with difficulty in walking, often after achieving independent ambulation. Strabismus, flaccid paraparesis, pyramidal signs, and a polyneuropathy are then noted. The child then regresses, becomes spastic, loses coordination, and develops dysarthria. Eventually, the child is bed bound in a rigid decerebrate or decorticate posture and dies before the end of the first decade.

Juvenile-and adult-onset forms of MLD are also encountered. The young adult with MLD may, in the beginning, show changes in personality, memory difficulties, and other intellectual deficits and later develops gait imbalance and pyramidal tract findings.

The cause of MLD is an accumulation of sulfatides that may be found to be increased in peripheral nerves as metachromatic granules. The diagnosis is most readily made by demonstration of a marked increase in urine sulfatide and by deficiency of leukocyte arylsulfatase A (sulfatidase) activity. In very rare instances, the disease is due not to a deficiency of arylsulfatase A but to a defect in the sphingolipid activator protein, saposin B, that participates with arylsulfatase A in the degradation of sulfatide. Another variant—mucosulfatidosis—is distinguished clinically by the presence of ichthyosis and features suggestive of a mucopolysaccharidosis as well as a leukodystrophy. In this disease, sulfatide and mucopolysaccharides accumulate, and there are deficiencies of multiple sulfatases. Mucosulfatidosis results from the failure of a post-transitional modification of all sulfatases in which the thiol group of a cysteine is oxidized.

The gene for arylsulfatase A is on chromosome 22 and for saposin B is on chromosome 10. A pseudodeficiency allele exists for arylsulfatase A, which is present in 7–15% of the population and can complicate the diagnosis of MLD and its carrier state.[66]

Adrenoleukodystrophy

Abnormalities of central myelin are a feature of many of the peroxisomal diseases. X-linked ALD is the most common.[67] ALD includes a wide range of phenotypes of which the childhood cerebral form is the most common. The affected boy is usually 4–8 years old when symptoms first appear. He becomes withdrawn, less verbal, and has difficulty with auditory and visual discrimination. He develops spastic paresis, incontinence, and feeding difficulty, often with rapid progression to a vegetative state.

The demyelination often first appears in the parieto-occipital regions on the MRI. Some patients may first present with Addison's disease, and, in others, adrenal insufficiency may be the only clinical manifestation. A juvenile and an adult cerebral form are also encountered, and, in 25% of cases, the disease involves mainly the spinal cord. This latter form, known as *adrenomyeloneuropathy*, has a mean age of onset of 27 years and progresses much more slowly than ALD.

The demyelination progresses in a caudorostral direction with the earliest MRI lesions in the occipital and posterior parietal white matter. The areas of demyelination are characterized by a striking perivascular inflammatory reaction consisting primarily of T-lymphocytes and macrophages. The cells of the adrenal cortex, brain macrophages, and Schwann's cells contain lamellar cytoplasmic inclusions that are composed of very-long-chain fatty acids. The diagnosis can be made in all variants by demonstrating elevations in plasma very-long-chain fatty acids.

The *ALD* gene codes for a peroxisomal membrane protein that is lacking in 70% of ALD patients. Dietary treatment restricting very-long-chain fatty acids and the use of Lorenzo's Oil have not significantly changed the natural history of the disease.[68] Substantial benefit has been obtained by bone marrow transplantation in presymptomatic and early symptomatic cases.[69]

Alexander's Disease

This primarily sporadic leukodystrophy was first reported by Alexander in 1949 in a 16-month-old boy with megalencephaly, hydrocephalus, and psychomotor retardation.[70] Infantile-, juvenile-, and adult-onset variants are recognized.[71] The infantile form is the most common.[72] It presents between birth and age 2 years with rapid head enlargement, frontal bossing, and loss of developmental milestones. Hydrocephalus and seizures sometimes occur. The child becomes quadriparetic and spastic, requires tube feeding, and may survive for a few years.

Children with the juvenile form develop symptoms between ages 4 years and adolescence.[71–74] They have signs of brain stem involvement, including speech and swallowing difficulties and also progressive spasticity, especially in the lower extremities. Cognitive decline may occur late in the course of the illness. Megalencephaly is not usually present. Their age of death is variable. The adult form is the least common. Progression is slow with dementia developing in some patients. Some cases may resemble multiple sclerosis.

On MRI, there is bilateral frontal white-matter involvement and abnormalities of the basal ganglia, especially the caudate and sometimes the thalami. Periventricular structures may appear swollen and, cystic changes can be seen.[73,75] Single-photon emission computed tomography[75] and positron emission tomography[74] scanning reveal diminished cerebral metabolism in the frontal white matter. The EEG often shows slow and sharp activity, especially over the anterior regions.[72] Brain stem–evoked potential studies show loss of the components following wave I with an increase in the I-V interval.[72] Visual-evoked potentials are usually normal.[72,76] The spinal component of the somatosensory-evoked potentials is abnormal.[76]

Pathologically, there is widespread myelin deficiency and, frequently, cystic degeneration and cavitation. The arcuate fibers may be spared, and there is relative sparing of the occipital lobes and cerebellum. Those with the infantile form may not myelinate properly, whereas, in older children, the white matter degenerates. Adult cases may have only patchy zones of myelin pallor or cavitation.

Microscopically, large numbers of Rosenthal fibers are present in all regions of the CNS but are especially concentrated in the subependymal, subpial, and perivascular regions; in the basal ganglia and thalamus; and in the brain stem. These are eosinophilic, refractile, often rod-shaped bodies found in astrocytic processes. Electron microscopic studies of these bodies disclose intracellular osmiophilic deposits.[77] Their primary constituents are *GFAP*, and the stress proteins αB-crystallin and heat shock protein 27.[78] An elevation in αB-crystallin and heat shock protein 27 is also found in CSF.[79]

A few familial cases have been reported (reviewed in reference 80), but the majority is sporadic. Males and females are affected in equal numbers. The idea that *GFAP* might be a candidate gene was first suggested by Becker and Teixeira,[81] but it was not examined until large numbers of Rosenthal fibers were found in transgenic mice carrying the human *GFAP* gene.[82] Heterozygous missense mutations in *GFAP* have now been found in 26 of 28 cases, almost all involving a change from an arginine to another neutral amino acid.[83,84] This produces a dominant gain-of-function that Messing et al.[80] believe could result in abnormal association of the mutant protein with other cellular constituents to form aggregates or, alternatively, interruption in the formation of normal filament networks causing a reactive increase in the synthesis and production of *GFAP*. The rare sibships affected could be owing to a mutation in a parental germinal stem cell resulting in gonadal mosaicism, but the mutation event in most cases probably occurs during embryogenesis. Amplification of exons 1, 4, and 8 will detect 93% of patients with *GFAP* mutations and is recommended for prenatal diagnosis of all further pregnancies in the families of patients with Alexander's disease.[84] Bone marrow transplantation in one patient failed to arrest the neurologic deterioration.[85]

Leukoencephalopathy with Vanishing White Matter

This fascinating, yet poorly understood, disease entity[86] is also known as *myelinopathia centralis diffusa*[87] and *childhood ataxia with diffuse central hypomyelination*.[88] It usually begins in early childhood, but severe infantile onset[89] and milder- and later-onset cases have also been described.[90] Development is initially normal or mildly delayed. The onset may be rapid, precipitated by fever, infection, or minor head trauma. The principal findings are cerebellar ataxia and spasticity with relative preservation of mental abilities. Seizures and optic atrophy may also occur.

MRI signal intensity of the brain white matter resembles that of CSF. The white matter appears swollen and the ventricles are enlarged. The gray matter structures appear normal, but cerebellar atrophy occurs. MR spectroscopy discloses an absence of nearly all metabolites in the lesions except for glucose and lactate.

On histopathologic examination, widespread rarefaction and cystic degeneration of white matter are observed. Some areas contain a meshwork of residual tissue strands. Better-preserved regions show signs of astrogliosis and proliferation of macrophages. The subcortical arcuate fibers, internal capsule, corpus callosum, anterior commissure, and cerebellar white matter are relatively preserved.

There is axonal loss, and the remaining myelin sheaths are thin. Although myelin lipid and protein are reduced, there is an increase in the number of oligodendroglia without mitotic activity.[90,91]

Brück et al.[87] have demonstrated that, in childhood ataxia with diffuse central hypomyelination, mature oligodendrocytes undergo apoptosis followed by recruitment of progenitor cells expressing PLP messenger RNA. They conclude that the death of mature oligodendrocytes is the critical event in this disease and speculate that some cytotoxic mediator, such as tumor necrosis factor-α or lymphotoxin or overexpression of the proto-oncogene p53, could trigger the oligodendrocyte apoptosis.

The gene for this presumably autosomal recessive condition has been mapped to chromosome 3q27.[92] Analysis of CSF amino acids has revealed a consistent elevation in glycine, but the glycine cleavage system was found to be normal.[93]

Vacuolating Megalencephalic Leukoencephalopathy

Progressive megalencephaly noted during the first year and a mild clinical course distinguish vacuolating megalencephalic leukoencephalopathy from the entity of vanishing white matter described earlier. It was first reported by Harbord et al[94] and has been described in many patients from Turkey[95] and India[96] but is being recognized worldwide.[97–99] It is characterized by a mild clinical course that includes ataxia, spastic paraparesis, and, occasionally, seizures. There is accelerated head growth during the first year and mild to moderate gross motor delay. Mental functioning is either normal or only mildly impaired with some decline occurring in the second decade.

The EEG findings reveal multifocal epileptiform discharges.[94,100,101] The MRI is remarkable for diffuse involvement of the supratentorial white matter with frontotemporal cysts and relative sparing of the occipital lobe white matter. The gray matter is preserved, but the gyri appear swollen and flattened. The signal intensity within the cysts resembles that of CSF in all sequences. There is variable involvement of the subcortical arcuate fibers, frequent involvement of the external capsules, and sparing of the internal capsules. Brain stem and cerebellar white matter are less involved.

In contrast to Canavan's disease, the *N*-acetylas-partate to creatinine ratio on MR spectroscopy is normal or slightly reduced.[97] Histologic studies indicate a spongiform leukoencephalopathy with a vacuolar change involving the outermost myelin lamellae.[101]

The appearance of this disorder in siblings and consanguinity among the parents in several families has suggested an autosomal mode of inheritance. No biochemical changes have been found to link this condition with other forms of inherited leukodystrophy. This disorder has been mapped to chromosome 22qtel.[102]

Secondary Demyelination

Congenital Muscular Dystrophy

A subset of patients with congenital muscular dystrophy is deficient in the laminin-α2 (LAMA2) chain of merosin by muscle immunocytochemistry.[103] These patients have severe muscle weakness and contractures, and only 25% achieve ambulation. Onset is at birth or in the first 6 months, but later-onset milder cases and even asymptomatic cases have been detected. Most are not walking by 2 years of age. In one-half of the patients, the weakness is slowly progressive, and, in others, it is static or improving. Between 8–20% have seizures. In more than 80% of cases, creatine kinase levels are elevated above 1,000 U/liter but vary and can decrease with age. Abnormalities in the electrocardiogram or echocardiogram, or both, have also been reported.

White-matter hypodensity is evident on cerebral MRI in approximately 90% of patients, as shown by an abnormally high T_2 signal in the periventricular and subcortical white matter.[104–106] However, in only 7–12% is there clinical evidence of mental retardation. A neuronal migration defect is present in 5%, and, in 6%, the MRI is normal.[103]

The *LAMA2* gene is located on chromosome 6q22.[107] Mutations in *LAMA2* have been identified in one-fourth of cases of LAMA2 deficiency, confirming that the deficiency is primary rather than secondary.[108] *LAMA2* mutations have been detected in cases in which the brain MRI was normal and, in only one of nine cases, reported to have a neuronal migration defect on MRI.[103] Secondary LAMA2 deficiency occurs in patients with Fukuyama congenital muscular dystrophy[109] and muscle-eye-brain disease.[110]

Sjögren-Larsson Syndrome

Sjögren-Larsson syndrome is an autosomal recessive disorder resulting from mutations in the gene for the microsomal enzyme fatty aldehyde dehydrogenase (FALDH). First described in 1957 by Sjögren and Larsson in a consanguineous cohort from the county of Vasterbotten in northern Sweden,[111] the worldwide prevalence of this panethnic disorder is probably less than 0.4 per 100,000.

Many of the patients are born preterm. Ichthyosis is present at birth. It is generalized and brownish-yellow in color and is associated with a severe pruritus. Within the first or second year, developmental delay and spasticity appear. The spasticity is more severe in the lower extremities and leads to contractures and eventually to wheelchair dependency. Cognition is impaired in most patients. Pseudobulbar dysarthria and delayed speech are common, and seizures occur in approximately 40%. Ophthalmologic abnormalities include photophobia, macular dystrophy, and decreased visual acuity. After several years, glistening white dots surround the macular region of the retina. Peripheral nerve function is normal.[112]

FALDH catalyzes the oxidation of medium- and long-chain fatty aldehydes to the corresponding carboxylic acids. As a consequence of the deficiency in FALDH first reported by Rizzo et al. in 1989,[113] free fatty acids are elevated in plasma and urinary concentrations of leukotriene B4, and 20-OH-leukotriene B4 is increased as well.[112] The accumulation of fatty alcohols or aldehyde-modified macromolecules is believed to disrupt the integrity of multilamellar membranes in skin and myelin.

The EEG shows symmetrical slow background activity without epileptiform patterns. Cerebral MRI studies reveal multifocal areas of delayed myelination, hyperintense signal abnormality in the periventricular zone, and mild ventricular enlargement in the oldest patients.[114,115] A sharp lipid peak is present on MR spectroscopy, which differs from that found in other white-matter diseases.[115] It is believed to arise from the accumulation of long-chain fatty alcohols or fatty aldehydes.

The few neuropathologic investigations performed have found a reduction in myelinated nerve fibers in cerebral and cerebellar white matter, loss of neurons in the cortex and basal ganglia, and deposition of pigments. In addition, in one patient who died at 8 years of age, Yamaguchi and Handa[116] found periodic acid-Schiff–positive lipoid substances in the subpial, subependymal, and perivascular glial layers and cerebral and cerebellar white matter, perivascular macrophages containing lipofuscin-like pigments, and spheroid bodies in the neuropil of several brain stem nuclei.

More than 40 mutations have been described in the *FALDH* gene that is localized to chromosome 17p11.2.[112,117] Nearly all are private mutations specific to only one or a small number of families. Two of the more common mutations—a 1297-1298 GA deletion and a 943 C→T base substitution—were present in a European population with frequencies of 17.2% and 8.6%, respectively.[118]

Treatment has been attempted with a low-fat diet supplemented with medium-chain fatty acids but was not successful.[119] Beneficial effects have recently been described using the leukotriene B4 synthesis inhibitor zileuton.[120]

Cockayne Syndrome

Central and peripheral nerve demyelinations occur in this rare autosomal recessive multisystem degenerative disease. CS was first reported by Cockayne in 1936 and 1946 in two brothers with dwarfism, deafness, retinal degeneration, and slowly progressive psychomotor retardation.[121,122] Symptoms in the classic type I form begin at the end of the first year or the beginning of the second year.[123] An earlier-onset type II variant and a later-onset form also exist.

There is growth failure that progresses to cachectic dwarfism. The child becomes microcephalic and assumes an unusual facial appearance with sunken orbits, a relatively large beak-like nose, and narrow mouth and chin. The hair is sparse and the skin is photosensitive and heals with scarring and pigmentary changes. Ophthalmic signs[124] include photophobia, poor pupillary dilatation, decreased lacrimation, cataracts, retinal pigmentary degeneration, optic atrophy, strabismus, and nystagmus. Oral manifestations include the absence of some permanent teeth, dental caries, a narrow palate, atrophy of the alveolar processes, and condylar hypoplasia. Neurologic findings consist of sensorineural hearing loss, dysarthria, tremor, ataxia, mental retardation, and a peripheral sensorimotor neuropathy. Skeletal anomalies and cryptorchidism are also encountered. Brain imaging studies reveal cerebral atrophy, increased ventricular size, and calcification of the basal ganglia. MRI T_2-weighted sequences demonstrate high-signal lesions in the periventricular and subcortical white matter.

Histopathologic changes in the cerebrum include patchy demyelination of the subcortical white matter and microscopic perivascular calcifications throughout the CNS. Within the peripheral nervous system there is segmental demyelination with decrease in the density of the small myelinated fibers. Remyelination is evident with onion bulb formation. Macrophages and Schwann's cells contain granular osmophilic material.

The molecular defect in CS involves a subpathway of nucleotide excision repair known as *transcription-coupled repair*. Normally, damage in the transcribed strand of transcriptionally active genes is repaired at a faster rate than in the coding nontranscribed strand. However, CS cells do not show this preferential strand-specific repair of transcriptionally active genes. Instead, the damage in active genes of CS cells is repaired at the same relatively slow rate as bulk DNA. This accounts for the fact that, after ultraviolet irradiation, RNA and DNA synthesis recovers rapidly in normal cells but not in CS cells.[125,126]

This delay in recovery of RNA and DNA synthesis has been used to demonstrate the presence of two complementation groups in CS, designated *CSA* and *CSB*. The ultraviolet sensitivity is corrected when cells from CS patients of different complementation groups are fused to form a heterodikaryon but not if the heterodikaryon is formed by two cell lines exclusively of the CSA group or the CSB group. The *CSA* gene maps to chromosome 5 and encodes a tryptophan aspartate (WD)–repeat protein.[127] The CSB protein is encoded by a gene designated *ERCC6* that is located on chromosome 10q11.[128] The CSA and CSB proteins interact with each other and with the transcription factor TFIIH. Eighty percent of CS patients have mutations in the *ERCC6* gene.[128] One 14-year-old patient has been described with low CSF levels of 5-hydroxyindole acetic acid. Although oral supplementation did not correct his CSF level of 5-hydroxyindole acetic acid, no further clinical deterioration was observed over a 2-year period.[129]

Cerebrotendinous Xanthomatosis

Cerebrotendinous xanthomatosis should always be considered in the differential diagnosis of a leukodystrophy, as it is a treatable condition. Symptoms appear in childhood or during the second decade. There may be difficulty in school owing to slowly progressive mental retardation. Behavioral problems and psychiatric symptoms also occur. Other manifestations include cataracts, tendon and tuberous xanthomata (especially of the Achilles tendon), diarrhea, osteoporosis, and bone fractures. Not all patients will manifest cataracts or Achilles tendon xanthomata. Neurologic findings include cerebellar and pyramidal tract signs, peripheral neuropathy, and seizures.[130–132] A variant with parkinsonism has also been described.[130]

Imaging studies disclose diffuse brain and spinal cord atrophy and brain white-matter hypodensity. The cerebellar white matter is especially involved, and there is hyperintensity of the dentate nuclei bilaterally on the fluid-attenuated inversion recovery sequence.[133] A mainly spinal cord syndrome can occur with white-matter abnormalities in the lateral and dorsal columns of the spinal cord.[134] MR spectroscopy has shown significant decreases in N-acetylaspartate and increases in lactate MR signals. These have been interpreted as indicative of widespread axonal damage and diffuse brain mitochondrial dysfunction.[133]

Menkes et al.[135] discovered that the brain of patients with cerebrotendinous xanthomatosis contained increased amounts of cholestanol. This 5-α-dihydro-derivative of cholesterol is normally present in minute amounts but is increased 10- to 100-fold in cerebrotendinous xanthomatosis. Its presence in plasma, urine, and CSF can be used to aid in the diagnosis.

Cholestanol accumulation is due to a block in bile acid synthesis caused by mutations in the *sterol 27-hydroxylase* gene located on human chromosome 2. At least 37 different mutations have been found, but because of phenotypic heterogeneity within families and among patients with the same mutation, no clearcut genotype-phenotype correlations have been found.[132]

The defective bile acid synthesis results in an absence of chenodeoxycholic acid in the bile and excretion of bile alcohols (bile acid precursors) in the bile and urine. Because of the absence of the end product, there is upregulation of endogenous bile acid synthesis. Long-term oral therapy with chenodeoxycholic acid (750 mg/day) has been shown to suppress the abnormal bile acid synthesis, correct the biochemical abnormalities, and reverse the progression of cerebrotendinous xanthomatosis.[136] Treatment is most effective in presymptomatic individuals, hence the importance of early detection and beginning treatment before neurologic symptoms develop.[137,138] Inhibitors of 3-hydroxy-3-methylglutaryl (HMG) coenzyme A reductase will also reduce serum cholesterol levels but need to be used with caution, because they can exacerbate the mitochondrial impairment.[137,139]

Cerebral Autosomal Dominant Arteriopathy with Subcortical Infarcts and Leukoencephalopathy

CADASIL is an autosomal dominant arteriopathy, which, in middle life, is distinguished by a subcortical dementia with diffuse leukoencephalopathy.[140] However, symptoms and MRI findings of patchy white-matter involvement may be noticed from childhood. It presents as migraine with or without aura. By the third or fourth decades, the white-matter lesions have coalesced. There are well-defined lesions of the basal ganglia, and patients may also manifest with strokes and psychosis. Patients may live into their 60s.

The major pathology is in small- and middle-sized arteries. The smooth muscle cells of the media are replaced with deposits of basophilic granular material that is electron dense (granular osmophilic bodies).[141] At least 26 separate mutations have been described in the defective gene, *Notch3,* which is coded on chromosome 19p13.[142,143] Most are clustered in exons 3 and 4. Mildly elevated protein levels are found in the CSF, but oligoclonal bands are absent. Acetazolamide has been helpful in reducing migraine attacks.[144] Other aspects of CADASIL are discussed in Chapter 10.

Glycogen Storage Disease Type IV

Glycogen storage disease type IV is an autosomal recessive disorder resulting from the deficient activity of the branching enzyme 1,4-glucan 6-glucosyltransferase mapped to chromosome 3. It usually presents in infancy with severe liver disease, causing cirrhosis, portal hypertension, and early death. Myopathy may be the presenting feature, and cardiomyopathy has been reported in some individuals.[145] A late-onset variant referred to as *adult polyglucosan storage disease* consists of progressive weakness and spasticity of the legs that may progress to quadriparesis, urinary incontinence, and a peripheral neuropathy.[146] Cognitive impairments[147] may be present, and a leukodystrophy[148] has been noted in many patients. Several mutations (Tyr329Ser) in the gene encoding the branching enzyme have been reported in patients with adult polyglucosan storage disease,[149] including a Tyr329Ser alteration in a series of Ashkenazi Jewish patients.[150]

Other Diseases with Secondary Demyelination

Other rare forms of secondary demyelinating diseases with identifiable molecular abnormalities have been described. One such disorder is *proximal myotonic myopathy*, an autosomal dominantly inherited disease characterized by myotonia, proximal muscle weakness, and cataracts. Mental changes include hypersomnia, parkinsonian features, stroke-like episodes, and seizures.[151] It is due to a CCTG repeat expansion (mean approximately 5,000 repeats) in intron 1 of the zinc finger protein 9.[152]

A mutation in the *SOX10* gene that eliminates a stop codon and results in a protein with an extended tail has been shown to produce a disease of central and peripheral myelin resembling PMD and Charcot-Marie-Tooth disease.[153] *SOX10* is a myelin-specific transcription factor that is preferentially expressed in the late embryonic glial cell lineage and in mature myelin-forming cells of the CNS and PNS. It also modulates other myelin-related transcription factors and is therefore important for both CNS and PNS myelin development and maintenance.

Leukodystrophies of Unknown Etiology

More than one-third of all leukodystrophies do not have a known etiology.[154] Attempts are being made to group familial cases with distinctive phenotypic characteristics so that genome-wide linkage analyses can be performed and causative genes identified. The following disorders are distinctive enough to suggest separate categories of leukodystrophy, but their exact etiology remains unknown.

Leukodystrophy with Ovarian Dysgenesis

Mild mental deficiency, frontal cortical atrophy, and ovarian failure have been described in four women with diffuse white-matter abnormalities with a frontal predominance. MR spectroscopy showed a reduction of choline-containing compounds in the affected white matter of all patients.[155]

Aicardi-Goutières Syndrome

Aicardi-Goutières syndrome, an autosomal recessive leukoencephalopathy, is associated with developmental arrest, intracerebral calcifications, and chronic CSF lymphocytosis.[156,157] A very early encephalopathy may be noted in the first month, or the onset may be delayed until 6–10 months with loss of acquired skills. These infants develop secondary microcephaly, spasticity, truncal hypotonia, and dystonic posturing. They are severely developmentally delayed, have no purposeful speech, and do not ambulate. Generalized seizures have occurred in 30% of patients.[158] Serial computed tomography scans demonstrate progressive periventricular, basal ganglia and subcortical calcifications, cerebral atrophy, and loss of white matter. Some of the calcific deposits are associated with infarcted areas or surround small vessels.[158] Some patients have developed swelling and acrocyanosis of the toes with peeling of the skin without coolness of the extremities. There is a persistent synthesis of CSF interferon alpha, but toxoplasmosis, rubella, cytomegalovirus, and herpes simplex virus studies are negative, and no infectious cause has been found. Linkage analysis in a study of 23 children from 13 families has suggested locus heterogeneity with one potential site on chromosome 3p21.[159]

Hereditary Leukoencephalopathy and Palmoplantar Keratoderma

Four affected siblings have been reported with early-onset palmoplantar keratoderma followed in adulthood by a cognitive impairment and a progressive tetrapyramidal syndrome.[160] The dermatosomal cadherin gene cluster, which includes a gene *DSG1* that is mutated in palmoplantar keratoderma, is coded on chromosome 18q12.1.[161] This raises the question of whether the affected siblings in this family may have had an interstitial deletion in the long arm of chromosome 18 involving both the *DSG1* gene at 18q12.1 and the *MBP* gene at 18q22.3. Indeed, another patient has been reported with the combination of a dermatologic condition (lichen sclerosis et atrophicus) and abnormal myelination who did have a deletion on the long arm of chromosome 18.[162] Leukodystrophy associated with a skin disorder, in this case oculocutaneous albinism, has been reported in a child with an 11q14 deletion.[163]

Numerous additional reports of individual families or small geographic isolates with unique forms of leukoencephalopathy can be found in the literature.[164]

References

1. Bielschowski M, Henneberg R. Über familiare diffuse sklerose (leukodystrophie cerebri progressiva hereditaria). J Psychol Neurol 1928;36:131–181.
2. Seitelberger F. Structural manifestations of leukodystrophies. Neuropediatrics 1984;15(Suppl):53–61.
3. Morell P, Wiesmann U. A correlative synopsis of the leukodystrophies. Neuropediatrics 1984;15(Suppl):62–65.
4. Menkes JH. The leukodystrophies. N Engl J Med 1990;322:54–55.
5. Lasbury N, Garg B, Edwards-Brown M, et al. Clinical correlates of white-matter abnormalities on head magnetic resonance imaging. J Child Neurol 2001;16:668–672.
6. Kristjansdottir R, Uvebrant P, Wiklund LM. Clinical characteristics of children with cerebral white matter abnormalities. Europ J Paediatr Neurol 2000;4:17–26.
7. van der Knapp MS, Valk J. Non-leukodystrophic white matter changes in inherited disorders. Intern J Neuroradiol 1995;1:56–66.
8. Filley CM, Kleinschmidt-DeMasters BK. Toxic leukoencephalopathy. N Engl J Med 2001;345:425–432.
9. Balslev T, Cortez MA, Blaser SI, Haslam RH. Recurrent seizures in metachromatic leukodystrophy. Pediatr Neurol 1997;17:150–154.
10. Filley CM. The behavioral neurology of cerebral white matter. Neurology 1998;50:1535–1540.
11. Riva D, Bova SM, Bruzzone MG. Neuropsychological testing may predict early progression of asymptomatic adrenoleukodystrophy. Neurology 2000;54:1651–1655.
12. Hüppi PS, Wardfield S, Kikinis R, et al. Quantitative magnetic resonance imaging of brain development in premature and mature newborns. Ann Neurol 1998;43:224–235.
13. Peterson BS, Ment LR. The necessity and difficulty of conducting magnetic resonance imaging studies on infant brain development. Pediatrics 2001;107:593–594.
14. Barkovich AJ, Ferriero DM, Bass N, Boyer R. Involvement of the pontomedullary corticospinal tracts: a useful finding in the diagnosis of X-linked adrenoleukodystrophy. AJNR Am J Neuroradiol 1997;18:95–100.
15. Folkerth RD. Abnormalities of developing white matter in lysosomal storage diseases. J Neuropathol Exp Neurol 1999;58:887–902.
16. Campagnoni AT, Skoff RP. The pathobiology of myelin mutants reveal novel biological functions of the MBP and PLP genes. Brain Pathol 2001;11:74–91.
17. Pelizaeus F. Uber eine eigentimiliche form spastischer Lahmung mit Zerebralerscheinungen auf hereditarer Grundlage multiple sklerose. Arch Psychiat Nervenkt 1885;16:698–710.
18. Merzbacher L. Eine eigenartige familiare Erkrankungsform (aplasia axialis extracorticalis congenita). Z Ges Neurol Psychiat 1910;3:1–138.
19. Seitelberger F. Die Pelizaeus-Merzbacher'sche Krankheit. Klinische und anatomische Untersuchungen zum Problem ihrer Stellung inter den diffusen Sklerosen. Wien Z Nhk 1954;9:128–289.
20. Saugier-Veber P, Munnich A, Bonneau D, et al. X-linked spastic paraplegia and Pelizaeus-Merzbacher disease are allelic disorders at the proteolipid protein locus. Nat Genet 1994;6:257–262.
21. Wang P-J, Young C, Liu H-M, et al. Neurophysiologic studies and MRI in Pelizaeus-Merzbacher disease: comparison of classic and connatal forms. Pediatr Neurol 1995;12:47–53.
22. Apkarian P, Koetsveld-Baart C, Barth PG. Visual evoked potential characteristics and early diagnosis of Pelizaeus-Merzbacher disease. Arch Neurol 1993;50:981–985.
23. Nezu A, Kimura S, Takeshita S, et al. An MRI and MRS study of Pelizaeus-Merzbacher disease. Pediatr Neurol 1998;18:334–337.
24. Koeppen AH. Pelizaeus-Merzbacher Disease: X-Linked Proteolipid Protein Deficiency in the Human Central Nervous System. In RE Martenson (ed), Myelin: Biology and Chemistry. Boca Raton: CRC Press, 1992;703–721.
25. Zeman W, DeMyer WE, Falls HF. Pelizaeus-Merzbacher disease: a study in nosology. J Neuropathol Exp Neurol 1964;23:334–354.
26. Koeppen AH, Ronca NA, Greenfield EA, Hans MB.

Defective biosynthesis of proteolipid protein in Pelizaeus-Merzbacher disease. Ann Neurol 1987;21:159–170.

27. Willard HF, Riordan JR. Assignment of the gene for myelin proteolipid protein to the X chromosome: Implications for X-linked myelin disorders. Science 1985;230:940–942.

28. Mattei MG, Alliel PM, Dautigny A, et al. The gene encoding for the major brain proteolipid (PLP) maps on the q-22 band of the human X-chromosome. Hum Genet 1986; 72:352–353.

29. Timsit S, Martinez S, Allinquant B, et al. Oligodendrocytes originate in a restricted zone of the embryonic ventral neural tube defined by DM-20 mRNA expression. J Neurosci 1995;15:1012–1024.

30. Boison D, Büssow H, D'Urso D, et al. Adhesive properties of proteolipid protein are responsible for the compaction of CNS myelin sheaths. J Neurosci 1995;15:5502–5513.

31. Bonavita S, Schiffman R, Moore DF, et al. Evidence for neuroaxonal injury in patients with proteolipid protein gene mutations. Neurology 2001;56:785–788.

32. Sistermans EA, de Coo RFM, De Wijs IJ, Van Oost BA. Duplication of the proteolipid protein gene is the major cause of Pelizaeus-Merzbacher disease. Neurology 1998; 50:1749–1754.

33. Woodward K, Kendall E, Vetrie D, Malcolm S. Pelizaeus-Merzbacher disease: Identification of Xq22 proteolipid protein duplications and characterization of breakpoints by interphase FISH. Am J Hum Genet 1998;63:207–217.

34. Gow A, Lazzarini RA. A cellular mechanism governing the severity of Pelizaeus-Merzbacher disease. Nat Genet 1996;13:422–428.

35. Cailloux F, Gauthier Barichard F, Mimault C, et al. Genotype-phenotype correlation in inherited brain myelination defects due to proteolipid protein gene mutations. Eur J Hum Genet 2000;8:837–845.

36. Johnston AW, McKusick VA. A sex-linked recessive form of spastic paraplegia. Am J Hum Genet 1962;14:83–94.

37. Kobayashi H, Hoffman EP, Marks HG. The rumpshaker mutation in spastic paraplegia. Nat Genet 1994;7:351–352.

38. Hobson GM, Davis AP, Stowell NL, et al. Mutations in noncoding regions of the proteolipid protein gene in Pelizaeus-Merzbacher disease. Neurology 2000;55:1089–1096.

39. Garbern J, Cambi F, Shy M, Kamholz J. The molecular pathogenesis of Pelizaeus-Merzbacher disease. Arch Neurol 1999;56:1210–1214.

40. Woodward K, Kirtland K, Dlouhy S, et al. X inactivation phenotype in carriers of Pelizaeus-Merzbacher disease: skewed in carriers of a duplication and random in carriers of point mutations. Eur J Hum Genet 2000;8:449–454.

41. de Grouchy J, Royer P, Salmon C, Lamy M. Délétion partielle de bras long du chromosome 18. Pathol Biol 1964; 12:579–582.

42. Schinzel A, Hayashi K, Schmid W. Structural aberrations of chromosome 18. II. The 18q– syndrome. Report of three cases. Humangenetik 1975;26:123–132.

43. Gay CT, Hardies LJ, Rauch RA, et al. Magnetic resonance imaging demonstrates incomplete myelination in 18q– syndrome: Evidence for myelin basic protein haploinsufficiency. Am J Med Genet 1997;74:422–431.

44. Miller G, Mowrey PN, Hopper KD, et al. Neurologic manifestations in 18q– syndrome. Am J Med Genet 1990; 37:128–132.

45. Ono J, Harada K, Yamamoto T, et al. Delayed myelination in a patient with 18q– syndrome. Pediatr Neurol 1994; 11:64–67.

46. Felding I, Kristoffersson U, Sjöström H, Norén O. Contribution to the 18q– syndrome. A patient with del (18) (q22.3qter). Clin Genet 1987;31:206–210.

47. Vogel H, Ulrich H, Horoupian DS, Wertelecki W. The brain in the 18q– syndrome. Dev Med Child Neurol 1990; 32:732–737.

48. Strathdee G, Sutherland R, Jonsson JJ, et al. Molecular characterization of patients with 18q23 deletions. Am J Hum Genet 1997;60:860–868.

49. Shine HD, Redhead C, Popko B, et al. Morphometric analysis of normal, mutant and transgenic CNS: correlation of myelin basic protein expression to myelinogenesis. J Neurochem 1992;58:342–349.

50. Chernoff GF. Shiverer: an autosomal recessive mutant mouse with myelin deficiency. J Hered 1981;72:128.

51. Kline AD, White ME, Wapner R, et al. Molecular analysis of the 18q– syndrome—and correlation with phenotype. Am J Hum Genet 1993;52:895–906.

52. Cleary MA, Walter JH, Wraith JE, et al. Magnetic resonance imaging in phenylketonuria: Reversal of cerebral white matter change. J Pediatr 1995;127:251–255.

53. Treacy E, Clow CL, Reade TR, et al. Maple syrup urine disease: interrelationships between branched-chain amino, oxo- and hydroxyacids; implications for treatment; associations with CNS dysmyelination. J Inherit Metab Dis 1992;15:121–135.

54. Poll BT, Duran M, Ruiter JPN, et al. Mild cerebral white matter disease associated with 2-methyl-3-hydroxybutyryl-CoA dehydrogenase deficiency. J Inherit Metab Dis 2001;24(Suppl 1):59.

55. Van Hove J, Jaeken J, Lagae L, et al. Multiple Acyl-CoA dehydrogenase deficiency: acquired leukodystrophy treated with D, L-3-hydroxybutyrate. J Inherit Metab Dis 2001; 24(Suppl 1):72.

56. Moroni I, Bizzi A, Bugiani M, et al. Diffuse leukodystrophy in patients with mitochondrial disorders. J Inherit Metab Dis 1999;22(Suppl 1):21.

57. deLonlay-Debeney P, von Kleist-Retzow J-C, Hertz-Pannier L, et al. Cerebral white matter disease in children may be caused by mitochondrial respiratory chain deficiency. J Pediatr 2000;136:209–214.

58. Harpey JP, Heron D, Prudent M, et al. Diffuse leukodystrophy in an infant with cytochrome-c oxidase deficiency. J Inherit Metab Dis 1998;21:748–752.

59. Topçu M, Saatci I, Apak RA, et al. Leigh syndrome in a 3-year-old boy with unusual brain MR imaging and pathologic findings. Am J Neuroradiol 2000;21:224–227.

60. Rahman S, Brown RM, Chong WK, et al. A SURF1 gene mutation presenting as isolated leukodystrophy. Ann Neurol 2001;49:797–800.

61. Schuelke M, Smeitink J, Mariman E, et al. Mutant NDUFV1 subunit of mitochondrial complex 1 causes leukodystrophy and myoclonic epilepsy. Nat Genet 1999;21:260–261.

62. Pinard JM, Marsac C, Barkaoui E, et al. Syndrome de

Leigh et leucodystrophie par deficit partiel en succinate deshydrogenase: regression sous riboflavine. Arch Pediatr 1999;6:421–426.

63. Nishino I, Spinazolla A, Hirano M. MNGIE: from nuclear DNA to mitochondrial DNA. Neuromuscul Disord 2001; 11:7–10.

64. van der Knapp MS, Wevers RA, Struys EA, et al. Leukoencephalopathy associated with a disturbance in the metabolism of polyols. Ann Neurol 1999;46:925–928.

65. Wenger DA, Suzuki K, Suzuki Y, Suzuki K. Galactosylceramide Lipidosis: Globoid Cell Leukodystrophy (Krabbe Disease). In R Scriver, AL Beaudet, WS Sly, D Valle (eds), The Metabolic & Molecular Bases of Inherited Disease. New York: McGraw-Hill, 2001;3669–3694.

66. von Figura K, Gieselmann V, Jaeken J. Metachromatic Leukodystrophy. In CR Scriver, AL Beaudet, WS Sly, D Valle (eds), The Metabolic and Molecular Bases of Inherited Disease. New York: McGraw-Hill, 2001;3695–3724.

67. Moser HW. Adrenoleukodystrophy: phenotype, genetics, pathogenesis and therapy. Brain 1997;120:1485–1508.

68. van Geel BM, Assies J, Haverkort EB, et al. Progression of abnormalities in adrenomyeloneuropathy and neurologically asymptomatic X-linked adrenoleukodystrophy despite treatment with "Lorenzo's oil." J Neurol Neurosurg Psychiatry 1999;67:290–299.

69. Shapiro E, Krivit W, Lockman L, et al. Long-term effect of bone-marrow transplantation for childhood-onset cerebral X-linked adrenoleukodystrophy. Lancet 2000;356:713–718.

70. Alexander WS. Progressive fibrinoid degeneration of fibrillary astrocytes associated with mental retardation in a hydrocephalic infant. Brain 1949;72:373–381.

71. Russo LS Jr., Aron A, Anderson PJ. Alexander's disease: a report and reappraisal. Neurology 1976;26:607–614.

72. Pridmore CL, Baraitser M, Harding B, et al. Alexander's disease: clues to diagnosis. J Child Neurol 1993;8:134–144.

73. Takanashi J-I, Sugita K, Tanabe Y, Niimi H. Adolescent case of Alexander disease: MR imaging and MR spectroscopy. Pediatr Neurol 1998;18:67–70.

74. Sawaishi Y, Hatazawa J, Ochi N, et al. Positron emission tomography in juvenile Alexander disease. J Neurol Sci 1999;165:116–120.

75. Bobele GB, Garnica A, Schaefer GB, et al. Neuroimaging findings in Alexander's disease. J Child Neurol 1990;5: 253–258.

76. DeMeirleir LJ, Taylor MJ, Logan WJ. Multimodal evoked potential studies in leukodystrophies of children. Can J Neurol Sci 1988;15:26–31.

77. Johnson AB. Alexander's Disease. In HW Moser (ed), Neurodystrophies and Neurolipidoses. Amsterdam: Elsevier 1996;701–710.

78. Johnson AD, Patel N, Chiu F-C. High molecular weight GFAP aggregates in Alexander's disease. J Neuropathol Exp Neurol 1998;57:483.

79. Ochi N, Kobayashi K, Maehara M, et al. Increment of αB-crystallin mRNA in the brain of patients with infantile type Alexander's disease. Biochem Biophys Res Commun 1991;179:1030–1035.

80. Messing A, Goldman JE, Johnson AB, Brenner M. Alexander disease: new insights from genetics. J Neuropathol Exp Neurol 2001;60:563–573.

81. Becker LE, Teixeira F. Alexander's Disease. In MD Norenberg, L Hertz, A Schousboe (eds), The Biochemical Pathology of Astrocytes. New York: Alan R Liss, Inc., 1988;179–190.

82. Messing A, Head MW, Galles K, et al. Fatal encephalopathy with astrocyte inclusions in GFAP transgenic mice. Am J Pathol 1998;152:391–398.

83. Brenner M, Johnson AB, Boespflug-Tanguy O, et al. Mutations in GFAP, encoding glial fibrillary acidic protein, are associated with Alexander disease. Nat Genet 2001;27:117–119.

84. Rodriquez D, Gauthier F, Bertini E, et al. Infantile Alexander disease: Spectrum of GFAP mutations and genotype-phenotype correlation. Am J Hum Genet 2001;69:1134–1140.

85. Staba MJ, Goldman S, Johnson FL, Huttenlocher PR. Allogenic bone marrow transplantation for Alexander's disease. Bone Marrow Transplant 1997;20:247–249.

86. van der Knapp MS, Barth PG, Gabreëls FJM, et al. A new leukoencephalopathy with vanishing white matter. Neurology 1997;48:845–855.

87. Brück W, Herms J, Brockmann K, et al. Myelinopathia centralis diffusa (vanishing white matter disease): evidence of apoptotic oligodendrocyte degeneration in early lesion development. Ann Neurol 2001;50:532–536.

88. Schiffman R, Moller JR, Trapp BD, et al. Childhood ataxia with diffuse central nervous system hypomyelination. Ann Neurol 1994;35:331–340.

89. Francalanci P, Eymard-Pierre E, Dionisi-Vici C, et al. Fatal infantile leukodystrophy. A severe variant of CACH/VWM syndrome, allelic to chromosome 3q27. Neurology 2001;57:265–270.

90. van der Knapp MS, Kamphorst W, Barth PG, et al. Phenotypic variation in leukoencephalopathy with vanishing white matter. Neurology 1998;51:540–547.

91. Rodriguez D, Gelot A, della Gaspera B, et al. Increased density of oligodendrocytes in childhood ataxia with diffuse central hypomyelination (CACH) syndrome: neuropathological and biochemical study of two cases. Acta Neuropathol 1999;97:469–480.

92. Leegwater PAJ, Könst AAM, Kuyt B, et al. The gene for leukoencephalopathy with vanishing white matter is located on chromosome 3q27. Am J Hum Genet 1999; 65:728–734.

93. van der Knapp MS, Wevers RA, Kure S, et al. Increased cerebrospinal fluid glycine: a biochemical marker for a leukoencephalopathy with vanishing white matter. J Child Neurol 1999;14:728–731.

94. Harbord MG, Hardin A, Harding B, et al. Megalencephaly with dysmyelination, spasticity, seizures and distinctive neurophysiological findings in two siblings. Neuropediatrics 1990;21:164–168.

95. Topçu M, Saatei T, Topçuoglu MA, et al. Megalencephaly and leukodystrophy with mild clinical course. A report on 12 new cases. Brain Dev 1998;20:142–153.

96. Singhal BS, Gursahani RD, Udani VP, Bioiwale AA. Megalencephalic leukodystrophy in an Asian Indian ethnic group. Pediatr Neurol 1996;14:294–296.

97. van der Knaap MS, Barth PG, Stroink H, et al. Leukoencephalopathy with swelling and a discrepantly mild clini-

cal course in eight children. Ann Neurol 1995;37:324–334.

98. Goutières F, Boulloche J, Bourgeois M, Aicardi J. Leukoencephalopathy, megalencephalopathy and mild clinical course. A recently individualized familial leukodystrophy. Report on five new cases. J Child Neurol 1996;11:439–444.

99. Bešenski N, Bošnjak V, Cop S, et al. Neuroimaging and clinically distinctive features in van der Knapp megalencephalic leukoencephalopathy. Int J Neuroradiol 1997;3:244–249.

100. Yalçinkaya C, Çomu S, Koçer N, et al. Siblings with cystic leukoencephalopathy and megalencephaly. J Child Neurol 2000;15:690–693.

101. van der Knapp MS, Barth PG, Vrensen GF, Valk J. Histopathology of an infantile-onset spongiform leukoencephalopathy with a discrepantly mild clinical course. Acta Neuropathol (Berl) 1996;92:206–212.

102. Topçu M, Gartioux C, Ribierre F, et al. Vacuolating megalencephalic leukoencephalopathy with subcortical cysts mapped to chromosome 22qtel. Am J Hum Genet 2000;66:733–739.

103. Jones KJ, Margan G, Johnston H, et al. The expanding phenotype of laminin α2 chain (merosin) abnormalities; case series and review. J Med Genet 2001;38:649–657.

104. van der Knaap MS, Smit LME, Barth PG, et al. Magnetic resonance imaging in classification of congenital muscular dystrophies with brain abnormalities. Ann Neurol 1997;42:50–59.

105. Farina L, Morandi L, Milanesi I, et al. Congenital muscular dystrophy with merosin deficiency: MRI findings in five patients. Neuroradiology 1998;40:807–811.

106. Philpot J, Cowan F, Pennock J, et al. Merosin-deficient congenital muscular dystrophy: the spectrum of brain involvement on magnetic resonance imaging. Neuromuscul Disord 1999;9:81–85.

107. Naom I, D'Alessandro M, Topaloglu H. Refinement of the laminin α2 locus to human chromosome 6q2 in severe and mild merosin deficient congenital muscular dystrophy. J Med Genet 1997;34:99–104.

108. Helbling-Leclerc A, Zhang X, Topaloglu H, et al. Mutations in the laminin α2 chain gene (LAMA2) cause merosin-deficient congenital muscular dystrophy. Nat Genet 1995;11:216–218.

109. Sunada Y, Saito F, Higuchi I, et al. Deficiency of a 180-kDa extracellular matrix protein in Fukuyama type congenital muscular dystrophy skeletal muscle. Neuromuscul Disord 2002;12:117–120.

110. Haltia M, Leivo I, Somer H, et al. Muscle-eye-brain disease: a neuropathological study. Ann Neurol 1997;41:173–180.

111. Sjögren T, Larsson T. Oligophrenia in combination with congenital ichthyosis and spastic disorders. Acta Psychiatr Neurol Scand 1957;32(Suppl 113):1–113.

112. Willemsen MAAP, IJlst L, Steijlen PM, et al. Clinical, biochemical and molecular genetic characteristics of 19 patients with the Sjögren-Larsson syndrome. Brain 2001;124:1426–1437.

113. Rizzo WB, Dammann AL, Craft DA, et al. Sjögren-Larsson syndrome: inherited defect in the fatty alcohol cycle. J Pediatr 1989;115:228–234.

114. DiRocco M, Filocamo M, Tortori-Donati P, et al. Sjögren-Larsson syndrome: nuclear magnetic resonance imaging of the brain in a 4-year-old-boy. J Inherit Metab Dis 1994;17:112–114.

115. van Domburg PHMF, Willemsen MAAP, Rotteveel JJ, et al. Sjögren-Larsson syndrome. Clinical and MRI/MRS findings in FALDH-deficient patients. Neurology 1999;52:1345–1352.

116. Yamaguchi K, Handa T. Sjögren-Larsson syndrome: Postmortem brain abnormalities: Pediatr Neurol 1998;18:338–341.

117. De Laurenzi V, Rogers GR, Hamrock DJ, et al. Sjögren-Larson syndrome is caused by mutations in the fatty aldehyde dehydrogenase gene. Nat Genet 1996;12:52–57.

118. IJlst L, Oostheim W, van Werkhoven M, et al. Molecular basis of Sjögren-Larsson syndrome: frequency of the 1297-1298 del GA and 943C→T mutation in 29 patients. J Inherit Metab Dis 1999;22:319–321.

119. Maaswinkel-Mooij PD, Brouwer OF, Rizzo WB. Unsuccessful dietary treatment of Sjögren-Larsson syndrome. J Pediatr 1994;124:748–750.

120. Willemsen MA, Rotteveel JJ, Steijlen PM, et al. 5-Lipoxygenase inhibition: a new treatment strategy for Sjögren-Larsson syndrome. Neuropediatrics 2000;31:1–3.

121. Cockayne EA. Dwarfism with retinal atrophy and deafness. Arch Dis Child 1936;11:1–8.

122. Cockayne EA. Dwarfism with retinal atrophy and deafness. Arch Dis Child 1946;21:52–54.

123. Nance MA, Berry SA. Cockayne syndrome: review of 140 cases. Am J Med Genet 1992;42:68–84.

124. Traboulsi EI, De Becker I, Maumenee IH. Ocular findings in Cockayne syndrome. Am J Ophthalmol 1993;114: 579–583.

125. Leaden SA, Cooper PK. Preferential repair of ionizing radiation-induced drainage in the transcribed strand of an active human gene is defective in Cockayne syndrome. Proc Natl Acad Sci U S A 1993; 90:10499–10503.

126. Lehmann AR, Thompson AF, Harcourt SA, et al. Cockayne's syndrome: correlation of clinical features with cellular sensitivity of RNA synthesis to UV irradiation. J Med Genet 1993;30:679–682.

127. Henning KA, Li L, Iyer N, et al. The Cockayne syndrome group A gene encodes a WD repeat protein that interacts with CSB protein and a subunit of RNA polymerase II TFIIH. Cell 1995;82:555–564.

128. Mallery DL, Tanganelli B, CoPella S, et al. Molecular analysis of mutations in the CSB (ERCC6) gene in patients with Cockayne syndrome. Am J Hum Genet 1998;62:77–85.

129. Ellaway CJ, Duggins A, Fung VS, et al. Cockayne syndrome associated with low CSF 5-hyfroxyindole acetic acid levels. J Med Genet 2000;37:553–557.

130. Berginer VM, Salen G, Shefer S. Cerebrotendinous xanthomatosis. Neurol Clin 1989;7:55–74.

131. Verrips A, Van Engelen BGM, Wevers RA, et al. Presence of diarrhea and absence of tendon xanthomas in patients with cerebrotendinous xanthomatosis. Arch Neurol 2000;57:520–524.

132. Verrips A, Hoefsloot LH, Steenbergen GCH, et al. Clinical and molecular genetic characteristics of patients with cerebrotendinous xanthomatosis. Brain 2000;123:908–919.

133. DeStefano N, Dotti MT, Mortilla M, Federico A. Magnetic resonance imaging and spectroscopic changes in brains of patients with cerebrotendinous xanthomatosis. Brain 2001; 124:121–131.

134. Verrips A, Lycklama à Nijeholt GJ, Barkhof F, et al. Spinal xanthomatosis: a variant of cerebrotendinous xanthomatosis. Brain 1999;122:1589–1595.

135. Menkes JH, Schimschock JR, Swanson PD. Cerebrotendinous xanthomatosis: The storage of cholestanol within the nervous system. Arch Neurol 1968;19:47–53.

136. Berginer VM, Salen G, Shefer S. Long-term treatment of cerebrotendinous xanthomatosis with chenodeoxycholic acid. N Engl J Med 1984;311:1649–1652.

137. Peynet J, Laurent A, DeLiege P, et al. Cerebrotendinous xanthomatosis: Treatments with simvastatin, lovastatin and chenodeoxycholic acid in 3 siblings. Neurology 1991;41: 434–436.

138. van Heijst AF, Verrips A, Wevers RA, et al. Treatment and follow-up of children with cerebrotendinous xanthomatosis. Eur J Pediatr1998;157:313–316.

139. Federico A, Dotti MT. Treatment of cerebrotendinous xanthomatosis. Neurology 1994;44:2218.

140. Dichgans M, Mayer M, Uttner I, et al. The phenotypic spectrum of CADASIL: clinical findings in 102 cases. Ann Neurol 1998;44:731–739.

141. Ruchoux MM, Maurage CA. CADASIL: cerebral autosomal dominant arteriopathy with subcortical infarcts and leukoencephalopathy. J Neuropathol Exp Neurol 1997;56: 947–964.

142. Bousser M-G, Tournier-Lasserve E. Cerebral autosomal arteriopathy with subcortical infarcts and leukoencephalopathy: from stroke to vessel wall physiology. J Neurol Neurosurg Psychiatry 2001;70:285–287.

143. de Lange RPJ, Bolt J, Reid E, et al. Screening British CADASIL families for mutations in the NOTCH3 gene. J Med Genet 2000;37:224–225.

144. Weller M, Dichgans J, Klockgether T. Acetazolamide-responsive migraine in CADASIL. Neurology 1998;50: 1505.

145. Servidei S, Riepe RE, Langston C, et al. Severe cardiopathy in branching enzyme deficiency. J Pediatr 1987;111:51–56.

146. Bruno C, Servidei S, Shanske S, et al. Glycogen branching enzyme deficiency in adult polyglucosan body disease. Ann Neurol 1993;33:88–93.

147. Rifai Z, Klitzke M, Tawil R, et al. Dementia of adult polyglucosan body disease. Evidence of cortical and subcortical dysfunction. Arch Neurol 1994;51:90–94.

148. Berkhoff M, Weis J, Schroth G, Sturzenegger M. Extensive white-matter changes in case of adult polyglucosan body disease. Neuroradiology 2001;43:234–236.

149. Ziemssen F, Sindern E, Schroder JM, et al. Novel missense mutations in the glycogen-branching enzyme gene in adult polyglucosan body disease. Ann Neurol 2000;47:536–540.

150. Lossos A, Meiner Z, Barash V, et al. Adult polyglucosan body disease in Ashkenazi Jewish patients carrying the Tyr329Ser mutation in the glycogen-branching enzyme gene. Ann Neurol 1998;44:867–872.

151. Hund E, Jansen O, Koch MC, et al. Proximal myotonic myopathy with MRI white matter abnormalities of the brain. Neurology 1997;48:33–37.

152. Liquori CL, Ricker K, Moseley ML, et al. Myotonic dystrophy type 2 caused by a CCTG expansion in intron 1 of ZNF9. Science 2001;293:864–867.

153. Inoue K, Tanabe Y, Lubski JR. Myelin deficiencies in both the central and peripheral nervous systems associated with a SOXIO mutation. Ann Neurol 1999;46:313–318.

154. Kristjansdottir R, Uvebrant P, Hagberg B, et al. Disorder of the cerebral white matter in children. The spectrum of lesions. Neuropediatrics 1996;27:295–298.

155. Schiffmann R, Tedeschi G, Kinkel RP, et al. Leukodystrophy in patients with ovarian dysgenesis. Ann Neurol 1997; 41:654–661.

156. Aicardi J, Goutières F. A progressive familial encephalopathy in infancy with calcifications of the basal ganglia and chronic cerebrospinal fluid lymphocytosis. Ann Neurol 1984;15:49–54.

157. Goutières F, Aicardi J, Barth PG, Lebon P. Aicardi-Goutières syndrome: an update and results of interferon alpha studies. Ann Neurol 1998;44:900–907.

158. Koul R, Chacko A, Joshi S, Sankhla D. Aicardi-Goutières syndrome in siblings. J Child Neurol 2001;16:759–761.

159. Crow YJ, Jackson AP, Roberts E, et al. Aicardi-Goutières syndrome displays genetic heterogeneity with one locus (AGS1) on chromosome 3p21. Ann J Hum Genet 2000; 67:213–221.

160. Lossos A, Cooperman H, Soffer D, et al. Hereditary leukoencephalopathy and palmoplantar keratoderma: A new disorder with increased skin collagen content. Neurology 1995;45:331–337.

161. Hunt DM, Rickman L, Whittock NV, et al. Spectrum of dominant mutations in the desmosomal cadherin desmoglein 1, causing the skin disease striate palmoplantar keratoderma. Eur J Hum Genet 2001;9:197–203.

162. Weiss BJ, Kamholz J, Ritter A, et al. Sequential spinal muscular atrophy and dermatological findings in a patient with chromosome 18q deletion. Ann Neurol 1991;30:419–423.

163. Coupry I, Taine L, Goizet C, et al. Leukodystrophy and oculocutaneous albinism in a child with an 11q14 deletion. J Med Genet 2001;38:35–39.

164. Black DN, Booth F, Watters GV, et al. Leukoencephalopathy among native Indian infants in Northern Quebec and Manitoba. Ann Neurol 1988;24:490–496.

Chapter 5

Multiple Sclerosis: A Prototypical Human Demyelinating Disease

Fernando Dangond

Inflammation plays an important role in many neurodegenerative disorders, including Alzheimer's disease and amyotrophic lateral sclerosis. Even Sandhoff disease, a neurometabolic inherited disorder traditionally thought to spare the immune system, was recently shown to be characterized by early activation of central nervous system (CNS) microglia.[1] These neurodegenerative disorders, however, are fairly distinct clinically and pathologically from the most common acquired disorder of myelin in humans—*multiple sclerosis* (MS), an inflammatory disease of the CNS characterized by neurodegeneration.

Our understanding of diseases that involve the immune system and the CNS is rapidly evolving with the advent of new technologies applicable to basic research and new standards for performing clinical treatment trials. In this chapter, I provide a brief historical account and discuss basic research and clinical aspects of MS, using it as a prototype for understanding features of other disorders of myelin.

Milestones in Multiple Sclerosis Research

- Jean Cruveilhier (1791–1874), first professor of pathology at the University of Paris, stated *"La phlebite domine toute la pathologie"* (phlebitis dominates all of pathology) and focused his attention on studying blood vessels in human disease. Cruveilhier has been credited with providing the first description of

MS symptoms in association with pathology (clinicoanatomic correlation).[2]
- Sir Robert Carswell (1793–1857), professor of pathologic anatomy at the University College London, became known for his detailed medical illustrations of postmortem tissues, including drawings of MS pathology.[3]
- Jean-Martin Charcot (1825–1893), working at La Salpêtrière, performed detailed clinicoanatomic correlations of MS in 1868[4] and coined the term *sclérose en plaques*, establishing MS as a unique pathologic entity. He recognized an MS clinical triad of nystagmus, intention tremor, and dysarthria.
- Carl Rokitansky (1804–1878) recognized tissue injury, which he described as "the disintegration of the brain tubes" in MS brain.[5]
- Friedrich Theodor von Frerichs (1819–1885), a German pathologist, recognized disease remissions, nystagmus, and mental deterioration as clinical features of MS.[6]
- Pio Del Rio-Hortega noticed *"glia de escasas radiaciones"* (glia with scarce radiations) and coined the term *oligodendroglia* in 1921.[7] He is also credited for the characterization of microglia and their role in brain pathology.
- Pierre Marie (1853–1940), Charcot's pupil at La Salpêtrière, was the first to postulate an infectious agent as a possible etiology for MS.[8]
- James Dawson at the University of Edinburgh in 1916 performed neuropathologic examinations of MS tissue with emphasis on the perivas-

cular distribution of inflammatory cells and the resulting finger-like appearance of veins and venules.[9] The term *Dawson's fingers* is now also used to describe the radiographic appearance of plaques arising from the corpus callosum and reflecting the perpendicular projection of the veins and venules in this region (see Figure 8-1A).

- Thomas Rivers at the Rockefeller Institute in New York in 1935 showed that brain tissue injections in mice induce experimental allergic (autoimmune) encephalomyelitis (EAE).
- Marjorie Lees and Jordi Folch-Pi discovered myelin proteolipid protein in 1951 (reviewed in reference 10).
- P. R. Carnegie reported in 1971 the complete amino acid sequence of human myelin basic protein (MBP).[11]
- Abnormal immunoglobulin G (IgG) production was shown in the cerebrospinal fluid (CSF) of MS patients by Elvin A. Kabat (1942), using electrophoresis.[8]
- Adrenocorticotropic hormone was shown by Rawson et al.[12] to speed optic neuritis recovery but not its long-term prognosis in a double-blind prospective study in 1966.
- In the 1960s, immunosuppressive agents, including cyclophosphamide, were used by clinical investigators in an effort to downregulate the immune system in MS. Important insights into the disease process have been gained from these studies and have ultimately led to the use of mitoxantrone for MS treatment.[13–18]
- Magnetic resonance imaging (MRI) rapidly gained widespread use as a diagnostic aid in MS and other demyelinating disorders after studies by Ian R. Young in 1981.[19]
- The Optic Neuritis Treatment Trial showed that intravenous methylprednisolone speeds optic neuritis recovery but does not affect its long-term outcome. It also showed that oral prednisone does not lead to faster recovery and may actually worsen the outcome for visual acuity.[20]
- Interferon beta-1b (IFN-β-1b) was found to be effective in early relapsing-remitting MS by the IFNB Multiple Sclerosis Study Group in 1993.[21,22]
- In 1996, IFN-β-1a and glatiramer acetate (previously known as *copolymer 1*) were added to the list of therapeutic options in MS.

Neuropathology

MS is a dynamic, inflammatory, demyelinating disease of the human brain and spinal cord. MS lesions are characterized by perivascular infiltration of activated monocytes and lymphocytes and appear as indurated foci in pathologic specimens—hence the term *sclérose en plaques* coined by Charcot. The lesions can be appreciated on the pial surface of the spinal cord or brain stem and around the ventricular zones on visual inspection. MS lesions appear as multifocal, often confluent areas of demyelination (Figure 5-1) associated with variable degrees of oligodendrocyte loss and gliosis on a background of edema and debris. In the advanced stages of lesion formation, myelin debris can be identified in the extracellular space in net-like or droplet-like accumulations or as clumps or rods within lipid-laden macrophages.[23] Not surprisingly, these "lipoid" macrophages are found adjacent to myelin-denuded axons.

Variable degrees of axonal loss can also occur (Figure 5-2), as demonstrated by both histopathologic and magnetic resonance spectroscopy studies. The exact sequence of immunopathologic events in plaque formation cannot be easily ascertained, as significant histopathologic heterogeneity is found in postmortem MS brains. Although some individuals exhibit lesions with predominant antibody or complement deposition, others have more pronounced oligodendrocyte loss, owing to apoptosis or to a "dying-back oligodendrogliopathy" with or without attempts at remyelination.[24–27] Attempts at remyelination by oligodendrocytes seem to be evident at the plaque border, where thinly myelinated axons are found leading to the term *shadow plaque*. Whether partial remyelination takes place owing to the action of oligodendrocyte progenitor cells (OPCs) present in the adult brain or of marginally affected oligodendrocytes, or both, is currently a subject of study.

Etiology

Viral Hypothesis

The reason for the triggering of immune cell activation in MS remains unclear. The initial targets of such activation are also undetermined. Despite intensive efforts at finding the cause of the disease, no single

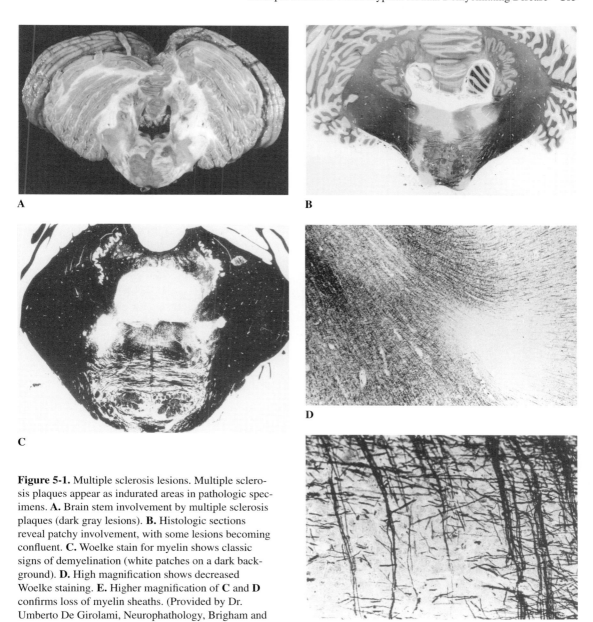

Figure 5-1. Multiple sclerosis lesions. Multiple sclerosis plaques appear as indurated areas in pathologic specimens. **A.** Brain stem involvement by multiple sclerosis plaques (dark gray lesions). **B.** Histologic sections reveal patchy involvement, with some lesions becoming confluent. **C.** Woelke stain for myelin shows classic signs of demyelination (white patches on a dark background). **D.** High magnification shows decreased Woelke staining. **E.** Higher magnification of **C** and **D** confirms loss of myelin sheaths. (Provided by Dr. Umberto De Girolami, Neurophathology, Brigham and Women's Hospital.)

etiologic agent for MS has been demonstrated. The fact that a retrovirus-associated disease—human T-cell lymphotropic virus type I–associated myelopathy/tropical spastic paraparesis—closely mimics the clinical presentation of primary progressive MS has led investigators to propose that MS may be viewed as a syndrome[28] of different etiologies, with a minor proportion of cases associated with a single

identifiable virus (e.g., human T-cell lymphotropic virus type I) and others possibly triggered or exacerbated by other environmental agents. In fact, only one in every four MS attacks is associated with an intercurrent viral infection, usually involving the upper respiratory tract. However, it is believed that such environmental triggers as viruses may solely serve as exacerbating factors in a more complex scenario of

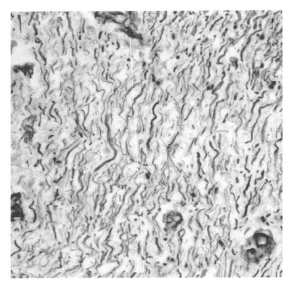

Figure 5-2. Multiple sclerosis lesions. Axonal loss is shown in multiple sclerosis brain. A Bodian stain is used to demonstrate fragmented axons traversing the white matter in multiple sclerosis.

genetic predisposition, hormonal imbalance, and immune system dysfunction. Over the last 100 years, multiple viruses have been implicated in the etiology of MS, including canine distemper virus, coronavirus, measles, parainfluenza, simian virus 5, and Epstein-Barr virus (EBV), among others.[29–33] Studies of the association of MS with prior infection with EBV[34] and persistence of IgM and IgA antibody levels against EBV in patients with relapses[35] suggest that prior EBV exposure may be a prerequisite for MS development, as previously suggested,[36] but these studies await confirmation. Other studies aimed at detecting protein targets for oligoclonal IgG in the CSF of MS patients have identified a peptide that shares homology with the EBV nuclear antigen[37,38] in a subset of patients; the significance of this finding is still unclear.

Recently, attention has focused on human herpesvirus 6 (HHV-6), variant A, the genomic DNA of which has been demonstrated in peripheral blood cells of some MS patients[39] and against which a proliferative cellular response is mounted.[40] Latency of HHV-6 infection in the CNS has been proven,[41] and elevated expression of the virus in active MS lesions[42] and elevated IgM titers in serum and CSF, suggesting an active recent infection,[43] have been demonstrated. However, elevated antibody titers against HHV-6 are not exclusive to

MS and have been reported in chronic fatigue syndrome.[44] Because other herpesviruses (i.e., EBV, herpes simplex virus type 1) seem to be reactivated during attacks, the true pathogenic significance of HHV-6 in MS remains undetermined.

Studies of enigmatic retrovirus-like particles isolated from MS tissues have resulted in the identification of endogenous retroviral sequences with reverse transcriptase activity of as yet unknown pathogenic significance.[36,45–51] However, we (F. Dangond, unpublished observations, 1995) and others[52] have not been able to demonstrate the presence of retroviral reverse transcriptase activity in MS-derived cell cultures. A retroviral etiology nevertheless seems attractive, because other retroviruses such as human T-cell lymphotropic virus type I in humans and visna virus in sheep,[53] among others, cause inflammatory demyelination. However, this phenomenon is not exclusive of retroviruses, as such other neurotropic viruses as Theiler picornavirus cause encephalomyelitis in mice.

Other Proposed Infectious Triggers

Besides viruses, other microorganisms such as *Chlamydia pneumoniae* have been implicated in MS pathogenesis,[54] but difficulty in reproducing these data has been reported.[55] The possibility of a secondary *Chlamydia* infection of an already injured MS brain tissue is acknowledged by the authors.[54] Other investigators have found a much smaller subset of patients with *Chlamydia* brain infection and MS.[56] The significance of these data is still uncertain.

Clinical Classification

MS most commonly afflicts individuals between the ages of 18–50 years; however, any age group can be affected. Clinical attacks in MS are neurologic deficits that typically last more than 24 hours and usually several days. MRI scans suggesting myelin loss in children should prompt a workup for inherited neurometabolic disorders (discussed in Chapter 4). MS can present in different forms, such as relapsing-remitting (70%), primary-progressive (15%), and relapsing-progressive (15%), depicted in Figure 5-3. At least two-thirds of patients with relapsing-remitting disease eventually develop a secondary-progressive form.

Figure 5-3. Clinical forms of multiple sclerosis. Patients may present with primary-progressive (PP), relapsing-remitting (RR), secondary-progressive (SP), or relapsing-progressive (RP) types. Evolution of clinical presentation over time is the main factor that helps to determine the clinical diagnosis.

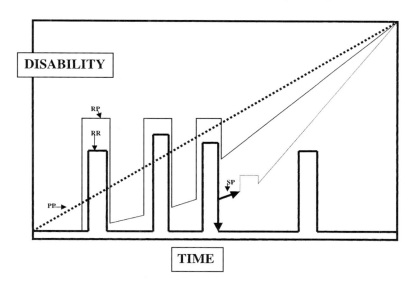

Relapsing-Remitting

Patients with relapsing-remitting MS have recurrent attacks followed by periods of total remission with partial sequelae or total improvement. They may accumulate disability after new attacks, and eventually their clinical presentation may become secondary progressive (continuous deterioration in the absence of new attacks). It is estimated that two-thirds of patients with relapsing-remitting MS will require unilateral assistance to walk (e.g., use of a cane) at 25 years from onset. By this time, most of these patients will have the secondary-progressive form of MS.

Primary-Progressive

Patients with the primary-progressive form of MS have the acute or subacute onset of symptoms that do not significantly improve with time, and disability accumulates gradually, often spreading to involve other anatomic regions. They experience no periods of recovery or stabilization, except for occasional plateaus.

Relapsing-Progressive

Patients with relapsing-progressive MS tend to present with recurrent attacks but accumulate significant disability (i.e., continue to progress) in the intervals between attacks. Patients with relapsing-progressive MS may experience partial or full recovery from exacerbations. Patients in this group may be difficult to distinguish from relapsing-remitting patients who exhibit an early conversion into a secondary-progressive phase.

Secondary-Progressive

Secondary-progressive MS patients have relapsing disease that then develops into a continuous, progressive course. These patients may continue to experience occasional attacks and may also experience occasional periods of stabilization or mild remission.[57]

Physiologic Basis for Multiple Sclerosis Symptomatology

Myelin is responsible for the increased resistance to the flow of ions through the axonal membrane; however, gaps at short interspersed axonal segments (nodes of Ranvier) allow the lowering of the capacitance per unit length of axon and thus facilitate local circuit dissemination. The influx of Na^+ through the voltage-gated Na^+ channels in the nodes of Ranvier is responsible for saltatory conduction (depolarization) of the electrical impulses. One oligodendrocyte can extend its processes to insulate different axons at variable distances from the cell body. In MS, diffuse and rapid demyelination results in loss of insulation for the current flow through the internodal regions, which results in simultaneous conduction block for multiple

axons, leading to MS symptomatology. The consequences of chronic or partial demyelination may
be exacerbated by changes in body temperature or
by mechanical strain resulting in such symptoms
as Uhthoff's phenomenon (worsening of MS
symptoms on exposure to hot temperatures) or
Lhermitte's phenomenon (electric shock-like sensations "down the spine" or "down the arms or legs"
on flexing the neck), respectively. It is also conceivable that any alteration of the axonal milieu
(i.e., due to inflammatory cell–derived cytokines
or due to the presence of inflammatory cells per
se) may result in impairment of conduction, which
may be corrected if such inflammatory cell presence is reversed. An alternative explanation for
heat-related symptoms in MS would be that a
latent infectious agent highly responsive to subtle
body temperature shifts would become rapidly
activated or released with increased body temperature, immediately triggering the immune system to
respond.

EBV[35] and herpes simplex virus type 1[58] reactivation during MS relapses, antibody titers to HHV-
6,[43] and a reported higher rate of herpes zoster
occurring at an earlier age in MS patients[58] suggest
that immune cell dysfunction in MS is preceded by
infections with viruses that become latent but can
be readily re-expressed. It is thus conceivable that
MS symptoms may occur not only after first exposure to environmental agents but also during recurrent immune system responses to latent viruses
(e.g., EBV, HHV-6, herpes simplex virus type 1, or
herpes zoster) on subclinical re-expression. Alternatively, the antiviral immune response may just be
an epiphenomenon of an unrelated disease-driven
immune reactivation.

Role of Genes and Environment

Prevalence

In the United States alone, MS has a prevalence
of nearly 350,000 cases. Every year, approximately 10,000 new U.S. patients are diagnosed
with various forms of the disease. More than 1
million patients are affected by MS worldwide.
Individuals of northern European ancestry living
in temperate climates seem more at risk of
developing MS. The highest reported incidence

of MS in the world seems to exist in southeast
Scotland (approximately 12.2 in 100,000).[59] The
incidence of MS in Asia, Africa, Mexico, the
Caribbean region, and northern South America is
considered low.[60,61]

The occurrence of an MS outbreak in the
Faroe Islands after the occupation by British
troops in 1940 led Kurtzke and Hyllested[62] to
propose that an exogenous environmental agent
had been introduced into the islands and had
been responsible for the outbreak. In 1943,
before the onset of the outbreak, no cases of MS
had been recognized in the islands; however, 24
cases appeared in the following two decades.
Another presumed outbreak of MS occurred in
Iceland in 1945.[63]

Migration after age 15 years from a high- to a
low-risk area for MS does not seem to lessen the
risk of developing MS (i.e., the risk of the country of origin is maintained); however, those who
migrate earlier than age 15 years decrease their
risk to that of the host country.[64] These observations are not conclusive but suggest that (1) hormonal or immune factors before or during
puberty may enhance susceptibility, regardless
of geographic residence, or (2) early exposure to
an environmental agent common to specific geographic areas may be a critical prerequisite for
developing the disease.

Sibling and Twin Studies

It has been estimated that the risk for a sibling of
an MS patient to develop MS is approximately
2.3–4.0%, but an increased frequency of head
MRI scans suggesting demyelination in asymptomatic relatives (up to 15%)[65] suggests that this
figure may be underestimated. The MS concordance rate among monozygotic twins is 20–
40%, suggesting the presence of predisposing
polygenic factors (nonmendelian inheritance).
The risk for dizygotic twins is the same as the
risk for other siblings (approximately 4%). Furthermore, the rate of MS for spouses of MS
patients is very low (0.17%), suggesting minimal or no common environmental factors in
adulthood responsible for triggering MS.[66] Thus,
familial aggregation in MS has been shown to
depend entirely on genetic factors.[67]

Gender Distribution

Although MS affects females more than males (1.6–2.0 to 1.0), the basis for this difference is unknown. This ratio is even higher (3 to 1) among patients with an atypical time of onset (i.e., less than 15 or more than 50 years of age), suggesting a hormonal component to the disease process. Although males have a higher tendency to develop progressive MS, females tend to have an earlier onset and experience more relapses.

Genome Screens for Linkage

A search for candidate genes using genome screens showed the 6p21 chromosomal region (harboring human leukocyte antigen [HLA] genes) as the localization with the strongest linkage; other regions were found in other chromosomal regions with a weaker linkage, but these results could not be replicated by all studies.[68–70] Others have mapped a putative MS vulnerability locus to 5p14-p12, a region that is known to be syntenic to a murine locus that confers susceptibility to EAE.[71] Although full genome screens for linkage in MS have so far been inconclusive—except for the association with the HLA region—it is expected that refinement of these techniques with the completion of the Human Genome Project will identify definitively at least two or three other regions of genetic susceptibility.

Genetic Polymorphisms

The hypotheses of MS causation include environmental agents (e.g., virus, bacteria, toxins) acting in concert with a specific genetic predisposition to result in immune dysfunction. The possibility that genetic factors play a role is supported by the fact that the disease is more common in white populations living in northern latitudes, whereas Native Americans and black individuals from these same regions have much lower risks. Different variants of genes normally found in the general population, commonly termed *polymorphisms*, may lead to different levels of expression of those genes and the proteins that they encode. Therefore, it is possible that an individual with a gain-of-function polymorphism within the promoter region of a gene that is involved in immune reactivity may generate an exaggerated response (i.e., elevated expression of a proinflammatory gene) to a given antigen, leading to uncontrolled immune cell proliferation and autoimmunity. The research of gene polymorphisms in MS is just beginning but promises to yield important clues about the pathogenesis of this disease.

HLA molecules are highly polymorphic cell-surface glycoproteins that play a prominent role in the normal immune response by serving as antigen presentation molecules, thus helping to shape the T-cell repertoire against antigens. HLA molecules include class I (HLA-A, -B, and -C) and class II (HLA-DR, -DQ, and -DP) and localize to chromosome 6. MS has been associated in whites with the HLA-DR2 allele, and linkage of MS to nearby genetic regions also suggests a component of genetic predisposition. However, there is no consensus as to which specific polymorphisms or individual genes within the region are actually responsible. Multiple studies point toward subregions of HLA-DR and -DQ as having a probable role in susceptibility[72,73]; however, multiple ethnic backgrounds and exposure to multiple different environmental triggering factors may modify the degree and pattern of risk conferred by these molecules. Besides containing class I and class II genes, the HLA region contains other genes collectively called *class III*, including the complement factors known as *C2*, *C4*, and *B* and *21-hydroxylase*. In addition, tumor necrosis factor-α (TNF-α) and genes involved in antigen transport (*TAP1* and *TAP2*) and antigen processing (*LMP1* and *LMP2*) are found in this region. It is possible that the known HLA region genes are markers of other nearby genes that truly mediate susceptibility and are cosegregated by linkage disequilibrium.[72,73] Recent associations of MS with polymorphic variants of the cytotoxic T lymphocyte–associated antigen 4 (CTLA4)[74]—a B7 costimulatory pathway immune attenuator—are provocative. Other studies suggest an association of interleukin-4 (IL-4) polymorphisms with age of MS onset.[75] Other genes under study include T-cell receptor (TCR) genes and MBP, but so far the results have been less convincing than the associations described earlier for HLA subregions.

Recent reports of mutations in the CD45 (T-cell differentiation–related) molecule in MS[76] further support the view that individuals with mutations or polymorphisms in genes associated with immune or CNS function may be at higher predisposition to develop MS on exposure to an, as yet, unknown array of environmental agents. HLA polymorphisms typically encode the antigenic peptide–binding region, suggesting that HLA-expressing antigen-presenting cells (APCs) from different individuals will have the capacity to bind different self or foreign peptides and therefore be capable of promoting distinct immune or autoimmune responses. Other molecules with polymorphisms that have been implicated in MS include adhesion molecules such as intercellular adhesion molecule-1,[77] proinflammatory cytokines such as lymphotoxin and TNF-α,[78] the antioxidant molecule glutathione S-transferase,[79] immunoglobulin heavy-chain genes,[80,81] and the vitamin D receptor[82] (see Table 18-2 for other non-HLA polymorphisms implicated in MS).

Immunopathogenesis

Adaptive and Innate Immune Systems

Two compartments of the immune system naturally act in defense of the organism: the adaptive and the innate compartments. The adaptive immune system is composed of T-lymphocytes that carry αβ chains in their TCRs and of antibodies. These adaptive effector cells and antibodies can encode for a wide diversity of antigens and therefore can provide selectivity in antigen binding. The innate immune response, which precedes the appearance of a response by the adaptive system by a few days, includes such cells as γδ T cells, macrophages-microglia, and natural killer cells, which function under less selective pressures and provide less specificity but recognize structures shared by common environmental antigens such as bacteria.[83] Cells from both compartments may adversely affect the outcome of an immune response if an autoimmune reaction is mounted in a susceptible individual, as these compartments are not fully independent of one another and may indeed cooperate in orchestrating tissue destruction.

T-Cell Specificity Generation

The TCR provides specificity to the response; however, TCRs are generated by random somatic rearrangements and thus have the potential for recognizing both foreign and self-antigens; therefore, a mechanism for controlling the populations of self-reactive T cells must exist to prevent autoimmunity. The thymus performs a surveillance role by deleting those T cells that recognize self-antigen. The self-reactive T cells that are able to escape the thymus may persist in the circulation but, owing to their inactivated state, do not attack self-antigens. However, if such antigens have been naturally sequestered (i.e., never exposed to immune cells) and later, after tissue injury, are exposed to the immune system, a self-reactive attack may develop. Whether early age-related changes in the thymus affect its ability to delete self-reactive T cells in MS or other autoimmune disorders remains to be investigated.

T-Cell Responsiveness

An activated T cell can become proliferative (i.e., divide into multiple, identical daughter cells with the same specificity in a process called *clonal expansion*) or cytotoxic (i.e., kill a target cell by releasing perforins, which are channel-forming molecules that allow the entry of granzymes and other toxic factors into the target cell). Different peptides presented by HLA molecules may induce differential responsiveness of T cells—that is, a T-cell clone originally found to be proliferative and cytotoxic in response to a given peptide may lose its proliferative but not its cytotoxic capabilities when exposed to a peptide that is the same size and differs in only one amino acid[84] or vice versa. This differential regulation of T-cell functions after such exquisite manipulations of the peptide being presented suggest that the adaptive immune system can respond to environmental triggers in diverse ways, and minimal amino acid differences between self-peptides and environmental peptides may lead to aberrant immune responses.

T-Cell Recognition of Antigen in the Context of Human Leukocyte Antigen Presentation

Antibodies can bind to specific soluble target proteins in the peripheral circulation. However, for a T cell to recognize an antigenic peptide, this peptide has to be presented bound to an HLA molecule on the surface of an APC (usually macrophages, microglia, or B cells). When a T cell comes in contact with an empty HLA molecule, it recognizes it as "self" tissue, and engagement and activation do not occur; however, if the HLA molecule is occupied by a foreign peptide, the T cell will recognize it as "nonself" and initiate an attack. During an autoimmune response and by reasons still poorly understood, T cells may also mount an attack against a self-peptide presented by HLA. Self-antigen assembly on HLA molecules is not, however, exclusive to disease states; therefore, other factors may play a role in promoting autoimmunity. It has been shown that besides interactions between the TCR and the HLA-antigen complex, other stimuli (i.e., costimulatory signals) must be present for T-cell activation to occur. The B7 family of costimulatory molecules on the APCs interacts with the CD28 surface molecule on T cells and promotes T-cell activation. In EAE studies, B7-1 engagement leads to an IFN-γ–producing, proinflammatory (Th1) phenotype during activation, whereas B7-2 seems to provide a stimulus for a proregulatory, prohumoral phenotype of T cells.[85] Manipulation of the Th1-Th2 cytokine balance has relevance in MS, as high expression of B7-1 and IL-12 (a potent Th1-promoting cytokine) has been shown in early formed MS plaques.[86,87] In addition, interactions between molecules on the surface of B and T cells such as CD40 and CD40 ligand may mediate elevation in levels of IL-12 in the circulation of MS patients.[88] Furthermore, higher IL-12 production by immune cells from progressive patients has been demonstrated[88,89] when compared to healthy controls. Finally, it has been shown that IFN-β may exert some of its disease-modifying effects by its ability to downregulate IL-12 production[90] and decrease expression of B7-1 on lymphocytes in vivo.[91]

Role of T Cells in Tissue Damage

Normal individuals have circulating self-reactive lymphocytes; however, these lymphocytes are not activated and therefore do not cause autoimmunity. In contrast, activated autoreactive T cells, presumably against myelin antigens, including MBP, are thought to underlie the pathogenesis of MS. This is supported by studies in EAE, a disease resembling MS that can be induced experimentally in animals on injection of myelin proteins and Freund's adjuvant. EAE studies have shown that radioactively labeled MBP-reactive T cells used to transfer the disease adoptively do not migrate far from the immediate perivenular space and are actually absent in relapses, supporting the concept that these autoreactive T cells may serve as initial orchestrators of the immune response, triggering the recruitment of inflammatory cells from the recipient animal.[92] In addition, MS patients with ongoing disease activity have been shown to harbor a high frequency of MBP-reactive T cells,[93] and in at least a subset of patients, the frequency may be as high as 1 in 300 T cells obtained from the peripheral circulation.[88] It has also been shown that a highly immunodominant and potentially encephalitogenic epitope of MBP—peptide 84-102—is presented by HLA-DR2+ cells.[94] On activation, T cells express surface adhesion molecules, such as very late antigen 4, which aid their entry through the blood-brain barrier.

Triggers of Multiple Sclerosis Attacks: Pathogen Invasion, Molecular Mimicry, Bystander Activation, or Epitope Spreading

Despite many recent advances in our understanding of MS, the identity of specific triggers that promote immune cell infiltration of brain tissue remains unclear. The molecular mimicry hypothesis states that viral or other environmental antigens may share epitopes with brain proteins, which may lead to erroneous activation and therefore accumulation of reactive immune cells in the target (brain) tissue. T-lymphocytes isolated from MS patients and known to react in vitro against myelin proteins have been shown also to recognize viral proteins that share similar amino acid sequences.[95] Some authors argue that there is significant heterogeneity of the disease process and that different patients may have developed MS under the influence of different initial triggers. The molecular mimicry model would also predict that patients may experience recurrent attacks based on exposure to a widely diverse number of antigens, and the genetic make up would thus generate a specific predisposition for each individual. For some patients, the trigger may need to be highly specific (i.e., a closely homologous amino acid sequence to be recognized by the TCR) and, for others, nonspecific (i.e., activation of the immune system by bacterial lipopolysaccharide or endogenous or exogenous superantigens, described later).

It is unknown whether the initial trigger of immune cell activation occurs in the brain (perivenular sites containing activated APCs such as microglia) or in the periphery (CNS-draining lymph nodes, where neural antigens or their molecular mimics could be transported) or simultaneously at these sites.

Soluble factors, such as proinflammatory cytokines released from the activated immune cells, may serve as the propagating agents for the mounting of a directed attack against the CNS with recruitment of additional T and B cells to the site of initial injury (i.e., phenomenon of bystander activation). It is conceivable that cells under the influence of such cytokines or undergoing an activation response may express viruses that would otherwise remain latent (e.g., endogenous retroviruses or exogenously acquired herpesviruses), and this may further amplify the exposure of new antigens to the immune system and trigger epitope spread and further inflammation. In this scenario, damage to myelin proteins may be secondary to propagation of a proinflammatory cytokine release cascade including TNF-α and IFN-γ that injures oligodendrocytes directly, or the damage may occur via cell-to-cell signaling pathways. In any case, myelin debris is engulfed by activated macrophages, which are then able to present myelin antigen to CNS-infiltrating or CNS-patrolling T-lymphocytes. As a result of myelin loss, impaired saltatory conduction through denuded axons manifests clinically as MS symptomatology.

Role of Microglial Cells as Central Mediators of Inflammation or Neurodegeneration

Microglial cells were shown in early studies to engulf myelin.[96] Phagocytic uptake of myelin may be mediated by its attachment to clathrin-coated pits, via Fc receptor binding on the surface of microglia-macrophage cells,[97] but other mechanisms of uptake may be playing a role, as the process can be blocked in vitro by immune complexes, by antibodies against complement receptor 3, and by adding oxidized low-density lipoprotein.[98] On the other hand, oxidation of plasma low-density lipoprotein and uptake of oxidized low-density lipoprotein by microglia-macrophages within MS lesions has been demonstrated,[99] underscoring the complexity of the demyelinating process in vivo.

Microglial cells are the predominant cell population in the brain with antigen presentation capabilities and have been shown to present myelin proteins to autoreactive T cells.[100,101] In addition, expression of B7 costimulatory molecules by human microglia has been demonstrated in vitro.[87,102] As stated, early MS plaques exhibit upregulated B7-1,[86] which delivers a proinflammatory stimulus to CD28-expressing T cells (i.e., stimulates T cells to secrete IFN-γ that, in turn, induces more B7-1 expression by microglial cells).

Activated microglia release IL-1α and acquire a phenotype consistent with the respiratory burst reaction of activated monocytes in which molecules of the cyclo-oxygenase pathway are upregulated and oxygen free radicals are released. Finally, microglia release matrix metalloproteinases (MMPs), which contribute to further tissue damage by allowing lymphocytes to traverse the extracellular matrix barrier and also secrete cytokines that alter the Th1-Th2 balance. Treatment aimed at neutralizing activated microglia would, in theory, have a beneficial effect in MS, as it would lead to a break in the antigen presentation–T-cell interaction cycle, protection of the integrity of the perivenular tissues, and a decrease in oxidative damage to neural tissue (axons). CNS resident microglial cell activation may also have an impact on axon integrity with the chronic release of axonal damaging factors possibly playing a role in the advanced stages of MS.

Role of B Cells

Elevated IgG in the CSF, which can be demonstrated by an electrophoretic pattern of oligoclonal bands (OCBs) (Figure 5-4), suggests an important humoral (B-cell activation) component. Variable degrees of infiltration by antibody-producing plasma cells and complement activation have been demonstrated in MS lesions.[103] Figure 5-5 presents a schematic representation of molecular mechanisms involved in the generation of MS lesions.

Role of Oligodendroglia

Oligodendrocytes may also play a direct role in the etiology of MS by harboring a, yet unidentified, etiologic agent or by expressing, yet unrecognized, self-antigens not necessarily derived from myelin. These cells are known to express class I major histocompatibility complex molecules[104] and elicit cytotoxicity mediated by HLA class I–restricted CD8+ T cells,[105,106] and they are potentially able to present antigen in vivo. Oligodendrocytes may also be attacked by γδ[107–110] and natural killer cells in vitro. In addition, their expression of heat shock proteins, particularly hsp65[111,112] under conditions of heat shock or cellular stress, may explain in part why there are high frequencies of γδ T cells in the CSF and infiltrating the brain parenchyma of MS patients.

CSF from active relapsing-remitting MS patients has been reported to harbor high levels of antibodies against AN2, an OPC-specific cell-surface glycoprotein.[113] Interference with precursor cell integrity, migration, or remyelinating ability by anti-AN2 antibodies may play a role in disease activity. In addition, interactions between fas and fas ligand molecules on the surface of oligodendrocytes and T cells have been implicated as possible triggers of oligodendrocyte programmed cell death (apoptosis).[114,115] Furthermore, apoptosis of oligodendrocytes has been shown in lesions of a subset of MS patients[27]; whether this apoptosis is primary (i.e., directly triggered by a virus or toxin) or secondary to the ongoing inflammation must be further investigated.

Proteases and Tissue Damage: Response of Astrocytes

Considerable attention has been focused recently on the role of proteases that may have an impact on the entry of lymphocytes through the blood-brain barrier. MMPs, as stated, facilitate T-cell entry from the perivenular spaces through the extracellular matrix by degrading extracellular matrix macromolecules. MMP-9 elevation in the CSF of MS patients has been demonstrated.[116] Studies in the EAE animal model have shown that MMP inhibition leads to significant reduction of lesions in experimentally induced demyelination.[117] Other proteases as well as basal membrane and endothelial cell proteins await further scrutiny for clarification of their role in MS. In addition, the role of astrocytes as potential APCs that have the ability to express B7 molecules[118,119] is under investigation.

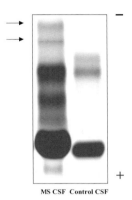

MS CSF   Control CSF

Figure 5-4. Oligoclonal bands in multiple sclerosis (MS). Cerebrospinal fluid (CSF) bands (as shown by *arrows*) are seen in at least 85% of MS patients.

Variable numbers of hypertrophic or fibrillary reactive astrocytes are found at the center or at the edge of MS lesions, and their role in gliotic lesion formation and in maintaining the integrity of the blood-brain barrier renders them candidate cells for playing an important role in MS.[120]

Role of Chemokines

Chemokines have recently received attention as potential propagators of the inflammatory response in MS. CCR5 stains periventricular monocytes in early active lesions.[121] Balashov et al.[122] showed an increase in CCR5(+) and CXCR3(+) T cells in MS and an increased expression of their ligands: macrophage inflammatory protein 1 alpha and IFN-γ–inducible protein 10 (IP-10) in MS lesions. This may have therapeutic significance, as both CCR5 and macrophage inflammatory protein 1 alpha are reduced by treatment with IFN-β-1a,[123] and anti–macrophage inflammatory protein 1 antibodies block EAE.[124] Other authors have shown high expression of CCR2, -3, and -5 in postmortem MS brain tissues[125]; elevated levels of RANTES (i.e., regulated upon activation, normal T-cell expressed and secreted)[121]; and increased expression of monocyte chemotactic protein-1 at the center of MS lesions.[126] Localization of these signals in different lesion areas is relevant, as it is known that as the MS plaque expands, the edge of the lesion gradually becomes the site of disease activity, and

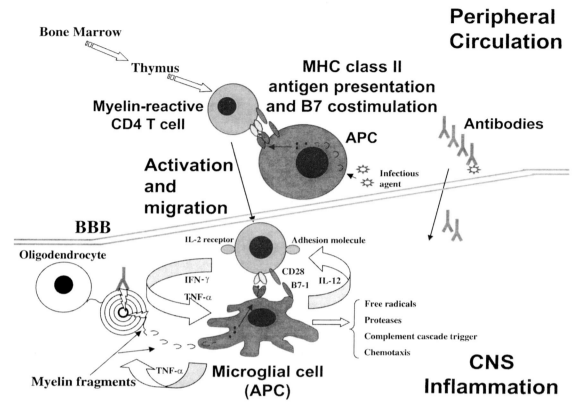

Figure 5-5. Molecular mechanisms in multiple sclerosis. Antigen-presenting cells (APCs), such as peripheral blood macrophages or B cells, present foreign antigen in the context of human leukocyte antigen molecules. If a costimulatory signal, such as that provided by the interaction of B7 and CD28 molecules, is delivered to the T cell, this T cell will become activated (e.g., express the interleukin-2 [IL-2] receptor) and may divide into multiple, identical daughter cells in a process known as *clonal expansion*. The T cell may also gain the ability to kill the APCs in a phenomenon known as *cytotoxicity*. In addition, activated T cells help in activating B cells that then become plasma cells and produce specific antibodies against that same antigen. These antibodies may be cross-reactive against myelin peptides. Activated, antigen-reactive T cells then are able to penetrate the blood-brain barrier (BBB) by their ability to express adhesion molecules such as very late antigen 4. Once in the perivenular space, they may release prodemyelinating (e.g., tumor necrosis factor-α [TNF-α]) and proinflammatory (e.g., interferon gamma [IFN-γ]) cytokines and lead to activation of residential macrophages, known as *microglial cells*. Activated microglial cells release IL-12, a potent proinflammatory cytokine, which in turn leads to more IFN-γ production by activated T cells. These activated microglial cells also release matrix metalloproteinases that damage the extracellular matrix and release oxygen free radicals that damage surrounding tissue. Microglial cells engulf myelin debris and express human leukocyte antigen and costimulatory molecules and have the capacity to present myelin antigens to the activated T cells infiltrating the perivenular space. Finally, activated microglial cells release glutamate and participate in complement activation, leading to further tissue damage. This is a simplistic view of a much more complex process involving multiple molecules, including proteins involved in immune activation, signal transduction, adhesion, apoptosis, and gene regulation. Antibody-producing plasma cells also become part of the cellular infiltrate and are responsible for the intrathecal production of oligoclonal bands. (CNS = central nervous system; MHC = major histocompatibility complex.) (Adapted from F Dangond. Multiple sclerosis. eMedicine Web site: Neurology. Available at: http://www.emedicine.com. Accessed February 2, 2002; Multimedia image courtesy of eMedicine.com, Inc. Copyright © 2001.)

the site of perivenular entry becomes inactive. This may also explain the presence of ring enhancement with gadolinium by MRI, indicating ongoing disease activity at the edge of the lesion.

Glutamate Excitotoxicity

As with primary neurodegenerative diseases, glutamate excitotoxicity has been implicated in MS. Glutamate can be released by neurons and astrocytes[127] and by activated immune cells, including microglia,[128–130] and may result in neuronal and oligodendrocyte injury. Earlier studies had shown that serum glutamate may be elevated several weeks before the onset of exacerbations, reaching a peak during the relapse.[131] More recent evidence of glutamatergic involvement in MS has come from the demonstration of elevated glutamate and aspartate in the CSF of MS patients, which seemed to correlate with the nature and severity of symptoms and disease course,[132] and from the demonstration that EAE can be significantly ameliorated by the use of alpha-amino-3-hydroxy-5-methylisoxazole-4-propionate (AMPA) receptor antagonists.[133,134]

Free Radical–Induced Tissue Damage

Nitrous oxide is a gaseous free radical, and inducible nitric oxide synthase has been shown to be elevated in MS brains[135] and in macrophages within active plaques.[136] Nitric oxide is transformed by superoxide to peroxynitrite, a highly toxic oxidant that leads to lipid peroxidation and tyrosine residue nitration. Extensive nitrotyrosine immunostaining has been identified in EAE brains, within the inflammatory plaques and in the parenchyma, and in a subset of microglia-macrophages.[137] Activated macrophages that phagocytize myelin release reactive oxygen species, and reactive oxygen species scavengers such as catalase prevent myelin uptake, suggesting that reactive oxygen species generation is a prerequisite for phagocytosis.[138] Further evidence that oxygen free radicals may play an important role in MS lesion formation is shown by the demonstration that uric acid, an antioxidant, ameliorates EAE.[139,140] EAE is also prevented by other specific scavengers of nitric oxide or peroxynitrite or by drugs that counteract other oxygen-reactive metabolites.[141,142]

Endogenous or Exogenous Superantigens

Superantigens are highly immunogenic microbial toxins that trigger widespread T-cell activation in the peripheral circulation by interacting simultaneously with the Vβ region of the TCR and with an HLA molecule on the APC. Although exogenous superantigens may be derived from microorganisms, endogenous superantigens may be encoded by retroviruses that have been integrated into the host genome throughout evolution but may still be infectious. For example, the mouse mammary tumor virus is transferred from female mice to offspring through milk. This retrovirus is tumorigenic and encodes for a superantigen that activates immune cells of the recipient mice. Owing to the massive stimulation of the immune system generally seen with superantigen stimulation, it would be interesting to investigate whether superantigen induction plays a role in cases of acute fulminant (Marburg variant) MS or in acute disseminated encephalomyelitis (ADEM).

Immunologic Parameters as Surrogate Markers of Disease Progression

The favorable clinical response to the newer immunomodulatory agents—*A*vonex (IFN-β-1a), *B*etaseron (IFN-β-1b), and *C*opaxone (glatiramer acetate) (ABC)—suggests that these medications work at least in part owing to their ability to counteract the proinflammatory cytokine phenotype of immune cells. There is evidence that an increase in immune cells expressing the activation markers CD25 (IL-2 receptor) and class II HLA correlates with an increase in the number of gadolinium-enhancing lesions in MS.[143] High levels of soluble intercellular adhesion molecule-1 in the circulation of MS patients have been shown to correlate in time with the onset of blood-brain barrier damage.[144–146] In addition, high levels of soluble intercellular adhesion molecule-1 and soluble TNF receptors have been shown to correlate with relapsing-progressive and progressive disease, respectively,[147] suggesting that factors released from activated immune cells can be used as markers of disease or disease progression.

Hormones and the Immune System: The Neuroendocrine-Immune Network

As disease activity for female MS patients seems to be modulated during and shortly after pregnancy and because women have a higher incidence of MS, it is believed that hormonal factors play a role in inducing immune system dysregulation. The hypothalamus-pituitary-adrenal axis links the neuroendocrine system with the immune system, and lymphocytes can express a variety of endocrine factors and receptors, including (among others) the progesterone receptor, pregnancy-specific beta-1 glycoprotein 4; thyroid-stimulating hormone[148]; the thyroid-stimulating hormone receptor[149]; luteinizing hormone-releasing hormone[150]; the adrenocorticotropic hormone receptor[151]; and the prolactin receptor.[152] Prolactin has been shown to enhance the immune response of monocytes and T and B cells,[153] suggesting that it may play a role in postpartum MS exacerbations. In addition, luteinizing hormone-releasing hormone is known to promote IL-2 receptor expression in lymphocytes, suggesting induction of activation.[154] More research is needed to understand the complex endocrine-immune system interactions and their possible role in EAE and MS; to date, no hormonal manipulations have been shown to ameliorate the disease course in humans.

Clinical Aspects of Multiple Sclerosis

MS attacks are characterized by the presence of new symptoms that reflect brain and spinal cord white-matter involvement. In some patients, the disease is characterized by a predominance of visual, cognitive, spinal cord, or cerebellar symptoms. MS symptoms are typically separated in time (usually weeks, months, or years) and in anatomic location (e.g., one or more limbs, optic nerve involvement, sensory symptoms, focal weakness), the latter reflecting the diffuse nature of the CNS involvement. The Schumacher criteria for the definite diagnosis of MS include (1) onset between ages 10–50 years, (2) CNS white-matter disease, (3) lesions disseminated in space and time, (4) objective clinical abnormalities,

(5) attacks lasting more than 1 day and spaced at least 1 month apart with a gradual or stepwise progression over 6 months, and (6) absence of an alternative diagnosis.[155]

Impact of Axonal Loss on Signs and Symptoms

It is now thought that MS patients reach a clinical threshold after which deterioration occurs continuously. Loss of myelin may secondarily lead to loss of trophic support for axons,[156] but inflammatory factors (cytokines, oxidative stress, and complement) may also adversely affect neurons. Other mechanisms that affect neuron viability but are not necessarily related to myelin integrity or the presence of inflammation may play a role in the disease process, but further research is needed to clarify what these mechanisms may be. The latter hypothesis is supported by the observations that (1) immunosuppression does not secondarily prevent neurodegeneration in MS,[157] and (2) in some patients, clinical deterioration may occur from onset without evidence of significant inflammatory-demyelinating lesion formation by MRI or recurrent attacks. MRI follow-up of these patients, however, often reveals early brain atrophy demonstrated as thinning of the corpus callosum and enlargement of the third ventricle, or it shows T_1 hypointensities (T_1 "holes"), indicative of aged lesions. In addition, N-acetylaspartate, which is assumed to be present only in neuronal cell bodies and axons, has been found to be significantly decreased in MS lesions and in surrounding, normal-appearing white matter as measured by magnetic resonance spectroscopy. N-acetylaspartate may be a surrogate marker for axonal loss as its measurement correlates well with disease load,[158] with the presence of T_1 holes,[159–161] and with neurologic disability.[162] A recent report brought attention to abnormalities of N-acetylaspartate in MS patients before the onset of disability, indicating early axonal loss.[163]

Chronic exposure of axons to the soluble factors released by proinflammatory immune cells may exact a heavy toll on their ability to cope with the disease process, and their destruction may be compounded by gliotic scarring. An intriguing possibility is that neurons undergoing degeneration or under the influence of IFN-γ may upregulate their surface expression of class I HLA molecules,[164] resulting in recognition by cytotoxic CD8+ T cells and in further damage. Axonal dropout has been shown to occur even in early MS lesions, and wallerian degeneration has been demonstrated histopathologically[165,166] and suggested by MRI.[167] Recent studies by Trapp et al.[168] have refocused the attention of MS investigators on the neurodegenerative nature of MS. Therefore, MS may be thought of as a primarily inflammatory but secondarily neurodegenerative disease of the CNS. This neurodegenerative process results in brain atrophy, which is usually clinically associated with cognitive decline and other abnormalities of mental function. Preventing atrophy in MS will probably become as important as preventing clinical exacerbations. This represents a challenge for the design of clinical trials, as one may envision interventions that prevent or counteract neuronal loss but do not significantly affect T-cell infiltration into the CNS. Therefore, imaging techniques or other tests that provide surrogate markers of neuronal integrity or myelin repair have to be developed. A recent report of correlation of the presence of urinary MBP-like material in MS patients with advanced disability, without relapses, and with secondary progression[169] will require further scrutiny as to its use in clinical practice and in clinical trials.

Although patients with the primary-progressive form tend to exhibit more involvement of the spinal cord by demyelination, there are MS cases in which clearly this does not apply. Primary-progressive MS patients do not respond to the current therapeutic options for MS, seem to accumulate disability faster than do relapsing-remitting MS patients, and tend to have a higher incidence of urinary incontinence. It remains to be demonstrated whether the primary-progressive form of MS is indeed a different syndrome characterized by a more pronounced axonal degeneration and therefore poor responsiveness to immunomodulatory treatment.

Clinical Spectrum of Multiple Sclerosis: From "Benign" to "Malignant"

The concepts of *benign* and *malignant* MS have not been well defined, and use of these terms remains controversial. Some clinicians apply the term *benign MS* to patients whose Expanded Disability Status Scale (EDSS) score remains less than 2 over several decades. However, the term *benign MS* may be misleading, as many patients with the least aggressive forms (i.e., least frequency of attacks) may still exhibit deterioration in other spheres manifesting as cognitive decline, short-term memory loss, alteration in visuospatial abilities, hypomania, pathologic laughing or crying, or evidence of atrophy by head or spinal cord MRI. MS patients with cognitive deficits perform poorly on multiple tests, including those that examine complex attention (Paced Auditory Serial Addition Test), processing speed (Symbol Digit Modalities Test), and verbal memory (Bushke Verbal Selective Reminding Test), and this deficit correlates with regional (frontoparietal) lesion burden, as assessed by volumetric MRI techniques.[170] If not properly sought in the history, on examination, or by MRI, the evidence for such manifestations may pass unnoticed. As the disease course is so unpredictable for an individual patient and because most patients will eventually develop significant disability with time,[171,172] the prospective use of the term *benign MS* should probably be discouraged. Although admittedly some patients may be assigned retrospectively to the benign MS category, the prospective use of this term often leads to false expectations of disease outcome, improper counseling, and inappropriate delay of treatment with disease-modifying medications.

The term *malignant MS* may be used to describe patients in whom the clinical attacks are fairly disabling from onset (paralysis, dementia, or sometimes coma and death), usually progressing over a short period and typically associated with a large number of gadolinium-enhancing lesions as seen on MRI. Most patients with such florid presentation respond poorly to the ABC immunomodulatory drugs; however, some patients who survive the initial attack may return to a classic, less malignant relapsing-remitting form, and these medications may then be helpful. Malignant MS should also be differentiated from patients who present initially with large demyelinating lesions on MRI but in whom, after follow-up, the lesions are found to decrease in size (Figure 5-6).

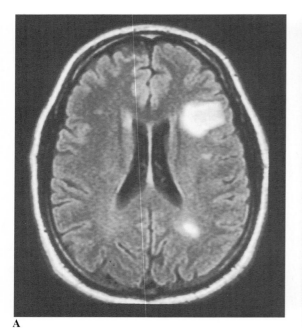
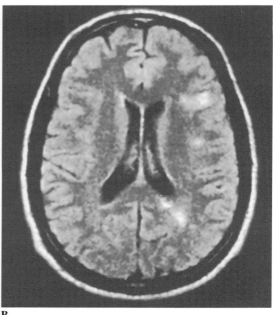

A   B

Figure 5-6. Magnetic resonance imaging (MRI) in a case of relapsing-remitting multiple sclerosis. **A.** Head MRI of a 35-year-old man with relapsing-remitting multiple sclerosis revealing multiple high T_2-signal intensity lesions. There is one large white-matter lesion. These demyelinating lesions may sometimes mimic brain tumors, owing to associated edema and inflammation. **B.** Head MRI of this patient performed 3 months later, showing a dramatic decrease in the size of lesions. See Chapter 8 for a detailed discussion of MRI findings in multiple sclerosis. (Adapted from F Dangond. Multiple sclerosis. eMedicine Web site: Neurology. Available at: http://www.emedicine.com. Accessed February 2, 2002; Multimedia image courtesy of eMedicine.com, Inc. Copyright © 2001.)

Interview and Physical Examination Findings in Multiple Sclerosis Patients

Fatigue is a common complaint of MS patients. By "fatigue," however, patients may mean either physical exhaustion or mental-cognitive slowing. Patients may feel particularly tired after taking a hot shower or after strenuous activity in heated environments. Fatigue symptoms are difficult to treat, but some patients may respond to newer medications, such as modafinil (Provigil) (Table 5-1).

Patients with an advanced, dementing illness (cerebral MS) may exhibit frontal release signs (snout, grasp, rooting, palmomental reflex increase). Another commonly overlooked manifestation of MS is the pseudobulbar affect, which manifests as uncontrolled laughing or weeping and may be absent during the examination. Behavioral-cognitive symptoms may also include social disinhibition, frank dementia, or depression. A higher tendency

for committing suicide (7.5-fold increased risk) in MS patients[173] is not solely related to a reactive depression, as this tendency seems to be higher than that of patients with other devastating neurologic disorders such as chronic inflammatory demyelinating polyradiculopathy. Patients with MS at higher risk of committing suicide are those with an EDSS disability score of approximately 4.5, they are more often male, they have had a disease onset before age 30 years, or they have MS diagnosed near the age of 40 years.[173] Bipolar disorder may be the first manifestation in patients with MS,[174] suggesting that the disease process may trigger an early imbalance of neuronal metabolism.

Optic neuritis (optic nerve inflammation) may occur as an isolated episode, as a prelude to developing MS, or during MS disease progression. Vision loss typically occurs over a 1-week period. If continued progression after this period is found, the physician should consider alternative

Table 5-1. Drugs Commonly Used for the Symptomatic Treatment of Multiple Sclerosis

Symptom	Treatment
Disease exacerbations that cause moderate to severe disability, including vision loss, persistent pain, sudden dysphagia, limb weakness, or gait instability	Intravenous methylprednisolone (Solumedrol), 1 g/day for 3–5 days to speed recovery
Depression	Fluoxetine (Prozac), sertraline (Zoloft), amitriptyline (Elavil), citalopram (Celexa), psychotherapy
Pseudobulbar affect	Haloperidol (Haldol), amitriptyline
Spasticity	Baclofen (Lioresal), tizanidine (Zanaflex), dantrolene (Dantrium), diazepam (Valium), clonazepam (Klonopin), botulinum toxin (Botox) injections, intrathecal baclofen delivered via a surgically implanted programmable pump
Painful tonic spasms	Baclofen, carbamazepine (Tegretol), gabapentin (Neurontin), phenytoin (Dilantin), valproate (Depakote), amitriptyline
Fatigue	Modafinil (Provigil), amantadine (Symmetrel), fluoxetine, methylphenidate (Ritalin), selegiline (Eldepryl), pemoline (Cylert)
Diplopia	Prisms, eye patch
Urinary dysfunction	Propantheline bromide (Pro-Banthine), tolterodine tartrate (Detrol), oxybutynin (Ditropan), imipramine (Tofranil), bethanechol (Urecholine), intermittent self-catheterization, condom catheter, Credé's maneuver, suprapubic tapping
Bowel dysfunction	Enemas, suppositories, laxatives, or high-fiber diets for constipation; anticholinergics or loperamide (Imodium) for incontinence
Tremors, ataxia	Clonazepam (Klonopin), primidone (Mysoline), propranolol (Inderal), weighted bracelets
Erectile dysfunction	Sildenafil citrate (Viagra), alprostadil (Muse), intracorporeal papaverine (not FDA-approved), penile prostheses, psychotherapy
Female sexual dysfunction	Lubricant gels (for dryness), local stimulants (for sensory loss), psychotherapy
Flu-like symptoms (treatment-associated)	Ibuprofen or other nonsteroidal anti-inflammatory drugs, acetaminophen (Tylenol)

FDA = U.S. Food and Drug Administration.

causes for the visual symptoms. Approximately 50% of MS patients will at some point develop optic neuritis symptoms. Optic neuritis may be identified as swelling of the optic nerve head (papillitis) seen on funduscopy. When the optic nerve head is not involved, the term *retrobulbar optic neuritis* is preferred. In such case, no funduscopic abnormalities may be evident. However, the clinician may be able to identify an afferent pupillary defect, also known as a *Marcus Gunn pupil*, in which alternative shining of a light (i.e., every 3 seconds) on each pupil leads to paradoxical dilatation in the affected side. Symptoms of optic neuritis include visual blurring, retro- or periorbital pain at rest and exacerbated by movement of the eye (more than 90% of patients), color desaturation (perception of red as gray or

orange), or contrast sensitivity. The pain tends to last only a few days. Visual field testing may reveal a cecocentral scotoma associated with involvement of the optic nerve. Altitudinal field defects, although typical of anterior ischemic optic neuropathy, may also be demonstrated. Optic neuritis may occur bilaterally and may recur several times in MS patients.

Once the acute or subacute disease stage is completed, the optic disk may become atrophic and pale, reflecting the fate of similarly affected regions in the brain parenchyma that culminate in atrophy, presumably the result of residual gliotic scarring and loss of axonal integrity. The lesions can sometimes extend to involve the optic chiasm. However, more than two-thirds of patients with optic neuritis experience nearly total resolution of their symptoms. Even despite resolution, symptoms of optic neuritis may recur after exposure to higher body temperatures (Uhthoff's phenomenon) or after strenuous exercise. Field defects of the homonymous type may occur in MS owing to involvement of optic radiations, but these are rarely found.

Direction-changing or pendular nystagmus, saccadic intrusions, square wave jerks, or internuclear ophthalmoplegia are signs often seen in MS. Internuclear ophthalmoplegia is the inability to adduct one eye (on the side of the lesion) while the other eye is fully abducted but exhibiting persistent horizontal nystagmus. The lesion is localized to the medial longitudinal fasciculus pathways in the brain stem; thus, internuclear ophthalmoplegia is not exclusively found in MS.

Bilateral facial weakness or trigeminal neuralgia strongly suggests the diagnosis of MS, but most commonly these symptoms are present in only one side. Linear lesions involving the intrapontine trigeminal root and mimicking herpetic lesions seen in experimental animals have been shown by MRI in MS.[175] Facial myokymia, or bag-of-worms–like undulating movements of facial muscles, may also be a manifestation of MS and may respond to botulinum toxin treatment.[176] However, facial myokymia as an isolated symptom can occur in other diseases, including brain stem gliomas.[177] Symptoms in MS that resemble isolated cranial neuropathies are instead the result of involvement of such nerves in their intraparenchymal (i.e., brain stem) course; therefore, the disease is still considered CNS specific.

Episodes of central vertigo are not uncommon, occurring in at least one-third of MS patients. The nystagmus that accompanies central vertigo symptoms has a rapid onset, does not fatigue easily, and changes with direction of gaze. CNS vertigo is usually accompanied by other neurologic complaints that can be directly attributed to cranial nerve or brain stem involvement (i.e., diplopia and dysarthria). Tinnitus may be a common manifestation of MS. MS-related acute deafness is less common and is usually the result of a demyelinating lesion in the eighth nerve, close to the pontomedullary junction.[178]

Motor symptoms include weakness and reflex contractions, and motor signs include hyperreflexia (Hoffman's sign, clonus, crossed-adductor hyperreflexia); other long-tract signs (upgoing toes); and spontaneous, paroxysmal spasms of limbs. These tonic spasms typically respond well to low doses of carbamazepine, although their natural course dictates their spontaneous disappearance with time. Most motor symptoms tend to begin asymmetrically and, except for the patients with primary-progressive MS, most symptoms of weakness reach maximum severity acutely or subacutely, reflecting the presence of an exacerbation. Weakness of hip flexion or the new onset of a foot drop is not unusual. Atrophy of muscles occurs secondarily to limb disuse rather than to true denervation. Occasionally, the enhanced tone may help affected patients to maintain their posture or their gait stability, and antispasticity agents must thus be used with caution. It is important to remind patients that exposure to high temperatures exacerbates not only optic neuritis–related symptoms but also other symptoms and signs of MS, including weakness.

Sensory dysfunction is the most common symptomatology attributed to MS, with practically all patients having experienced some degree of numbness, tingling, "pins and needles," hyper- or hypoalgesia, loss of vibration, or loss of position sense. It is not unusual to demonstrate a sensory level or autonomic manifestations such as limb discoloration or swelling suggesting reflex sympathetic dystrophy. A history of sciatica-like radicular pains may be elicited, and it is believed that these symptoms arise as the result of dorsal root entry zone involvement by MS lesions. Bilateral symptoms circumscribed to discrete anatomic pathways of the spinal cord such as marked loss of proprioception and vibration sense in the lower extremities (suggesting posterior column involvement) should alert the physician to explore other diagnostic possibilities, including vitamin B_{12} deficiency or human immunodeficiency virus myelopathy.

Cerebellar manifestations also include end-of-intention tremor, central or appendicular ataxia, dysarthria sometimes progressing to anarthria, head titubation, frank truncal instability, and inability to fixate gaze. The examination may reveal hypotonia, incoordination of fine finger movements, dysmetria, and abnormal heel-to-shin maneuver. More subtle cerebellar deficits may be detected by asking affected patients to tap each foot several times successively against the examiner's hand, with the loss of rhythmicity on one foot suggesting ipsilateral cerebellar pathway dysfunction.

Multiple Sclerosis and Pregnancy

As stated, MS can be exacerbated during the postpartum period presumably by hormonal changes. A lower rate of attacks during pregnancy, especially during the third trimester, has also been demonstrated.[179,180] In studies involving small numbers of patients,[181,182] intravenous immunoglobulin has been reported to eliminate postpartum exacerbations. In the long term, multiparous women do not seem to acquire a higher risk of disability from the disease in comparison to nulliparous women also affected with MS.[183] Others have suggested that women who become pregnant after MS onset tend to progress less rapidly to assignment of a disability score of 6.[184]

Patients who want to become pregnant should stop administration of the ABC immunomodulatory drugs. These medications may be resumed a few weeks after delivery; however, patients should not breast-feed after the medications are restarted.

Optic Neuritis and the Risk of Developing Multiple Sclerosis

The risk of developing clinically definite MS after a first episode of optic neuritis has been calculated at 30% in 5 years, but risk ranges from 16% in patients without lesions seen by MRI to 51% or more in patients with three or more MRI lesions.[20] Some consider isolated optic neuritis a forme fruste of MS, as both occur more commonly in women and in northern latitudes and share similarities in HLA data, family history, CSF and serum findings, pathology, and incidence.[185] Some studies have noted that the earlier the age at which optic neuritis develops, the higher the risk for developing MS,[186] but this is not supported by other reports.[187] The presence of OCBs in patients with optic neuritis also correlates with a significantly greater risk of developing MS.[188]

Transverse Myelitis and Risk of Multiple Sclerosis

The acute or subacute onset of symptoms indicative of isolated spinal cord involvement signals an episode of transverse myelitis. This myelitis can be categorized as complete or incomplete (partial). For patients with complete transverse myelitis, the risk for devel-

oping clinically definite MS is approximately 8%, much lower than that for patients with incomplete myelopathic signs, 20% of whom go on to develop MS even in the absence of cranial MRI-revealed lesions.[189] These risks increase in the presence of OCBs or of multiple lesions as seen by cranial or spinal cord MRI.

Measuring Disability

Kurtzke's EDSS[190] is used as a disease progression measure by assigning a severity score (0–9.5) to patients' clinical status (10 is death due to MS). Although the scale is not linear with relation to the natural progression rate of MS patients (scores from 4 to 7 correlate better with ability to walk, upper extremity function is not well addressed, and patients with scores of more than 4 progress more rapidly than do those with lower scores), its widespread use and ease of implementation allow its use as a standardization measure for clinical trials (Table 5-2). The Multiple Sclerosis Functional Composite is a new measure that includes scores for arm dexterity, walking speed, and cognition and is gaining acceptance for use as an outcome measure in MS clinical trials.[191]

Diagnostic Studies

Cerebrospinal Fluid Examination

OCBs are demonstrated in CSF samples of at least 85% of MS patients. OCBs are distinct electrophoretic patterns that reflect substantial elevation of positively charged IgG produced by clonally derived plasma cells of restricted but unknown specificity. Recent reports suggest that some OCBs in MS may represent responses to several different common viruses such as rubella, mumps, or varicella zoster.[192] However, it is not known whether some of these bands represent a response to an infectious agent highly relevant to the disease process. Some authors have suggested that the absence of CSF OCBs may signal a more benign course for MS.[193]

The CSF IgG index is often elevated. This index is derived from the following formula:

$$\text{IgG index} = \frac{\text{CSF IgG}/\text{CSF albumin}}{\text{Serum IgG}/\text{Serum albumin}}$$

Table 5-2. Kurtzke's Expanded Disability Status Scale

Grade	Definition
0	Normal neurologic examination (all grade 0 in FS, cerebral grade 1 acceptable)
1.0	No disability, minimal signs in one FS (one grade 1 excluding cerebral grade 1)
1.5	No disability, minimal signs in more than one FS (more than one grade 1 excluding cerebral grade 1)
2.0	Minimal disability in one FS (one FS grade 2, others 0 or 1), 2.5 minimal disability in two FS (two FS grade 2, others 0 or 1)
3.0	Moderate disability in one FS (one FS grade 3, others 0 or 1) or mild disability in three or four FS (three to four FS grade 2, others 0 or 1)
3.5	Fully ambulatory but with moderate disability in one FS (one grade 3 and one or two FS grade 2); or two FS grade 3, others 0 or 1; or five FS grade 2, others 0 or 1
4.0	Fully ambulatory without aid, self-sufficient, up and about some 12 hrs/day despite relatively severe disability consisting of one FS grade 4 (others 0 or 1) or combinations of lesser grades exceeding limits of previous steps; able to walk without aid or rest some 500 m (0.3 mi)
4.5	Fully ambulatory without aid, up and about much of the day, able to work a full day, may otherwise have some limitation of full activity or require minimal assistance; characterized by relatively severe disability, usually consisting of one FS grade 4 (others 0 or 1) or combinations of lesser grades exceeding limits of previous steps; able to walk without aid or rest for some 300 m (975 ft)
5.0	Ambulatory without aid or rest for approximately 200 m (650 ft); disability severe enough to impair full daily activities (e.g., to work full day without special provisions) (usual FS equivalents: one grade 5 alone, others 0 or 1; or combinations of lesser grades usually exceeding specifications for step 4.0)
5.5	Ambulatory without aid or rest for approximately 100 m (325 ft); disability severe enough to impair full daily activities (usual FS equivalents: one grade 5 alone, others 0 or 1; or combinations of lesser grades usually exceeding specifications for grade 4.0)
6.0	Intermittent or constant unilateral assistance (cane, crutch, brace) required to walk approximately 100 m (325 ft) with or without resting (usual FS equivalents: combinations with more than two FS grade 3+)
6.5	Constant bilateral assistance (canes, crutches, braces) required to walk approximately 20 m (65 ft) (usual FS equivalents: combinations with more than two FS grade 3+)
7.0	Unable to walk beyond approximately 5 m (16 ft) even with aid, essentially restricted to wheelchair; wheels self in standard wheelchair a full day and transfers alone; up and about in wheelchair some 12 hrs/day (usual FS equivalents: combinations with more than one FS grade 4+; very rarely pyramidal grade 5 alone)
7.5	Unable to take more than a few steps; restricted to wheelchair; may need aid in transfers, wheels self but cannot carry on in standard wheelchair a full day; may require motorized wheelchair (usual FS equivalents: combinations with more than one FS grade 4+)
8.0	Essentially restricted to bed or chair or perambulated in wheelchair, but may be out of bed much of the day; retains many self-care functions; generally has effective use of arms (usual FS equivalents: combinations, generally grade 4+ in several systems)
8.5	Essentially restricted to bed for much of the day; has some effective use of one or both arms; retains some self-care functions (usual FS equivalents: combinations, generally grade 4+ in several systems)
9.0	Helpless bed patient; can communicate and eat (usual FS equivalents: combinations, mostly grade 4)
9.5	Totally helpless bed patient; unable to communicate effectively or eat and swallow (usual FS equivalents: combinations, almost all grade 4+)
10.0	Death due to multiple sclerosis

FS = functional system.

Source: Reprinted with permission from JF Kurtzke. Rating neurologic impairment in multiple sclerosis: an expanded disability status scale (EDSS). Neurology 1983;33:1444–1452.

Although the range of detection may vary among various laboratories, a normal CSF IgG is typically less than 4.7 mg/dl (less than 12% of total protein), and the normal IgG index is less than 0.8. Most MS patients exhibit an elevated IgG index higher than 1.7. Other chronic infections such as subacute sclerosing panencephalitis, Lyme neuroborreliosis, neurosyphilis, human T-cell lymphotropic virus type I–associated myelopathy/tropical spastic paraparesis, as well as autoimmune neuropathies may test positive for the presence of CSF OCBs.

MBP is a major component of the myelin sheath and may be elevated in the CSF of MS patients.[194] However, its clinical use as a marker of presumed demyelination or disease activity is limited and therefore not widely used.

CSF glucose is usually normal. CSF protein can be normal or slightly elevated; a protein count higher than 100 mg/dl should strongly raise suspicion about other inflammatory diseases. White blood cells in the CSF can be slightly to moderately elevated, and the majority are T-lymphocytes. However, it is not unusual for MS patients to present with normal CSF cell counts. Cell counts higher than 100 or the presence of neutrophils should raise strong suspicion about other inflammatory conditions.

Role of Magnetic Resonance Imaging and Newer Imaging Techniques

Lesion formation in MS occurs constantly, and the clinical course leads to progressive physical disability. This dynamic nature of the disease can be demonstrated by serial MRI investigations (see Chapter 8). MRI shows high T_2-signal intensity lesions of variable location in the white matter of the brain, brain stem, optic nerves, or spinal cord. T_2 hyperintensities in MS may comprise several different types of lesions including new plaques, resolving inflammation, or more chronic lesions. Brain lesions tend to occur in periventricular areas or in the corpus callosum. The administration of gadolinium reveals that blood-brain barrier disruption occurs early during lesion initiation, and this is consistent with the histopathologic demonstration of interstitial and perivascular edema or immune cell infiltration. It is estimated that for every 8–10 new lesions seen by MRI, only one to two clinical manifestations can be demonstrated. This discrepancy may be explained by (1) the appearance of lesions in "silent" brain regions or (2) by small cellular infiltrates that can be detected by MRI but are not large enough to cause dysfunction. Conversely, clinical attacks that have no MRI correlates may be explained by cellular infiltrates in the white matter that localize to particularly vulnerable "nonsilent" regions but that are too small to be detected

by MRI (see Color Plate 10 for an example of a small MS infiltrate by histology). Relapsing-remitting MS patients with active disease may have an average of 2–6 new lesions per year and one or two clinical exacerbations, but patients with more active disease may develop more than 10 lesions and numerous attacks. Newer MRI techniques, which include magnetization transfer, fluid-attenuated inversion recovery, and magnetic resonance spectroscopy, promise to yield important information regarding MS clinical heterogeneity, prognostic factors, presence of disease in otherwise normal-appearing white matter, and treatment effects (see Chapter 8).

Electrophysiologic Tests

The measurement of electrical events in the brain as a response to visual, auditory, or somatosensory stimuli can be recorded in an evoked potential laboratory. With the advent of MRI, evoked potentials are rarely used now and are reserved for the detection of chronic, subtle lesions in the spinal cord or optic nerves—anatomic regions in which MRI may not be as sensitive. The visual-evoked potentials are the most sensitive (50–85% sensitivity) and are followed in sensitivity by the somatosensory evoked potentials (50–70% sensitivity). Brain stem auditory-evoked responses have a sensitivity of 50–65% in detecting the presence of CNS lesions. These electrophysiologic tests are discussed in Chapter 7.

Histopathology

Rarely, demyelinating inflammatory lesions may present as large masses mimicking brain tumors, and a brain biopsy is performed to rule out a malignancy. Histopathologic examination reveals the typical perivenular infiltration of lymphocytes (most of which are CD4[+] T cells) and macrophages, with some series reporting variable degrees of demyelination.[195] An acute presentation with only one or a few large inflammatory lesions and no evidence of further progression over the years does not represent MS but may rather be a variant of ADEM. Transected axons may be found in chronic (and sometimes in acute) MS lesions.[168]

Differential Diagnosis

Other diseases may resemble MS clinically or by imaging techniques. The presence of systemic symptoms such as diffuse skin rash, recurrent fevers, or malaise should make the clinician suspect diseases other than MS. These diseases are discussed more extensively in Chapter 10. Briefly, disorders thought to be closely related to MS are mentioned here.

Multiple Sclerosis Variants versus Distinct Disorders

- Rare cases of optic nerve involvement are accompanied by a necrotizing myelopathy (Devic's disease, neuromyelitis optica) in which cystic, necrotic lesions and prominent vascularization can be demonstrated.[196] Some authors consider Devic's disease a variant of MS.
- MS may also present in an acute and clinically fulminant form (termed *Marburg's variant* of MS), which may lead to coma or death within a few days or weeks.[197,198]
- ADEM is an isolated postinfectious or postvaccinial autoimmune attack on the CNS, often devastating. In its most fulminant form, ADEM presents with hemorrhagic lesions, and the terms *acute hemorrhagic encephalomyelitis* or *Hurst hemorrhagic leukoencephalitis* are used.[199,200] Rare cases of forme fruste ADEM presenting with unifocal or unihemispheric lesions may be a challenge for diagnosis, but a carefully obtained patient history documenting prior exposure to an infectious agent or immunization should help to clarify it.[201]
- Schilder's disease is characterized in children and young adolescents by massive and often asymmetric demyelination (often occupying an entire lobe region). It follows a malignant course (i.e., deterioration over months or a few years with cortical blindness or hemi- or paraplegia). Some cases, however, may respond to corticosteroids and immunosuppressive therapy.
- Baló's concentric sclerosis is considered by some authors to be a variant of Schilder's disease, with lesions shown by MRI as a characteristic alternating pattern of sparing and damage that suggests progression of the disease process

from the periventricular regions outward. Baló's concentric sclerosis is usually associated with a more inflammatory CSF and a more fulminant course than those seen in typical MS.[202]

Treatment

Therapeutic intervention with disease-modifying drugs is discussed in Chapter 9. This section covers issues pertaining to palliative, medical (see Table 5-1), and consultative options for patients with MS and is followed by a description of potential new therapeutic approaches in MS.

Medical-Palliative Care

Patients with MS have multiple needs, and it is the neurologist's responsibility to seek a comprehensive team approach, which includes physical therapy and access to rehabilitation and orthotic equipment. Support from family members in helping to accomplish goals, pursue interests, and maintain fundamental values is key for the patient's mental well-being; however, many patients with advanced forms of the disease may have already lost the support of family and friends and constantly require psychiatric and nursing assistance. These patients create a challenge for the physician who is not trained in handling these demanding aspects of medical care.

Treatment of weakness is difficult and largely relies on physical therapy aid and rehabilitation measures. The physical therapist should devise an individualized treatment program that considers the patient's degree of mobility in bed and need for adaptive equipment and should assess tone, strength and conditioning, coordination, and balance as well as teach sensory compensation techniques. 3,4-Diaminopyridine has been shown to improve leg strength significantly; however, this medication does not seem to alter the EDSS score and is associated with side effects such as paresthesias, abdominal pain, confusion, and, less frequently, seizures.[203] More clinical trials of 3,4-diaminopyridine in MS are required to define better such issues as compliance, impact on quality of life, adverse effects, and long-term efficacy.

In addition, neurologists should not underestimate the impact of fatigue symptoms on the patient's ability to perform daily activities. Treatment with amantadine (Symmetrel) or modafinil should be attempted. Other conditions that may present as fatigue or asthenia such as hypothyroidism, anemia, depression, drug use or abuse, or a chronic concomitant illness should also be considered. Patients should receive recommendations to plan daily activities, take naps or periods of rest at specific times, and exercise regularly.

Consultations

MS patients may require multiple consultations to rule out other causes for their symptoms. For example, dysphonia symptoms may merit an evaluation by an otolaryngologist to rule out laryngeal lesions unrelated to MS. Significant dysarthria or dysphagia merits a rehabilitative team approach. The neurologist should always consider the possibility of concomitant peripheral neuropathy, herpes zoster radiculopathy, or other illnesses that may cause pain. Aids such as home and motor vehicle alterations are aimed to improve the quality of life of MS patients.

The most common consultant services used at our MS clinic are listed here:

- Gastroenterology
- Urology
- Ear, nose, and throat
- Ophthalmology
- Neuropsychology
- Psychiatry
- Physical or occupational therapy and rehabilitation
- Rheumatology
- Orthopedics

Surgical Care

Surgical procedures that relate to MS are primarily directed to help alleviate symptoms such as dysphagia (gastrojejunal tube placement), significant limb spasticity or contractures (adductor leg muscle tendon release), urinary dysfunction (supravesical diversion, transurethral external sphincterotomy), or severe neuropathic pain (rhizotomy). The surgical implantation of pumps for intrathecal delivery of antispasticity medications (e.g., baclofen) has

also proven to be beneficial. MS patients with weakness, vertigo, or ataxia and multiple falls may sustain fractures, especially if suffering from chronic corticosteroid–induced osteoporosis; these cases commonly require orthopedic consultation.

Diet

MS patients are encouraged to eat a balanced diet, but there are no specific restrictions known to change the course of the illness. Any balanced diet that the patient acknowledges as contributing to his or her well-being should be encouraged by the physician.

Effects of Activity, Emotional Stress, Heat, and Trauma

Patients are encouraged to exercise regularly but to avoid strenuous exercise that may lead to exhaustion and excessive heat exposure, as increased body temperature has been associated with triggering MS symptoms. Although sunlight by itself is not considered to be deleterious, it is conceivable that excessive exposure and warming may mimic the effects seen with hot showers. The impact of stress on MS exacerbations is thought to be minimal or noncontributory, and trauma has no real impact on triggering attacks or affecting disease course.[204]

Management of Urinary Symptoms

Urinary retention, hesitancy, or incontinence are common symptoms in MS affecting up to 78%.[205–207] The management of urinary symptoms of patients is especially challenging, because the symptomatology may change over time as is seen with other symptoms of the disease. Patients may also be more prone to urinary tract infections, and acidification of the urine with cranberry juice or vitamin C may be worthwhile. Urodynamic studies are required to establish the best possible treatment approach, because, in more than one-half of cases, the patient's complaints do not correlate with the actual pathophysiologic mechanisms uncovered by these studies.[208] A postvoid residual can be determined using straight catheterization or ultrasound techniques. An acceptable postvoid residual is less than 100 ml. Urodynamic studies (subtracted filling, voiding cystometry, external sphincter electromyography) in MS are most often consistent with detrusor hyper-reflexia, which manifests clinically as urgency and may respond to anticholinergics. Voluntary changes in voiding schedule (delaying or prompting), behavioral modification, and avoidance of caffeine or alcohol should be recommended. If these fail, surgical procedures such as augmentation cystoplasty and selective sacral rhizotomy, may be required.[209]

Detrusor sphincter dyssynergia occurs when there is loss of the normal reflex relaxation of the bladder neck that precedes detrusor contraction, which results in the simultaneous contraction of sphincter and detrusor. Detrusor sphincter dyssynergia accompanies detrusor hyperreflexia. Dyssinergia may respond to antispasticity agents, anti–alpha-adrenergic agents, or anticholinergics used in conjunction with intermittent catheterization.[210] If these measures fail, surgical interventions such as external sphincterotomy, indwelling urethral stent, or urinary diversion may be required.[209]

Detrusor areflexia leads to a large, flaccid bladder that does not empty well. Detrusor areflexia is rare in MS, does not respond well to Credé's or Valsalva's maneuvers or to drugs, and often is treated surgically with urinary diversion. The neurologist should be aware that the presence of genital-sacral hypoesthesia may impair the patient's ability to perceive fullness of the bladder and may therefore exacerbate overflow incontinence. Some patients have limitations of manual dexterity or vision that prevent their compliance with self-catheterization. Acute urinary retention should be treated with catheterization or, if there is documented outflow obstruction, relief by surgical measures.

Management of Bowel Symptoms

Bowel habit changes may occur, usually owing to constipation, but bowel incontinence is a rare complaint in MS patients. When it occurs, however, it tends to be socially and psychologically devastating. An examination should be undertaken to document neurologic involvement of the sacral-anorectal region; the physician should be aware of alterna-tive reasons for incontinence, including chronic diarrhea, anatomic defects, history of pelvic trauma, postsurgical complications, and anal sphincter or puborectalis muscle dysfunction associated with obstetric injury. Stool bulk–forming agents and diet modification may be tried. Surgical procedures to correct anatomic defects (i.e., rectocele) may be required. A rare but treatable cause of fecal incontinence in MS and other neurologic disorders is pneumatosis coli, a condition characterized by collections of encysted gas within the submucosa or subserosa of the colon and rectum, which may respond to continuous oxygen therapy.[211]

Management of Sexual Dysfunction

The management of sexual dysfunction in MS patients is especially challenging. A wide range of symptoms in men with MS, including erectile dysfunction, premature ejaculation, impaired genital sensation, loss of libido, or the inability to interact physically with the sexual partner owing to painful leg adductor muscle spasms, has been reported. New drug options for erectile dysfunction have significantly improved the management of male MS patients (see Table 5-1).

Women with MS most commonly complain of impaired genital sensation, vaginal dysesthesias, decreased vaginal lubrication, orgasmic dysfunction, and loss of libido. Depression, fatigue, drug effects, and menopause may contribute to these symptoms. More research is needed to understand better the mechanisms of sexual dysfunction in women with MS so that appropriate therapies can be instituted. Comprehensive care of male and female MS patients should address sexual dysfunction issues, and efforts to treat expeditiously should be implemented, as improvement may have a significant impact on patients' self-esteem and quality of life.

Interventions Based on Current Knowledge of Immune Mechanisms

Although some controversy still exists regarding the autoimmune nature of MS, pathologic studies unquestionably show that it is a CNS disease with a prominent inflammatory component. Several treatments have thus been designed on the basis of our current understanding of immune cell interactions in MS and of the demonstrated impact of cytokine imbalance in triggering or maintaining disease. Studies using IFN-γ[212,213] in MS patients led to the demonstration that proinflammatory factors may exacerbate the disease and suggested that agents that would counteract these factors would be beneficial for MS patients. The presumed modes of action of the ABC immunomodulatory drugs are summarized in Table 5-3. These medications and their use in clinical trials are discussed in Chapter 9.

Treatment of "presumed MS" with immunomodulatory drugs is not indicated. The neurologist should have a fairly reasonable diagnosis based at least on patient history, clinical examination, and MRI findings. Treatment based on suspicion but not on a definitive diagnosis can lead to unnecessary emotional and long-term financial costs for the patient and relatives and should be avoided. An exception should be considered: Recent results of the Controlled High Risk Avonex Multiple Sclerosis[214] and Early Treatment of MS trials suggest that IFN-β-1a may be beneficial in patients with an isolated clinical attack and with MRI findings highly suggestive of MS. The Controlled High Risk Avonex Multiple Sclerosis trial found significantly fewer new lesions in treated patients as compared with those receiving placebo and found an adjusted reduction of 51% in the occurrence of a second attack. In the Early Treatment of MS study, the reduction was approximately 24%. It is, therefore, suggested that only patients with a classic MRI picture of MS may be treated after the first attack, as more than 60% of patients with a first attack and an MRI scan highly suggestive of MS will go on to develop ongoing disease manifestations. However, postinfectious demyelination or other diseases that mimic MS should be considered carefully. Follow-up should be performed to ascertain whether the episode was self-limited. In patients with stereotyped and vague symptomatology, it is not unusual to encounter other conditions such as migraine headaches, a history of childhood meningoencephalitis, or other antecedent illness that may explain MS-mimicking lesions seen by MRI. Recently, new guidelines for the diagnosis of MS have been released by an international panel, and the reader is encouraged to review these detailed recommendations.[215] On the basis of the

Table 5-3. U.S. Food and Drug Administration–Approved Avonex, Betaseron, and Copaxone (ABC) Immunomodulators and Some Known Modes of Action*

Interferon beta-1a (Avonex) and interferon beta-1b (Betaseron)
Reduce T-cell proliferation
Downregulate major histocompatibility complex expression and antigen presentation
Downregulate B7-1 expression
Downregulate tumor necrosis factor-α production
Downregulate macrophage inflammatory protein-1α
Downregulate interferon gamma production
Downregulate CCR5
Upregulate interleukin-10 secretion
Modulate expression of adhesion molecules, metalloproteinases, chemokines
Counteract viral protein synthesis
Glatiramer acetate (Copaxone)
Widespread induction of suppressor immune cells
Competition with myelin basic protein for antigen presentation
Modulation of macrophage function

*Although the effects listed in this table should potentially have an impact on multiple sclerosis progression or rate of relapses, many still undiscovered mechanisms could be playing a role. All ABC drugs reduce clinical relapse rate and variably inhibit the development of new gadolinium-enhancing lesions by magnetic resonance imaging in multiple sclerosis. A shift from production of Th1 proinflammatory cytokines such as interferon gamma and tumor necrosis factor-α to a Th2 (immunoregulatory, prohumoral) phenotype may play a key role in the immunomodulatory action of these drugs. Whether glatiramer acetate actually competes with myelin proteins remains a controversial issue.

Controlled High Risk Avonex Multiple Sclerosis and Early Treatment of MS trials, there is increasing impetus for clinicians to start early therapy for MS even after a single attack; therefore, new drugs tested in clinical trials will have to contend with the fact that most early patients will already have started treatment.

It is imperative to prevent disease progression by using available medications, especially for patients with MS diagnosed early and probably responsive to treatment. Drugs that not only prevent relapses but also prevent disability are needed in MS. Several recently proposed treatments have been initially disappointing, and others still hold significant promise. These potential therapies are discussed next (Table 5-4).

Table 5-4.   Potential New Treatments for Multiple Sclerosis*

T-cell receptor peptide vaccination

Myelin peptides/mimics by different routes of administration or with different dosing schedules

Combination therapy with disease-modifying drugs

Different routes of administration for disease-modifying drugs

Cancer treatment adapted for multiple sclerosis treatment

Intravenous immunoglobulin

Hormonal manipulation

Extracorporeal removal of serum factors or cells

Stem cell– or oligodendrocyte progenitor–based transplantation, growth factors, myelin repair–inducing agents

Antibody therapies against adhesion molecules, against matrix metalloproteinases, against proinflammatory soluble or surface molecules, against costimulatory molecules (treatment with cytotoxic T lymphocyte–associated antigen 4 fusion protein immunoglobulin [CTLA4Ig] or anti-B7 antibodies), against antigens that interfere with remyelination

Macrophage activation blockers

Manipulation of complement pathways

Soluble anti-inflammatory factors, including Th2 phenotype–promoting cytokines

Soluble receptors for inflammatory cytokines

Small molecules

Targeted manipulation of specific cells of the immune system

Targeted manipulation of blood-brain barrier permeability

Prevention of glutamate and oxygen free radical injury

Antiviral compounds

Gene therapy via implantation of genetically modified stem cells or via other vectors

Bone marrow transplant

*Most of these treatments are under investigation.

Antibodies Against Integrins

Antibodies against α4β1 integrin (very late antigen 4)—a leukocyte receptor that binds vascular cell adhesion molecule 1 on the surface of endothelial cells—significantly decrease disease activity in the guinea pig EAE model.[216,217] Humanized monoclonal antibodies against α4β1 integrin (natalizumab [Antegren]) have been used in patients with MS. Initial studies have shown that at least in the short term, administration of natalizumab leads to a statistically significant reduction in the number of new lesions.[218] More studies are being conducted to assess the response to long-term administration and the safety profile of this treatment.

Lymphocyte-Depleting Antibodies

Treatment with anti-CD52 (Campath-1H)—a humanized antibody that depletes peripheral blood mononuclear cells—significantly reduces inflammation in the brain of MS patients, as evidenced by the presence of fewer gadolinium-enhancing lesions. However, this treatment has led to exacerbation of MS symptoms after the first dose,[157] and up to one-third of patients develop autoimmune thyroiditis, indicating a switch from a Th1 cellular phenotype to a Th2 humoral phenotype.[157] In addition, the treatment did not prevent the progression of brain and spinal cord atrophy in these patients.[219]

Transforming Growth Factor β Pathway

Transforming growth factor β has properties that would make it the ideal candidate for MS therapy: It is a potent immunosuppressor that downregulates microglial activation and proliferation and counteracts the effects of IFN-γ (i.e., upregulation of HLA class II and Fc receptor by microglia)[220] and the production of TNF-α.[221] However, serious adverse effects, including tissue fibrosis and renal insufficiency, have made this potential treatment less appealing than originally thought. Perhaps more subtle transforming growth factor β pathway manipulations that minimize side effects could bring new opportunities for treatment.

Tumor Necrosis Factor-α Pathway

A soluble, recombinant TNF receptor—Fc fusion protein (etanercept [Enbrel])—which is highly effective in rheumatoid arthritis and theoretically should be helpful in MS, has been unexpectedly associated with a higher incidence of MS-like lesions in patients treated for rheumatoid arthritis.

Mucosal Tolerance Pathway

The concept of and experimental evidence for oral tolerance dates back to 1911, when H. Gideon Wells[222] at the University of Chicago demonstrated that oral ovalbumin administration prevented fatal hyperergic reactions to intravenously administered ovalbumin in experimental animals; these experiments were later followed by Merrill W. Chase's demonstration in 1946[223] at the Rockefeller Institute that oral administration of 2DNP-benzene prevented the allergic skin reaction triggered by the intracutaneous injection of the same chemical. Higgins and Weiner[224] proposed and demonstrated that the concept of oral tolerance could be expanded to include the administration of self-antigens, such as myelin proteins, as tolerogens. A series of sound observations later suggested that in the EAE model, oral myelin may lead to the generation of a suppressor type of lymphocyte, actively secreting transforming growth factor β.[225] Besides inducing active suppression, oral tolerance may also lead to clonal anergy and clonal deletion of immune cells. Reports from investigators around the world confirmed that several different models of autoimmunity (i.e., collagen-induced arthritis, S-antigen–induced uveitis) seem to respond dramatically to oral tolerance induction with target organ–specific peptides.[226,227]

After the demonstration that oral tolerance treatment in humans was safe,[228] a double-blind phase III study of bovine myelin in relapsing-remitting MS with daily dosing for a 2-year period was conducted. Patients were randomly assigned prospectively by gender and HLA-DR type. Against expectations, no difference in the primary end point (relapse rate) or in disability scales could be demonstrated in this large-scale study, although a statistically significant decrease in T_2-lesion volume correlated with oral myelin treatment in a subset of male DR2(–) MS patients. Several reasons for the apparent failure of oral tolerance induction in humans are possible:

1. The dose used in the study may have been suboptimal.
2. A strong placebo effect seen in this study may have "blurred" the distinction between a modest positive effect with oral myelin versus no myelin.
3. The method of preparation for myelin may need a special adaptation for oral delivery in humans.

It is theoretically possible that oral myelin may help in MS if used in combination with other drugs or adjuvants; however, the disappointing results of the clinical trial have hampered the initial enthusiasm for this form of treatment. Recent studies of oral administration of glatiramer acetate in EAE showing induction of protective, regulatory immune cells and ongoing trials with oral glatiramer acetate in MS patients may lead to further understanding of the mechanisms of oral tolerance that operate in humans.[229,230]

Altered Peptide Ligands

Recent reports have shown disappointing results with altered peptide ligands in the treatment of MS,[231,232] with some patients responding with an increased rate of relapses. There may be a multitude of reasons for such failure; however, most likely the explanation lies in the now-proven promiscuity of the TCR (i.e., specificity is relative), leading T cells stimulated by the altered peptide to cross-react with native myelin.

Attempts at Promoting Remyelination or Replacing Neurons

OPCs can be recognized with antibodies against a sulfated proteoglycan, NG2,[233–235] and against the platelet-derived growth factor alpha receptor.[236,237] The widespread presence of NG2+ OPCs in both gray and white matter of the adult human brain suggests that attempts at remyelination may be successful once the potential ability of these cells is harnessed and targeted specifically in MS patients. A few technical issues will need to be solved: Investigators need to (1) optimize the minimal number of oligodendrocyte precursors needed to achieve remyelination, (2) recognize the cytokine milieu that facilitates the proper differentiation of these cells into oligodendrocytes, (3) identify the factors that can enhance such differentiation and could thus be added as part of the drug treatment, (4) replace natural factors derived from injured axons that stimulate remyelination with exogenous agents, and (5) establish the ideal route of administration of exogenous OPCs.

A future intervention that seems to hold promise is the use of neural stem cells, which in animal models has opened the possibility of repopulation of neurons and oligodendrocytes, previously unthinkable goals of therapy. Furthermore, these stem cells could be genetically engineered to deliver anti-inflammatory cytokines or neuronal growth factors that could counteract the disease process. An interesting candidate for gene replacement (via stem cells or viral vectors) is nerve growth factor, which has been found to be elevated in the CSF during MS relapses[238] and has been shown to ameliorate anti-myelin oligodendrocyte glycoprotein antibody–associated EAE in marmosets.[239] Nerve growth factor increases IL-6 in phytohemagglutinin-stimulated peripheral blood mononuclear cells and IL-10 production by astrocytes[240] and decreases HLA expression by microglia,[240] all of which should, in theory, counteract mechanisms leading to MS. Finally, replacement therapy with genes that counteract oxidative stress or neuronal/oligodendroglial apoptosis needs to be tested in the EAE animal model.

Prognosis

MS causes considerable suffering and psychosocial distress in the working-age population group. If untreated, at least 60% of relapsing-remitting MS patients will develop significant physical disability within 25 years from onset. This prognosis may change for MS patients with the advent of new treatments.

People with MS usually die of concurrent illnesses, including recurrent infections, especially in the advanced cases in which the patient is bedridden, may have received long-term immunosuppression, and is prone to skin ulceration. With advances in the care of chronic, neurologically disabled patients, life expectancy in MS approaches that of the general population. Male patients with primary-progressive MS have the worst prognosis, as they respond less favorably to treatment and continuously accumulate disability. The higher incidence of spinal cord lesions in primary-progressive MS also contributes to the rapid development of disability. Among patients with relapsing-remitting MS, those with more frequent early attacks seem to carry a higher risk for rapid development of disability and worse prognosis. Corticospinal and cerebellar clinical presentations have a higher tendency to affect gait and cause significant disability with higher EDSS scores and therefore are considered predictors of worse outcomes.

It is imperative to remind patients that early treatment with some agents may possibly help to counteract the progressive brain atrophy seen on MRI[241]; however, more studies are needed, as there is controversy about the definitive interpretation of these reports and about the long-term efficacy of these agents in preventing neuronal loss. A recent report has revealed that in progressive MS patients who have reached an EDSS score of 4, the presence of superimposed relapses did not shorten the time interval to reach the assignment of a score of 6[242] as compared with patients with progressive disease without relapses. This study suggests that once a critical clinical threshold has been reached, the use of disease-modifying drugs (which are known to prevent relapses) may be of marginal, if any, benefit in secondarily delaying disability.

Patient Education

Patients may benefit from referral to professional organizations and Web sites that are dedicated to the prevention and treatment of MS. Among these, the National Multiple Sclerosis Society Web site (http://www.nmss.org) is highly recommended for obtaining information on current hypotheses, ongoing research, general patient resources, and new educational programs.

Conclusions

MS is an enigmatic disease that has puzzled investigators for more than a century. We have witnessed for the first time the advent of disease-modifying drugs and modern ways of monitoring disease progression by using immunologic and imaging studies. However, despite considerable advances in our knowledge of the immune and nervous systems during the last few decades, no consensus has been reached regarding MS etiology. Clinically and pathologically, the disease is clearly heterogeneous, and a wide spectrum of manifestations range from the so-called benign to malignant extreme variants, with more classic presentations resembling those cases described by Charcot and Cruveilhier more than a century ago. The impact of genetic and environmental factors is evident; thus, people from different genetic and environmental backgrounds may develop common MS-related manifestations under different triggers and through different immunopathogenic mechanisms. The approach to treatment will require understanding these concepts so that combined therapies and even individualization of treatment for patients with different genetic backgrounds may be applied in future interventions. Finally, the prospects of enhancing myelin repair, implementing neuronal replacement, and modifying disease via gene therapy are promising, but it will require years of exhaustive research for these techniques to become available, safe, and widely accepted.

References

1. Wada R, Tifft CJ, Proia RL. Microglial activation precedes acute neurodegeneration in sandhoff disease and is suppressed by bone marrow transplantation. Proc Natl Acad Sci U S A 2000;97:10954–10959.
2. Cruveilhier J. Anatonile pathologique du corps humain. Paris: Bailliere, 1842.
3. Carswell R. Pathological Anatomy: Illustrations of the Elementary Forms of Disease. London: Longman, 1838.
4. Charcot J-M. Histologie de la sclérose en plaques. Paris: Gazette Hospital, 1868;41:554–555, 557–558, 566.
5. Rokitansky C. Handbuch der pathologischen anatornic. Bei Braumuller & Seidel, 1846.
6. Fredrikson S, Kam-Hansen S. The 150-year anniversary of multiple sclerosis: does its early history give an etiological clue? Perspect Biol Med 1989;32:237–243.
7. Del Rio-Hortega P. La glia de escasa radiaciones (oligodendroglia) and subdivided. Bulletin de la real sociedad Espanola de historia natural 1921;21:63.
8. Lamer AJ. Aetiological role of viruses in multiple sclerosis: a review. J R Soc Med 1986;79:412–417.
9. Dawson JW. The histology of disseminated sclerosis. Trans R Soc Edinburgh 1916;50:517–740.
10. Lees MB, Sakura JD, Sapirstein VS, Curatolo W. Structure and function of proteolipids in myelin and non-myelin membranes. Biochim Biophys Acta 1979;559:209–230.
11. Carnegie PR. Amino acid sequence of the encephalitogenic basic protein from human myelin. Biochem J 1971;123:57–67.
12. Rawson MD, Liversedge LA, Goldfarb G. Treatment of acute retrobulbar neuritis with corticotrophin. Lancet 1966;2:1044–1046.
13. Mauch E, Kornhuber HH, Krapf H, et al. Treatment of multiple sclerosis with mitoxantrone. Eur Arch Psychiatry Clin Neurosci 1992;242:96–102.
14. Millefiorini E, Gasperini C, Pozzilli C, et al. Randomized placebo-controlled trial of mitoxantrone in relapsing-remitting multiple sclerosis: 24-month clinical and MRI outcome. J Neurol 1997;244:153–159.
15. Noseworthy JH, Hopkins MB, Vandervoort MK, et al. An open-trial evaluation of mitoxantrone in the treatment of progressive MS. Neurology 1993;43:1401–1406.
16. Bastianello SC, Pozzilli F, D'Andrea E, et al. A controlled trial of mitoxantrone in multiple sclerosis: serial MRI evaluation at one year. Can J Neurol Sci 1994;21:266–270.
17. Edan G, Miller D, Clanet M, et al. Therapeutic effect of mitoxantrone combined with methylprednisolone in multiple sclerosis: a randomised multicentre study of active disease using MRI and clinical criteria. J Neurol Neurosurg Psychiatry 1997;62:112–118.
18. Cursiefen S, Flachenecker P, Toyka KV, Rieckmann P. Escalating immunotherapy with mitoxantrone in patients with very active relapsing-remitting or progressive multiple sclerosis. Eur Neurol 2000;43:186–187.
19. Young IR, Hall AS, Pallis CA, et al. Nuclear magnetic resonance imaging of the brain in multiple sclerosis. Lancet 1981;2:1063–1066.
20. Beck RW, Cleary PA, Anderson MM, Jr., et al. A randomized, controlled trial of corticosteroids in the treatment of acute optic neuritis. The Optic Neuritis Study Group. N Engl J Med 1992;326:581–588.
21. Interferon beta-1b is effective in relapsing-remitting multiple sclerosis. I. Clinical results of a multicenter, randomized, double-blind, placebo-controlled trial. The IFNB Multiple Sclerosis Study Group. Neurology 1993;43:655–661.
22. Paty DW, Li DK. Interferon beta-1b is effective in relapsing-remitting multiple sclerosis. II. MRI analysis results of a multicenter, randomized, double-blind, placebo-controlled trial. UBC MS/MRI Study Group and the IFNB Multiple Sclerosis Study Group. Neurology 1993;43:662–667.
23. Raine CS. The Dale E. McFarlin Memorial Lecture: the immunology of the multiple sclerosis lesion. Ann Neurol 1994;36:S61–S72.
24. Lucchinetti CF, Noseworthy JH, Rodriguez M. Promotion of endogenous remyelination in multiple sclerosis. Mult Scler 1997;3:71–75.
25. Lucchinetti CF, Brueck W, Rodriguez M, Lassmann H. Multiple sclerosis: lessons from neuropathology. Semin Neurol 1998;18:337–349.
26. Lucchinetti C, Bruck W, Parisi J, et al. A quantitative analysis of oligodendrocytes in multiple sclerosis lesions. A study of 113 cases. Brain 1999;122:2279–2295.
27. Lucchinetti C, Bruck W, Parisi J, et al. Heterogeneity of multiple sclerosis lesions: implications for the pathogenesis of demyelination. Ann Neurol 2000;47:707–717.
28. Hafler DA. The distinction blurs between an autoimmune versus microbial hypothesis in multiple sclerosis. J Clin Invest 1999;104:527–529.
29. Johnson RT. Viral Aspects of Multiple Sclerosis. In JC Koester, PJ Vinken, GW Bruyn, HL Klawans (eds), Handbook of Clinical Neurology. Amsterdam: Elsevier Sciences, 1985;319–336.
30. Cook SD, Dowling PC. Multiple sclerosis and viruses: an overview. Neurology 1980;30:80–91.

31. Meulen VT, Koprowski H, Iwasaki Y, Kackell YM. Fusion of cultured multiple-sclerosis brain cells with indicator cells: presence of nucleocapsids and virions and isolation of parainfluenza-type virus. Lancet 1972;2:1–5.

32. Mitchell DN, Porterfield JS, Micheletti R, et al. Isolation of an infectious agent from bone-marrows of patients with multiple sclerosis. Lancet 1978;2:387–391.

33. Prasad I, Broome JD, Pertschuk LP, et al. Recovery of Paramyxovirus from the jejunum of patients with multiple sclerosis. Lancet 1977;1:1117–1119.

34. Ascherio A, Munch M. Epstein-Barr virus and multiple sclerosis. Epidemiology 2000;11:220–224.

35. Wandinger K, Jabs W, Siekhaus A, et al. Association between clinical disease activity and Epstein-Barr virus reactivation in MS. Neurology 2000;55:178–184.

36. Haahr S, Sommerlund M, Christensen T, et al. A putative new retrovirus associated with multiple sclerosis and the possible involvement of Epstein-Barr virus in this disease. Ann N Y Acad Sci 1994;724:148–156.

37. Rand KH, Houck H, Denslow ND, Heilman KM. Epstein-Barr virus nuclear antigen-1 (EBNA-1) associated oligoclonal bands in patients with multiple sclerosis. J Neurol Sci 2000;173:32–39.

38. Rand KH, Houck H, Denslow ND, Heilman KM. Molecular approach to find target(s) for oligoclonal bands in multiple sclerosis. J Neurol Neurosurg Psychiatry 1998;65:48–55.

39. Kim JS, Lee KS, Park JH, et al. Detection of human herpesvirus 6 variant A in peripheral blood mononuclear cells from multiple sclerosis patients. Eur Neurol 2000;43:170–173.

40. Soldan SS, Leist TP, Juhng KN, et al. Increased lymphoproliferative response to human herpesvirus type 6A variant in multiple sclerosis patients. Ann Neurol 2000;47:306–313.

41. Herndon RM. Herpesviruses in multiple sclerosis [editorial]. Arch Neurol 1996;53:123–124.

42. Challoner PB, Smith KT, Parker JD, et al. Plaque-associated expression of human herpesvirus 6 in multiple sclerosis. Proc Natl Acad Sci U S A 1995;92:7440–7444.

43. Berti R, Soldan SS, Akhyani N, et al. Extended observations on the association of HHV-6 and multiple sclerosis. J Neurovirol 2000;6(Suppl):S85–S87.

44. Ablashi DV, Eastman HB, Owen CB, et al. Frequent HHV-6 reactivation in multiple sclerosis (MS) and chronic fatigue syndrome (CFS) patients. J Clin Virol 2000;16:179–191.

45. Perron H, Geny C, Laurent A, et al. Leptomeningeal cell line from multiple sclerosis with reverse transcriptase activity and viral particles. Res Virol 1989;140:551–561.

46. Perron H, Firouzi R, Tuke P, et al. Cell cultures and associated retroviruses in multiple sclerosis. Collaborative Research Group on MS. Acta Neurol Scand Suppl 1997;169:22–31.

47. Perron H, Garson JA, Bedin F, et al. Molecular identification of a novel retrovirus repeatedly isolated from patients with multiple sclerosis. The Collaborative Research Group on Multiple Sclerosis. Proc Natl Acad Sci U S A 1997;94:7583–7588.

48. Christensen T, Jensen AW, Munch M, et al. Characterization of retroviruses from patients with multiple sclerosis. Acta Neurol Scand Suppl 1997;169:49–58.

49. Christensen T, Dissing P, Sorensen H, et al. Expression of sequence variants of endogenous retrovirus RGH in particle form in multiple sclerosis [letter] [published erratum in Lancet 1998;352(9134):1154]. Lancet 1998;352:1033.

50. Christensen T, Tonjes RR, zur Megede J, et al. Reverse transcriptase activity and particle production in B lymphoblastoid cell lines established from lymphocytes of patients with multiple sclerosis. AIDS Res Hum Retroviruses 1999;15:285–291.

51. Christensen T, Dissing P, Sorensen H, et al. Molecular characterization of HERV-H variants associated with multiple sclerosis. Acta Neurol Scand 2000;101:229–238.

52. Höllsberg P, Moller-Larsen A, Skou Pedersen F, et al. Search for a retrovirus in long-term cultured cerebrospinal fluid cells and peripheral blood mononuclear cells from patients with multiple sclerosis. Acta Neurol Scand 1989;80:603–609.

53. Georgsson G, Martin JR, Klein J, et al. Primary demyelination in visna. An ultrastructural study of Icelandic sheep with clinical signs following experimental infection. Acta Neuropathol 1982;57:171–178.

54. Sriram S, Stratton CW, Yao S, et al. Chlamydia pneumoniae infection of the central nervous system in multiple sclerosis. Ann Neurol 1999;46:6–14.

55. Boman J, Roblin PM, Sundstrom P, et al. Failure to detect *Chlamydia pneumoniae* in the central nervous system of patients with MS. Neurology 2000;54:265.

56. Layh-Schmitt G, Bendl C, Hildt U, et al. Evidence for infection with Chlamydia pneumoniae in a subgroup of patients with multiple sclerosis. Ann Neurol 2000;47:652–655.

57. Lublin FD, Reingold SC. Defining the clinical course of multiple sclerosis: results of an international survey. National Multiple Sclerosis Society (USA) Advisory Committee on Clinical Trials of New Agents in Multiple Sclerosis. Neurology 1996;46:907–911.

58. Ferrante P, Mancuso R, Pagani E, et al. Molecular evidences for a role of HSV-1 in multiple sclerosis clinical acute attack. J Neurovirol 2000;6(Suppl 2):S109–S114.

59. Rothwell PM, Charlton D. High incidence and prevalence of multiple sclerosis in south east Scotland: evidence of a genetic predisposition. J Neurol Neurosurg Psychiatry 1998;64:730–735.

60. Kurtzke JF. A reassessment of the distribution of multiple sclerosis. Part one. Acta Neurol Scand 1975;51:110–136.

61. Gorelick PB. Clues to the mystery of multiple sclerosis. Postgrad Med 1989;85:125–128, 131–134.

62. Kurtzke JF, Hyllested K. Multiple sclerosis in the Faroe Islands: I. Clinical and epidemiological features. Ann Neurol 1979;5:6–21.

63. Kurtzke JF, Gudmundsson KR, Bergmann S. Multiple sclerosis in Iceland: 1. Evidence of a postwar epidemic. Neurology 1982;32:143–150.

64. Kurtzke JF, Dean G, Botha DP. A method for estimating the age at immigration of white immigrants to South Africa, with an example of its importance. S Afr Med J 1970;44:663–669.

65. Sadovnick AD, Ebers GC. Epidemiology of multiple sclerosis: a critical overview. Can J Neurol Sci 1993;20:17–29.

66. Ebers GC, Yee IM, Sadovnick AD. Conjugal multiple sclerosis: population-based prevalence and recurrence risks in offspring. Canadian Collaborative Study Group. Ann Neurol 2000;48:927–931.

67. Ebers GC, Sadovnick AD, Risch NJ. A genetic basis for familial aggregation in multiple sclerosis. Canadian Collaborative Study Group. Nature 1995;377:150–151.

68. Ebers GC, Kukay K, Bulman DE, et al. A full genome search in multiple sclerosis. Nat Genet 1996;13:472–476.

69. Haines JL, Ter-Minassian M, Bazyk A, et al. A complete genomic screen for multiple sclerosis underscores a role for the major histocompatability complex. The Multiple Sclerosis Genetics Group. Nat Genet 1996;13:469–471.

70. Sawcer S, Jones HB, Feakes R, et al. A genome screen in multiple sclerosis reveals susceptibility loci on chromosome 6p21 and 17q22. Nat Genet 1996;13:464–468.

71. Kuokkanen S, Sundvall M, Terwilliger JD, et al. A putative vulnerability locus to multiple sclerosis maps to 5p14-p12 in a region syntenic to the murine locus Eae2. Nat Genet 1996;13:477–480.

72. Hillert J, Olerup O. Multiple sclerosis is associated with genes within or close to the HLA-DR-DQ subregion on a normal DR15,DQ6,Dw2 haplotype. Neurology 1993;43:163–168.

73. Olerup O, Hillert J, Fredrikson S, et al. Primarily chronic progressive and relapsing/remitting multiple sclerosis: two immunogenetically distinct disease entities. Proc Natl Acad Sci U S A 1989;86:7113–7117.

74. Ligers A, Xu C, Saarinen S, et al. The CTLA-4 gene is associated with multiple sclerosis. J Neuroimmunol 1999;97:182–190.

75. Vandenbroeck K, Martino G, Marrosu M, et al. Occurrence and clinical relevance of an interleukin-4 gene polymorphism in patients with multiple sclerosis. J Neuroimmunol 1997;76:189–192.

76. Jacobsen M, Schweer D, Ziegler A, et al. A point mutation in PTPRC is associated with the development of multiple sclerosis. Nat Genet 2000;26:495–499.

77. Mycko MP, Kwinkowski M, Tronczynska E, et al. Multiple sclerosis: the increased frequency of the ICAM-1 exon 6 gene point mutation genetic type K469. Ann Neurol 1998;44:70–75.

78. Mycko M, Kowalski W, Kwinkowski M, et al. Multiple sclerosis: the frequency of allelic forms of tumor necrosis factor and lymphotoxin-alpha. J Neuroimmunol 1998;84:198–206.

79. Mann CL, Davies MB, Boggild MD, et al. Glutathione S-transferase polymorphisms in MS: their relationship to disability. Neurology 2000;54:552–557.

80. Hashimoto LL, Walter MA, Cox DW, Ebers GC. Immunoglobulin heavy chain variable region polymorphisms and multiple sclerosis susceptibility. J Neuroimmunol 1993;44:77–83.

81. Walter MA, Gibson WT, Ebers GC, Cox GC. Susceptibility to multiple sclerosis is associated with the proximal immunoglobulin heavy chain variable region. J Clin Invest 1991;87:1266–1273.

82. Niino M, Fukazawa T, Yabe I, et al. Vitamin D receptor gene polymorphism in multiple sclerosis and the association with HLA class II alleles. J Neurol Sci 2000;177:65–71.

83. Janeway CA, Jr. The immune system evolved to discriminate infectious nonself from noninfectious self. Immunol Today 1992;13:11–16.

84. Höllsberg P, Weber WE, Dangond F, et al. Differential activation of proliferation and cytotoxicity in human T-cell lymphotropic virus type I Tax-specific CD8 T cells by an altered peptide ligand. Proc Natl Acad Sci U S A 1995;92:4036–4040.

85. Kuchroo VK, Das MP, Brown JA, et al. B7-1 and B7-2 costimulatory molecules activate differentially the Th1/Th2 developmental pathways: application to autoimmune disease therapy. Cell 1995;80:707–718.

86. Windhagen A, Newcombe J, Dangond F, et al. Expression of costimulatory molecules B7-1 (CD80), B7-2 (CD86), and interleukin 12 cytokine in multiple sclerosis lesions. J Exp Med 1995;182:1985–1996.

87. Dangond F, Windhagen A, Groves CJ, Hafler DA. Constitutive expression of costimulatory molecules by human microglia and its relevance to CNS autoimmunity. J Neuroimmunol 1997;76:132–138.

88. Balashov KE, Smith DR, Khoury SJ, et al. Increased interleukin 12 production in progressive multiple sclerosis: induction by activated CD4+ T cells via CD40 ligand. Proc Natl Acad Sci U S A 1997;94:599–603.

89. Comabella MK, Balashov S, Issazadeh D, et al. Elevated interleukin-12 in progressive multiple sclerosis correlates with disease activity and is normalized by pulse cyclophosphamide therapy. J Clin Invest 1998;102:671–678.

90. Wang X, Chen M, Wandinger KP, et al. IFN-beta-1b inhibits IL-12 production in peripheral blood mononuclear cells in an IL-10-dependent mechanism: relevance to IFN-beta-1b therapeutic effects in multiple sclerosis. J Immunol 2000;165:548–557.

91. Genc K, Dona DL, Reder AT. Increased CD80(+) B cells in active multiple sclerosis and reversal by interferon beta-1b therapy. J Clin Invest 1997;99:2664–2671.

92. Cross AH, Cannella B, Brosnan CF, Raine CS. Homing to central nervous system vasculature by antigen-specific lymphocytes. I. Localization of 14C-labeled cells during acute, chronic, and relapsing experimental allergic encephalomyelitis. Lab Invest 1990;63:162–170.

93. Allegretta MJ, Nicklas A, Sriram S, Albertini RJ. T cells responsive to myelin basic protein in patients with multiple sclerosis. Science 1990;247:718–721.

94. Ota K, Matsui M, Milford EL, et al. T-cell recognition of an immunodominant myelin basic protein epitope in multiple sclerosis. Nature 1990;346:183–187.

95. Wucherpfennig KW, Strominger JL. Molecular mimicry in T cell-mediated autoimmunity: viral peptides activate human T cell clones specific for myelin basic protein. Cell 1995;80:695–705.

96. Prineas JW, Raine CS. Electron microscopy and immunoperoxidase studies of early multiple sclerosis lesions. Neurology 1976;26:29–32.

97. Raine CS, Scheinberg LC. On the immunopathology of plaque development and repair in multiple sclerosis. J Neuroimmunol 1988;20:189–201.

98. Cuzner ML. Molecular Biology of Microglia. In WC Russell (ed), Molecular Biology of Multiple Sclerosis. New York: John Wiley & Sons, Inc., 1997;97–120.

99. Newcombe J, Li H, Cuzner ML. Low density lipoprotein uptake by macrophages in multiple sclerosis plaques: implications for pathogenesis. Neuropathol Appl Neurobiol 1994;20:152–162.

100. Aloisi F, Ria F, Columba-Cabezas S, et al. Relative efficiency of microglia, astrocytes, dendritic cells and B cells in naive CD4+ T cell priming and Th1/Th2 cell restimulation. Eur J Immunol 1999;29:2705–2714.

101. Matsumoto Y, Ohmori K, Fujiwara M. Immune regulation by brain cells in the central nervous system: microglia but not astrocytes present myelin basic protein to encephalitogenic T cells under in vivo-mimicking conditions. Immunology 1992;76:209–216.

102. Williams K, Ulvestad E, Antel JP. B7/BB-1 antigen expression on adult human microglia studied in vitro and in situ. Eur J Immunol 1994;24:3031–3037.

103. Cross AH, Trotter JL, Lyons J. B cells and antibodies in CNS demyelinating disease. J Neuroimmunol 2001; 112:1–14.

104. Grenier Y, Ruijs TC, Robitaille Y, et al. Immunohistochemical studies of adult human glial cells. J Neuroimmunol 1989;21:103–115.

105. Jurewicz A, Biddison WE, Antel JP. MHC class I-restricted lysis of human oligodendrocytes by myelin basic protein peptide-specific CD8 T lymphocytes. J Immunol 1998;160:3056–3059.

106. Ruijs TC, Freedman MS, Grenier YG, et al. Human oligodendrocytes are susceptible to cytolysis by major histocompatibility complex class I-restricted lymphocytes. J Neuroimmunol 1990;27:89–97.

107. Zeine R, Pon R, Ladiwala U, et al. Mechanism of gammadelta T cell-induced human oligodendrocyte cytotoxicity: relevance to multiple sclerosis. J Neuroimmunol 1998;87:49–61.

108. Freedman MS, Ruijs TC, Selin LK, Antel JP. Peripheral blood gamma-delta T cells lyse fresh human brain-derived oligodendrocytes. Ann Neurol 1991;30:794–800.

109. Freedman MS, D'Souza S, Antel JP. Gamma delta T-cell-human glial cell interactions. I. In vitro induction of gammadelta T-cell expansion by human glial cells. J Neuroimmunol 1997;74:135–142.

110. Freedman MS, Bitar R, Antel JP. Gamma delta T-cell-human glial cell interactions. II. Relationship between heat shock protein expression and susceptibility to cytolysis. J Neuroimmunol 1997;74:143–148.

111. Selmaj K, Brosnan CF, Raine CS. Colocalization of lymphocytes bearing gamma delta T-cell receptor and heat shock protein hsp65+ oligodendrocytes in multiple sclerosis. Proc Natl Acad Sci U S A 1991;88:6452–6456.

112. Selmaj K, Brosnan CF, Raine CS. Expression of heat shock protein-65 by oligodendrocytes in vivo and in vitro: implications for multiple sclerosis. Neurology 1992; 42:795–800.

113. Niehaus A, Shi J, Grzenkowski M, et al. Patients with active relapsing-remitting multiple sclerosis synthesize antibodies recognizing oligodendrocyte progenitor cell surface protein: implications for remyelination. Ann Neurol 2000;48:362–371.

114. Sabelko-Downes KA, Russell JH, Cross AH. Role of Fas—FasL interactions in the pathogenesis and regulation of autoimmune demyelinating disease. J Neuroimmunol 1999;100:42–52.

115. D'Souza SD, Bonetti B, Balasingam V, et al. Multiple sclerosis: Fas signaling in oligodendrocyte cell death. J Exp Med 1996;184:2361–2370.

116. Sellebjerg F, Madsen HO, Jensen CV, et al. CCR5 delta32, matrix metalloproteinase-9 and disease activity in multiple sclerosis. J Neuroimmunol 2000;102:98–106.

117. Liedtke W, Cannella B, Mazzaccaro RJ, et al. Effective treatment of models of multiple sclerosis by matrix metalloproteinase inhibitors. Ann Neurol 1998;44:35–46.

118. Soos JM, Ashley TA, Morrow J, et al. Differential expression of B7 co-stimulatory molecules by astrocytes correlates with T cell activation and cytokine production. Int Immunol 1999;11:1169–1179.

119. Soos JM, Morrow J, Ashley TA, et al. Astrocytes express elements of the class II endocytic pathway and process central nervous system autoantigen for presentation to encephalitogenic T cells. J Immunol 1998;161:5959–5966.

120. Lee SC, Brosnan CF. Molecular Biology of Glia: Astrocytes. In WC Russell (ed), Molecular Biology of Multiple Sclerosis. New York: John Wiley & Sons, Inc., 1997;71–96.

121. Sorensen TL, Tani M, Jensen J, et al. Expression of specific chemokines and chemokine receptors in the central nervous system of multiple sclerosis patients. J Clin Invest 1999;103:807–815.

122. Balashov KE, Rottman JB, Weiner HL, Hancock WW. CCR5(+) and CXCR3(+) T cells are increased in multiple sclerosis and their ligands MIP-1alpha and IP-10 are expressed in demyelinating brain lesions. Proc Natl Acad Sci U S A 1999;96:6873–6878.

123. Zang YC, Halder JB, Samanta AK, et al. Regulation of chemokine receptor CCR5 and production of RANTES and MIP-1alpha by interferon-beta. J Neuroimmunol 2001;112:174–180.

124. Karpus WJ, Lukacs NW, McRae BL, et al. An important role for the chemokine macrophage inflammatory protein-1 alpha in the pathogenesis of the T cell-mediated autoimmune disease, experimental autoimmune encephalomyelitis. J Immunol 1995;155:5003–5010.

125. Simpson J, Rezaie P, Newcombe J, et al. Expression of the beta-chemokine receptors CCR2, CCR3 and CCR5 in multiple sclerosis central nervous system tissue. J Neuroimmunol 2000;108:192–200.

126. McManus C, Berman JW, Brett FM, et al. MCP-1, MCP-2 and MCP-3 expression in multiple sclerosis lesions: an immunohistochemical and in situ hybridization study. J Neuroimmunol 1998;86:20–29.

127. Holopainen I, Kontro P, Oja SS. Release of taurine from cultured cerebellar granule cells and astrocytes: co-release with glutamate. Neuroscience 1989;29:425–432.

128. Koutsilieri E, Sopper S, Heinemann T, et al. Involvement of microglia in cerebrospinal fluid glutamate increase in

SIV-infected rhesus monkeys (Macaca mulatta). AIDS Res Hum Retroviruses 1999;15:471–477.

129. Hegg CC, Thayer SA. Monocytic cells secrete factors that evoke excitatory synaptic activity in rat hippocampal cultures. Eur J Pharmacol 1999;385:231–237.

130. Noda M, Nakanishi H, Akaike N. Glutamate release from microglia via glutamate transporter is enhanced by amyloid-beta peptide. Neuroscience 1999;92:1465–1474.

131. Westall FC, Hawkins A, Ellison GW, Myers LW. Abnormal glutamic acid metabolism in multiple sclerosis. J Neurol Sci 1980;47:353–364.

132. Barkhatova VP, Zavalishin IA, Askarova L, et al. Changes in neurotransmitters in multiple sclerosis. Neurosci Behav Physiol 1998;28:341–344.

133. Smith T, Groom A, Zhu B, Turski L. Autoimmune encephalomyelitis ameliorated by AMPA antagonists. Nat Med 2000;6:62–66.

134. Pitt D, Werner P, Raine CS. Glutamate excitotoxicity in a model of multiple sclerosis. Nat Med 2000;6:67–70.

135. Bo L, Dawson TM, Wesselingh S, et al. Induction of nitric oxide synthase in demyelinating regions of multiple sclerosis brains. Ann Neurol 1994;36:778–786.

136. De Groot CJ, Ruuls SR, Theeuwes JW, et al. Immunocytochemical characterization of the expression of inducible and constitutive isoforms of nitric oxide synthase in demyelinating multiple sclerosis lesions. J Neuropathol Exp Neurol 1997;56:10–20.

137. van der Veen RC, Hinton DR, Incardonna F, Hofman FM. Extensive peroxynitrite activity during progressive stages of central nervous system inflammation. J Neuroimmunol 1997;77:1–7.

138. van der Goes A, Brouwer J, Hoekstra K, et al. Reactive oxygen species are required for the phagocytosis of myelin by macrophages. J Neuroimmunol 1998;92:67–75.

139. Spitsin SV, Scott GS, Kean RB, et al. Protection of myelin basic protein immunized mice from free-radical mediated inflammatory cell invasion of the central nervous system by the natural peroxynitrite scavenger uric acid. Neurosci Lett 2000;292:137–141.

140. Hooper DC, Scott GS, Zborek A, et al. Uric acid, a peroxynitrite scavenger, inhibits CNS inflammation, blood-CNS barrier permeability changes, and tissue damage in a mouse model of multiple sclerosis. FASEB J 2000;14:691–698.

141. Hooper DC, Bagasra O, Marini JC, et al. Prevention of experimental allergic encephalomyelitis by targeting nitric oxide and peroxynitrite: implications for the treatment of multiple sclerosis. Proc Natl Acad Sci U S A 1997;94:2528–2533.

142. Malfroy B, Doctrow SR, Orr PL, et al. Prevention and suppression of autoimmune encephalomyelitis by EUK-8, a synthetic catalytic scavenger of oxygen-reactive metabolites. Cell Immunol 1997;177:62–68.

143. Khoury SJ, Guttmann CR, Orav EJ, et al. Changes in activated T cells in the blood correlate with disease activity in multiple sclerosis. Arch Neurol 2000;57:1183–1189.

144. Tsukada N, Miyagi K, Matsuda M, Yanagisawa N. Increased levels of circulating intercellular adhesion molecule-1 in multiple sclerosis and human T-lymphotropic virus type I-associated myelopathy. Ann Neurol 1993;33:646–649.

145. Hartung HP, Michels M, Reiners K, et al. Soluble ICAM-1 serum levels in multiple sclerosis and viral encephalitis. Neurology 1993;43:2331–2335.

146. Sharief MK, Noori MA, Ciardi M, et al. Increased levels of circulating ICAM-1 in serum and cerebrospinal fluid of patients with active multiple sclerosis. Correlation with TNF-alpha and blood-brain barrier damage. J Neuroimmunol 1993;43:15–21.

147. Khoury SJ, Orav EJ, Guttmann CR, et al. Changes in serum levels of ICAM and TNF-R correlate with disease activity in multiple sclerosis. Neurology 1999;53:758–764.

148. Kimoto Y. A possibility of all mRNA expression in a human single lymphocyte. Hum Cell 1996;9:367–370.

149. Bagriacik EU, Klein JR. The thyrotropin (thyroid-stimulating hormone) receptor is expressed on murine dendritic cells and on a subset of CD45RBhigh lymph node T cells: functional role for thyroid-stimulating hormone during immune activation. J Immunol 2000;164:6158–6165.

150. Azad N, La Paglia N, Jurgens KA, et al. Immunoactivation enhances the concentration of luteinizing hormone-releasing hormone peptide and its gene expression in human peripheral T-lymphocytes. Endocrinology 1993;133:215–223.

151. Clarke BL, Bost KL. Differential expression of functional adrenocorticotropic hormone receptors by subpopulations of lymphocytes. J Immunol 1989;143:464–469.

152. Matera L, Muccioli G, Cesano A, et al. Prolactin receptors on large granular lymphocytes: dual regulation by cyclosporin A. Brain Behav Immun 1988;2:1–10.

153. Zhu XH, Zellweger R, Wichmann MW, et al. Effects of prolactin and metoclopramide on macrophage cytokine gene expression in late sepsis. Cytokine 1997;9:437–446.

154. Batticane N, Morale MC, Gallo F, et al. Luteinizing hormone-releasing hormone signaling at the lymphocyte involves stimulation of interleukin-2 receptor expression. Endocrinology 1991;129:277–286.

155. Schumacher GA, Beebe GW, Kibler RF. Problems of experimental trials of therapy in multiple sclerosis: report by the panel on the evaluation of experimental trials of therapy in multiple sclerosis. Ann N Y Acad Sci 1965;122:552–568.

156. Trapp BD, Ransohoff R, Rudick R. Axonal pathology in multiple sclerosis: relationship to neurologic disability. Curr Opin Neurol 1999;12:295–302.

157. Coles AJ, Wing MG, Molyneux P, et al. Monoclonal antibody treatment exposes three mechanisms underlying the clinical course of multiple sclerosis. Ann Neurol 1999;46:296–304.

158. Gonen O, Catalaa I, Babb JS, et al. Total brain N-acetylaspartate: a new measure of disease load in MS. Neurology 2000;54:15–19.

159. Richards TL. Proton MR spectroscopy in multiple sclerosis: value in establishing diagnosis, monitoring progression, and evaluating therapy. AJR Am J Roentgenol 1991;157:1073–1078.

160. Larsson HB, Christiansen P, Jensen M, et al. Localized in vivo proton spectroscopy in the brain of patients with multiple sclerosis. Magn Reson Med 1991;22:23–31.

161. Simone IL, Tortorella C, Federico F, et al. Axonal damage in multiple sclerosis plaques: a combined magnetic resonance imaging and 1H-magnetic resonance spectroscopy study. J Neurol Sci 2001;182:143–150.

162. Bjartmar C, Kidd G, Mork S, et al. Neurological disability correlates with spinal cord axonal loss and reduced N-acetyl aspartate in chronic multiple sclerosis patients. Ann Neurol 2000;48:893–901.

163. De Stefano N, Narayanan S, Francis GS, et al. Evidence of axonal damage in the early stages of multiple sclerosis and its relevance to disability. Arch Neurol 2001;58:65–70.

164. Neumann H, Cavalie A, Jenne DE, Wekerle H. Induction of MHC class I genes in neurons. Science 1995;269:549–552.

165. Weller RO. Pathology of Multiple Sclerosis. In WB Matthews, ED Acheson, JR Batchelor, et al. (eds) McAlpine's Multiple Sclerosis. London: Churchill Livingstone, 1985; 301–343.

166. Adams RD, Kubik CS. The morbid anatomy of the demyelinative diseases. Am J Med 1952;12:510–546.

167. Simon JH, Kinkel RP, Jacobs L, et al. A Wallerian degeneration pattern in patients at risk for MS. Neurology 2000;54:1155–1160.

168. Trapp BD, Peterson J, Ransohoff RM, et al. Axonal transection in the lesions of multiple sclerosis. N Engl J Med 1998;338:278–285.

169. Whitaker JN, Wolinsky JS, Narayana PA, et al. Relationship of urinary myelin basic protein-like material with cranial magnetic resonance imaging in advanced multiple sclerosis. Arch Neurol 2001;58:49–54.

170. Sperling R, Guttmann CRG, Hohol MJ, et al. Regional magnetic resonance imaging lesion burden and cognitive function in multiple sclerosis. Arch Neurol 2001;58:115–121.

171. Runmarker B, Andersson C, Oden A, Andersen O. Prediction of outcome in multiple sclerosis based on multivariate models. J Neurol 1994;241:597–604.

172. Hawkins SA, McDonnell GV. Benign multiple sclerosis? Clinical course, long term follow up, and assessment of prognostic factors. J Neurol Neurosurg Psychiatry 1999; 67:148–152.

173. Sadovnick AD, Eisen K, Ebers GC, Paty DW. Cause of death in patients attending multiple sclerosis clinics. Neurology 1991;41:1193–1196.

174. Hutchinson M, Stack J, Buckley P. Bipolar affective disorder prior to the onset of multiple sclerosis. Acta Neurol Scand 1993;88:388–393.

175. Nakashima I, Fujihara K, Kimpara T, et al. Linear pontine trigeminal root lesions in multiple sclerosis. Arch Neurol 2001;58:101–104.

176. Sedano MJ, Trejo JM, Macarron JL, et al. Continuous facial myokymia in multiple sclerosis: treatment with botulinum toxin. Eur Neurol 2000;43:137–140.

177. Selvapandian S, Rajshekhar V. Facial myokymia as the presenting symptom of a pontine glioma. Neurol India 1999;47:241–242.

178. Jabbari B, Marsh EE, Gunderson CH. The site of the lesion in acute deafness of multiple sclerosis—contribution of the brain stem auditory evoked potential test. Clin Electroencephalogr 1982;13:241–244.

179. Nelson LM, Franklin GM, Jones MC. Risk of multiple sclerosis exacerbation during pregnancy and breast-feeding. JAMA 1988;259:3441–3443.

180. Korn-Lubetzki I, Kahana E, Cooper G, Abramsky O. Activity of multiple sclerosis during pregnancy and puerperium. Ann Neurol 1984;16:229–231.

181. Orvieto R, Achiron R, Rotstein Z, et al. Pregnancy and multiple sclerosis: a 2-year experience. Eur J Obstet Gynecol Reprod Biol 1999;82:191–194.

182. Achiron A, Rotstein Z, Noy S, et al. Intravenous immunoglobulin treatment in the prevention of childbirth-associated acute exacerbations in multiple sclerosis: a pilot study. J Neurol 1996;243:25–28.

183. Worthington J, Jones R, Crawford M, Forti A. Pregnancy and multiple sclerosis—a 3-year prospective study. J Neurol 1994;241:228–233.

184. Runmarker B, Andersen O. Pregnancy is associated with a lower risk of onset and a better prognosis in multiple sclerosis. Brain 1995;118:253–261.

185. Ebers GC. Optic neuritis and multiple sclerosis. Arch Neurol 1985;42:702–704.

186. Rizzo JF, Lessell S. Risk of developing multiple sclerosis after uncomplicated optic neuritis: a long-term prospective study. Neurology 1988;38:185–190.

187. Kurland LT, Beebe GW, Kurtzke JF, et al. Studies on the natural history of multiple sclerosis. 2. The progression of optic neuritis to multiple sclerosis. Acta Neurol Scand 1966;42:157+.

188. Stendahl-Brodin L, Link H. Optic neuritis: oligoclonal bands increase the risk of multiple sclerosis. Acta Neurol Scand 1983;67:301–304.

189. Morrissey SP, Miller DH, Kendall BE, et al. The significance of brain magnetic resonance imaging abnormalities at presentation with clinically isolated syndromes suggestive of multiple sclerosis. A 5-year follow-up study. Brain 1993;116:135–146.

190. Kurtzke JF. Rating neurologic impairment in multiple sclerosis: an expanded disability status scale (EDSS). Neurology 1983;33:1444–1452.

191. Cutter GR, Baier ML, Rudick RA, et al. Development of multiple sclerosis functional composite as a clinical trial outcome measure. Brain 1999;122:871–872.

192. Sindic CJ, Monteyne P, Laterre EC. The intrathecal synthesis of virus-specific oligoclonal IgG in multiple sclerosis. J Neuroimmunol 1994;54:75–80.

193. Zeman AZ, Kidd D, McLean BN, et al. A study of oligoclonal band negative multiple sclerosis. J Neurol Neurosurg Psychiatry 1996;60:27–30.

194. Gupta MK, Whitaker JN, Johnson C, Goren H. 1988. Measurement of immunoreactive myelin basic protein peptide (45-89) in cerebrospinal fluid. Ann Neurol 23:274–280.

195. Bakshi R, Glass J, Louis DN, Hochberg FH. Magnetic resonance imaging features of solitary inflammatory brain masses. J Neuroimaging 1998;8:8–14.

196. Mandler RN, Davis LE, Jeffery DR, Kornfeld M. Devic's neuromyelitis optica: a clinicopathological study of 8 patients. Ann Neurol 1993;34:162–168.

197. Wood DD, Bilbao JM, O'Connors P, Moscarello MA. Acute multiple sclerosis (Marburg type) is associated with

developmentally immature myelin basic protein. Ann Neurol 1996;40:18–24.

198. Mendez MF, Pogacar S. Malignant monophasic multiple sclerosis or "Marburg's disease." Neurology 1988;38:1153–1155.

199. Hurst EW. Acute hemorrhagic leucoencephalitis: a previously undefined entity. Med J Aust 1941;1:1–6.

200. Baker AB. Hemorrhagic encephalitis. Am J Pathol 1935; 11:185–236.

201. Dangond F, Lacomis D, Schwartz RB, et al. Acute disseminated encephalomyelitis progressing to hemorrhagic encephalitis. Neurology 1991;41:1697–1698.

202. Castaigne P, Escourolle R, Chain F, et al. Baló's concentric sclerosis. Rev Neurol 1984;140:479–487.

203. Bever CT, Jr., Anderson PA, Leslie J, et al. Treatment with oral 3,4 diaminopyridine improves leg strength in multiple sclerosis patients: results of a randomized, double-blind, placebo-controlled, crossover trial. Neurology 1996;47:1457–1462.

204. Goodin DS, Ebers GC, Johnson KP, et al. The relationship of MS to physical trauma and psychological stress. Report of the therapeutics and technology assessment subcommittee of the American Academy of Neurology. Neurology 1999;52:1737–1745.

205. Piazza DH, Diokno AC. Review of neurogenic bladder in multiple sclerosis. Urology 1979;14:33–35.

206. Blaivas JG, Bhimani G, Labib KB. Vesicourethral dysfunction in multiple sclerosis. J Urol 1979;122:342–347.

207. Bradley WE, Logothetis JL, Timm GW. Cystometric and sphincter abnormalities in multiple sclerosis. Neurology 1973;23:1131–1139.

208. Blaivas JG. Management of bladder dysfunction in multiple sclerosis. Neurology 1980;30(7 Pt 2):12–18.

209. Miller A, Bourdette D, Cohen JA, et al. Multiple sclerosis. Continuum 1999;5:128.

210. Swierzewski SJ III, Gormley EA, Belville WD, et al. The effect of terazosin on bladder function in the spinal cord injured patient. J Urol 1994;151:951–954.

211. Snape J, Hulman G, Reddy PR, Panto PN. Pneumatosis coli: an uncommon but treatable cause of faecal incontinence. Int J Clin Pract 1998;52:501–503.

212. Panitch HS, Hirsch RL, Haley AS, Johnson KP. Exacerbations of multiple sclerosis in patients treated with gamma interferon. Lancet 1987;1:893–895.

213. Panitch HS, Hirsch RL, Schindler J, Johnson KP. Treatment of multiple sclerosis with gamma interferon: exacerbations associated with activation of the immune system. Neurology 1987;37:1097–1102.

214. Jacobs LD, Beck RW, Simon JH, et al. Intramuscular interferon beta-1a therapy initiated during a first demyelinating event in multiple sclerosis. CHAMPS Study Group. N Engl J Med 2000;343:898–904.

215. McDonald WI, Compston A, Edan G. Recommended diagnostic criteria for multiple sclerosis: guidelines from the International Panel on the diagnosis of multiple sclerosis. Ann Neurol 2001;50:121–127.

216. Kent SJ, Karlik SJ, Cannon C, et al. A monoclonal antibody to alpha 4 integrin suppresses and reverses active experimental allergic encephalomyelitis. J Neuroimmunol 1995;58:1–10.

217. Kent SJ, Karlik SJ, Rice GP, Horner HC. A monoclonal antibody to alpha 4-integrin reverses the MR-detectable signs of experimental allergic encephalomyelitis in the guinea pig. J Magn Reson Imaging 1995;5:535–540.

218. Tubridy N, Behan PO, Capildeo R, et al. The effect of anti-alpha4 integrin antibody on brain lesion activity in MS. The UK Antegren Study Group. Neurology 1999;53:466–472.

219. Paolillo A, Coles AJ, Molyneux PD, et al. Quantitative MRI in patients with secondary progressive MS treated with monoclonal antibody Campath 1H. Neurology 1999;53:751–757.

220. Loughlin AJ, Woodroofe MN, Cuzner ML. Modulation of interferon-gamma-induced major histocompatibility complex class II and Fc receptor expression on isolated microglia by transforming growth factor-beta 1, interleukin-4, noradrenaline and glucocorticoids. Immunology 1993;79:125–130.

221. Suzumura A, Sawada M, Yamamoto H, Marunouchi T. Transforming growth factor-beta suppresses activation and proliferation of microglia in vitro. J Immunol 1993;151:2150–2158.

222. Wells HG. Studies on the chemistry of anaphylaxis (III). Experiments with isolated proteins, especially those of the hen's egg. J Infect Dis 1911;8:147.

223. Chase MW. Inhibition of experimental drug allergy by prior feeding of the sensitizing agent, Proc Soc Exp Biol Med (N Y) 1946;61:257.

224. Higgins PJ, Weiner HL. Suppression of experimental autoimmune encephalomyelitis by oral administration of myelin basic protein and its fragments. J Immunol 1988;140:440–445.

225. Chen Y, Kuchroo VK, Inobe J, et al. Regulatory T cell clones induced by oral tolerance: suppression of autoimmune encephalomyelitis. Science 1994;265:1237–1240.

226. Nussenblatt RB, Caspi RR, Mahdi R, et al. Inhibition of S-antigen induced experimental autoimmune uveoretinitis by oral induction of tolerance with S-antigen. J Immunol 1990;144:1689–1695.

227. Zhang ZY, Lee CS, Lider O, Weiner HL. Suppression of adjuvant arthritis in Lewis rats by oral administration of type II collagen. J Immunol 1990;145:2489–2493.

228. Weiner HL, Mackin GA, Matsui M, et al. Double-blind pilot trial of oral tolerization with myelin antigens in multiple sclerosis. Science 1993;259:1321–1324.

229. Teitelbaum D, Arnon R, Sela M. Immunomodulation of experimental autoimmune encephalomyelitis by oral administration of copolymer 1. Proc Natl Acad Sci U S A 1999;96:3842–3847.

230. Weiner HL. Oral tolerance with copolymer 1 for the treatment of multiple sclerosis. Proc Natl Acad Sci U S A 1999;96:3333–3335.

231. Bielekova B, Goodwin B, Richert N, et al. Encephalitogenic potential of the myelin basic protein peptide (amino acids 83-99) in multiple sclerosis: results of a phase II clinical trial with an altered peptide ligand. Nat Med 2000;6:1167–1175.

232. Kappos L, Comi G, Panitch H, et al. Induction of a non-encephalitogenic type 2 T helper-cell autoimmune response in multiple sclerosis after administration of an altered

peptide ligand in a placebo-controlled, randomized phase II trial. Nat Med 2000;6:1176–1182.

233. Levine JM. Increased expression of the NG2 chondroitin-sulfate proteoglycan after brain injury. J Neurosci 1994; 14:4716–4730.

234. Levine JM, Stallcup WB. Plasticity of developing cerebellar cells in vitro studied with antibodies against the NG2 antigen. J Neurosci 1987;7:2721–2731.

235. Keirstead HS, Levine JM, Blakemore WF. Response of the oligodendrocyte progenitor cell population (defined by NG2 labelling) to demyelination of the adult spinal cord. Glia 1998;22:161–170.

236. Nishiyama A, Lin XH, Giese N, et al. Interaction between NG2 proteoglycan and PDGF alpha-receptor on O2A progenitor cells is required for optimal response to PDGF. J Neurosci Res 1996;43:315–330.

237. Nishiyama A, Lin XH, Giese N, et al. Co-localization of NG2 proteoglycan and PDGF alpha-receptor on O2A progenitor cells in the developing rat brain. J Neurosci Res 1996;43:299–314.

238. Laudiero LB, Aloe L, Levi-Montalcini R, et al. Multiple sclerosis patients express increased levels of beta-nerve growth factor in cerebrospinal fluid. Neurosci Lett 1992; 147:9–12.

239. Villoslada P, Hauser SL, Bartke I, et al. Human nerve growth factor protects common marmosets against autoimmune encephalomyelitis by switching the balance of T helper cell type 1 and 2 cytokines within the central nervous system. J Exp Med 2000;191:1799–1806.

240. Neumann H, Misgeld T, Matsumuro K, Wekerle H. Neurotrophins inhibit major histocompatibility class II inducibility of microglia: involvement of the p75 neurotrophin receptor. Proc Natl Acad Sci U S A 1998;95:5779–5784.

241. Rudick RA, Fisher E, Lee JC, et al. Use of the brain parenchymal fraction to measure whole brain atrophy in relapsing-remitting MS. Multiple Sclerosis Collaborative Research Group. Neurology 1999;53:1698–1704.

242. Confavreux C, Vukusic S, Moreau T, Adeleine P. Relapses and progression of disability in multiple sclerosis. N Engl J Med 2000;343:1430–1438.

Chapter 6

Experimental Autoimmune Encephalomyelitis and Multiple Sclerosis: From Bench to Bedside

Karim Makhlouf, Jaime Imitola, and Samia J. Khoury

Multiple sclerosis (MS) is the most common demyelinating disorder in humans. It is also the most common neurologic disease of young adults. Most of the research in MS has focused on the immunologic aspects of the disease. Indeed, within the last 15 years, we have developed a new understanding of the underlying immunologic mechanisms of MS, and new treatments have become available.

Although MS is clinically and pathologically heterogenous, demyelination is a key feature of the disease. However, very early in the course of the disease, axonal damage occurs[1] and leads to the irreversible clinical symptoms of the chronic phase of MS. MS is considered an immune mediated disease, but genetic and environmental factors (such as viral infections) may also play a pathogenic role. Experimental autoimmune encephalomyelitis (EAE) is the most widely used animal model for studying the pathogenic and therapeutic mechanisms of MS.

Definition of Experimental Autoimmune Encephalomyelitis

EAE is an inflammatory, demyelinating disease of the central nervous system (CNS) that can be induced in several mammalian species, such as rodents, dogs, or primates. There are several models of EAE that differ from one another by the species in which EAE is induced, by the specific antigen used during immunization, and by the way it mimics the human disease: No single EAE model can be expected to reflect every aspect of the clinical and pathologic pictures of MS.[2] For example, an acute monophasic disease can be induced in the Lewis rat, characterized by the absence of relapses and almost no demyelination, one of the hallmarks of MS, but it still presents major pathologic similarities with MS, such as a perivascular mononuclear cell infiltration of the brain and the spinal cord. It is also possible to induce a chronic, relapsing EAE in the same rat strain or in other species, such as guinea pigs or marmosets, with relapses and remissions and demyelination foci following the same distribution patterns as those in MS. In the SJL mouse strain, EAE is manifested clinically by relapses and remissions. Therefore, each model may be useful to study one particular aspect of the human disease.

Historically, the EAE model was developed in the first half of the twentieth century, after the observation of spinal cord inflammation and clinical paralysis after rabies immunization in humans: The paralytic accidents were due to immunization against brain tissue, which was used for growing the attenuated rabies virus.[3,4] The development of Freund's adjuvant made it possible to induce EAE reproducibly in many animal strains after a single injection of CNS extract. See Chapter 1 for a his-

Table 6-1. Comparisons Among Clinical, Genetic, and Pathologic Features in Multiple Sclerosis (MS) and Experimental Autoimmune Encephalomyelitis (EAE)

Feature	MS	EAE
Relapses and remissions	Present	Present
Paralysis	Present	Present
Visual impairment	Present	Present
Ataxia	Present	Present
MHC-linked susceptibility	Yes	Yes
Female predominance	Yes	Yes
Myelin-reactive T cells	Present	Present
Inflammation in CNS	Present	Present
Myelin antibodies	Present	Present
Demyelination	Present	Present
Axonal dystrophy	Present	Present
Epitope spreading	Present	Present

CNS = central nervous system; MHC = major histocompatibility complex.

torical perspective on the development of the EAE model.

EAE can be induced in two major ways: either by injection of whole white matter or single myelin proteins, such as proteolipid protein, myelin basic protein (MBP), myelin oligodendrocyte glycoprotein (MOG), myelin-associated glycoprotein and others, in susceptible animal strains, or by transfer of cellular components from affected animals into naïve recipients. Also important is the concept of epitope spreading, which refers to the process of broadening of the immune response against one epitope on the inducing myelin antigen to the recognition of other (±) dominant epitopes on the same molecule or other myelin antigens (intra- or intermolecular spreading).[5,6]

Similar to what is seen is MS, there is a clear relationship between the animals' major histocompatibility complex (MHC) class II background and the disease susceptibility. The interactions between the MHC class II molecule and the presented antigenic peptide are of prime importance for immunogenicity and encephalitogenicity.[7]

Even if imperfect, the EAE model shares major clinical, genetic, and pathologic similarities with MS (Table 6-1), which renders it one of the best available tools for studying the mechanisms of the disease at the cellular and molecular levels. Although EAE is by far the most frequently used model of MS, it is not the only one: A demyelinating disease induced by the Theiler murine encephalomyelitis virus (TMEV) has emerged during the last 20 years as a very interesting model for exploring the viral hypothesis in MS. Theiler's virus, a murine picornavirus, induces in mice a neurologic disease characterized by an acute encephalomyelitis wherein TMEV-specific T cells cross the blood-brain barrier (BBB) to attack virally infected glial cells and macrophages in the white matter.[8] This is followed by a chronic phase, involving the activation of myelin-reactive T cells.[9] This late demyelinating disease, which lasts for the life of the animals, is studied as a model for MS because of its chronicity and similarity of the lesions' histology to those of MS.

The classic description of the demyelinating process in MS involves T cells, immunoglobulins (Igs), and complement, but recent evidence shows that cytokines, chemokines, adhesion molecules, metalloproteinases, nitric oxide, and oxygen metabolites all participate in the effector stages of the disease and can, therefore, be potential therapeutic targets. Oligodendrocytes, which are a key target of the demyelinating process, are addressed in Chapters 2 and 3.

Role of T Cells

The Bench

Describing in detail the role of T cells in EAE/MS is beyond the scope of this chapter. A few key concepts are addressed because of their potential therapeutic applications. As mentioned, the adoptive transfer of myelin-specific T cells from affected animals into naive ones has confirmed that EAE is a T-cell–mediated autoimmune disease.[10] In fact, it is also possible to generate encephalitogenic T cells (i.e., capable of inducing EAE) from peripheral blood lymphocytes in vitro.[11] This indicates that autoreactive T cells are part of the normal T-cell repertoire, suggesting that they can escape the thymic negative selection, and this has been shown in animals as well as in humans.[12,13] What transforms "normal" autoreactive T cells into "pathogenic" autoaggressive T cells is unknown. One hypothesis is that an infectious event (systemic or in the CNS) might induce an initial activation of myelin-reactive

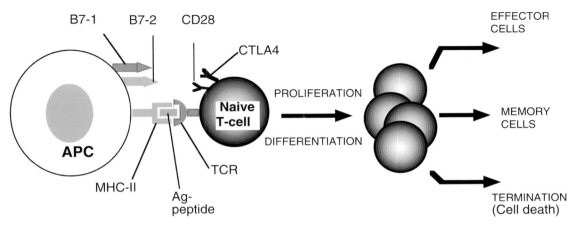

Figure 6-1. Molecules involved in costimulation between a naïve T cell and an antigen-presenting cell (APC). The first signal is given by the contact between the T-cell receptor (TCR) and the complex made of the antigen-peptide (Ag-peptide) and the major histocompatibility complex (MHC) molecule. The second signal is delivered by the contact between B7-1 and B7-2 on one side and CD28 and cytotoxic T lymphocyte–associated antigen 4 (CTLA4) on the other side. New molecules involved in costimulation are being characterized. After stimulation, T cells proliferate, differentiate, and end up as effector or memory cells or may die as a consequence of the regulation of the immune response.

T cells because of some molecular mimicry between the putative infectious agent (a virus) and a myelin antigen.[14] This initial event would be followed by epitope spreading and recognition of multiple CNS myelin proteins. Recent data regarding the TMEV model have demonstrated that after viral CNS infection, myelin antigen can indeed be processed and presented by microglial cells to naive T cells to activate them.[15] Another somehow related hypothesis contends that molecular mimicry events could be more frequent, owing to a reduced number of pathogen-specific memory T cells in individuals living in developed societies, where pathogen exposure is both reduced and delayed during life (and where MS prevalence is higher than in developing countries). This would lead to a relatively limited repertoire, which would induce overshooting responses to an infectious agent, which in turn would stimulate resting, cross-reactive, low-affinity T cells.[16]

It is currently believed that it is the CNS antigen-reactive T cells that provide the organ specificity of the pathogenic process in EAE and recruit antigen-nonspecific lymphocytes and monocytes, by upregulating adhesion molecules, proinflammatory cytokines, and chemokines. These lymphocytes and monocytes, which normally do not cross the BBB, act as effector cells by releasing myelinotoxic substances. Almost all the T cells involved in EAE/MS

are CD4+ and, therefore, recognize antigen only when presented by MHC class II molecules (termed *MHC class II restriction*). Although CD8+ cells (which are MHC-class I restricted) have been detected in MS plaques,[17] their role in MS pathogenesis is not known.

The Bedside

For a T cell to react to antigen (i.e., to become activated), the antigen has to be presented by MHC molecules and recognized by the T-cell receptor (Figure 6-1). When CD4+ T cells specific for a particular peptide antigen recognize that antigen presented by a competent antigen-presenting cell (APC), such as monocytes or B cells, these T cells become activated and proliferate. However, if these same T cells first encounter a variant mutated form of that antigen in which the residues in contact with the T-cell receptor are slightly altered, the T cells may become anergic (i.e., they will not become activated) or they may downregulate their proinflammatory cytokine profile even on later presentation of the original peptide antigen.[18] The variant form of the antigen is called *altered peptide ligand* and represents a mechanism by which T-cell activation can be regulated in physiologic, pathologic, or even therapeutic situations. Glatiramer acetate, which is a synthetic polypeptide made of the random sequence of four amino acids (glutamate, tyrosine, alanine, lysine) and is believed to act as a "universal altered peptide ligand,"[19] is a drug currently used to reduce the relapse rate in MS and is a good example of a therapeutic approach that originated from the EAE model. Recombinant interferon beta (IFN-β), the other major drug in MS therapy, was actually first shown to be clinically effective in relapsing MS before it was shown to ameliorate EAE.

Role of Costimulation

To become activated and proliferate after contact with a specific antigen, a T cell requires two signals from the APC: the first is antigen-specific and delivered by the recognition of the antigen peptide–MHC complex on the APC by the T-cell receptor; the second signal, termed *costimulatory*, is delivered by the contact between several soluble or membrane-bound molecules (see Figure 6-1). Some of the most important costimulatory molecules are CD28 and cytotoxic T lymphocyte–associated antigen 4 (CTLA4) (also named CD152) on the surface of T cells, which bind to B7-1 (also named *CD80*) and B7-2 (also named *CD86*), expressed on the surface of APCs.[20] Unlike the process with CD28, binding of B7 molecules to CTLA4 provides a negative signal, leading to T-cell death or anergy.[21]

The Bench

The B7-CD28-CTLA4 costimulatory system plays a critical role in EAE and is, therefore, a promising therapeutic target in MS. CD28 costimulation is crucial for the development of actively induced EAE, as shown in CD28-deficient mice, which are resistant to EAE.[22] Blockade of CD28 signaling with the CD28 Fab antibody fragments ameliorates MBP-induced EAE.[23] CTLA4Ig, a fusion protein that binds and blocks B7-1 and B7-2 signaling, prevents the adoptive transfer of chronic relapsing EAE in mice[24] and inhibits actively induced disease.[25,26] Systemic injection of APCs treated ex vivo with the p71-90 peptide of MBP and CTLA4Ig before immunization protected rats from clinical EAE.[27]

There is evidence for separate roles of B7-1 and B7-2 in EAE induction and progression. Thus, B7-1 blockade was reported to exacerbate or protect from disease, depending on the timing of administration.[28,29] Initial studies using specific anti–B7-1 or anti–B7-2 blocking monoclonal antibodies to prevent EAE showed that administration of anti–B7-1 was effective in preventing disease, whereas administration of anti–B7-2 worsened the disease.[30] Further studies from our group using a mutant form of CTLA4Ig that binds and blocks only B7-1 did not support these findings and showed that in the murine and Lewis rat models of EAE, systemic B7-1 blockade was detrimental.[31,32] Furthermore, B7-1 is expressed in the CNS during remission from EAE and not during relapses[33] at the time when expression of CTLA4 expression is increased, suggesting a potential regulatory role for B7-1–CTLA4 interaction.[31] We have recently shown that EAE can be induced in CD28-deficient animals by blocking B7-1.[34] These data suggest an important regulatory role for B7-1 and B7-2, but further understanding of the function of these molecules is needed.

A new costimulatory molecule, ICOS ("*inducible co*stimulatory") has recently been described, which is structurally and functionally related to CD28.[35] ICOS expression on the surface of T cells requires induction, unlike CD28, which is constitutively expressed. An ICOS ligand has also been identified on murine B cells and macrophages, called *B7h*, *B7RP-1*, or *LICOS*, which has 20% homology with B7 molecules and stimulates T cells in a CD28-independent manner.[36]

The Bedside

Using reverse transcriptase–polymerase chain reaction and immunocytochemistry, Windhagen et al.[37] showed in human brain biopsy samples that expression of B7-1 is increased in acute MS plaques as compared to inflammatory infarcts, whereas B7-2 is constitutively expressed in all samples (MS and non-MS). The number of circulating B7-1–positive B cells is increased in the blood in active MS but not in stable MS, and IFN-β-1b reduces this number, whereas it increases the number of B7-2–positive circulating monocytes.[38] B7-1 is also increased in the cerebrospinal fluid (CSF) of relapsing-remitting MS patients.[39]

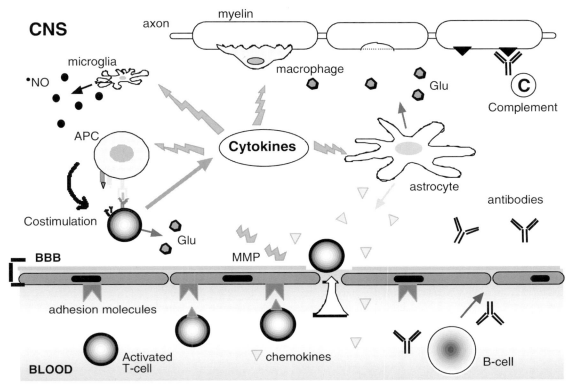

Figure 6-2. Overview of the immunopathogenic mechanisms involved in demyelination in multiple sclerosis. (APC = antigen-presenting cell; BBB = blood-brain barrier; C = complement; CNS = central nervous system; Glu = L-glutamate; MMP = matrix metalloproteinase; ˙NO = nitric oxide.)

As a therapeutic approach, administration of CTLA4Ig appears to be promising, although there is still no report of its use in MS. Phase 1 clinical trials have shown that CTLA4Ig treatment of patients with psoriasis vulgaris is well tolerated and results in clinical improvement.[40] Other human autoimmune diseases and cancers may benefit from CTLA4Ig treatment after successful attempts with animal models, such as murine lupus,[41] collagen-induced arthritis,[42] and metastatic prostate cancer.[43] Phase I trials with MS patients are in preparation.

Role of Cytokines

The Bench

Many cytokines are involved in EAE and MS. These signaling molecules are produced by lymphocytes and macrophages, the effector cells in EAE (Figure 6-2). After antigenic stimulation, CD4+ T cells differentiate into two distinct populations, each producing its own set of cytokines and mediating separate effector functions.[44] Type 1 T helper (Th1) cells produce interleukin-2 (IL-2), tumor necrosis factor-β (TNF-β), and IFN-γ and mediate activation of macrophages and induction of delayed-type hypersensitivity responses. Th2 cells produce IL-4, -5, -10, and -13, which provide help for B-cell function. These two cell populations mutually regulate each other's function.[45] Th2 cytokines have been shown to suppress cell-mediated immunity.[46] Recently, several studies in autoimmune and transplantation models showed that tolerance induction is sometimes associated with a state of immune deviation toward predominantly Th2-cell function, with inhibition of Th1 and upregulation of Th2 cytokines in the target organ.

EAE is induced by autoreactive Th1 cells,[47–49] whereas regulatory T cells that suppress the development of EAE produce Th2 cytokines.[30,50,51] In addition, recovery from EAE is associated with expression of Th2 cytokines in the CNS.[52–54] However, recent data have raised some concerns by suggesting that Th2 cytokines may cause worsening of disease.[55,56]

Complicating the picture further, induction of EAE in single cytokine knockout mice has not provided conclusive results as to the role of Th1 versus Th2 cells in disease. Disruption of the IFN-γ gene does not prevent EAE in susceptible mouse strains[57] and renders mice that are normally resistant to EAE susceptible to disease.[58] Some studies in mice deficient in IL-4 report that these mice have more severe EAE but recover at the same time as wild-type mice, suggesting that the absence of IL-4 does not induce chronic disease.[59] However, other studies suggested that IL-4 plays no role in the severity or recovery from EAE[60] and is not as critical as IL-10 in protection from EAE.[61] Therefore, disruption of a single cytokine gene may not give definitive answers on the role of that cytokine because of redundancy of function shared by other cytokines.

It is important to keep a critical view on the results obtained with genetically manipulated animals, first because the effects of such manipulations and their possible consequences on the animal's development are far from being understood. For example, TNF-α and lymphotoxin double-deficient mice have no lymph nodes, have defective T cells, and have abnormal spleen architecture.[62] Second, in many of the experiments using cytokine gene overexpression, the gene of interest is overexpressed in only one system (i.e., the CNS) and not in the rest of the organism, which renders it questionable whether this represents appropriate conditions under which to study a gene function and make conclusions about its role in EAE.[63] Third, many of the targeted cytokine-receptors have redundant functions. Therapeutic attempts aiming at a single effector pathway may have limited efficacy or no efficacy at all, if parallel pathways are still at work.

Direct parenteral administration of a cytokine or of an antibody has been used to study the role of cytokines in EAE. Thus, EAE can be induced by administration of IL-12[64] and prevented by anti–IL-12 antibodies.[65] Systemic administration of IFN-γ confers resistance to EAE.[66] Treatment of both TNF-β–deficient and TNF-α–overexpressing mice with TNF-α reduces disease severity,[67] sug-

gesting a protective role for this cytokine. However, TNF-α in vitro can damage myelin and injure oligodendrocytes in culture,[68] and it has also been shown that an antibody to TNF (and lymphotoxin) prevents transfer of EAE in mice.[69] These data demonstrate that a given cytokine may have different and even opposite effects at different time points and when studied in different systems or environments (i.e., in vivo vs. in vitro, transgenic vs. wild-type). An interesting new development is IFN-tau, a bovine molecule that seems to possess all the functions of the type 1 IFNs (such as IFN-β) but not their toxic effects and that can be used to prevent EAE.[70]

The Bedside

On the basis of results obtained with EAE, several cytokines or cytokine-related products have been tried in MS patients. Some have proven to be ineffective, including Lenercept,[71] a recombinant soluble TNF receptor p55 Ig fusion protein, which protects against EAE.[72] Others have had deleterious effects, such as IFN-γ, which induced severe relapses in MS patients.[73] Thus, although EAE is a useful model for MS, one cannot always extrapolate therapeutic benefits from the animal model to the human disease. There is now increasing evidence that IL-12 plays a major role in the pathogenesis of MS.[74] Salbutamol, a β$_2$-agonist that decreases IL-12 through an increase of intracellular cyclic adenosine monophosphate[75] and is mostly used for treatment of bronchospasm, decreases IL-12 in chronic MS patients when given orally[76] and induces a Th2 shift.[76] IL-12 is expressed in human MS brains.[37] Several treatments used in MS, such as IFN-β, do in fact decrease IL-12,[77] and we have previously shown that pulsed cyclophosphamide normalizes IL-12 in chronic MS patients.[78] A humanized monoclonal antibody to IL-12 is in clinical trials for treating inflammatory bowel disease and will be considered for treatment of MS.

Role of Chemokines

Chemokines, or chemoattractant cytokines, are molecules secreted by various cell types that have the ability to activate leukocytes and induce their homing or migration in a particular direction (see Figure 6-2). They are also involved in cell-mediated and humoral immune reactions and in cell adhesion. They act on receptors that are expressed on their target cells, including various leukocyte types and primary CNS cells (i.e., neurons and glia).[79]

The Bench

As the recruitment of inflammatory cells into the CNS is critical for EAE development, chemokines may have a necessary—but not sufficient—role in its induction, as their main action is to attract antigen-specific T cells and other nonspecific macrophages through the BBB. This may result in multifocal inflammation and myelin damage.[80] The chemokines that most closely correlate with the clinical onset and severity of inflammation seem to be macrophage inflammatory protein 1 alpha in chronic EAE[80] and RANTES (regulated upon activation, normal T-cell expressed and secreted) in monophasic EAE.[81] Both these two cytokines are produced by CNS-infiltrating leukocytes. In chronic EAE, several chemokines are upregulated during relapses, such as macrophage inflammatory protein 1 alpha, RANTES, but also monocyte chemotactic protein-1 (MCP-1), IFN inducible protein-10 (IP-10), and growth-regulated oncogene alpha, which are produced by astrocytes around the inflammatory foci.[82] Interestingly, anti–macrophage inflammatory protein 1 alpha antibodies can inhibit the development of acute EAE,[80] whereas anti–MCP-1 antibodies reduce only the severity of relapsing EAE. Another approach has been tried successfully in EAE, using vaccination with naked DNA encoding a particular group of chemokines.[83] Chemokines are not only responsible for the migration of leukocytes to the inflammatory site but also locally stimulate these leukocytes to release proteases,[84] which can cleave proteins, including MBP, into peptides that can generate autoreactive responses[85] (reviewed in reference 86).

The Bedside

Similar to that in EAE, the demyelination process occurring in the brain of MS patients is thought to be mainly due to an inflammatory response in which CD4[+] T cells and macrophages cross the BBB and infiltrate the white matter under the influence of chemokines. Several chemokines are overexpressed in the brains of MS patients, such as MCP-1, MCP-2, MCP-3,[87,88] with a predominant localization to astrocytes and mononuclear cells. Similarly, there is also an increase in the expression of chemokine receptors in white blood cells obtained from the CSF, as compared with the peripheral blood of MS patients.[89] Balashov et al.[90] found that CXCR3(+) T cells were increased in the blood of relapsing-remitting MS patients and that both CCR5(+) and CXCR3(+) T cells were increased in the blood of progressive MS patients as compared with controls. Furthermore, peripheral blood CCR5(+) T cells secreted high levels of IFN-γ in these patients.

By their capacity to attract leukocytes into the CNS and stimulate the secretion of enzymes that can cleave MBP or other myelin proteins that trigger autoreactive responses, chemokines and their receptors are interesting potential targets for immune-based therapy in MS.

Autoantibodies and Complement in Multiple Sclerosis

The Bench

Evidence for a significant role of autoantibodies in the pathogenesis of MS stems from EAE data: The incidence of demyelination in T-cell–mediated EAE is dramatically increased if anti-MOG antibodies are given at the onset of the process.[91] However, only the complement-activating anti-MOG antibodies can induce an inflammatory demyelination in EAE.[92] It has recently been demonstrated in the marmoset EAE as well as in human MS that MOG autoantibodies play a role in the formation of disrupted myelin sheaths.[93] MOG, a minor (less than 0.05%) myelin glycoprotein exposed on the outer surface of oligodendrocytes and of myelin sheaths, is easily accessible to antibodies and is the only antigen in the CNS that can trigger both encephalitogenic T-cell response and the generation of demyelinating antibodies.[94] On the other hand, MBP is a cytosolic protein, and proteolipid protein and myelin-associated glycoprotein are buried deep into the myelin membrane:

They are, therefore, not readily accessible to antibodies. Nonetheless, anti-MBP, anti-proteolipid protein, and anti–myelin–associated glycoprotein antibodies are detected in the CSF of MS patients. Some autoantibodies may play a beneficial role in EAE/MS. Rodriguez et al.[95,96] showed that the transfer of serum directed against spinal cord homogenate into TMEV-infected mice resulted in an important increase of CNS remyelination and confirmed that this effect was due to the IgG contained within this anti–spinal cord homogenate serum. Also in the TMEV model, Warrington et al.[97] recently showed that human monoclonal antibodies reactive to oligodendrocytes promoted remyelination, further challenging the assumption that antibodies that bind oligodendrocytes are necessarily pathogenic.

The mechanism by which autoantibodies may enhance myelin repair is unknown; they might stimulate mature or immature oligodendrocytes to differentiate, divide, or produce myelin, or they might act indirectly by promoting the production of oligodendrocyte survival factors by astrocytes or microglia. They could also inhibit lymphocyte or macrophage activation or even neutralize cytokines interfering with complete remyelination.[98]

The Bedside

One of the hallmarks of MS is the intrathecal synthesis of Igs and the presence of oligoclonal IgG in the CSF of most of the patients. Yet, there is no definite "causative" autoantibody that is pathogenic in the disease, although many autoantibodies have been described in MS (reviewed in reference 99). Igs are found not only in the CSF but also in the actively demyelinating areas (or plaques). A colocalization between Igs and C3d was observed in macrophages in the most active lesions.[100]

Based on the fact that when given in excess, Igs have, via various mechanisms of action, a reliable therapeutic effect in several autoimmune diseases (such as Guillain-Barré syndrome, myasthenia, and other nonneurologic diseases), intravenous Ig administration was also tried in MS patients, with variable success. Recent studies suggest that intravenous Ig may be effective to some degree in patients with relapsing-remitting MS.[101,102] Because

of differences in methodologic design and patient populations, as well as the relatively small number of patients in some of these studies, a definitive role of intravenous Ig in MS therapy has not been established.

T-cell vaccination with myelin-reactive irradiated T-cell lines from the patients' own peripheral blood showed that it could promote an effective depletion of T cells that were reactive against different myelin antigens.[103]

Role of Adhesion Molecules

The Bench

Adhesion molecules promote cell-cell and cell–extracellular matrix interactions and, as such, are involved in many steps of the immune response, including the migration of inflammatory cells through the BBB (see Figure 6-2). They are classified into three families according to their structure: Ig superfamily members, integrins, and selectins. It is now well documented that the expression of some adhesion molecules, such as intercellular cell adhesion molecule-1 (ICAM-1) and vascular cell adhesion molecule-1, is upregulated on microvessel endothelial cells in active lesions of MS[104] as is the expression of their respective receptors on leukocytes: leukocyte function antigen 1 for ICAM-1, and very late antigen 4, also named α4 integrin, for vascular cell adhesion molecule-1.

Adhesion molecules can be found either as cell surface–anchored or as soluble, circulating molecules. Thus, possible therapeutic targets include the molecules themselves, their receptors, and the enzymes responsible for cleavage and shedding of the circulating form. The use of an anti–α4 integrin monoclonal antibody reduced cellular infiltration in the CNS and inhibited development of EAE in rats and guinea pigs[105,106] and reversed the ongoing disease process in the guinea pig.[107] Anti–ICAM-1 monoclonal antibodies inhibited EAE in rats,[108] although in another study, neither anti–ICAM-1 nor anti–leukocyte function antigen 1 antibodies could alter the course of EAE.[109] However, ICAM-1–deficient mice develop a more severe EAE than in controls, suggesting that ICAM-1 plays an important role in downregulating autoimmune inflammation in the CNS.[110]

The Bedside

Besides ICAM-1 and vascular cell adhesion molecule-1, other adhesion molecules are upregulated in MS.[111] Circulating ICAM-1 is the most studied in MS. Its serum levels are constantly elevated in active relapsing-remitting MS, and these levels also correlate with magnetic resonance imaging (MRI) disease activity.[112,113]

In 1999, a randomized, double-blind, placebo-controlled trial of a humanized anti–α4 integrin antibody was performed on 72 patients with relapsing-remitting and secondary progressive MS.[114] This study showed a significant reduction in the number of new active lesions on MRI. The drug was given intravenously and was well tolerated, but the study was not designed to look at the effect on the relapse rate.

Role of Matrix Metalloproteinases

Matrix metalloproteinases (MMPs) are enzymes that can degrade any protein component in the extracellular matrix, including but not limited to membrane-bound adhesion molecules, cytokine precursors and receptors, and proforms of MMP. Most MMPs are secreted by a wide range of cell types as proenzymes that must be cleaved to become activated. Except for the membrane-type MMPs, all other MMPs are secreted into the extracellular space, including that of the CNS (see Figure 6-2), where their lytic activity needs to be finely regulated to avoid potential tissue destruction.

The Bench

In animal models, MMPs are involved in the demyelinating process either as direct effectors, because they can degrade MBP, at least in vitro,[115] or as indirect effectors, by damaging the BBB, thus allowing autoreactive inflammatory cells to enter the CNS. The injection of MMP-7, -8, and -9 in the brain parenchyma of rats with a delayed-type hypersensitivity model of MS is followed by a BBB breakdown and leukocyte recruitment into the CNS.[116] MMPs, and in particular MMP-9, are shown to promote in vitro the trans–basement membrane migration of T cells.[117] In EAE, the messenger RNA encoding for MMP-7 and -9 is dramatically upregulated at the peak of clinical disease.[118] On the other hand, some MMP inhibitors can suppress the development of EAE in rats[119]; they can even reverse ongoing clinical EAE by restoring the damaged BBB without influencing the degree of inflammation and demyelination.[120] It is also interesting that the adhesion molecule α4 integrin (or very late antigen 4) induces the activation of MMP-2.[121]

The Bedside

There is evidence that MMPs are also involved in the BBB breakdown in MS patients; thus, MMP-9 is increased in the CSF of MS patients during clinical relapses.[122] High serum MMP-9 levels are significantly associated with more T_1-weighted gadolinium-enhancing MRI lesions.[123] Treatment with high-dose methylprednisolone (which is known to downregulate MMP) is shown to reduce both MRI gadolinium-enhancing lesions and CSF levels of MMP-9 in MS patients.[124] There are no ongoing trials with MMP inhibitors in MS, but such drugs are being tested in other autoimmune diseases and cancers.[125] Naturally occurring MMP inhibitors, called *tissue inhibitors of metalloproteases*, are involved in the regulation of MMP expression, and it has been suggested that an abnormality in the inhibitory response to MMP might play an etiologic role in the chronicity of MS.[123]

Role of Nitric Oxide and Other Reactive Oxygen Species

The free radical nitric oxide ($^{\bullet}$NO) is produced from the oxidation of L-arginine into L-citrulline by large enzymes called *nitric oxide synthases* (NOS), which are either constitutively expressed in endothelial cells, skeletal muscle cells, and neurons (respectively, eNOS and nNOS), or inducible by different immunologic stimuli and produced by macrophages and microglia (iNOS; see Figure 6-2). $^{\bullet}$NO mediates various biological functions; it acts as a vasodilator, a secondary messenger, and a neurotransmitter and can induce apoptosis.[126] It is not highly toxic by itself, but it reacts very rapidly with other molecules (half-life, less than 5 seconds), and this results in the formation of more damaging products, such as peroxynitrite, which is highly cytotoxic through several mechanisms, including the induction of DNA damage, and in the inhibition of various intracellular enzymes and of the mitochondrial respiratory chain.

The Bench

·NO is an important mediator of inflammation in EAE[127,128] and other demyelinating disorders.[129] The p40 subunit of IL-12, one of the key cytokines in the pathogenesis of EAE and MS, has recently been shown to induce NOS in mice microglia.[130] Elevated levels of iNOS messenger RNA are detected in the CNS of animals during acute EAE.[127] In contrast, mice lacking the *NOS2* gene develop an exacerbated form of EAE,[131] suggesting that iNOS might also have a protective role in demyelination. The effect of NOS inhibitors, such as aminoguanidine, on EAE has also been controversial, as some studies showed that this inhibitor ameliorated EAE induced by T-cell transfer in mice,[132] whereas other groups showed a worsening of the disease in rats.[133] A study by Okuda et al.[134] suggested that the timing of administration of aminoguanidine in relation to time of EAE induction may be crucial. Another NOS inhibitor, uric acid, which is a naturally occurring scavenger of peroxynitrite, prevents development of EAE in mice when given before the clinical onset of the disease and promotes recovery from already active EAE.[135]

Oligodendrocytes seem to be more sensitive to ·NO damage than other CNS cells.[136] Reactive oxygen species affect both lipid and protein components of the myelin sheath. In vitro studies have demonstrated that incubation of myelin with reactive oxygen species results in lipid peroxidation and decompaction of myelin lamellae along the intraperiod line.[137] Both types of degradation were also detected in MS lesions.[138] Recent reports have shown that ·NO blocks axonal conduction in vivo in rats.[139]

The Bedside

The presence of activated macrophages expressing high levels of iNOS and evidence of peroxynitrite formation have been demonstrated in plaque areas of postmortem brain tissue from MS patients.[140] A few cross-sectional studies of MS patients have detected increased levels of ·NO in the CSF,[141] serum,[142] and urine,[143] but this is not specific for MS, as high ·NO levels in body fluids are also detected in other inflammatory neurologic and nonneurologic diseases. It is interesting to note that in a survey of 20 million outpatient database records searched for MS, gout (hyperuricemia), or both, 36,000 patients had gout, 34,000 had MS, but only four had both conditions, although the distributions of MS and gout in the studied population should have led to approximately 60 patients with both diseases,[135] suggesting that the two diseases tend to be mutually exclusive. The same report showed that in 46 MS patients and 46 age- and gender-matched controls with other neurologic disease who were placed on the same diet for 5 days, levels of serum uric acid were significantly lower in MS patients than in controls, suggesting that high serum uric acid levels may protect against the development of MS.

However, the exact role of ·NO and other reactive oxygen species in the pathogenesis of MS is still unknown. These compounds, and in particular ·NO, may have both protective and deleterious effects on the disease, depending on its stage. There are no current trials of NOS inhibitors in humans.

Role of Excitotoxicity

L-Glutamate (Glu) is the most widespread excitatory transmitter system in the vertebrate CNS. In addition to its role as a synaptic neurotransmitter, Glu induces long-lasting changes in neuronal excitability, synaptic structure and function, neuronal migration during development, and neuronal viability. These effects are mediated by two general classes of receptors, those that form ion channels (or "ionotropic"), such as the kainate, alpha-amino-3-hydroxy-5-methylisoxazole-4-propionic acid (AMPA), and *N*-methyl-D-aspartate receptors, and those that are linked to G proteins (or "metabotropic"). Glu is not only produced by neurons and glial cells but also by cells of the immune system, such as macrophages and T cells (see Figure 6-2), and Glu receptors are expressed both in neuronal and glial membranes.

The term *excitotoxicity* simply refers to the cellular toxicity induced by elevated glutamate or other excitatory neurotransmitter, such as aspartate, and mediated by its receptors.

The Bench

Activated immune cells release large amounts of Glu in the murine CNS[144] and, like neurons, oligodendrocytes are highly sensitive to AMPA–kainate receptor–mediated death.[145] Based on these facts, two groups simultaneously and independently showed that 1,2,3,4-tetrahydro-6-nitro-2,3-dioxobenzo(f)quinoxaline-7-sulfonamide disodium, an AMPA-kainate receptor antagonist, substantially improved clinical EAE and increased oligodendrocyte survival without reducing the lesion size or the degree of CNS inflammation, both in SJL mice[146] and in Lewis rats,[147] suggesting that Glu excitotoxicity is an important mechanism in autoimmune demyelination. This is in accordance with the fact that Glu degradation is downregulated in astrocytes during EAE, due to glutamine synthetase– and glutamate dehydrogenase–reduced expression, thus leading to an increase of Glu in the CNS.[148]

The Bedside

There is an increased level of Glu in the CSF of patients during acute attacks of MS,[149] and this might be explained by the increased ·NO and peroxynitrite generation in the disease.[150] Increased CSF Glu level is not specific for MS, as it is also demonstrated in patients with encephalitis and with stroke.[151] Serum Glu is also elevated during relapses.[152] AMPA antagonists are now being tested in stroke patients. There is no report yet on the use of Glu or Glu receptor antagonists in MS patients.

Conclusions

Demyelination is one of the most important pathologic processes occurring in MS, an extremely complex and heterogenous disease of the human CNS. With the help of modern biotechnology, it has been possible during the last few decades to examine in detail many of the mechanisms involved in the pathogenesis of the disease, to conceive new rational therapeutic strategies based on these mechanisms, and to test them in dependable animal models. Although it is not always straightforward to extrapolate from animal results to humans, EAE and other animal models of MS have helped to bring to MS patients new effective treatments and new hopes for their disease.

References

1. Trapp BD, Peterson J, Ransohoff RM, et al. Axonal transection in the lesions of multiple sclerosis. N Engl J Med 1998;338:278–285.
2. Martin R, McFarland HF. Immunology of Multiple Sclerosis and Experimental Allergic Encephalomyelitis. In CS Raine, HF McFarland, WW Tourtellotte (eds), Multiple Sclerosis: Clinical and Pathogenetic Basis. London: Chapman & Hall, 1997;221–242.
3. Kabat EA, Wolf A, Bezer AL. The rapid production of acute disseminated encephalomyelitis in Rhesus monkeys by injection of heterologous and homologous brain tissue with adjuvants. J Exp Med 1947;85:117–129.
4. Rivers TM, Schwentker FF. Encephalomyelitis accompanied by myelin destruction experimentally produced in monkeys. J Exp Med 1935;61:689–702.
5. Lehmann PV, Forsthuber T, Miller A, Sercarz EE. Spreading of T-cell autoimmunity to cryptic determinants of an autoantigen. Nature 1992;358:155–157.
6. Tuohy VK, Yu M, Yin L, et al. The epitope spreading cascade during progression of experimental autoimmune encephalomyelitis and multiple sclerosis. Immunol Rev 1998;164:93–100.
7. Greer JM, Sobel RA, Sette A, et al. Immunogenic and encephalitogenic epitope clusters of myelin proteolipid protein. J Immunol 1996;156:371–379.
8. Miller SD, Gerety SJ. Immunologic aspects of Theiler's murine encephalomyelitis virus (TMEV)-induced demyelinating disease. Semin Virol 1990;1:263–272.
9. Miller SD, Vanderlugt CL, Begolka WS, et al. Persistent infection with Theiler's virus leads to CNS autoimmunity via epitope spreading. Nat Med 1997;3:1133–1136.
10. Zamvil SS, Steinman L. The T lymphocyte in experimental allergic encephalomyelitis. Annu Rev Immunol 1990; 8:579–621.
11. Schluesener HJ, Wekerle H. Autoaggressive T lymphocyte lines recognizing the encephalitogenic region of myelin basic protein: in vitro selection from unprimed rat T lymphocyte populations. J Immunol 1985;135:3128–3133.
12. Burns J, Rosenzweig A, Zweiman B, Lisak RP. Isolation of myelin basic protein-reactive T-cell lines from normal human blood. Cell Immunol 1983;81:435.
13. Ota K, Matsui M, Milford EL, et al. T cell recognition of an immunodominant myelin basic protein epitope in multiple sclerosis. Nature 1990;346:183–187.

14. Fujinami RS, Oldstone MBA. Amino acid homology between the encephalitogenic site of myelin basic protein and virus: mechanism for autoimmunity. Science 1985;230:1043–1046.

15. Katz-Levy Y, Neville KL, Girvin AM, et al. Endogenous presentation of self myelin epitopes by CNS-resident APCs in Theiler's virus-infected mice. J Clin Invest 1999;104:599–610.

16. Kaufman MD. Do microbes with peptides mimicking myelin cause multiple sclerosis if the T cell response to their unique peptides is limited? J Theor Biol 1998; 193:691–708.

17. Jurewicz A, Biddison WE, Antel JP. MHC class I-restricted lysis of human oligodendrocytes by myelin basic protein peptide-specific CD8 T lymphocytes. J Immunol 1998;160:3056–3059.

18. Nicholson LB, Greer JM, Sobel RA, et al. An altered peptide ligand mediates immune deviation and prevents autoimmune encephalomyelitis. Immunity 1995;3:397–405.

19. Duda PW, Schmied MC, Cook SL, et al. Glatiramer acetate (Copaxone) induces degenerate, Th2-polarized immune responses in patients with multiple sclerosis. J Clin Invest 2000;105:967–976.

20. Abbas AK, Lichtman AH, Pober JS. Cellular and Molecular Immunology. Philadelphia: Saunders, 1997.

21. Krummel MF, Allison JP. CD28 and CTLA-4 have opposing effects on the response of T cells to stimulation. J Exp Med 1995;182:459–465.

22. Oliveira-dos-Santos AJ, Ho A, Tada Y, et al. CD28 costimulation is crucial for the development of spontaneous autoimmune encephalomyelitis. J Immunol 1999;162: 4490–4495.

23. Perrin PJ, June CH, Maldonado JH, et al. Blockade of CD28 during in vitro activation of encephalitogenic T cells or after disease onset ameliorates experimental autoimmune encephalomyelitis. J Immunol 1999;163: 1704–1710.

24. Perrin PJ, Scott D, Quigley L, et al. Role of B7:CD28/CTLA-4 in the induction of chronic relapsing experimental allergic encephalomyelitis. J Immunol 1995;154: 1481–1490.

25. Cross AH, Girard TJ, Giacoletto KS, et al. Long-term inhibition of murine experimental autoimmune encephalomyelitis using CTLA-4-Fc supports a key role for CD28 costimulation. J Clin Invest 1995;95:2783–2789.

26. Khoury SJ, Akalin E, Chandraker A, et al. CD28-B7 costimulatory blockade by CTLA4Ig prevents actively induced experimental autoimmune encephalomyelitis and inhibits Th1 but spares Th2 cytokines in the central nervous system. J Immunol 1995;155:4521–4524.

27. Khoury SJ, Gallon L, Verburg RR, et al. Ex vivo treatment of antigen-presenting cells with CTLA4Ig and encephalitogenic peptide prevents experimental autoimmune encephalomyelitis in the Lewis rat. J Immunol 1996;157: 3700–3705.

28. Perrin PJ, Scott D, June CH, Racke MK. B7-mediated costimulation can either provoke or prevent clinical manifestations of experimental allergic encephalomyelitis. Immunol Res 1995;14:189–199.

29. Racke MK, Scott DE, Quigley L, et al. Distinct roles for B7-1 (CD-80) and B7-2 (CD-86) in the initiation of experimental allergic encephalomyelitis. J Clin Invest 1995; 96:2195–2203.

30. Kuchroo VK, Das MP, Brown JA, et al. B7-1 and B7-2 costimulatory molecules differentially activate the TH1/TH2 developmental pathways: Application to autoimmune disease therapy. Cell 1995;80:707–718.

31. Gallon L, Chandraker A, Issazadeh S, et al. Differential effects of B7-1 blockade in the rat experimental autoimmune encephalomyelitis model. J Immunol 1997;159:4212–4216.

32. Schaub M, Issazadeh S, Stadlbauer TH, et al. Costimulatory signal blockade in murine relapsing experimental autoimmune encephalomyelitis. J Neuroimmunol 1999; 96:158–166.

33. Issazadeh S, Navikas V, Schaub M, et al. Kinetics of expression of costimulatory molecules and their ligands in murine relapsing experimental autoimmune encephalomyelitis in vivo. J Immunol 1998;161:1104–1112.

34. Chitnis T, Najafian N, Abdallah KA, et al. CD28-independent induction of experimental autoimmune encephalomyelitis. J Clin Invest 2001;107:575–583.

35. Hutloff A, Dittrich AM, Beier KC, et al. ICOS is an inducible T-cell co-stimulator structurally and functionally related to CD28. Nature 1999;397:263–266.

36. Yoshinaga SK, Whoriskey JS, Khare SD, et al. T-cell costimulation through B7RP-1 and ICOS. Nature 1999;402: 827–832.

37. Windhagen A, Newcombe J, Dangond F, et al. Expression of costimulatory molecules B7-1 (CD80), B7-2 (CD86), and interleukin 12 cytokine in multiple sclerosis lesions. J Exp Med 1995;182:1985–1996.

38. Genc K, Dona DL, Reder AT. Increased CD80(+) B cells in active multiple sclerosis and reversal by interferon beta-1b therapy. J Clin Invest 1997;99:2664–2671.

39. Svenningsson A, Dotevall L, Stemme S, Andersen O. Increased expression of B7-1 costimulatory molecule on cerebrospinal fluid cells of patients with multiple sclerosis and infectious central nervous system disease. J Neuroimmunol 1997;75:59–68.

40. Abrams JR, Lebwohl MG, Guzzo CA, et al. CTLA4Ig-mediated blockade of T-cell costimulation in patients with psoriasis vulgaris. J Clin Invest 1999;103:1243–1252.

41. Finck BK, Linsley PS, Wofsy D. Treatment of murine lupus with CTLA4Ig. Science 1994;265:1225–1227.

42. Webb LM, Walmsley MJ, Feldmann M. Prevention and amelioration of collagen-induced arthritis by blockade of the CD28 co-stimulatory pathway: requirement for both B7-1 and B7-2. Eur J Immunol 1996;26:2320–2328.

43. Kwon ED, Foster BA, Hurwitz AA, et al. Elimination of residual metastatic prostate cancer after surgery and adjunctive cytotoxic T lymphocyte-associated antigen 4 (CTLA-4) blockade immunotherapy. Proc Natl Acad Sci U S A 1999;96:15074–15079.

44. Mosmann TR, Cherwinski H, Bond MW, et al. Two types of murine helper T cell clone. I. Definition according to profiles of lymphokine activities and secreted proteins. J Immunol 1986;136:2348–2357.

45. Paul WE, Seder RA. Lymphocyte responses and cytokines. Cell 1994;76:241–251.

46. Powrie F, Coffman RL. Cytokine regulation of T-cell function: potential for therapeutic intervention. Immunol Today 1993;14:270–274.

47. Zamvil S, Nelson P, Trotter J, et al. T-cell clones specific for myelin basic protein induce chronic relapsing paralysis and demyelination. Nature 1985;317:355–358.

48. Vandenbark AA, Gill T, Offner H. A myelin basic protein-specific T lymphocyte line that mediates experimental autoimmune encephalomyelitis. J Immunol 1985;153: 223–228.

49. Kuchroo VK, Martin CA, Greer JM, et al. Cytokines and adhesion molecules contribute to the ability of myelin proteolipid protein-specific T cell clones to mediate experimental allergic encephalomyelitis. J Immunol 1993; 151:4371–4382.

50. Chen Y, Kuchroo VK, Inobe J-I, et al. Regulatory T cell clones induced by oral tolerance: suppression of autoimmune encephalomyelitis. Science 1994;265:1237–1240.

51. Cua DJ, Hinton DR, Stohlman SA. Self-antigen-induced Th2 responses in experimental allergic encephalomyelitis (EAE)-resistant mice. Th2-mediated suppression of autoimmune disease. J Immunol 1995;155:4052–4059.

52. Khoury SJ, Hancock WW, Weiner HL. Oral tolerance to myelin basic protein and natural recovery from experimental autoimmune encephalomyelitis are associated with down-regulation of inflammatory cytokines and differential upregulation of transforming growth factor-β and prostaglandin E expression in the brain. J Exp Med 1992;176:1355–1364.

53. Kennedy MK, Torrance DS, Picha KS, Mohler KM. Analysis of cytokine mRNA expression in the central nervous system of mice with experimental autoimmune encephalomyelitis reveals that IL-10 mRNA expression correlates with recovery. J Immunol 1992;149:2496–2505.

54. Issazadeh S, Lorentzen JC, Mustafa MI, et al. Cytokines in relapsing experimental autoimmune encephalomyelitis in DA rats: persistent mRNA expression of proinflammatory cytokines and absent expression of interleukin-10 and transforming growth factor-beta. J Neuroimmunol 1996; 69:103–115.

55. Genain CP, Abel K, Belmar N, et al. Late complications of immune deviation therapy in a nonhuman primate. Science 1996;274:2054–2057.

56. Lafaille JJ, Keere FV, Hsu AL, et al. Myelin basic protein-specific T helper 2 (Th2) cells cause experimental autoimmune encephalomyelitis in immunodeficient hosts rather than protect them from the disease. J Exp Med 1997;186: 307–312.

57. Ferber IA, Brocke S, Taylor-Edwards C, et al. Mice with a disrupted IFN-gamma gene are susceptible to the induction of experimental autoimmune encephalomyelitis (EAE). J Immunol 1996;156:5–7.

58. Krakowski M, Owens T. Interferon-gamma confers resistance to experimental allergic encephalomyelitis. Eur J Immunol 1996;26:1641–1646.

59. Falcone M, Rajan AJ, Bloom BR, Brosnan CF. A critical role for IL-4 in regulating disease severity in experimental allergic encephalomyelitis as demonstrated in IL-4-deficient C57BL/6 mice and BALB/c mice. J Immunol 1998;160:4822–4830.

60. Liblau R, Steinman L, Brocke S. Experimental autoimmune encephalomyelitis in IL-4-deficient mice. Int Immunol 1997;9:799–803.

61. Bettelli E, Das MP, Howard ED, et al. IL-10 is critical in the regulation of autoimmune encephalomyelitis as demonstrated by studies of IL-10- and IL-4-deficient and transgenic mice. J Immunol 1998;161:3299–3306.

62. Eugster HP, Muller M, Karrer U, et al. Multiple immune abnormalities in tumor necrosis factor and lymphotoxin-alpha double-deficient mice. Int Immunol 1996;8:23–36.

63. Steinman L. Some misconceptions about understanding autoimmunity through experiments with knockouts. J Exp Med 1997;185:2039–2041.

64. Smith T, Hewson AK, Kingsley CI, et al. Interleukin-12 induces relapse in experimental allergic encephalomyelitis in the Lewis rat. Am J Pathol 1997;150:1909–1917.

65. Leonard JP, Waldburger KE, Goldman SJ. Prevention of experimental autoimmune encephalomyelitis by antibodies against interleukin 12. J Exp Med 1995;181:381–386.

66. Krakowski M, Owens T. Interferon-gamma confers resistance to experimental allergic encephalomyelitis. Eur J Immunol 1996;26:1641–1646.

67. Liu J, Marino MW, Wong G, et al. TNF is a potent anti-inflammatory cytokine in autoimmune-mediated demyelination. Nat Med 1998;4:78–83.

68. Selmaj K, Raine CS. Tumor necrosis factor mediates myelin damage in organotypic cultures of nervous tissue. Ann N Y Acad Sci 1988;540:568–570.

69. Ruddle NH, Bergman CM, McGrath KM, et al. An antibody to lymphotoxin and tumor necrosis factor prevents transfer of experimental allergic encephalomyelitis. J Exp Med 1990;172:1193–1200.

70. Soos JM, Subramaniam PS, Hobeika AC, et al. The IFN pregnancy recognition hormone IFN-tau blocks both development and superantigen reactivation of experimental allergic encephalomyelitis without associated toxicity. J Immunol 1995;155:2747–2753.

71. TNF neutralization in MS: results of a randomized, placebo-controlled multicenter study. The Lenercept Multiple Sclerosis Study Group and The University of British Columbia MS/MRI Analysis Group. Neurology 1999;53: 457–465.

72. Klinkert WE, Kojima K, Lesslauer W, et al. TNF-alpha receptor fusion protein prevents experimental autoimmune encephalomyelitis and demyelination in Lewis rats: an overview. J Neuroimmunol 1997;72:163–168.

73. Panitch HS, Hirsch RL, Haley AS, Johnson KP. Exacerbations of multiple sclerosis in patients treated with gamma interferon. Lancet 1987;1:893–895.

74. Trembleau S, Germann T, Gately MK, Adorini L. The role of IL-12 in the induction of organ-specific autoimmune diseases. Immunol Today 1995;16:383–386.

75. Panina-Bordignon P, Mazzeo D, Lucia PD, et al. Beta2-agonists prevent Th1 development by selective inhibition of interleukin 12. J Clin Invest 1997;100:1513–1519.

76. Makhlouf K, Comabella M, Imitola J, et al. Oral salbutamol decreases IL-12 expression in monocytes of patients with multiple sclerosis. J Neuroimmunol 2001;117:156–165.

77. Karp CL, Biron CA, Irani DN. Interferon beta in multiple sclerosis: is IL-12 suppression the key? Immunol Today 2000;21:24–28.

78. Comabella M, Balashov K, Issazadeh S, et al. Elevated interleukin-12 in progressive multiple sclerosis correlates with disease activity and is normalized by pulse cyclophosphamide therapy. J Clin Invest 1998;102:671–678.

79. Luster AD. Chemokines—chemotactic cytokines that mediate inflammation. N Engl J Med 1998;338:436–445.

80. Karpus WJ, Lukacs NW, McRae BL, et al. An important role for the chemokine macrophage inflammatory protein-1 alpha in the pathogenesis of the T cell-mediated autoimmune disease, experimental autoimmune encephalomyelitis. J Immunol 1995;155:5003–5010.

81. Miyagishi R, Kikuchi S, Takayama C, et al. Identification of cell types producing RANTES, MIP-1 alpha and MIP-1 beta in rat experimental autoimmune encephalomyelitis by in situ hybridization. J Neuroimmunol 1997;77:17–26.

82. Glabinski AR, Tani M, Strieter RM, et al. Synchronous synthesis of alpha- and beta-chemokines by cells of diverse lineage in the central nervous system of mice with relapses of chronic experimental autoimmune encephalomyelitis. Am J Pathol 1997;150:617–630.

83. Youssef S, Wildbaum G, Maor G, et al. Long-lasting protective immunity to experimental autoimmune encephalomyelitis following vaccination with naked DNA encoding C-C chemokines. J Immunol 1998;161:3870–3879.

84. Proost P, Wuyts A, van Damme J. The role of chemokines in inflammation. Int J Clin Lab Res 1996;26:211–223.

85. Opdenakker G, Van Damme J. Cytokine-regulated proteases in autoimmune diseases. Immunol Today 1994;15:103–107.

86. Zhang GX, Baker CM, Kolson DL, Rostami AM. Chemokines and chemokine receptors in the pathogenesis of multiple sclerosis. Mult Scler 2000;6:3–13.

87. Van Der Voorn P, Tekstra J, Beelen RH, et al. Expression of MCP-1 by reactive astrocytes in demyelinating multiple sclerosis lesions. Am J Pathol 1999;154:45–51.

88. McManus C, Berman JW, Brett FM, et al. MCP-1, MCP-2 and MCP-3 expression in multiple sclerosis lesions: an immunohistochemical and in situ hybridization study. J Neuroimmunol 1998;86:20–29.

89. Sorensen TL, Tani M, Jensen J, et al. Expression of specific chemokines and chemokine receptors in the central nervous system of multiple sclerosis patients. J Clin Invest 1999;103:807–815.

90. Balashov KE, Rottman JB, Weiner HL, Hancock WW. CCR5(+) and CXCR3(+) T cells are increased in multiple sclerosis and their ligands MIP-1alpha and IP-10 are expressed in demyelinating brain lesions. Proc Natl Acad Sci U S A 1999;96:6873–6878.

91. Linington C, Bradl M, Lassmann H, et al. Augmentation of demyelination in rat acute allergic encephalomyelitis by circulating mouse monoclonal antibodies directed against a myelin/oligodendrocyte glycoprotein. Am J Pathol 1988;130:443–454.

92. Piddlesden SJ, Lassmann H, Zimprich F, et al. The demyelinating potential of antibodies to myelin oligodendrocyte glycoprotein is related to their ability to fix complement. Am J Pathol 1993;143:555–564.

93. Genain CP, Cannella B, Hauser SL, Raine CS. Identification of autoantibodies associated with myelin damage in multiple sclerosis. Nat Med 1999;5:170–175.

94. Bernard CC, Johns TG, Slavin A, et al. Myelin oligodendrocyte glycoprotein: a novel candidate autoantigen in multiple sclerosis. J Mol Med 1997;75:77–88.

95. Rodriguez M, Lennon VA, Benveniste EN, Merrill JE. Remyelination by oligodendrocytes stimulated by antiserum to spinal cord. J Neuropathol Exp Neurol 1987;46:84–95.

96. Rodriguez M, Lennon VA. Immunoglobulins promote remyelination in the central nervous system. Ann Neurol 1990;27:12–17.

97. Warrington AE, Asakura K, Bieber AJ, et al. Human monoclonal antibodies reactive to oligodendrocytes promote remyelination in a model of multiple sclerosis. Proc Natl Acad Sci U S A 2000;97:6820–6825.

98. Lucchinetti CF, Noseworthy JH, Rodriguez M. Promotion of endogenous remyelination in multiple sclerosis. Mult Scler 1997;3:71–75.

99. Kieseier BC, Storch MK, Archelos JJ, et al. Effector pathways in immune mediated central nervous system demyelination. Curr Opin Neurol 1999;12:323–336.

100. Gay D, Esiri M. Blood-brain barrier damage in acute multiple sclerosis plaques. An immunocytological study. Brain 1991;114:557–572.

101. Sorensen PS, Wanscher B, Schreiber K, et al. A double-blind, cross-over trial of intravenous immunoglobulin G in multiple sclerosis: preliminary results. Mult Scler 1997;3:145–148.

102. Achiron A, Gabbay U, Gilad R, et al. Intravenous immunoglobulin treatment in multiple sclerosis. Effect on relapses. Neurology 1998;50:398–402.

103. Correale J, Lund B, McMillan M, et al. T cell vaccination in secondary progressive multiple sclerosis. J Neuroimmunol 2000;107:130–139.

104. Cannella B, Raine CS. The adhesion molecule and cytokine profile of multiple sclerosis lesions. Ann Neurol 1995;37:424–435.

105. Yednock TA, Cannon C, Fritz LC, et al. Prevention of experimental autoimmune encephalomyelitis by antibodies against alpha 4 beta 1 integrin. Nature 1992;356:63–66.

106. Kent SJ, Karlik SJ, Cannon C, et al. A monoclonal antibody to alpha 4 integrin suppresses and reverses active experimental allergic encephalomyelitis. J Neuroimmunol 1995;58:1–10.

107. Keszthelyi E, Karlik S, Hyduk S, et al. Evidence for a prolonged role of alpha 4 integrin throughout active experimental allergic encephalomyelitis. Neurology 1996;47:1053–1059.

108. Archelos JJ, Jung S, Maurer M, et al. Inhibition of experimental autoimmune encephalomyelitis by an antibody to the intercellular adhesion molecule ICAM-1. Ann Neurol 1993;34:145–154.

109. Cannella B, Cross AH, Raine CS. Anti-adhesion molecule therapy in experimental autoimmune encephalomyelitis. J Neuroimmunol 1993;46:43–55.

110. Samoilova EB, Horton JL, Chen Y. Experimental autoimmune encephalomyelitis in intercellular adhesion molecule-1-deficient mice. Cell Immunol 1998;190:83–89.

111. Archelos JJ, Hartung HP. Adhesion Molecules in Multiple Sclerosis: A Review. In A Siva, J Kesselring, AJ Thomp-

son (eds), Frontiers in Multiple Sclerosis II. London: Martin Dunitz Ltd., 1999;85–116.

112. Giovannoni G, Lai M, Thorpe J, et al. Longitudinal study of soluble adhesion molecules in multiple sclerosis: correlation with gadolinium enhanced magnetic resonance imaging. Neurology 1997;48:1557–1565.

113. Khoury SJ, Orav EJ, Guttmann CR, et al. Changes in serum levels of ICAM and TNF-R correlate with disease activity in multiple sclerosis. Neurology 1999;53:758–764.

114. Tubridy N, Behan PO, Capildeo R, et al. The effect of anti-alpha4 integrin antibody on brain lesion activity in MS. The UK Antegren Study Group. Neurology 1999;53:466–472.

115. Chandler S, Coates R, Gearing A, et al. Matrix metalloproteinases degrade myelin basic protein. Neurosci Lett 1995;201:223–226.

116. Anthony DC, Miller KM, Fearn S, et al. Matrix metalloproteinase expression in an experimentally-induced DTH model of multiple sclerosis in the rat CNS. J Neuroimmunol 1998;87:62–72.

117. Leppert D, Waubant E, Galardy R, et al. T cell gelatinases mediate basement membrane transmigration in vitro. J Immunol 1995;154:4379–4389.

118. Kieseier BC, Kiefer R, Clements JM, et al. Matrix metalloproteinase-9 and -7 are regulated in experimental autoimmune encephalomyelitis. Brain 1998;121:159–166.

119. Hewson AK, Smith T, Leonard JP, Cuzner ML. Suppression of experimental allergic encephalomyelitis in the Lewis rat by the matrix metalloproteinase inhibitor Ro31-9790. Inflamm Res 1995;44:345–349.

120. Gijbels K, Galardy RE, Steinman L. Reversal of experimental autoimmune encephalomyelitis with a hydroxamate inhibitor of matrix metalloproteases. J Clin Invest 1994;94:2177–2182.

121. Graesser D, Mahooti S, Haas T, et al. The interrelationship of alpha4 integrin and matrix metalloproteinase-2 in the pathogenesis of experimental autoimmune encephalomyelitis. Lab Invest 1998;78:1445–1458.

122. Leppert D, Ford J, Stabler G, et al. Matrix metalloproteinase-9 (gelatinase B) is selectively elevated in CSF during relapses and stable phases of multiple sclerosis. Brain 1998;121:2327–2334.

123. Lee MA, Palace J, Stabler G, et al. Serum gelatinase B, TIMP-1 and TIMP-2 levels in multiple sclerosis. A longitudinal clinical and MRI study. Brain 1999;122:191–197.

124. Rosenberg GA, Dencoff JE, Correa N Jr., et al. Effect of steroids on CSF matrix metalloproteinases in multiple sclerosis: relation to blood-brain barrier injury. Neurology 1996;46:1626–1632.

125. Brown PD. Ongoing trials with matrix metalloproteinase inhibitors. Expert Opin Investig Drugs 2000;9:2167–2177.

126. Moncada S, Higgs A. The L-arginine-nitric oxide pathway. N Engl J Med 1993;329:2002–2012.

127. Koprowski H, Zheng YM, Heber-Katz E, et al. In vivo expression of inducible nitric oxide synthase in experimentally induced neurologic diseases [published erratum appears in Proc Natl Acad Sci U S A 1993;90(11):5378]. Proc Natl Acad Sci U S A 1993;90:3024–3027.

128. Lin RF, Lin TS, Tilton RG, Cross AH. Nitric oxide localized to spinal cords of mice with experimental allergic encephalomyelitis: an electron paramagnetic resonance study. J Exp Med 1993;178:643–648.

129. Smith KJ, Kapoor R, Felts PA. Demyelination: the role of reactive oxygen and nitrogen species. Brain Pathol 1999;9:69–92.

130. Pahan K, Sheikh FG, Liu X, et al. Induction of nitric oxide synthase and activation of NF-kappaB by interleukin-12 p40 in microglial cells. J Biol Chem 2001;276:7899–7905.

131. Fenyk-Melody JE, Garrison AE, Brunnert SR, et al. Experimental autoimmune encephalomyelitis is exacerbated in mice lacking the NOS2 gene. J Immunol 1998;160:2940–2946.

132. Cross AH, Misko TP, Lin RF, et al. Aminoguanidine, an inhibitor of inducible nitric oxide synthase, ameliorates experimental autoimmune encephalomyelitis in SJL mice. J Clin Invest 1994;93:2684–2690.

133. Zielasek J, Jung S, Gold R, et al. Administration of nitric oxide synthase inhibitors in experimental autoimmune neuritis and experimental autoimmune encephalomyelitis. J Neuroimmunol 1995;58:81–88.

134. Okuda Y, Sakoda S, Fujimura H, Yanagihara T. Aminoguanidine, a selective inhibitor of the inducible nitric oxide synthase, has different effects on experimental allergic encephalomyelitis in the induction and progression phase. J Neuroimmunol 1998;81:201–210.

135. Hooper DC, Spitsin S, Kean RB, et al. Uric acid, a natural scavenger of peroxynitrite, in experimental allergic encephalomyelitis and multiple sclerosis. Proc Natl Acad Sci U S A 1998;95:675–680.

136. Mitrovic B, Ignarro LJ, Montestruque S, et al. Nitric oxide as a potential pathological mechanism in demyelination: its differential effects on primary glial cells in vitro. Neuroscience 1994;61:575–585.

137. Bongarzone ER, Pasquini JM, Soto EF. Oxidative damage to proteins and lipids of CNS myelin produced by in vitro generated reactive oxygen species. J Neurosci Res 1995;41:213–221.

138. LeVine SM, Wetzel DL. Chemical analysis of multiple sclerosis lesions by FT-IR microspectroscopy. Free Radic Biol Med 1998;25:33–41.

139. Shrager P, Custer AW, Kazarinova K, et al. Nerve conduction block by nitric oxide that is mediated by the axonal environment. J Neurophysiol 1998;79:529–536.

140. Hooper DC, Bagasra O, Marini JC, et al. Prevention of experimental allergic encephalomyelitis by targeting nitric oxide and peroxynitrite: implications for the treatment of multiple sclerosis. Proc Natl Acad Sci U S A 1997;94:2528–2533.

141. Giovannoni G. Cerebrospinal fluid and serum nitric oxide metabolites in patients with multiple sclerosis. Mult Scler 1998;4:27–30.

142. Giovannoni G, Heales SJ, Silver NC, et al. Raised serum nitrate and nitrite levels in patients with multiple sclerosis. J Neurol Sci 1997;145:77–81.

143. Giovannoni G, Silver NC, O'Riordan J, et al. Increased urinary nitric oxide metabolites in patients with multiple sclerosis correlates with early and relapsing disease. Mult Scler 1999;5:335–341.

144. Piani D, Frei K, Do KQ, et al. Murine brain macrophages induced NMDA receptor mediated neurotoxicity in vitro by secreting glutamate. Neurosci Lett 1991;133: 159–162.

145. McDonald JW, Althomsons SP, Hyrc KL, et al. Oligodendrocytes from forebrain are highly vulnerable to AMPA/ kainate receptor-mediated excitotoxicity. Nat Med 1998; 4:291–297.

146. Pitt D, Werner P, Raine CS. Glutamate excitotoxicity in a model of multiple sclerosis. Nat Med 2000;6:67–70.

147. Smith T, Groom A, Zhu B, Turski L. Autoimmune encephalomyelitis ameliorated by AMPA antagonists. Nat Med 2000;6:62–66.

148. Hardin-Pouzet H, Krakowski M, Bourbonniere L, et al. Glutamate metabolism is down-regulated in astrocytes during experimental allergic encephalomyelitis. Glia 1997;20:79–85.

149. Stover JF, Pleines UE, Morganti-Kossmann MC, et al. Neurotransmitters in cerebrospinal fluid reflect pathological activity. Eur J Clin Invest 1997;27:1038–1043.

150. Gurwitz D, Kloog Y. Peroxynitrite generation might explain elevated glutamate and aspartate levels in multiple sclerosis cerebrospinal fluid [letter]. Eur J Clin Invest 1998;28:760–761.

151. Launes J, Siren J, Viinikka L, et al. Does glutamate mediate damage in acute encephalitis? Neuroreport 1998;9:577–581.

152. Westall FC, Hawkins A, Ellison GW, Myers LW. Abnormal glutamic acid metabolism in multiple sclerosis. J Neurol Sci 1980;47:353–364.

Chapter 7

Clinical Neurophysiology of Central and Peripheral Demyelinating Disorders

Steven A. Greenberg

Clinical neurophysiologic studies are useful in the diagnosis of both central and peripheral demyelinating disorders. Nerve conduction studies (NCSs) and electromyography (EMG) are principally helpful in characterizing peripheral nervous system diseases, and evoked potentials (EPs) are principally useful with central nervous system diseases, although either category of studies may be helpful with either anatomic location. Several less commonly used techniques, including magnetic EPs and event-related potentials, have been studied and are of limited value.

Nerve Conduction Studies and Electromyography

NCSs and EMG are principally useful in the diagnosis of disorders of the peripheral nervous system. EMG may also be useful in the diagnosis of upper motor neuron disorders. NCSs of value in demyelinating nerve diseases generally consists of sensory NCSs, motor NCSs, and the late-response F-waves and H-reflexes.

Sensory NCSs are typically performed on the median, ulnar, radial, sural, and superficial peroneal sensory nerves. For the median and ulnar, a common technique involves stimulation at the wrist and recording with ring electrodes on the second and fifth digits, respectively. For the other nerves, a bar electrode is often used. Other less commonly used techniques are available for other

sensory nerves. These studies allow for the measurement of sensory nerve action potential (SNAP) amplitudes and sensory nerve conduction velocities. The amplitude of the SNAP is the summation of the individual nerve action potentials of the axons in the nerve and thus reflects the number of intact conducting axons in the nerve. Reductions in SNAP amplitude generally imply axonal loss. The conduction velocity may be reduced in both axonal and demyelinating disorders, although marked reductions occur only in the latter.

Motor NCSs are typically performed for median, ulnar, peroneal, and tibial nerves and less commonly in others. Recordings are made over a muscle, and the resulting study allows for the measurement of a compound muscle action potential (CMAP) amplitude, distal motor latency (DML), and motor conduction velocity. As in sensory studies, reductions in CMAP generally reflect axonal loss, and prolongations in DML and motor conduction velocity, when marked, reflect demyelination.

F-wave studies are performed by supramaximal stimulation of a motor nerve recording over the muscle, as in motor nerve studies. Antidromic motor axon conduction of action potentials into the anterior gray matter of the spinal cord appears to result in activation of a variable pool of motor neurons that then conduct orthodromic potentials to the muscle and result in a small CMAP reflecting the activity of a handful of motor units. F-wave studies provide one of few means to assess proximal conduction of peripheral nerve. The parameters of interest are the minimum F-wave latency (sometimes the average is used), the chronodispersion, or range of latencies, and the persistence, typically defined as the number of F-waves obtained with 10 stimuli.

H-reflex studies are also useful for the assessment of proximal conduction. A number of muscles may be used, but typically a recording is made from the soleus, and the tibial nerve at the knee is stimulated. At an appropriate submaximal stimulus, conduction of sensory afferents to the spinal cord results in reflex motor conduction to the muscle, and a muscle action potential is recorded. After optimizing this response, a direct tibial-soleus supramaximal CMAP is recorded, the M-response. The H-reflex minimum latency and the H/M amplitude ratio are of clinical value.

Electrodiagnostic Criteria for Peripheral Nerve Demyelination

The hallmarks of peripheral nerve demyelination are the presence of conduction block, temporal dispersion, and reduced nerve conduction velocities. The concept of conduction block refers to the failure of transmission of an intact motor or sensory axon. The term *partial conduction block* applies to a nerve and implies conduction block of one or more, but not all, axons in the nerve. Complete conduction block implies conduction block of all axons in the nerve. Partial or complete conduction block persisting for more than 1 week implies focal demyelination.[1] The time criterion is important to distinguish acute focal axonal injury, such as nerve infarction or transection, which may produce "pseudo-conduction block" initially but is then followed by wallerian degeneration and loss of the distal evoked CMAP.

Temporal dispersion results from the range of nonidentical conduction velocities in the population of axons constituting a single nerve. Simultaneously generated impulses at a single site in a population of axons will conduct at differing velocities and arrive at a different site along the nerve at differing times. The range of arrival times is greater as the distance traveled by the impulse increases, and it is this range that is conceptualized in the term *temporal dispersion*. Physiologic temporal dispersion is thus a normal phenomenon, whereas disease processes that increase the range of conduction velocities in populations of axons may produce abnormal temporal dispersion. A significant degree of temporal dispersion occurring focally along a short segment of a nerve is diagnostic of focal demyelination.[1]

The electrophysiologic correlates of conduction block and temporal dispersion are controversial,[2–10] although recent consensus criteria have been developed for conduction block.[1] The electrophysiologic correlates of reduced conduction velocities are clearer and include reductions in motor and sensory nerve conduction velocities, increases in DMLs, and increases in minimum F-wave and H-reflex latencies.

Recent development of consensus criteria by an American Association of Electrodiagnostic Medicine panel may prove to be a valuable addition to our understanding of these correlates (Table 7-1).[1] Consideration of the consensus criteria for conduction block involves several technical points. Marked axonal loss or temporal dispersion precludes the confident recognition of conduction block. The criteria are thus applicable only to nerves with distal CMAP amplitude of at least 20% of the lower limit of normal (LLN) and CMAP duration changes of less than 60% increases in the proximal as compared to the distal site. The criteria are also more restrictive for the radial, peroneal, and tibial nerves than for the median and ulnar nerves. In addition, very proximal stimulation is limited in value. Stimulation at Erb's point and the sciatic notch were not considered sufficiently reliable in producing supramaximal stimulation to be included in the criteria unless certain stimulator requirements are present, and nerve root stimulation, by needle or magnetic coil, is not sufficiently technically reliable to have been included at all. The criteria are the most conservative published to date and would be expected to produce a high degree of confidence when abnormal (i.e., high specificity).

Similar consensus criteria for abnormal temporal dispersion have not been explicitly developed, although a limit of 30% increase in CMAP duration with proximal versus distal stimulation has been commonly set forth and is supported by limited normal studies.[11] These limits may be made tighter through the use of regression models with variables of age and length of nerve segments.[11]

Similarly, the electrophysiologic correlates of reduced conduction velocity, including reduced sensory and motor nerve velocity, and prolonged DML and minimum F-wave latency, vary across studies without clear consensus.[2–6,8–10,12] These criteria are noteworthy in their dependence on the distal CMAP amplitude. Reduction in CMAP amplitude from axonal loss may result in reduction in nerve conduction velocities without the presence of demyelination of intact axons, so more stringent velocity and latency requirements are used in this setting.[1,5]

The practical application of these electrophysiologic parameters has generally taken the form of a required number of abnormalities chosen from a "menu," as shown in Table 7-2. Although idealized as broad criteria for peripheral nerve demyelination,[8] such criteria may be more appropriately applicable to only specific diseases. For example, criteria developed for chronic inflammatory demyelinating polyneuropathy (CIDP) may perform very poorly for the diagnosis of acute inflammatory demyelinating polyneuropathy (AIDP).[2]

Electrophysiology in Common Peripheral Nerve Diseases

Guillain-Barré Syndrome

Guillain-Barré syndrome (GBS) is a common cause of acute flaccid paralysis, resulting in progressive weakness, sensory loss, and areflexia. A number of variants, or subtypes, have been recognized. The range of pathophysiology among these variants is extensive and includes predominant demyelination, predominant axonal loss, or a mixture, and uncertain localizations that may include the central nervous system as well, as has been hypothesized in some patients with the Miller-Fisher variant. Electrophysiologic studies can be of great use in the evaluation of patients with acute flaccid paralysis, can add to the categorization of GBS variants, and can provide prognostic information in patients with GBS.

GBS is a disease that typically evolves over several weeks; electrophysiologic studies differ, depending on when in the course of the disease they are performed. The electrodiagnostic abnormalities may also differ among the variants of GBS. This variability in both the spectrum of disease, and

Table 7-1. Consensus Amplitude Reduction Criteria for Partial Conduction Block*

Nerve or Segment	Temporal Dispersion <30%		Temporal Dispersion 31–60%	
	Definite (%)	Probable (%)	Definite (%)	Probable (%)
Median				
Forearm	>50	40–50	—	>50
Arm	>50	40–50	—	>50
Proximal	—	>40	—	>50
Ulnar				
Forearm	>50	40–50	—	>50
Across elbow	>50	40–50	—	>50
Arm	>50	40–50	—	>50
Proximal	—	>40	—	>50
Radial				
Forearm	—	>50	—	>60
Arm	—	>50	—	>60
Proximal	—	>50	—	>60
Peroneal				
Leg	>60	50–60	—	>60
Across fibula	>50	40–50	—	>50
Thigh	—	>50	—	>60
Tibial				
Leg	>60	50–60	—	>60
Thigh	—	>50	—	>60

*Criteria for area reduction always of magnitude 10% less than amplitude (e.g., amplitude/area = 50%/40%).

point in evolution when studied may account for varying prevalences of abnormalities reported in the literature.[2–4,6,8,13]

The earliest NCS abnormalities in GBS are generally absent or prolonged minimum F-wave or H-reflex responses.[4,11] EMG studies of weak muscles will usually show abnormalities of recruitment typical of motor unit disorders, even when NCSs are normal and, when present, immediately confirm disease of the peripheral motor nerves as a cause of paralysis. Prolongation of DMLs may also be an early finding,[8] suggesting that physiologic evidence of demyelination initially occurs proximally and distally along nerve fibers, with midlimb abnormalities appearing later.

Electrophysiologic evidence for demyelination is apparent in approximately 50% of patients by the second week and 85% of patients by the third week[3]

Table 7-2. Electrodiagnostic Criteria for Demyelination in Chronic Inflammatory Demyelinating Polyneuropathy

---

At least three of the following:
  In two or more nerves
    Amplitude >80% LLN ⇒ conduction velocity <80% LLN
    Amplitude <80% LLN ⇒ conduction velocity <70% LLN
  In two or more nerves
    Amplitude >80% LLN ⇒ distal motor latency >125% ULN
    Amplitude <80% LLN ⇒ distal motor latency >150% ULN
  In one or more nerves
    Conduction block as defined by amplitude reduction >20%
    or
    Temporal dispersion as defined by proximal-distal duration increase of 15% or more
  In two or more nerves
    Amplitude >80% LLN ⇒ minimum F-wave latency >120% ULN
    Amplitude <80% LLN ⇒ minimum F-wave latency >150% ULN

LLN = lower limit of normal; ULN = upper limit of normal.

and consists of combinations of conduction block, temporal dispersion, and reduced motor and sensory nerve conduction velocities. Reduction in SNAP and CMAP amplitudes may occur as well and may be the consequence of distal conduction block, temporal dispersion, or axonal loss. In the acute motor axonal neuropathy and acute motor-sensory axonal neuropathy variants, these reductions may occur early in the course of disease and may be the predominant electrodiagnostic abnormalities.[14]

Fibrillation potentials and positive waves are particularly common in the acute motor axonal neuropathy and acute motor-sensory axonal neuropathy variants but may be present throughout the GBS spectrum, although generally not appearing until relatively late in the course. Their prevalence in proximal muscles peaks at 6–10 weeks and in distal muscles at 11–15 weeks.[4] Reduction of CMAP amplitudes, as reflected in a mean of several motor studies, to less than 10–20% of the LLN is a powerful predictor of poor outcome.[4,8]

Attempts to develop accurate (i.e., highly sensitive and specific) electrophysiologic criteria for GBS

have met with varying success. Early criteria suggestive of demyelination in GBS required at least one of the following in two or more nerves: (1) if amplitude greater than 50% of LLN, then conduction velocity less than 95% LLN; if amplitude less than 50% LLN, then conduction velocity less than 85% LLN; (2) if amplitude normal, then distal latency greater than 110% upper limit of normal (ULN); if amplitude less than normal, then distal latency greater than 120% ULN; (3) conduction block as defined by amplitude reduction of greater than 30% or the presence of temporal dispersion as defined by proximal-distal duration increase of 30% or more; and (4) minimum F-wave response latency greater than 120% ULN.[3] These criteria were met by 87% of patients with a diagnosis of GBS in a retrospective evaluation, although some of these diagnoses were made with the results of electrodiagnostic studies in mind.

These criteria were subsequently made more stringent, likely because of poor specificity.[4] Three, instead of two, abnormalities were required; the conduction velocity limits were changed to 90% and 80% LLN (for amplitudes greater or less than 50%, respectively), the distal latency limits were changed to 115% and 125% ULN, and the minimum F-wave response latency was changed to 125% ULN. In addition, nerve segments that are common compression sites (median at the wrist, ulnar at the elbow, and peroneal across the fibular head) could not be used to meet these criteria. These modified criteria were not evaluated in the original set of patients. In a later evaluation of patients with clinical diagnoses of GBS by separate investigators, the original criteria had a 72% sensitivity, whereas the modified criteria had a 37% sensitivity.[2]

Subsequent criteria for peripheral nerve demyelination were proposed and applied to both GBS and CIDP, although without published evaluation.[5,8] These criteria when subsequently evaluated performed fairly poorly,[1] identifying only 21% of patients with the AIDP subtype of GBS, the subgroup in which one would expect the criteria to perform best. These criteria are outlined in Table 7-2.

Several other lists of criteria have been proposed.[10,14,15] The sensitivity of these criteria ranges between 47–63%. The specificity and accuracy of such electrodiagnostic criteria for GBS do not appear to have been studied. Hence, the principal clinical use of electrodiagnostic studies in patients with suspected

GBS is providing evidence against other causes of acute generalized weakness, such as spinal cord, muscle, or neuromuscular junction disorders. A normal thorough electrodiagnostic study in a patient with clinically suspected early GBS may serve to strengthen, not diminish, confidence in this diagnosis.

Chronic Inflammatory Demyelinating Polyneuropathy

CIDP is an immune-mediated neuropathy characterized by relapsing or progressive proximal and distal symmetric weakness. Progression occurs over at least 2 months, typically longer, distinguishing this disorder from AIDP. Motor and sensory involvement is most common, but variants with pure motor or sensory involvement as well as asymmetric or markedly multifocal variants all occur commonly.

As focal demyelination is the prominent pathophysiologic process in both AIDP and CIDP, proposed electrodiagnostic criteria for these diagnoses are analogous in their attempts to capture the electrodiagnostic correlates of reduced conduction velocities, conduction block, and temporal dispersion. Criteria put forth by Albers and Kelly[4] are as follows. Three of the following in motor nerves are required: (1) conduction velocity in two or more nerves less than 75% LLN; (2) conduction block defined as at least 30% proximal-distal CMAP amplitude reduction or temporal dispersion in one or more nerves; (3) prolonged DML in two or more nerves greater than 130% ULN; and (4) prolonged minimum F-wave latency in one or more nerves of greater than 130% LLN. These criteria are significantly different from the ones proposed by the same authors for AIDP. There is no dependency on amplitude limits; nerves with marked axonal loss can still be considered as providing evidence of demyelination. The limits of abnormality were slightly tightened as well; for example, reductions in conduction velocity of only 90% or 80% LLN, depending on amplitudes, were proposed for AIDP.

The subsequent American Academy of Neurology (AAN) criteria, initially published as criteria for peripheral nerve demyelination in the context of GBS and later published as research criteria for CIDP, are shown in Table 7-2.[5] These criteria do not appear to have been evaluated before publication. In the only prospective evaluation published

to date, the Albers-Kelly and AAN criteria showed similar sensitivities of 50% and 46%, respectively, and 100% specificity when applied to patients with CIDP, diabetic neuropathy, and motor neuron disease as a combined group.[7] These sensitivities depended on the number of nerves studied and improved to 64% and 60% when only patients with more thorough electrodiagnostic evaluations were analyzed. In fact, a much simpler criterion, requiring only reduction in conduction velocity to less than 70% of LLN in a single nerve, appeared to have a sensitivity of 66% and specificity of 100% in this study. Alternatively, modifying the Albers-Kelly criteria (1 and 3) to require only one instead of two nerves to meet the specifications results in a similar improvement. This later modification would likely perform better than the simple single-nerve reduced conduction velocity criterion for patients with inherited demyelinating polyneuropathies.

More recent criteria have been proposed (see Table 7-2).[12] These criteria are similar to the AAN's but replace the partial conduction block criteria with those of the American Association of Electrodiagnostic Medicine consensus panel and require only two of four rather than three of four abnormalities from the list (see Table 7-1). These proposed criteria have not been prospectively evaluated in a patient population, although they seem rational and reflect clinical practice by neuromuscular specialists more cautious in interpreting proximal CMAP amplitude reductions.

In summary, thorough examination to include bilateral median, ulnar, peroneal, and tibial motor and F-wave studies can improve diagnostic accuracy. However, there remain a substantial percentage of patients with clinically defined CIDP who do not meet electrodiagnostic criteria.

Inherited Demyelinating Neuropathies

Our understanding of inherited demyelinating polyneuropathies is changing rapidly in the current era of molecular diagnosis. The dramatic developments in our understanding of the human genome offer enormous opportunity for very precise delineation of diagnostic categories among the inherited demyelinating polyneuropathies and for much tighter correlation of electrodiagnostic studies with these syndromes.

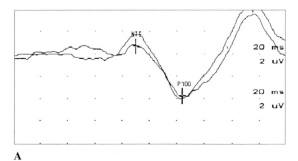

A

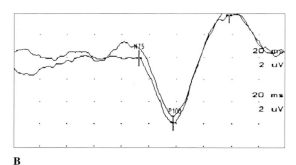

B

Figure 7-1. Visual-evoked potentials in a 41-year-old woman with prior episodes of optic neuritis in each eye. Note good reproducibility of waveforms with marked P100 latency prolongation. Right P100 latency is 124 ms **(A)** and left P100 latency **(B)** is 118 ms. The laboratory normal upper limit is 105 msec (mean, + 2 standard deviations).

A now classic study[16] demonstrated important distinctions in electrophysiology between inherited and acquired demyelinating polyneuropathies. In general, in inherited neuropathies with the exception of hereditary neuropathy with liability to pressure palsies, conduction velocities are uniformly reduced, and conduction block and abnormal temporal dispersion are not present. Uniform conduction slowing implies similar reductions in nerve conduction velocities, distal latencies, and minimum F-wave latencies in comparable nerves and segments.

The situation now appears more complex.[17] The syndromes of Charcot-Marie-Tooth disease type 1a, Dejerine-Sottas disease, and hereditary neuropathy with liability to pressure palsies typically have a duplication of the peripheral myelin protein 22 (PMP22), a deletion of *PMP22*, or a *PMP22* mutation, respectively. However, patients with mutations within the same gene may differ both in electrodiagnostic parameters and in clinical classification. For example, point mutations in either the *PMP22* gene

or the myelin protein zero gene may result in syndromes of either Charcot-Marie-Tooth disease type 1 or Dejerine-Sottas disease. Some patients with *PMP22* point mutations may have hereditary neuropathy with liability to pressure palsies. Some patients with connexin 32 mutations, the most common cause of X-linked hereditary motor and sensory neuropathy, and some patients with myelin protein zero mutations may even have nerve conduction velocities that do not fall into the demyelinating range of Charcot-Marie-Tooth disease type 1 but are clearly reduced in comparison to strictly axonal inherited neuropathies (e.g., Charcot-Marie-Tooth disease type 2) and have been termed *intermediate*.

Evoked Potentials

EPs are time-locked electrical responses of the nervous system to external stimuli. They are the principal electrophysiologic tools used in the study of the central nervous system, although sometimes they are helpful in the diagnosis of peripheral nervous system lesions. They are especially useful in the diagnosis of demyelinating disorders of the central nervous system, of which multiple sclerosis (MS) is the most common, and may provide definitive evidence for subclinical lesions. Although the advent of magnetic resonance imaging has reduced the need for electrophysiologic demonstration of subclinical lesions in MS and resulted in a reduction in the use of EPs,[18] EPs remain valuable diagnostic tools in a number of settings.

Several different EP studies exist.[19–21] Visual EPs (VEPs) are highly sensitive studies of the anterochiasmatic visual pathways (Figure 7-1). Their value in the diagnosis of retrochiasmatic lesions is controversial. Brain stem auditory EPs (BAEPs) are useful in the diagnosis of lesions of the cochlear nerves and brain stem affecting auditory pathways. They are especially useful in evaluating hearing loss in infants and young children. Somatosensory EPs (SEPs) allow for the study of central somatosensory pathways and are occasionally useful in peripheral nerve disorders, such as nerve root avulsion.

EPs are small signals recorded with repeated averaging at the scalp or spine or, in the case of upper extremity SEPs, the brachial plexus as well. Multiple recordings at different locations are made simultaneous to stimulation, and a high degree of attention to technical factors is required. As a rule, the latency of an EP is far more valuable than the amplitude in clinical diagnosis, except when an EP is absent.

Visual-Evoked Potentials

VEPs can be elicited by a number of stimuli, but the most common is a monocular stimulus consisting of a checkerboard pattern reversal shown at 4 Hz or less for two sets of 500 stimuli each. Recording electrodes are placed either at the left-occipital, midline-occipital, and right-occipital locations (under the Queen Square System) or at O1, Oz, and O2 locations (under the International 10–20 System) and at the midline-frontal (MF) and auricular A1 or A2 sites. The typical montage used has four channels as follows: left occipital–MF, midline occipital–MF, right occipital–MF, and MF-A1.[20]

In normal subjects, four major responses are noted: the N75, P100, and N145 in the occipital regions and the N100 in the midfrontal region. The P100 is the most consistent peak and is the principal peak from which interpretations of the VEP are made. Several derived measures are important and include the interocular latency difference, the difference in the P100 latency at the midline-occipital site to left and right eye stimulation. Prolongation of the interocular latency difference is probably the most sensitive electrophysiologic indicator of optic nerve lesions.[21]

The AAN has provided an evidence-based practice parameter on the use of EPs in patients with suspected MS. In this review, VEPs were found to be "probably useful" in identifying patients at risk of developing clinically definite MS.[22] In addition to MS, VEPs may be abnormal in patients with compressive lesions of the anterior visual pathways, Friedreich's ataxia, and vitamin B_{12} deficiency. Although as a rule they are not helpful in the diagnosis of retrochiasmatic visual pathway lesions, partial field stimulation and recording from laterally placed electrodes may demonstrate some value.[21]

Brain Stem Auditory–Evoked Potentials

BAEPs are typically evoked by auditory clicks with a broad-band in which the acoustic energy is spread over a wide range of frequencies. Stimulus rates of 8–10/second delivered monaurally in two sets of 1,000 stimuli each are recommended. Electrode placement is typically at Cz and either at both earlobes, A1 and A2, or at both mastoid processes, M1 and M2. The recording montage is typically vertex-ipsilateral (Cz-Ai or Cz-Mi) and vertex contralateral (Cz-Ac or Cz-Mc).[20]

In normal subjects, five waveforms are of interest (termed *waves I–V*), and most attention is paid to waves I, III, and V. Waves VI and VII have been noted but are so often absent in normal individuals that they are of uncertain value. Of most interest are the absolute peak latencies of waves I, III, and V; the three interpeak latencies I–III, III–V, and I–V; and wave I amplitude, wave V amplitude, and the wave V/I amplitude ratio. The anatomic source of these waves has been the subject of intense study.[21]

Abnormalities in BAEPs are common in MS, occurring in more than 50% of patients with definite MS in some series. Some data have suggested that BAEPs are more sensitive than magnetic resonance imaging for demonstrating demyelination in the posterior fossa. However, the AAN review of the evidence concluded that there is currently insufficient evidence to recommend BAEPs as a useful test to identify patients with clinically suspected MS at risk for developing clinically definite MS.[22]

BAEP abnormalities have also been noted in other demyelinating disorders: leukodystrophies, spinocerebellar degenerations, and vitamin B_{12} deficiency.[21]

Somatosensory-Evoked Potentials

SEPs are typically generated by peripheral nerve stimulation at 3–5 Hz with an intensity adequate to produce a consistent but tolerable muscle twitch. Several hundred to several thousand stimuli in each of two trials are usually applied to ensure clear and reproducible waveforms. Recording locations depend on the nerve studied.

For the upper extremity, median nerve stimulation is typically used, although ulnar nerve stimulation, with separate normal values, may be used. A minimal recording includes electrodes at CPc, Cpi, C5S (over the fifth cervical vertebra), Epi (the ipsilateral Erb's point), and a noncephalic reference, often Epc. A typical montage consists of four channels: CPc-Cpi, Cpi–reference site (REF), C5S-REF, and Epi-REF.[20] Other montages and recording locations are also effective. The principal components of median SEP recordings are EP, resulting from a propagated volley under Erb's point; N13, a stationary neck recorded potential; the P14 and N18, subcortically generated far-field potentials; and N20, reflecting activation of the primary somatosensory cortex. Note that under the foregoing montage, N20 is typically a bipolar recording to subtract the far-field potentials P14 and N18.

These five obligate waveforms are all present in a normal upper extremity SEP study. The peak latencies of EP, P14, and N20 and the interpeak latencies EP to P14 (reflecting brachial plexus to lower brain stem conduction), P14 to N20 (reflecting lower brain stem to cortex conduction), and EP to N20 (reflecting brachial plexus to cortex conduction) are all measured. Absence of an obligate waveform or prolongation of an interpeak latency constitutes an abnormality.

For the lower extremity, the posterior tibial nerve at the ankle or the common peroneal nerve at the knee may be used and have separate normal values. Recording is performed at a lumbar site, typically T12S, and at C5S, Fpz, CPz, and CPi. A typical montage consists of four channels: CPi-Fpz, CPz-Fpz, Fpz-C5S, and T12S-REF.[20] The principal components of a lower-extremity posterior tibial nerve SEP are the LP (lumbar potential), P31 and N34 (subcortical far-field potentials), and P37 (sometimes called *P40*) cortical response.

The peak and interpeak latencies are evaluated as in upper extremity SEPs. Definite abnormalities are the absence of any of the obligate waveforms LP, P31, N34, and P37 and prolongation of the LP-P37 interpeak latency.

Abnormalities in upper and lower extremity SEPs are also common in patients with MS. A frequently encountered abnormality is loss of the C5S with intact P14 and N20 responses with upper-limb SEPs. As with other EPs, the advent of magnetic resonance imaging has largely replaced the use of SEPs in the diagnosis of MS. Little correlation between clinical deficit and EP abnormalities exists. The AAN review for SEPs concluded that they are possibly useful in identifying patients with suspected MS at risk for developing clinically definite MS.[22,23]

SEPs may be abnormal in leukodystrophies, spinocerebellar degenerations, Friedreich's ataxia, hereditary spastic paraplegia, and vitamin B_{12} deficiency, as well as structural lesions of the spinal cord.[21] A number of investigators have reported SEP abnormalities in patients with amyotrophic lateral sclerosis, despite the absence of clinical sensory involvement in this disorder.[24–28] The significance of this finding remains uncertain. The value of SEPs in the diagnosis of peripheral nerve disease is not established, although it appears they may be useful in assessing proximal conduction of sensory nerves in patients with suspected GBS when NCSs, including F-wave studies, are normal.[13]

Other Techniques

A number of other techniques have been described and are either investigational or of unproven value. Dermatomal SEPs involve stimulation of a single nerve root and have been studied largely in relation to lumbosacral root disease. Their specific use in demyelinating disorders has not been established. Event-related potentials are long-latency cortical responses that have been studied as a reflection of cognitive impairment and are insensitive measures of cognitive dysfunction in patients with MS.[18] Motor EPs involve stimulation of cerebral motor cortex and cervical nerve roots with magnetic fields and recording of limb muscle action potentials in response. The use of motor EPs allow for the determination of central motor conduction time, which has been shown to be frequently abnormal in demyelinating disorders of the central nervous system. However, marked central motor conduction slowing has also been demonstrated in patients with the D90A CuZn-SOD familial amyotrophic lateral sclerosis mutation.[27] The clinical value of recording central motor conduction time in patients with suspected MS is not established.

References

1. Olney RK. Consensus criteria for the diagnosis of partial conduction block. Muscle Nerve 1999;22(Suppl 8):S225–S229.
2. Alam TA, Chaudhry V, Cornblath DR. Electrophysiological studies in the Guillain-Barré syndrome: distinguishing subtypes by published criteria. Muscle Nerve 1998;21(10):1275–1279.

3. Albers JW, Donofrio PD, McGonagle T. Sequential electrodiagnostic abnormalities in acute inflammatory demyelinating polyradiculoneuropathy. Muscle Nerve 1985;8: 528–539.

4. Albers JW, Kelly JJ Jr. Acquired inflammatory demyelinating polyneuropathies: clinical and electrodiagnostic features. Muscle Nerve 1989;12(6):435–451.

5. American Academy of Neurology. Research criteria for diagnosis of chronic inflammatory demyelinating polyneuropathy (CIDP). Report from an Ad Hoc Subcommittee of the American Academy of Neurology AIDS Task Force. Neurology 1991;41(5):617–618.

6. Asbury AK, Cornblath DR. Assessment of current diagnostic criteria for Guillain-Barré syndrome. Ann Neurol 1990;27(Suppl):S21–S24.

7. Bromberg MB. Related Articles. Comparison of electrodiagnostic criteria for primary demyelination in chronic polyneuropathy. Muscle Nerve 1991;14(10):968–976.

8. Cornblath DR. Electrophysiology in Guillain-Barré syndrome. Ann Neurol 1990;27(Suppl):S17–S20.

9. Cornblath DR, Sumner AJ, Daube J, et al. Conduction block in clinical practice. Muscle Nerve 1991;14(9):869–871.

10. Meulstee J, van der Meche FG. Electrodiagnostic criteria for polyneuropathy and demyelination: application in 135 patients with Guillain-Barré syndrome. Dutch Guillain-Barré Study Group. J Neurol Neurosurg Psychiatry 1995; 59(5):482–486.

11. Taylor PK. CMAP dispersion, amplitude decay, and area decay in a normal population. Muscle Nerve 1993;16(11): 1181–1187.

12. Saperstein D, Katz J, Amato A, Barohn R. Clinical spectrum of chronic acquired demyelinating polyneuropathies. Muscle Nerve 2001;24:311–324.

13. Olney RK, Aminoff MJ. Electrodiagnostic features of the Guillain-Barré syndrome: the relative sensitivity of different techniques. Neurology 1990;40:471–475.

14. Ho TW, Mishu B, Li CY, et al. Guillain-Barré syndrome in northern China. Relationship to *Campylobacter jejuni* infection and anti-glycolipid antibodies. Brain 1995;118 (Pt 3):597–605.

15. The Italian Guillain-Barré Study Group. The prognosis and main prognostic indicators of Guillain-Barré syndrome. A multicentre prospective study of 297 patients. Brain 1996;119(Pt 6):2053–2061.

16. Lewis RA, Sumner AJ, Shy ME. Electrophysiological features of inherited demyelinating neuropathies: a reappraisal in the era of molecular diagnosis. Muscle Nerve 2000;23(10):1472–1487.

17. Lewis RA, Sumner AJ. The electrodiagnostic distinctions between chronic familial and acquired demyelinative neuropathies. Neurology 1982;32(6):592–596.

18. Leocani L, Comi G. Neurophysiological investigations in multiple sclerosis. Curr Opin Neurol 2000;13(3):255–261.

19. American Association of Electrodiagnostic Medicine. Guidelines for somatosensory evoked potentials. Muscle Nerve 1999;22(Suppl 8):S123–S138.

20. American Electroencephalographic Society. Guideline nine: guidelines on evoked potentials. J Clin Neurophysiol 1994;11(1):40–73.

21. Chiappa K. Evoked Potentials in Clinical Medicine. Philadelphia: Raven Press, 1997.

22. Kraft GH, Aminoff MJ, Baran EM, et al. Somatosensory evoked potentials: clinical uses. AAEM Somatosensory Evoked Potentials Subcommittee. American Association of Electrodiagnostic Medicine. Muscle Nerve 1998;21(2): 252–258.

23. Gronseth GS, Ashman EJ. Practice parameter: the usefulness of evoked potentials in identifying clinically silent lesions in patients with suspected multiple sclerosis (an evidence-based review): report of the Quality Standards Subcommittee of the American Academy of Neurology. Neurology 2000;54(9):1720–1725.

24. Bosch EP, Yamada T, Kimura J. Somatosensory evoked potentials in motor neuron disease. Muscle Nerve 1985; 8(7):556–562.

25. Radtke RA, Erwin A, Erwin CW. Abnormal sensory evoked potentials in amyotrophic lateral sclerosis. Neurology 1986;36(6):796–801.

26. Zanette G, Polo A, Gasperini M, et al. Far-field and cortical somatosensory evoked potentials in motor neuron disease. Muscle Nerve 1990;13(1):47–55.

27. Weber M, Eisen A, Stewart H, et al. The physiological basis of conduction slowing in ALS patients homozygous for the D90A CuZn-SOD mutation. Muscle Nerve 2001;24:89–97.

28. Cosi V, Poloni M, Mazzini L, Callieco R. Somatosensory evoked potentials in amyotrophic lateral sclerosis. J Neurol Neurosurg Psychiatry 1984;47(8):857–861.

Chapter 8

Magnetic Resonance Imaging in Disease Progression in Multiple Sclerosis

Anthony Traboulsee and Donald W. Paty

Multiple sclerosis (MS) research and individual patient care have greatly benefited from the application of magnetic resonance imaging (MRI) techniques over the last 15 years. The ability to reveal MS lesions in a noninvasive way and to follow the evolution of those lesions over time has been provided by MRI. Conventional MRI and subsequent MR techniques provide a powerful approach by which to characterize and quantify objectively the evolving pathology in MS patients.

MR techniques have three major roles in the field of MS: as diagnostic tools, outcome measures for clinical trials of new therapies, and research tools for the in vivo study of MS pathogenesis. This chapter emphasizes the role of conventional MRI and of the new MR techniques for studying disease progression.

MRI has revolutionized the approach to diagnosis in MS and has also been established as an objective measure of following disease activity and natural history studies[1,2] and in clinical trials.[3,4] In addition to these major contributions, MR techniques now have the promise of revealing the actual tissue characteristics of MS in vivo pathology as it evolves.[5]

Clinical Parameters of Disease Progression

MS is both a phasic and a chronic progressive disorder of the central nervous system. The clinical hallmarks of the disease are episodes or attacks (relapse) of neurologic dysfunction caused by inflammatory demyelination, followed by complete or partial recovery (remission). There is marked heterogeneity among patients in terms of severity, location, frequency, and degree of recovery from these clinical attacks. These clinical attacks are often associated with new lesions seen on MRI.

The majority of patients begin with the relapsing-remitting form of MS (RRMS or early MS). Approximately 30% will run a benign course, with repeated relapses but without accumulating any significant disability 10 years after the onset of their disease. However, the majority of RRMS patients eventually enter a progressive phase of the disease, whereby they slowly accumulate irreversible deficits in the absence of new attacks (secondary-progressive or SPMS). Finally, there is a group of patients who slowly progress from the onset with no evidence of relapses throughout the course of their disease (primary-progressive or PPMS).

Clinical outcome measures remain the gold standard for following natural history studies and clinical trials of new therapies for MS patients and predate the use of MRI for monitoring disease progression by several decades. The important clinical measures are relapses and degree of disability.

Most MS patients have subacute attacks of demyelination (relapses). These attacks can be documented as annual frequency, severity, need for hospitalization, and steroid use. On average, MS patients have one clinical relapse per year, although this can be fairly variable among individuals and for any one patient.

Progressive disability occurs as a result of incomplete recovery from relapses or independent of relapses as a slow, relentless process. Disability has been traditionally measured on the 10-point Kurtzke's Expanded Disability Status Scale (EDSS) (see Table 5-2).[6] This scale can have significant inter- and intrarater variability and tends to neglect cognitive dysfunction and fatigue. Many alternative clinical scales have been used, including the Scripps Neurological Disability Rating Scale,[7,8] Ambulation Index,[9] and more recently the Multiple Sclerosis Functional Composite Score that incorporates a cognitive function measure.[10,11]

MRI is sensitive for detecting new central nervous system lesions at the time of a clinical relapse. Furthermore, it is extremely sensitive for detecting clinically silent disease activity that is occurring throughout the course of the disease. As will be seen, the advantages of MRI-derived measurements over clinical scales include greater objectivity, sensitivity, and reproducibility. Clinical scales are biased to lesions affecting locomotion.

However, the use of MRI in research into the basic mechanisms of a disease may have different requirements than its use in a clinical trial setting.[12] Newer MRI techniques are being developed to study further in vivo pathologic changes beyond the resolution of conventional MRI techniques.[13]

application of MRI to this field. There is strong correlation between the pathology of MS and conventional MRI abnormalities.[16] In addition, MRI has become an important outcome measure for clinical trials of new therapeutic agents. MRI demonstrates disease activity in the absence of clinical findings, thereby permitting more effective evaluation of patients and facilitating objective determination of the efficacy of therapy.[12]

There are presently many MR measures that can aid the assessment of damage to the brain. The conventional MRI techniques for monitoring disease progression are the markers of new MS lesions (gadolinium-enhancing lesions, new or enlarging T_2 or proton density [PD] lesions) and markers of chronic disease (T_2 burden of disease [BOD] and, more recently, atrophy). Newer MRI techniques include burden of chronic T_1 "black holes," magnetization transfer imaging, T_2 relaxation times, diffusion imaging, MR spectroscopy, and functional MRI. These methods have the potential for improving the specificity of MR with respect to the underlying pathology.

This chapter illustrates how MR techniques have shown that MS is extremely active in the absence of obvious new clinical symptoms or signs and that normal-appearing brain (on conventional MRI) has evidence of disease activity.

Magnetic Resonance Imaging Parameters of Disease Progression

MR techniques have had a major impact in our understanding and managing of MS.[14] MR images of MS were first published in the early 1980s,[15] and the exquisite ability of MRI to identify asymptomatic lesions disseminated in space in the absence of clinical findings has led to its widespread use in diagnosis.

Although the lesions of MS can be visualized with computed tomography (CT) in many patients, CT lacks sensitivity for the burden of lesions commonly seen on MRI. T_2-weighted brain imaging remains the standard diagnostic tool but, in some instances, it is usefully complemented with gadolinium enhancement and spinal imaging. However, the diagnosis of MS remains primarily a clinical one.

Much has been learned about the complex pathogenesis of MS since the 1980s, owing to the

Principles of Magnetic Resonance Imaging

MR machines are large magnets with a field strength ranging from 0.02 to 8.0 tesla (T).[17] Signal-to-noise ratio is proportional to the square root of the field strength, with larger magnets having the best resolution. However, most clinical and research magnets are currently around 1.0–1.5 T, with a usual resolution of 1 mm × 1 mm.[18]

There are several excellent reviews of MRI physics that go beyond the scope of this chapter.[19–21] MRI is a measurement of the magnetism (spin) inherent in some nuclear isotopes, especially protons (hydrogen atoms) found in water molecules. A strong magnetic field aligns the spins within the patient. A second, rotating magnetic field (radiofrequency pulse) is applied intermittently, causing temporary excitation followed by magnetization decay.

Tissues, both normal and pathologic, are characterized by their individual spin density and by the T_1 and T_2 time constants. Varying the repetition and echo times of the pulse sequence will cause an image to be T_1-, T_2-, or PD-weighted. This optimizes the contrast between various tissues.

In living tissues, water and fat have the greatest abundance of protons (H nuclei), and the signal from protons forms a conventional MRI image. Different tissues, normal or pathologic, are discriminated by differences in the density and macromolecular environment of their mobile protons. In the brain, these are almost all water protons. The signal intensity of tissues is influenced by three main parameters: T_1 and T_2 relaxation times and PD. Relaxation times refer to the rate at which the MR signal decays after the radiofrequency excitation pulse ceases. Various strategies allow one or other to have a major influence on the image and are termed *weighting of the image.*

The pathologic features of both acute and chronic MS lesions most likely account for the remarkable sensitivity of MRI for identifying the dynamic changes in MS lesions. It has been known for a long time that the lipid content of demyelinated plaques is reduced by approximately 75% and that this lipid is replaced by water.[22] It is the increase in mobile water content that causes the lesions to appear as white spots on conventional proton MRI.

The standard sequences used in MRI monitoring usually include dual-echo T_2, with one echo time (PD) revealing the cerebrospinal fluid (CSF) as dark when compared to white matter. The second (longer) echo will usually show the CSF as bright. In addition, a pre- and a postgadolinium infusion T_1-weighted scan will reveal chronic black holes, acute black holes, and disease activity identified by the breakdown in the blood-brain barrier (BBB), as determined by gadolinium enhancement.

Conventional MRI techniques acquire signals mainly from differences in relaxation properties and density of free water protons. MRI techniques have a high sensitivity in detecting lesions, but pathologic specificity is low.[23] Conventional MRI techniques focus on tissue structure. Some newer techniques are able to determine changes in the chemical composition of tissues, whereas other techniques assess functional connectivity.

Conventional MRI refers to T_1-, T_2-, PD-weighted images and their variants (fluid-attenuated inversion recovery, fast-spin echo, rapid acquisition with refocused echoes). It also includes the use of

gadolinium contrast enhancement of T_1-weighted images. Atrophy and T_1-weighted black holes can be applied systematically in parallel with other T_2-weighted MRI sequences. Newer MR techniques include MR spectroscopy, magnetization transfer ratio (MTR), diffusion-weighted imaging (DWI), and functional MRI.

Early on, it was discovered that PD- and T_2-weighted images were more sensitive than T_1-weighted images in detecting MS lesions.[24] PD- and T_2-weighted sequences are more sensitive for detecting lesions in the periventricular regions because of improved contrast between high-signal MS lesions and low-signal CSF. Typical MS lesions detected by conventional MR images are demonstrated in Figure 8-1.

Modifications of conventional spin-echo techniques such as fast-spin echo, turbo-spin echo, and fluid-attenuated inversion recovery can improve the detection of some lesions or reduce the overall scanner time. Fluid-attenuated inversion recovery is somewhat more sensitive for hemispheric lesions. However, PD- or T_2-weighted (PD/T_2-weighted) images are better for infratentorial lesions.

The sensitivity of conventional MRI has evolved with improvements in software and magnet strength. A comparison of images from a 1.5-T and a 4-T MR machine showed that images obtained with the stronger 4-T magnet detected on average 45% more lesions.[25] All of the lesions were less than 5 mm and were typically aligned along perivascular spaces. MRI at 4 T can depict white-matter abnormalities in MS patients not detectable at 1.5 T through higher resolution with comparable signal to noise ratios and imaging times.

One of the problems with MRI has been that people older than 45 years gradually develop nonspecific white-matter lesions.[26] Specificity features for MS on MRI include large lesions, oval lesions[27] and corpus callosum lesions,[28] and infratentorial lesions. Assessment of spinal cord damage using MR still lags behind the development of brain methodologies.[29]

MRI allows sequential quantitative in vivo studies of the pathologic evolution of MS without any risk for tissue damage to the patient. One of the practical applications of this method of following disease activity has been the use of MRI in clinical trials.

Acute dynamic changes can be detected by frequent systematic scanning to identify the number of new, enlarging, stable, or enhancing lesions.[30] More

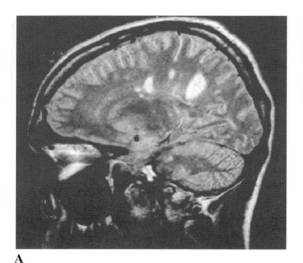

A

Figure 8-1. Typical magnetic resonance imaging findings in multiple sclerosis. **A.** Lesions in the corpus callosum on sagittal image. **B.** Proton density–weighted image of three white-matter bright lesions, one of which is enhancing with gadolinium on the corresponding T_1-weighted image (**C**, *arrows*), characteristic of an acute multiple sclerosis lesion with breakdown of the blood-brain barrier.

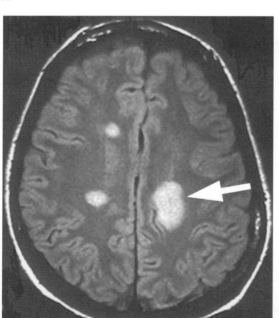

B

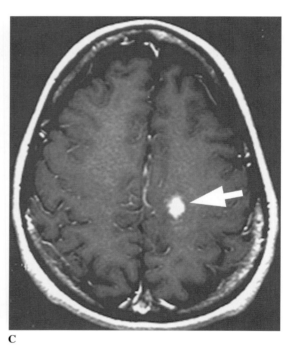

C

significant chronic changes can be estimated by measuring the total extent of the pathologic process at selected points using baseline comparisons.

Image analysis techniques used to analyze MRI data include quantification of the MRI BOD (burden of disease or lesion load) and coregistration of multiple MR images. MRI data can be stored electronically, and lesion load can be measured manually (reproducibility, 94%) as performed at the University of British Columbia MS/MRI research unit.[4] Semiautomated methods have also been developed with similar reproducibility and are also time consuming. Fully automated techniques are also available but not yet validated. The accuracy of lesion load measurement is improved by obtaining thinner slices due to the reduction in partial volume errors. Three-dimensional fast-spin echo will allow more accurate lesion quantification with thin image slices. This will also help to minimize error due to poor repositioning for serial studies.[31]

Reproducibility of MRI BOD measurements can be influenced by such factors as biological activity, pulse sequences, slice thickness, accuracy in repositioning, use of different MR machines, and inter- and intraobserver variability. Whereas intraobserver agreement typically is near 98–99%, this can drop to 91% with the use of different MR machines.[32] Studies of the precision of measurements have shown that most of the techniques have reasonable reproducibility,[33] particularly when taking into consideration the extreme variability in the biological aspects of lesion extent and activity. Interscanner variation in brain MRI lesion load measurement limits the usefulness of interpreting serial scans for individual patients or could have an impact on the interpretation of clinical trial data from multiple centers.

MR data from serial studies or from different MR methods (MTR, MR spectroscopy, etc.) can be compared using coregistration techniques. Several methods are available, including the use of standardized stereotaxic atlas of the brain and three-dimensional fast-spin echo sequences.[12]

Conventional Magnetic Resonance Imaging and Disease Progression: Gadolinium-Enhancing Lesions

Gadolinium enhancement is a common finding in new MS lesions.[2] The typical new MS lesion is first seen as a spot of gadolinium enhancement in a previously unaffected area of white matter. Enhancement has been correlated with the acute inflammatory phase of lesion development in MS and disruption of the BBB.[34–36] The enhancement often is solid with fresh lesions and has the form of a ring with lesions several weeks old. Enhancing lesions persist for at least 4 or 5 weeks.[37] Enhancement usually lasts fewer than 4 weeks and is sensitive to steroids and other anti-inflammatory treatments. Higher ("triple") doses of gadolinium have been shown to increase not only the number of enhancing MS lesions by approximately 28% but also the intensity of some lesions.[38] Many of these acute lesions are also seen on the unenhanced T_1-weighted image as acute black holes that may completely resolve.

Most evidence points to disruption of the BBB as the initial event in the development of the lesion in MS. It is thought that antigen-specific T cells enter the nervous system, recognize antigen, and begin a cytokine cascade that mediates disruption of the BBB seen on contrast-enhanced MRI. Subsequently, the inflammatory response is amplified, and the effector stage leading to myelin damage is initiated.[39] The BBB disruption allows leakage of immunocompetent cells, macrophages, and other inflammatory components into brain substance to produce a reversible inflammatory lesion that can be seen on the PD/T_2-weighted MRI scan.[35,40]

The importance of the BBB integrity has been shown in a rat model of central pontine myelinolysis by Adler and colleagues.[41] In this condition, demyelination is caused by rapid correction of chronic hyponatremia. MRI monitored the integrity of the BBB, and demyelination was confirmed on histopathology. Disruption of the BBB during the first 24 hours of sodium correction was associated with a 70% risk of developing demyelination, compared to only an 8% risk if the BBB was intact.

A few days or hours after enhancement develops, a new lesion can be seen on the PD/T_2 scan. After the appearance of a bright lesion on the PD/T_2 image, the lesion will then enlarge to a variable extent. After a period of enlargement, the lesion will become smaller.[42,43] At some point, that same lesion will reactivate, usually by re-enhancing and re-enlarging.[2,44] This cycle of repeated breakdown of the BBB and inflammation is probably repeated several times before significant demyelination occurs.[45]

Further activation of an MS lesion can manifest as recurrent enhancement or enlargement or both. In many instances, the enhancement that occurs is at the margin of the lesion or as a round enlarging area budding off the side of the previously stable lesion.[46]

Gadolinium-enhancing lesions correlate with the occurrence of relapses, CSF myelin breakdown products and, in patients with RRMS, with higher EDSS. However, the predictive value of the frequency of enhancement for changes in EDSS is only weak.[47]

Conventional Magnetic Resonance Imaging and Disease Progression: Proton Density–T_2 Lesion Dynamics

The characteristic abnormalities consist of periventricular lesions in the cerebral hemispheres seen in T_2-weighted images. Additional common sites

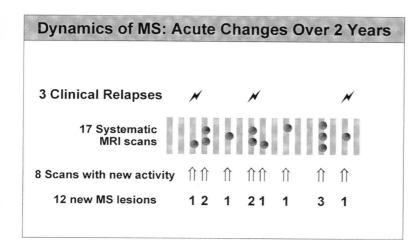

Figure 8-2. The dynamics of multiple sclerosis (MS) pathology as revealed by monthly magnetic resonance imaging (MRI) scans over a 2-year period. MRI detects a significant frequency of clinically silent MS relapses and the accumulation of T_2 lesion load.

include other parts of the cerebral white matter, optic nerves, internal capsule, corpus callosum, middle cerebellar peduncles, brain stem, and spinal cord.[48] MS lesions appear as hypointense or isointense on T_1-weighted images and are typically larger and more extensive on T_2-weighted images.

Typically, the new PD/T_2-weighted lesion will increase in size over several weeks, probably owing to increasing inflammation. After approximately 4 weeks, this new and enlarging lesion will shrink in size to be visualized as a smaller stable lesion. The stable lesion probably represents permanent demyelination. In time (months), this stable lesion will be seen to reactivate by additional enhancement, enlargement, or most likely both. In the meantime, the pathology within the apparent stable lesion is probably maturing to include gliosis and axonal loss. Eventually, after many reactivations, the evolving lesion will fuse with its neighbors to form confluent lesions. Thus, what may have started out as several small lesions may end up forming one large confluent lesion.[49]

The dynamic nature of T_2 lesions is elegantly illustrated at the Harvard Medical School Whole Brain Atlas Web site (http://www.med.harvard.edu/AAN-LIB/home.html), where one can follow the Multiple Sclerosis link under "Inflammatory diseases" for a time-lapse movie. Some lesions do not develop in this dynamic way but grow steadily. These slowly enlarging lesions probably represent the chronic active lesion identified in classic MS pathology.

In the early 1980s, pathologic correlation studies[50] showed that MRI could identify the chronic lesions

of MS with precision. The PD/T_2 lesion, although sensitive for detecting MS plaques, is not specific for underlying pathology. Barnes and colleagues[51] showed that chronic plaques seen on MRI were pathologically heterogeneous. Most lesions (87%) had an expanded extracellular space. It is possible that T_2 lesions overestimated the extent of the pathology due to the edema and other forms of increased water content without specific pathology.[52]

It was apparent early on that MRI could detect many neurologically asymptomatic lesions. At the time of diagnosis, the average number of lesions present on the PD/T_2-weighted image is approximately five. This indicates that there is a preclinical phase in which MRI lesions accumulate before the clinical onset of the disease. The rate of accumulation of new lesions over time is a least four to five new lesions per year.[30] Therefore, approximately 80% of the active MRI lesions seen on scans of the head are neurologically asymptomatic.

The strategy for showing the exquisite sensitivity of MR to detect clinical silent lesions is illustrated in Figure 8-2. In a series of patients, serial MRI was performed every 6 weeks for 2 years.[4] During that time, the average patient had three clinical relapses. Of the 17 MRI scans performed, a number of scans would show new PD/T_2 lesions coinciding with the clinical relapses. However, the frequent MRI scanning also showed many more new MS lesions in the absence of clinical relapses (silent lesions). Untreated MS patients are expected to increase in yearly lesion load by 5–10%.[53]

The location and morphology of MS lesions on the coronal MR image is reminiscent of the classic appearance of periventricular demyelination seen at autopsy. Immediate postmortem imaging of the brain in situ and subsequent imaging of formalin-fixed tissue has shown that individual demyelinated lesions identifiable on both pathology and the MRI scan correlate extremely well in terms of size and location.[50,54] The overall correlation between the degree of involvement on the MRI slice and the extent of pathology visualized grossly on the same slice can be fairly variable. Well-positioned comparative slices usually correlate fairly well (r = 0.80–0.94).

Most new MRI lesions are neurologically silent. The factors that determine neurologic expression are probably a combination of location and the intensity of pathology in the active lesion. Approximately 1 in 10 MRI active lesions hits an eloquent neurologic tract and causes specific neurologic symptoms such as a clinical relapse. The severity of the pathologic process in that lesion will affect the severity of the symptoms. Lesions that occur in relatively nonspecific areas of the brain such as the frontal lobes and the temporal lobes probably cause very subtle cognitive and emotional changes without necessarily producing specific neurologic syndromes.

A number of studies have shown correlation between individual MS lesions and clinical symptoms.[55] However, the confusing aspect of clinical-MRI or pathologic correlation is that after recovery from an acute deficit, such as vision loss in optic neuritis, the functional vision can return to near normal in the face of a markedly prolonged visual evoked potential and a significant residual MRI optic nerve lesion. Recovery of function has not been extensively studied in MS,[56] but it is clear that there are factors such as plasticity and redundancy that support recovery of function in spite of persistent pathology.[57] These factors are probably important in explaining the lack of strong correlation between various neurologic deficits and the rate and extent of MRI abnormalities.

Cognitive dysfunction in MS is relatively common and is associated with significantly higher unemployment than in noncognitively impaired MS patients having the same degree of physical disability.[58] Cognitive abnormalities, including poor memory, poor word finding, and impaired executive function, correlate well with the extent of involvement on the standard axial MRI image.[59] The total extent of MS lesions in the cerebral hemispheres, particularly those lesions related to the corpus callosum, seem to correlate fairly well with cognitive aspects of MS.[60] A study of 39 MS patients[61] suggests that subcortical white-matter disease is more important than total lesion load or cerebral atrophy. This probably relates to disruption of subcortical association fibers.

The correlations between the total extent of MRI abnormalities and global neurologic status as measured on Kurtzke's EDSS scale have usually been positive but of low to modest degree, as shown in the large interferon beta study.[62] However, some studies have shown a higher correlation.[63] The correlation coefficient between the clinical measures (EDSS) and the various conventional T_2-weighted MRI measures has been between 0.2–0.6. Although these correlations have been highly statistically significant, the strength of the correlation has been weak to modest at best. The correlation is limited by the poor sensitivity of clinical measures and by the inherent lack of tissue specificity of T_2-weighted images.[47]

MRI measures are rarely used for prognosis because of the poor correlation with clinical outcome factors. One exception is in a group of patients at high risk of developing MS. The number and extent of PD/T_2-weighted MRI abnormalities at first presentation with a clinically isolated syndrome suggestive of demyelination strongly predicts the risk of developing clinically definite MS (CDMS) in the next few years.[14] In addition to being important in predicting diagnosis of CDMS, it is also predictive of the degree of neurologic impairment at both 5 and 10 years.[64] In a 10-year follow-up study of 81 patients who had a baseline T_2-weighted MRI at presentation, 67% had an initial scan that was abnormal.[64] Of those with an initial abnormal MRI scan, 83% had progressed to CDMS, compared to only 11% of those with a normal MRI scan at first presentation. A normal early scan also appears to predict a more benign course, although the numbers are fairly small.

MRI is the best paraclinical test for detecting asymptomatic dissemination in space and for predicting the diagnosis of CDMS. In a University of British Columbia MS Clinic prospective study of 200 suspected MS patients who did not meet diagnostic criteria, 67% had an abnormal MRI at presentation.[65] One-half of these patients went on to develop CDMS within 2 years, compared to only 5% of those with a normal MRI at baseline. The MRI criteria used for an MRI strongly suggestive of MS included a scan with four lesions or a scan with three lesions if one is periventricular. Lesions were greater than 3 mm, bright on T_2-weighted images, and located in the white matter.[66]

The Optic Neuritis Treatment Trial[67] enrolled 448 patients with acute optic neuritis. Eighty-seven percent of these patients did not have a diagnosis of MS at the time of their episode of optic neuritis. Most (88%) completed a 5-year follow-up phase and, of those patients who did not initially fulfill diagnostic criteria, 27% had progressed to CDMS. However, 51% of patients with an abnormal baseline MRI (three or more lesions) at the time of their episode of optic neuritis developed MS within 5 years, compared to only 16% of patients with a normal MRI at baseline.[68]

Another interesting aspect of MRI in MS is that the pattern of MRI activity seems to vary with the clinical syndrome. For example, benign MS patients tend to have much fewer active lesions than do patients with a clinically aggressive course.[69] Patients with PPMS have very low levels of MRI activity,[70] compared to SPMS patients. The PPMS patients, who tend to have chronic spinal syndromes clinically, have a pattern of cerebral involvement that tends to be limited to chronic periventricular lesions only, without significant MRI evidence for dynamic activity.

A large cross-sectional study (N = 188) showed similar patterns of lesion load, size, and location of lesions between RRMS and PPMS patients. SPMS patients showed significantly larger lesion loads and, as compared to PPMS patients, tended to develop more BOD when correlated to duration of disease. The lesion load in SP patients had a modest correlation with EDSS ($r = 0.52$).[71] MR abnormalities vary for the different subgroups of MS, with RRMS and SPMS probably representing different ends of the same spectrum of the disease. Other groups have found poor or no correlation with EDSS and T_2 BOD.[72]

Patients with PPMS or transitional-progressive MS have been shown to have low brain T_2 and T_1 lesion loads and slow rates of new lesion formation with minimal gadolinium enhancement, despite their accumulating disability. Stevenson et al.[73] followed up a group of 167 MS patients with serial imaging of brain and spinal cord 1 year apart. There was an increase in median percentage changes of T_2 BOD of 7.3–10.8%, with a greater increase in T_1 lesion load of 12.6% in a subset of patients. Fewer new lesions were seen in the spinal cord; however, there was a median change of 3.8–4.9% over 1 year in the cord cross sectional area.

The brain tends to have more T_2 activity than does the spinal cord. A small serial study with monthly MRI scans over the course of 1 year on 19 patients with either PPMS or SPMS found 132 active lesions in the brain and only 6 in the cord.[74] The majority (85%) of the new brain lesions occurred in the SPMS cohort, especially in those who had superimposed relapses. There was no correlation with MRI activity and change in disability over the year of follow-up. Despite the lack of disease activity, the cross sectional spinal cord area continued to decrease over the year in these patients, suggesting another mechanism besides relapses is leading to progressive disability.

Conventional Magnetic Resonance Imaging: Treatment Effects

MRI monitoring was crucial for several MS clinical trials to justify regulatory approval of the drugs under study. These include the interferon beta-1a and beta-1b trials (Avonex, Betaseron, Betaferon, Rebif). There have also been several studies of agents monitored by MRI that did not show a therapeutic effect: interferon alpha,[75] cyclosporine,[76] and others. One study, using very low doses of interferon beta-1a, showed that an MRI effect could be clearly shown at low doses, where there was no significant clinical treatment effect.[77] Copaxone has recently been shown to have a modest MRI treatment effect. There have been some clinical trials in which both clinical activity and MRI activity were accelerated by proposed treatments, including monoclonal antibodies against tumor necrosis factor[78] and tumor necrosis factor–soluble receptor used to block the effects to tumor necrosis factor.[79] There have been clinical trials in which the degree of gadolinium enhancement was suppressed by treatments that did not show a clear-cut clinical benefit, including antilymphocyte monoclonal antibodies[80] and immunosuppressants such as cladribine.[81] However, the most dramatic effects seen in the reduction of MRI activity (PD/T_2 lesions, gadolinium enhancement) are with the use of interferon beta at the higher doses. Suppression of active lesions and new lesion formation in these studies were in the range of 80–90%.[82]

The average number of lesions on a PD/T$_2$ MRI at the onset of MS is five. The average number of new lesions per year is four. All forms of interferon beta therapy had beneficial effects on the disease process measured by brain MRI. The treatment effect for new T$_2$ lesions is a 75% reduction from four new lesions per year to one new lesion per year. After 5 years of MS, the expected number of lesions would increase from 5 to 25, whereas on interferon beta treatment, the total number of lesions at 5 years would be 10. From an MRI standpoint, that treatment effect is very significant, with implications for long-term follow-up based on the findings of O'Riordan et al.[64]

The suppression of the inflammatory component of the total MRI BOD is fairly significant and detectable within the first few months of treatment. The lower doses of interferon beta seem to have a more modest effect,[83,84] and higher doses seem to be more effective up to what may be a therapeutic ceiling of approximately 80–90% reduction.[82]

Conventional Magnetic Resonance Imaging: Conclusions

Conventional MRI techniques refer to PD/T$_2$-weighted MR images and gadolinium-enhanced T$_1$-weighted images. These were the first MR parameters applied systematically to the in vivo study of MS. MRI has become an important diagnostic and prognostic tool for patients who have had a single event of demyelination and are therefore at risk of developing CDMS.

Natural history studies have shown that MS lesions are common and accumulate over the course of the disease. Most new lesions appear in the absence of clinical activity. At the time of diagnosis, the average patient will have five lesions detected by MRI. They will develop four to five new lesions per year, with an increase of overall volume of lesion burden of 5–10% per year.

Individual lesions, as detected by MRI, are dynamic, with the ability to enlarge, disappear, then reappear or re-enhance. Pathologic correlation demonstrates that gadolinium-enhancing lesions repre-

sent new, acute inflammatory lesions. However, T$_2$-weighted images lack pathologic specificity, except in the very chronic stage, where they correlate fairly precisely with demyelination and axonal loss.[54]

Conventional MRI measures correlate weakly with clinical scales of disability, and the lack of pathologic specificity has driven the search for new MR techniques for in vivo investigation of the complex pathogenesis of MS. However, the main problem is the poor correlation between the extent of pathology and the clinical manifestations.

Atrophy: Background

Although conventional MRI has greatly increased the understanding of the pathophysiology of MS, its relationship to the development of disability is complex. More pathologically specific imaging markers have, therefore, been sought to try to understand the underlying process that is responsible for the progressive disability seen in MS. Of these, the simplest to understand conceptually is the measurement of atrophy, which most probably represents axonal loss. Although atrophy measures are not new, they are being applied to MS with great vigor.

Brain atrophy had been noted on autopsy even before neuroimaging techniques were widely available. Conventional CT studies were the first neuroimaging tools used in the assessment of MS patients,[85] and a comprehensive CT study of 100 MS patients in 1978 demonstrated atrophy as a feature of MS brains and also demonstrated that it was progressive in a small subset of patients followed up for up to 21 months.[86]

Because of new developments in imaging analysis, atrophy measures are more reliable and reproducible. Hence, the measurement of atrophy now provides an objective marker by which to evaluate putative treatment aimed at preventing disability in MS.[87] Several research groups have looked at atrophy measures in the search for an MRI parameter that correlates strongly with clinical disability. Different methods have been used, including ventricular size, corpus callosum area, spinal cord cross-sectional area, measuring selected brain slices, or segmentation of the entire brain to calculate a brain parenchymal volume or fraction.

MS patients have less brain parenchymal volume than do age-matched controls.[88,89] Atrophy was found in 47–100% of RRMS and SPMS patients, including evidence of atrophy in the brain stem, cerebellum, cervical cord, cerebral white matter, and corpus callosum area of approximately 20% as compared to controls.[90–92] In a large cohort of MS patients (N = 188), the degree of atrophy was greatest for SPMS patients.[71] However, it can also be an early finding in patients who have had their first attack of demyelination and subsequently go on to develop MS.[93] Spinal cord atrophy (decrease in cross-sectional area compared to controls) was seen in 41% of SPMS patients and in only two patients with more benign disease.[94]

Atrophy is progressive during the course of MS. The presence of atrophy probably is due to a combination of the loss of myelin, loss of axons, and shrinkage of the glial scar (gliosis). Factors that would increase brain volume would be inflammation and edema. Therefore, anti-inflammatory treatments that decrease the inflammation could likely accelerate the appearance of atrophy. Patients with RRMS tended to lose 17.3 ml per year of brain parenchymal volume as compared to 23.6 ml per year for SPMS.[88] In another study using registered serial scans, MS patients had a rate of cerebral atrophy of 0.8% per year as compared to 0.3% for controls, whereas the rate of ventricular enlargement was five times that for controls.[89]

The Queen Square group[95] found that progressive atrophy could be detected in 55% of MS patients followed up serially with monthly scans over an 18-month period. There was a higher rate of atrophy in the subset of patients who clinically deteriorated as compared to those who did not have sustained disability. There was no correlation in this small cohort (N = 29) for atrophy with T_2 lesion load at baseline, change in T_2 lesion load over 18 months, and the volume of new gadolinium-enhancing lesions. In another study, brain atrophy worsened without clinical disease activity for many patients with early RRMS.[96]

In one cross-sectional study, RRMS patients had significantly lower brain volumes and corpus callosum areas than did healthy control subjects. Although there was no correlation between atrophy and T_2 lesion load, modest correlations were found between brain volume and corpus callosum area ($r = 0.58$) and T_1-hypointense lesion load ($r = 0.48$).[91] Brain atrophy is an early MRI finding in RRMS and is closely related to black hole burden rather than T_2 lesion load.

There was a modest correlation for atrophy with EDSS in the SPMS patients, with a correlation factor of –0.69. There was no correlation with T_2 lesion volume (BOD).[88] In another small group of 28 SPMS patients, a correlation with EDSS and atrophy also was shown, but investigators were unable to show any correlation with T_1 or T_2 lesion load.[72] However, another group looking at a small cohort of 30 patients showed a modest correlation with T_2 lesion volume.[97] In another study, there was a suggestion that atrophy (enlargement of the third ventricle) may be correlated to the number of gadolinium-enhancing lesions at baseline.[98]

The Queen Square group, in their earlier work, did not find any correlation with atrophy to baseline T_2 lesion load, change in T_2 lesion load, and volume of new gadolinium-enhancing lesions on monthly scans.[95] Further work looking at the spinal cord area using a technique with good reproducibility demonstrated a strong ($r = -0.7$) correlation between spinal cord area and disability measured by the Kurtzke EDSS.[99] At a mildly impaired EDSS of 3, the average cord area was reduced by 12%, whereas, at a severe level of disability (EDSS of 8), the average cord area was reduced by 35%.

Correlation with disability (EDSS or Scripps) was modest (range, $r = -0.37$ to 0.49)[90] in a study by Liu et al. The T_2 lesion load did correlate modestly with some atrophy measures, including ventricular enlargement and corpus callosum area ($r = 0.5$). In another study by the same group, cervical spinal cord atrophy had a stronger correlation with EDSS ($r = -0.5$) and disease duration ($r = -0.39$) than did cerebellar or brain stem volume. These latter measures had a modest correlation with the Scripps Neurological Disability Rating Scale scores ($r = 0.49$ and $r = 0.34$, respectively).[100] Furthermore, significant correlation between ventricular measures of atrophy and impaired cognitive function has been demonstrated.[101]

There is an apparent treatment effect on brain atrophy with one of the interferon beta-1a agents, demonstrated by a post hoc analysis. The rate of brain atrophy in the actively treated cohort was slower than that of the placebo group.[96] However, anti-inflammatory drugs used concomitantly with interferons may falsely increase the degree of apparent atrophy. Therefore, the scenario might be that the more potent the anti-inflammatory treatment, the less likely a therapeutic effect on atrophy would be seen. Perhaps a strategy of examining the anti-inflammatory effect (PD/T$_2$ BOD) and the degree of atrophy in parallel would help to understand the interaction of these phenomena.

Progressive cerebral atrophy is an important feature of MS. In addition to accumulation of relatively nonspecific PD/T$_2$ lesions, longitudinal evaluations have found that patients with only mild to modest disability are already developing significant cerebral atrophy. Atrophy, in both brain and spinal cord, occurs early in the clinical disease course, correlates with worsening disability, and gives additional information to that obtained with conventional MRI. Cerebral atrophy measures lack specificity for the type of brain tissue being lost and probably reflect a combination of myelin loss, axonal and neuronal loss, and scarring.

Atrophy changes can be detected within 1 year and may have potential as a marker of progression in monitoring therapeutic trials.[89] The effect of putative therapies aimed at preventing disability could be objectively assessed by atrophy measures.

Atrophy has a stronger correlation with clinical disability and may prove to be a valuable MRI measure for serial studies and treatment trials. It requires standardization and is unlikely to be helpful to the individual patient with multiple, unregistered MRI scans from several different scanners.

Black Holes in Disease Progression

MS lesions appear as areas of high signal (bright) on conventional PD/T$_2$-weighted MRI. Most PD/T$_2$ bright MS lesions are isointense, with normal-appearing white matter (NAWM) on the unenhanced T$_1$-weighted conventional MR image. However, a proportion of the MS lesions will appear as hypointense (black holes).[102] Most gadolinium-enhancing lesions will become PD/T$_2$ bright lesions, and 80% will appear as acute black holes. However, only 36% will progress to become chronic black holes,[103] with the remainder becoming isointense on serial T$_1$-weighted images.

Longer T$_1$ relaxation times occur in pathologic tissues, with expanded extracellular space indicating loss of tissue structure. Chronic hypointense MS lesions also have lower MTRs (putative marker of tissue destruction) than do isointense lesions.[104] It is likely that the subset of MS lesions that appear as black holes or hypointensity on T$_1$-weighted images have more significant tissue destruction.

Postmortem studies show that chronic black holes may be in vivo markers of axonal loss.[47] One study of the black holes seen on the unenhanced T$_1$-weighted images and the postmortem pathology correlated fairly well with the more severe elements of pathology, such as demyelination and axonal loss.[105] However, it is likely to be a complex relationship.

A large cross-sectional study of 91 MS patients by Nijeholt et al.[106] found that SPMS patients had more T$_1$ lesion load (black holes), increased ventricular size (atrophy), and more spinal cord atrophy than did RRMS patients. Furthermore, EDSS correlated well with T$_1$ lesion load and atrophy measures for the RRMS and SPMS patients. For T$_1$ black holes, a correlation up to 0.81 has been reported for SPMS patients.

In another series of SPMS patients, Brex and colleagues[107] looked at the N-acetylaspartate (NAA) signal in chronic T$_2$ lesions. Those lesions that were hypointense on T$_1$-weighted images had a lower NAA concentration as compared to lesions that were isointense on T$_1$-weighted images. Because NAA is a marker of axonal and neuronal damage, this finding suggests that the subset of MS lesions that appear as chronic black holes has more severe pathology, including axonal damage.

New Magnetic Resonance Imaging Techniques

New MRI techniques are developing to identify pathology that is not detected by conventional MRI techniques. Several studies using new MRI techniques have shown pathologic abnormalities within the NAWM. Some of these abnormalities begin several months before the development of a new gadolinium-enhancing lesion in that same area of NAWM.[108]

Magnetic Resonance Spectroscopy for Monitoring Axonal Disease in Multiple Sclerosis

MS is primarily a disease of myelin, although the degeneration of neurons and axons is receiving considerably more interest as a major factor contributing to disability. MR spectroscopy provides chemical information of tissue metabolites, whereas conventional MRI provides structural information.

Several atomic nuclei will resonate and can be studied by MR spectroscopy. The resolution for conventional MRI is approximately 1 mm × 1 mm when the signal is obtained from water (^{1}H protons). MR sensitivity for protons is far greater than it is for phosphorous, carbon, fluoride, and sodium, which will produce much lower resolution images. Suppression of signal from surrounding brain tissue is used to isolate the metabolite of interest. Small voxels (1–2 ml) and long acquisition times produce relatively low signal-to-noise ratios.

With suppression of the water signal from brain, four major resonances are revealed by MR spectroscopy using long echo times. These include choline, creatinine, NAA, and lactate peaks. The choline peak represents phospholipids. The concentration of creatinine is relatively constant in the brain, so the height of the creatinine peak serves as an internal control. The NAA peak is extremely important as a marker of in vivo axonal and neuronal damage.[109] NAA measures can be reported for MS lesions, NAWM, and whole brain. The lactate peak is normally barely visible above the base line noise. In certain pathologic conditions causing anaerobic metabolism (ischemia, inflammation), the lactate signal will increase.

Decreases in brain NAA are associated with neuronal loss or dysfunction. NAA is the second most abundant amino acid in the central nervous system.[110] It is contained almost entirely within neurons and axons. Its function is uncertain, but it is a putative marker of axonal integrity as loss of axons occurs in acute and chronic MS lesions and may be an important cause of irreversible disability.[109,111]

Shorter echo times are better for detecting lipids, myoinositol, glutamate, and γ-aminobutyric acid. Little nuclear MR signal is obtained from lipids of intact myelin because of their immobility. The ability to detect mobile lipid resonances within MS lesions on proton MR spectroscopy provides a noninvasive tool with which to monitor myelin breakdown directly.[112]

An interesting study from Queen Square[113] compared the NAA peak in the cerebellar white matter of MS patients with and without cerebellar signs. In addition to a normal control group, they also compared the NAA signal to a group of eight patients with autosomal dominant cerebellar ataxia,

known to have marked cerebellar atrophy due to neuronal and axonal degeneration. The MS group with cerebellar signs and the autosomal dominant cerebellar ataxia group both showed cerebellar atrophy on conventional MRI and a significant reduction in the NAA peak as compared to the control subjects and MS patients without ataxia.

MR spectroscopy was performed before stereotactic biopsies of suspicious lesions in three patients, which eventually were determined to be demyelinating lesions. There was strong correlation with the degree of NAA loss and reduction in axonal density in the demyelinating lesions. A concomitant increase in choline and myoinositol corresponded to glial proliferation, and inflammation was associated with elevated lactate signal.[114,115] Thus, MR spectroscopy can provide in vivo markers of key pathologic features accompanying demyelinative diseases, including axonal loss.

MS patients have NAA metabolite concentration abnormalities in acute and chronic lesions and in the white-matter tracts that appear normal on conventional PD/T_2-weighted MRI (NAWM). In the acute gadolinium-enhancing MS lesion, the NAA peak is substantially reduced, and there is an increase in inositol compounds as compared to normal white matter. Although there may be recovery in the signal, it is only partial. Both the decline and recovery of NAA have been found to correlate strongly with alterations in neurologic impairment observed in MS patients. The acute lesion also shows an increase in lactate concentration that is most likely a transient phenomenon due to edema, inflammation, and macrophage invasion.[116] Also, increase in the neutral fat (seen at short-echo times) is a marker for active demyelination. This reinforces the hypothesis that axonal dysfunction is associated with neurologic dysfunction and its subsequent recovery in the acute phase of MS.

Narayana and colleagues[117] performed serial imaging on a group of 25 MS patients for 2 years. They included gadolinium-enhanced images in their protocol as well as conventional T_2-weighted images and MR spectroscopy. Several interesting points came out of this study. First, metabolic changes were observed in some patients before the appearance of lesions on conventional MRI. Second, the regional changes in the metabolite levels were dynamic and reversible in some cases. An acute plaque could have a transient NAA decrease;

indicating that an acutely reduced NAA level does not necessarily imply axonal loss. Third, strong lipid peaks could occur in the absence of gadolinium enhancement, suggesting that breakdown products of demyelination can occur independent of perivenous inflammatory changes.

In general, MS lesions have a similar decrease in NAA concentration regardless of the type of MS (RRMS, SPMS, or PPMS) as compared to the normal white matter of control subjects. These abnormalities were not found in the chronic lesions or NAWM of patients with benign MS (minimal deficit after 10 years of disease).[118–120]

Part of the focus of these new techniques is looking for evidence of specific pathologies in NAWM on conventional T_2-weighted MRI. Postmortem studies have confirmed substantial axonal loss occurring in the NAWM.[121] In the corpus callosum, the normal density of axons of patients with MS was less than one-half that of control brains.

The NAWM of the internal capsule in MS patients has lower NAA levels than control subjects.[122] There is a significant reduction in NAA concentration in the NAWM of RRMS and SPMS patients as compared to controls.[123] This reduction was more evident in the progressive patients and correlated with EDSS as well as T_2 lesion load.[124] However, the NAA spectra were not sufficient to distinguish between PPMS and SPMS patients.[125] The decrease in NAA concentration in the NAWM of patients with PPMS suggests that axonal loss occurring in the NAWM in PPMS may well be a mechanism for disease progression in this subgroup of MS patients who deteriorate in the absence of clinical relapses.[126]

To determine at what stage the loss of NAA occurs, Brex et al.[127] measured the NAA concentration in 20 patients with their first attack of demyelination (clinically isolated syndrome) and so at risk of developing CDMS. As expected, the T_2 lesions showed a decrease in the NAA concentration. In contrast to CDMS patients, there was no significant reduction of the NAA concentration in the NAWM as compared to age-matched controls. This finding suggests that more widespread axonal changes are not yet detectable at this early clinical stage.

NAA abnormalities are progressive. A group of RRMS patients with disease duration for at least 5 years had a significant decrease in whole-brain NAA. When correlated to age, the rate of decline of NAA in this small cohort was estimated to be 0.8% per year, 10 times faster than the control group.[128] This suggests that progressive neuronal loss is occurring and could be a new marker of treatment efficacy.

Arnold and colleagues[129] followed up a group of MS patients over an 18-month period with MR spectroscopy, MRI, and EDSS every 6 months. Compared to control subjects, all MS patients had decreased NAA concentration at baseline. Furthermore, all MS patients had a progressive decrease in NAA for a central brain volume. For patients with relapses, changes in NAA were strongly correlated ($r = -0.74$) with changes in lesion volume on conventional MR images.

Fu and colleagues[130] followed up a group of MS patients over a 30-month period, performing serial imaging every 6–8 months. Their cohort included 11 patients with RRMS and 17 with SPMS. The NAA of NAWM for RRMS patients decreased by 15.6% over the 30-month period. MS lesions in these patients had decreased NAA as compared to NAWM. This decrease was greater for RRMS patients (15.3%) as compared to SPMS (8.8%). However, this difference is due to a decrease in NAA in the NAWM of SPMS rather than a difference in the MS lesions of the two cohorts. Furthermore, the decrease in NAA in NAWM correlated strongly with changes in disability in the RRMS group. Axonal damage or loss may be responsible for the chronic functional impairments in MS. The accumulation of secondary axonal damage in the NAWM may be of particular significance for understanding chronic disability in this disease.

Although NAA alterations have been emphasized, MS lesions also show changes in other metabolites,[112] including increases in choline representing the phospholipid pool (membrane breakdown) and lactate (inflammation and edema). Spectra with short echo times improve the sensitivity of detecting increases in myoinositol and lipids. The serial changes in MR spectroscopy in acute, gadolinium-enhancing MS lesions were studied by Davie and colleagues.[131] They looked at short-echo (lipid) and long-echo (NAA) proton spectra. Eight patients with enhancing lesions had serial MR spectroscopy images at 1- to 2-month intervals for up to 9 months. The acute MS lesion had a decrease in NAA signal. In some cases, there was recovery in the NAA signal. There was an increase in the lipid peak in the lesions that had been enhancing for less than 1 month and remained elevated for an average of 5 months. This suggests that MR spectroscopy can detect myelin breakdown products as well as axonal damage (NAA) associated with acute inflammatory MS lesions.

Recent pathologic studies[111] and the use of MR spectroscopy to measure the axonal marker NAA has emphasized the fact that substantial axonal damage occurs in MS in addition to demyelination. The axonal damage is present in both lesions and NAWM, progresses over time, and correlates best with clinical disability.[132] This has led to the hypothesis that incomplete recovery from axonal damage may be responsible for a significant proportion of the chronic irreversible disability that occurs in MS.

The mechanisms of axonal loss are uncertain. It may involve axonal degeneration secondary to demyelination or damage to the axonal cytoskeleton. Inflammatory mediators, including cytokines and proteolytic enzymes, may contribute to axonal damage, as may nitric oxide. Axonal destruction may also be due to immune attack directed at axonal components. The realization that axonal degeneration is a fundamental component of MS that may occur early in the disease course should alter the approach to management and open avenues to a more targeted immunotherapy aimed at reducing the progression of disability.[133]

MR spectroscopy provides a unique opportunity to isolate and study in vivo one component of the complex pathology of MS, specifically, axonal integrity, and in active demyelination, the appearance of neutral fat.[112,134]

Magnetization Transfer Imaging and Tissue Destruction in Multiple Sclerosis

Magnetization transfer imaging is another tool for investigating pathologic tissue changes that are beyond the resolution of conventional MRI. Eighty percent of the water protons in the brain are free or mobile and contribute to the conventional MR image. The immobile pool of water protons is tightly bound to macromolecular structures, such as proteins and lipid membranes. They have extremely short T_2 relaxation times and are not visible on conventional MR images.[135] The bound pool of water protons can be selectively saturated with magnetiza-

tion by applying an additional radiofrequency pulse to a traditional MR sequence. This reduces the signal arising from the mobile pool, proportional to the complexity of the intact macromolecules. The MTR between bound and unbound protons reflects the amount and complexity of macromolecular structure present. Pathologic processes would be expected to decrease the macromolecule pool and thus decrease the MTR. Myelin is the most complex macromolecular structure present in normal white matter, and a decrease in the MTR may reflect demyelination.

MTR measurements are quantitative and highly reproducible and can be obtained in 10–20 minutes with good resolution.[136–138] Magnetization transfer is a method for monitoring destructive pathologic features in MS lesions.

The MTR values of MS lesions are decreased, and lesions vary in their MTR values. MTR values are lowest in chronic (nonenhancing) T_1-hypointense lesions and in acute (ring-enhancing) lesions. In one study, the acute lesions had dynamic, reversible MTR changes as compared to T_1-hypointense lesions. Nonenhancing isointense lesions and nodular enhancing lesions had less severe MTR abnormalities.[139] Furthermore, the MTR of the NAWM is also decreased as compared to control subjects.[140,141]

A small cross-sectional study of 18 MS patients ranging from benign to SPMS showed a significant correlation between the reduction in MTR and NAA concentration in the NAWM of SPMS patients.[120] PPMS patients also have abnormal white-matter MTR as compared to control subjects.[142] Patients with benign MS have relative preservation of NAA and MTR values.

Several longitudinal studies have demonstrated that there is a progressive decline in MTR values during the course of MS.[143,144] They discovered progressive MTR changes in the NAWM that would eventually develop a lesion. This abnormality was distinct from abnormalities elsewhere in NAWM and may have developed up to 2 years before the appearance of the lesion.[145]

Magnetization transfer imaging measures, when corrected for brain volume, correlate with disease duration. There were nonsignificant correlations with EDSS and ambulation index, although there was correlation with neuropsychological tests.[146] In one study, brain MTR histogram peak showed a stronger correlation with atrophy than did burden of T_2 lesion load, suggesting that the MTR histogram may be a better indicator of global disease burden than T_2 lesion volume.[97]

The correlation with spinal cord MTR abnormalities and EDSS has been weak, with a correlation coefficient of 0.25.[147] Spinal cord cross-sectional area, a marker of atrophy, was modestly better in correlating with EDSS ($r = -0.46$). There was no correlation between spinal cord MTR and atrophy in this group of 65 MS patients.

The amount and severity of MS pathology in the cervical cord is probably greater in the progressive forms of the disease, as SPMS and PPMS patients have lower average MTR of the cervical cord when compared to control subjects.[148] RRMS patients had values similar to the control group. The cervical cord MTR abnormalities did not correlate with brain lesion load.

No large cohorts have been looked at for evidence of a treatment effect with the disease-modifying interferon therapies on these new MR parameters. A very small study of eight RRMS patients on interferon beta-1b demonstrated a drug effect on T_2 lesion load by 15% and decreased enhancing lesions by 91% but did not have any apparent effect on whole-brain MTR.[149] In a group of eight early RRMS patients, Kita and colleagues[150] looked at MTR changes in acute MS lesions before and after initiating interferon beta-1a therapy. The MTR abnormalities were the same in new acute lesions regardless of treatment. However, MTR abnormalities improved at a faster rate while on therapy.

T_2 Relaxation

The T_2 decay curve is a plot of MR signal versus echo time, and it can be obtained accurately in vivo from a multiecho imaging sequence. T_2 decay curve trajectories differ for different normal brain structures as well as for different MS lesions. The differences are believed to arise from changes in microscopic tissue structure.

In normal brain, T_2 relaxation studies reveal at least three different water environments corresponding to water compartmentalized between myelin bilayers (T_2 less than 50 ms), cytoplasmic-extracellular water (T_2 between 70–90 ms), and CSF (T_2 more than 2 seconds). In MS lesions, these T_2 reservoirs shift in proportion.

The short T_2 component (T_2 less than 50 ms), which is believed to arise from water in normal myelin,[151] provides the possibility of measuring myelin content in vivo and thereby characterizing the demyelination process in MS. Studies on fixed brain have shown good correspondence between the decrease of the short T_2 component and the intensity of Luxol fast blue stain for myelin.[54] In vivo studies showed that MS lesions had reduced myelin water content (decrease in short T_2 component).[152]

In addition to myelin water content, the total water content can be estimated from the sum of all the T_2 components. MS lesions generally have 7% greater water content than the surrounding tissue. Furthermore, T_2 decay curves provide valuable information on MS pathology by characterizing the microscopic water environment and potentially differentiating among edema, inflammation, and gliosis.[153] The short T_2 component is a marker of myelin water, and a decrease in this signal reflects myelin damage.

Diffusion-Weighted Imaging and Structural Changes Caused by Multiple Sclerosis

MS and other pathologic processes that modify tissue integrity can result in abnormal diffusion of water molecules detectable by DWI. Two parameters are obtained with this new MR technique: apparent diffusion coefficient (ADC) and anisotropy. These provide structural information about tissues.

Water will diffuse through the brain, depending on the size, shape, and orientation of water spaces within the brain. The highest diffusion coefficient occurs in free water and is reduced when water is confined to small spaces. Using MR techniques, the ADC measures the movement of free water in the brain. Pathologic processes will affect the structural organization of the brain, altering the ADC measurement.[154] DWI sequences require large field gradients and are very susceptible to artefacts caused by patient motion.[155]

Information is also obtained on the orientation and anisotropy of the diffusion spaces. Normal white-matter tracts reveal that diffusion along the fiber tracts is greater than diffusion perpendicular to the fibers (anisotropic diffusion). For example, parallel flow in the corpus callosum is three to four times greater than perpendicular flow.

Several groups have shown increased diffusion of water (ADC) and decrease in anisotropy in MS lesions as compared to NAWM.[156–158] The highest ADC values were found in acute gadolinium-enhancing lesions and chronic, nonenhancing T_1-hypointense lesions (black holes). The diffusion value for T_1-hypointense lesions (black holes) was significantly higher than for those lesions that were T_1-isointense. The NAWM of MS patients also had a slightly higher ADC and lower anisotropy than white matter of healthy control subjects.[159,160]

As yet, the ADC values of lesion and NAWM do not clearly distinguish between patients with different clinical courses of MS, and there was no correlation with disability.[161–163] In a longitudinal study of five MS patients who had monthly MRI for 1 year, Werring and colleagues[164] collected data on average ADC before, during, and after new lesion formation. Before the appearance of a new gadolinium-enhancing lesion, there was an increase in the ADC of the prelesion NAWM. This was followed by a more rapid and marked increase at the time of gadolinium enhancement, followed by a slower decrease in ADC once enhancement disappears. This suggests that there are subtle, progressive alterations in tissue integrity that precede the appearance of new focal lesions and frank BBB leakage seen on conventional MR images.

In MS, MR studies of diffusion appear promising as a means of assessing the structural integrity of white-matter tracts. An alteration in the ADC and the degree of anisotropy might occur in the presence of demyelination or axonal loss (or both).[18]

Summary: Multiple Sclerosis Pathogenesis as Revealed by Various Magnetic Resonance Techniques

On conventional MR (PD/T_2) and gross pathology, plaques are the obvious manifestation of MS and had been the major focus of research studies and treatment trials. More recent quantitative pathologic studies and new MR techniques demonstrate that the disease process is much more widespread and diffuse than would be suspected clinically. Summarized here are the known and presumptive pathologic changes occurring in MS lesions and the brain as a whole. Table 8-1 summarizes the MR parameters used in MS and the pathology they possibly represent.

Evolution of the New Multiple Sclerosis Lesion

Breakdown of the BBB is probably the earliest clear-cut pathologic change to occur in new lesion development in RRMS and SPMS, and this usually correlates with active inflammation and myelin breakdown. Breakdown in the BBB appears as a gadolinium-enhanced lesion on the T_1-weighted image. Both processes contribute to conduction block and functional loss. When the inflammation subsides, edema resolves, and conduction is restored, probably as a result of the expansion of sodium channels into the demyelinated axon. Remyelination is not essential to remission. Some interesting abnormalities, as revealed by MTR and DWI, suggest that a chronic disease process is already underway in the tissue destined to be a lesion, as early as 2 years before the new lesion appears.

This enhanced area is followed in days by a new lesion that can be seen on the PD/T_2-weighted scan. Most of these PD lesions are permanent. Changes in the amount of water in the lesion and the inflammatory extent of the lesion can be revealed by changes in the PD/T_2-weighted scan. Sometimes, the acute new lesion can initially appear as a T_1-hypointense lesion (an acute black hole) that reflects edema and inflammation rather than severe tissue destruction, as in the chronic lesion.

New lesions will show a dynamic increase in size over several weeks and then a decrease in size to become residual stable lesions for many months or years, with reactivation at some later time. This stable area of abnormality (PD/T_2 white spot) probably represents chronic demyelination with some residual inflammatory component. Dynamic changes can also be seen with NAA and lipid peaks and MTR changes in the acute, new lesion, possibly reflecting a component of reversible axonal dysfunction and tissue disruption. Axonal loss and gliosis are probably also present in these early lesions.

Reactivation of lesions can produce an enlargement of a stable lesion or re-enhancement or both. After lesions mature in their pathology, they become chronic, and a proportion of these will become visible on the unenhanced T_1-weighed scan as a chronic black hole. These low-intensity areas represent the most severe destruction, as indicated by a drop in NAA, MTR, and histopathology. A number of acute MR changes are reversible, but the chronic persis-

Table 8-1. Magnetic Resonance (MR) Parameters That Identify and Measure the Specific Pathologies of Multiple Sclerosis (MS)*

MR Measure	MR Technique	Macroscopic Pathology	Microscopic Pathology
Proton density–T_2 bright lesion	Conventional MRI	Acute and chronic MS lesions	Nonspecific (abnormal tissue water)
Gadolinium-enhancing T_1 lesion	Conventional MRI	Acute MS lesion	Blood-brain barrier disruption
T_1-hypointense lesion or black hole	Conventional MRI	Acute MS lesion, chronic MS lesion	Edema, inflammation, severe tissue destruction
BPF, ventricle size	Conventional MRI	Atrophy	Generalized tissue loss
NAA peak	MR spectroscopy	Lesions and NAWM	Axonal loss or dysfunction (or both)
Lipid peak	MR spectroscopy	Lesion	Active demyelination
Lactate peak	MR spectroscopy	Lesion	Inflammation
MTR ROI and histogram analysis	MTI	Lesions and NAWM	Tissue destruction
ADC and anisotropy	DWI	Lesions and NAWM	Abnormal water diffusion
Short T_2 component	Relax	Lesions and NAWM	Loss of myelin water

ADC = apparent diffusion coefficient; BPF = brain parenchymal fraction; DWI = diffusion-weighted imaging; MRI = MR imaging; MTI = magnetization transfer imaging; MTR = magnetization transfer ratio; NAA = *N*-acetylaspartate; NAWM = normal-appearing white matter (on conventional MRI); Relax = T_2 relaxation analysis; ROI = region of interest.
*See text for details and references.

tent abnormalities in a number of MR parameters, such as reduced NAA, low MTRs, atrophy, and T_1-hypointensity, suggest the presence of demyelination and axonal degeneration in many chronic lesions.[14] Wallerian degeneration may be an important factor contributing to irreparable deficits.[57]

Based on observations from MRI studies, the natural history of the MS lesion appears to be progression from an acute enhancing lesion, corresponding to the early inflammatory stage, with evolution to a chronic T_2-hyperintense lesion, which is a nonspecific "footprint" of the prior event.

Global Brain Abnormalities

The brain has diffuse abnormalities revealed by other MR techniques. The most striking (grossly) is generalized atrophy and ventricular enlargement that can be detected at the earliest stages of MS. Abnormalities are also seen in NAA concentrations, DWI, T_2 relaxation, and MTR of the white matter that appears normal on conventional MRI (NAWM). Furthermore, these changes are progressive and may be independent of new lesion formation or the total burden of T_2 lesions.

Brain atrophy occurs early and may be independent of inflammation. It increases during the RRMS disease stage without concurrent disability progression. This suggests that compensatory mechanisms maintain neurologic function despite progressive brain tissue loss during the early stages of the disease.[165] However, anti-inflammatory treatment may reduce lesion size and, therefore, mimic atrophy. Therefore, one must be careful in interpreting the relationship between treatment effects and atrophy. A partially effective anti-inflammatory treatment may not have as much of an effect on brain volume as a more effective anti-inflammatory treatment. Consequently, a lack of short-term benefit on an atrophy measure in a treatment trial may be the result of a superimposed apparent atrophy in the treated group due to the anti-inflammatory drug effect on lesions.

Magnetic Resonance Imaging and the Dynamics of Disease Progression

Color Plate 11 and Figure 8-3 illustrate the dynamic in vivo changes detected by MR techniques over the life span of a "typical" MS patient. Several points can be made:

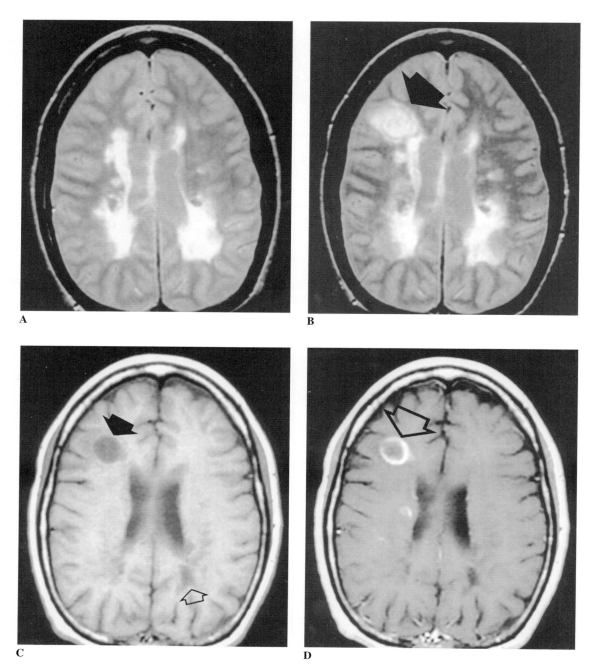

Figure 8-3. **A.** Baseline proton density–weighted magnetic resonance image demonstrates multiple "bright" white-matter multiple sclerosis (MS) lesions or plaques. **B.** Follow-up proton density–weighted image 1 month later shows several new and enlarging lesions (*arrow*). On average, MS patients accumulate five new lesions per year. **C.** Some of the proton density T_2 lesions are chronic hypointense black holes on the corresponding T_1-weighted image (*open arrow*). The corresponding T_1 image demonstrates an acute black hole (*closed arrow*). Unlike the chronic black hole, this is reversible and represents acute edema rather than severe tissue destruction. In long-standing MS, chronic black holes and atrophy with ventricular enlargement are commonly seen. Gadolinium enhancement is a common finding in new MS lesions (**D,** *open arrow*). These may or may not be associated with new clinical symptoms or signs.

1. Clinically, most patients have a presymptomatic phase before their MS is diagnosed. Occasionally, they will have had some mild, nonspecific symptoms during this period. Once their MS is diagnosed, the majority of patients will follow a relapsing-remitting course, with a variable number of relapses per year and complete or incomplete recovery from these. Eventually, these patients will enter a chronic or secondary-progressive phase, whereby they slowly deteriorate in the absence of frank clinical relapses. They may or may not have relapses in addition to the progressive deterioration.

2. Conventional MRI (PD/T_2) demonstrates that on average, patients with newly diagnosed MS will already have five lesions on their diagnostic MRI. Annually, they will develop four new lesions, most in the absence of clinical relapses. This accumulation of new lesions continues throughout the later (secondary-progressive) phase of their disease.

3. Markers of disease burden, such as PD/T_2 lesion extent (BOD), acute and chronic T_1 black holes, atrophy, NAA decline, and MTR abnormalities, will progress from an early stage, even before diagnosis.

Conclusions

MRI is a sensitive tool for monitoring in vivo progression of pathology in MS. Many new PD/T_2 lesions are clinically silent and accumulate annually, contributing to the patient's overall MRI BOD. T_2 lesions correlate well with plaques seen on postmortem examination, but lack specificity for the heterogeneity of MS plaques. The new MRI techniques allow for specific distinctions of pathologic changes that occur in normal-appearing brain tissue as well as MS lesions. MR techniques serve three major roles in the field of MS.

Magnetic Resonance Imaging as a Diagnostic Tool

The major use of MRI in MS is for diagnosis. The reason that MRI is so useful in the diagnosis of MS is that it reveals many asymptomatic lesions disseminated in space in the absence of clinical findings. T_2-weighted brain imaging remains the standard diagnostic tool but, in some instances, it is usefully complemented with gadolinium-enhancement and spinal imaging. However, the diagnosis of MS remains primarily a clinical one.

Magnetic Resonance Imaging as an Outcome Measure for Clinical Trials of New Therapies

Serial MR has become an important tool in monitoring treatment efficacy. It provides data that can be readily analyzed in a blinded fashion and that directly inspect the pathologic evolution. It also enables a rapid and sensitive measure of treatment outcome in early RRMS and SPMS. It can demonstrate ongoing disease activity even in patients who are stable clinically.

Today, many clinical trials use MRI as a primary or secondary outcome measure. Phase II trials frequently use MRI as a primary outcome measure, particularly MRI activity rates.[166] Conventional MRI remains a secondary outcome measure in phase III clinical trials because of insufficient correlation with clinical disability scales. MRI monitoring in MS is the best of the currently used surrogate outcomes in neurologic disease. The techniques used for MRI studies in evaluating clinical trials will vary according to the goals of the trial even though the optimal MRI measure to monitor the destructive pathologic process is uncertain.

Magnetic Resonance Imaging as a Research Tool for the In Vivo Study of Multiple Sclerosis Pathology

MR techniques have supplied us with important measurable and reproducible tools that have provided vital insights into the evolving pathology of MS. The basic aspects of the pathologic lesions in MS, such as edema, membrane disruption, demyelination, gliosis, cellular infiltration, and axonal loss, can be studied more precisely by combining MR techniques, which should better describe the destructive process. In the future, the systematic and parallel use of several MR techniques will help to identify specific pathologies as they evolve. Further work is needed to address issues of quality control in serial studies, statistical calculation of appropriate sample sizes, and optimization of the nature and frequency of MR outcomes measured.

The goal is to be able to understand the evolution of the pathology in individual lesions and also to identify where various therapies might work in modifying the evolution of that pathology. Systematic studies of natural history and clinical trials will hopefully help to answer some of these very important questions. The future of MR in helping to understand MS is very exciting because of these possibilities.

References

1. Paty DW. Multiple sclerosis: assessment of disease progression and effects of treatment. Can J Neurol Sci 1987;14(3 Suppl):518–520.

2. Miller DH, Rudge P, Johnson G, et al. Serial gadolinium enhanced magnetic resonance imaging in multiple sclerosis. Brain 1988;111(Pt 4):927–939.

3. Miller DH, Barkhof F, Nauta JJ. Gadolinium enhancement increases the sensitivity of MRI in detecting disease activity in multiple sclerosis. Brain 1993;116(Pt 5):1077–1094.

4. Paty DW, Li DK. Interferon beta-1b is effective in relapsing-remitting multiple sclerosis. II. MRI analysis results of a multicenter, randomized, double-blind, placebo-controlled trial. UBC MS/MRI Study Group and the IFNB Multiple Sclerosis Study Group. Neurology 1993;43(4):662–667.

5. Paty DW. MRI as a method to reveal in-vivo pathology in MS. J Neural Transm Suppl 1997;49:211–217.

6. Kurtzke JF. Rating neurologic impairment in multiple sclerosis: an expanded disability status scale (EDSS). Neurology 1983;33(11):1444–1452.

7. Sipe JC, Knobler RL, Braheny SL, et al. A neurologic rating scale (NRS) for use in multiple sclerosis. Neurology 1984;34(10):1368–1372.

8. Sipe JC, Romine JS, Koziol JA, et al. Cladribine in treatment of chronic progressive multiple sclerosis. Lancet 1994;344(8914):9–13.

9. Hauser SL, Dawson DM, Lehrich JR, et al. Intensive immunosuppression in progressive multiple sclerosis. A randomized, three-arm study of high-dose intravenous cyclophosphamide, plasma exchange, and ACTH. N Engl J Med 1983;308(4):173–180.

10. Rudick R, Antel J, Confavreux C, et al. Clinical outcomes assessment in multiple sclerosis. Ann Neurol 1996;40(3):469–479.

11. Cohen JA, Fischer JS, Bolibrush DM, et al. Intrarater and interrater reliability of the MS functional composite outcome measure. Neurology 2000;54(4):802–806.

12. Evans AC, Frank JA, Antel J, Miller DH. The role of MRI in clinical trials of multiple sclerosis: comparison of image processing techniques. Ann Neurol 1997;41(1):125–132.

13. Grossman RI. Application of magnetization transfer imaging to multiple sclerosis. Neurology 1999;53(5 Suppl 3):S8–S11.

14. Miller DH, Grossman RI, Reingold SC, McFarland HF. The role of magnetic resonance techniques in understanding and managing multiple sclerosis. Brain 1998;121(Pt 1):3–24.

15. Young IR, Hall AS, Pallis CA, et al. Nuclear magnetic resonance imaging of the brain in multiple sclerosis. Lancet 1981;2(8255):1063–1066.

16. Jacobs L, Kinkel WR, Polachini I, Kinkel RP. Correlations of nuclear magnetic resonance imaging, computerized tomography, and clinical profiles in multiple sclerosis. Neurology 1986;36(1):27–34.

17. Bourekas EC, Christoforidis GA, Abduljalil AM, et al. High resolution MRI of the deep gray nuclei at 8 Tesla. J Comput Assist Tomogr 1999;23(6):867–874.

18. Miller DH, Kesselring J, McDonald WI, et al. Magnetic Resonance in Multiple Sclerosis. Cambridge, UK: Cambridge University Press, 1997.

19. Pipe JG. Basic spin physics. Magn Reson Imaging Clin N Am 1999;7(4):607–627.

20. Duerk JL. Principles of MR image formation and reconstruction. Magn Reson Imaging Clin N Am 1999;7(4):629–659.

21. Mugler JP 3rd. Overview of MR imaging pulse sequences. Magn Reson Imaging Clin N Am 1999;7(4): 661–697.

22. Tourtellotte WW, Parker JA. Postmortem evaluation of the blood-brain barrier in multiple sclerosis. J Neuropathol Exp Neurol 1968;27(1):159–163.

23. Clanet M, Berry I. Magnetic resonance imaging in multiple sclerosis. Curr Opin Neurol 1998;11(4):299–303.

24. Ormerod IE, Miller DH, McDonald WI, et al. The role of NMR imaging in the assessment of multiple sclerosis and isolated neurological lesions. A quantitative study. Brain 1987;110(Pt 6):1579–1616.

25. Keiper MD, Grossman RI, Hirsch JA, et al. MR identification of white matter abnormalities in multiple sclerosis: a comparison between 1.5 T and 4 T. AJNR Am J Neuroradiol 1998;19(8):1489–1493.

26. Fazekas F, Offenbacher H, Fuchs S, et al. Criteria for an increased specificity of MRI interpretation in elderly subjects with suspected multiple sclerosis. Neurology 1988;38(12):1822–1825.

27. Horowitz AL, Kaplan RD, Grewe G, et al. The ovoid lesion: a new MR observation inpatients with multiple sclerosis. AJNR Am J Neuroradiol 1986;10:303–305.

28. Simon JH, Schiffer RB, Rudick RA, Herndon RM. Quantitative determination of MS-induced corpus callosum atrophy in vivo using MR imaging. AJNR Am J Neuroradiol 1987;8(4):599–604.

29. Grossman RI, Barkhof F, Filippi M. Assessment of spinal cord damage in MS using MRI. J Neurol Sci 2000;172 (Suppl 1):S36–S39.

30. Paty DW. Magnetic resonance imaging in the assessment of disease activity in multiple sclerosis. Can J Neurol Sci 1988;15(3):266–272.

31. Goodkin DE, Ross JS, Medendorp SV, et al. Magnetic resonance imaging lesion enlargement in multiple sclerosis. Disease-related activity, chance occurrence, or measurement artifact? Arch Neurol 1992;49(3):261–263.

32. Filippi M, van Waesberghe JH, Horsfield MA, et al. Inter-scanner variation in brain MRI lesion load measurements in MS: implications for clinical trials. Neurology 1997; 49(2):371–377.

33. Cover KS, Petkau J, Li DK, Paty DW. Lesion load repro-ducibility and statistical sensitivity of clinical trials in multiple sclerosis [letter]. Neurology 1999;52(2):433–435.

34. Nesbit GM, Forbes GS, Scheithauer BW, et al. Multiple sclerosis: histopathologic and MR and/or CT correlation in 37 cases at biopsy and three cases at autopsy. Radiol-ogy 1991;180(2):467–474.

35. Katz D, Taubenberger JK, Cannella B, et al. Correlation between magnetic resonance imaging findings and lesion development in chronic, active multiple sclerosis. Ann Neurol 1993;34(5):661–669.

36. Rodriguez M, Scheithauer BW, Forbes G, Kelly PJ. Oli-godendrocyte injury is an early event in lesions of multi-ple sclerosis. Mayo Clin Proc 1993;68(7):627–636.

37. Kermode AG, Tofts PS, Thompson AJ, et al. Heterogene-ity of blood-brain barrier changes in multiple sclerosis: an MRI study with gadolinium-DTPA enhancement. Neurol-ogy 1990;40(2):229–235.

38. Filippi M, Yousry T, Campi A, et al. Comparison of triple dose versus standard dose gadolinium-DTPA for detection of MRI enhancing lesions in patients with MS. Neurology 1996;46(2):379–384.

39. McFarland HF. The lesion in multiple sclerosis: clinical, pathological, and magnetic resonance imaging consider-ations. J Neurol Neurosurg Psychiatry 1998;64(Suppl 1):S26–S30.

40. Barnes D, McDonald WI, Landon DN, Johnson G. The characterization of experimental gliosis by quantitative nuclear magnetic resonance imaging. Brain 1988;111(Pt 1):83–94.

41. Adler S, Martinez J, Williams DS, Verbalis JG. Positive association between blood brain barrier disruption and osmotically-induced demyelination. Mult Scler 2000; 6(1):24–31.

42. Willoughby EW, Grochowski E, Li DK, et al. Serial mag-netic resonance scanning in multiple sclerosis: a second prospective study in relapsing patients. Ann Neurol 1989; 25(1):43–49.

43. Koopmans RA, Li DK, Oger JJ, et al. Chronic progressive multiple sclerosis: serial magnetic resonance brain imag-ing over six months. Ann Neurol 1989;26(2):248–256.

44. Koopmans RA, Li DK, Oger JJ, et al. The lesion of multi-ple sclerosis: imaging of acute and chronic stages. Neurol-ogy 1989;39(7):959–963.

45. Prineas JW, Barnard RO, Revesz T, et al. Multiple sclero-sis. Pathology of recurrent lesions. Brain 1993;116(Pt 3):681–693.

46. McDonald WI, Miller DH, Barnes D. The pathological evolution of multiple sclerosis. Neuropathol Appl Neuro-biol 1992;18(4):319–334.

47. Barkhof F. MRI in multiple sclerosis: correlation with expanded disability status scale (EDSS). Mult Scler 1999;5(4):283–286.

48. Gilman S. Imaging the brain. Second of two parts. N Engl J Med 1998;338(13):889–896.

49. Koopmans RA, Li DK, Grochowski E, et al. Benign ver-sus chronic progressive multiple sclerosis: magnetic reso-nance imaging features. Ann Neurol 1989;25(1):74–81.

50. Stewart WA, Hall LD, Berry K, Paty DW. Correlation between NMR scan and brain slice data in multiple scle-rosis [letter]. Lancet 1984;2(8399):412.

51. Barnes D, Munro PM, Youl BD, et al. The longstanding MS lesion. A quantitative MRI and electron microscopic study. Brain 1991;114(Pt 3):1271–1280.

52. Newcombe J, Hawkins CP, Henderson CL, et al. Histopa-thology of multiple sclerosis lesions detected by magnetic resonance imaging in unfixed postmortem central nervous system tissue. Brain 1991;114(Pt 2):1013–1023.

53. Paty DW, Li DK, Oger JJ, et al. Magnetic resonance imag-ing in the evaluation of clinical trials in multiple sclerosis. Ann Neurol 1994;36(Suppl):S95–S96.

54. Moore GRW, Leung E, MacKay AL, et al. A pathology-MRI study of the short-T2 component in formalin-fixed multiple sclerosis brain. Neurology 2000;55(10):1506–1510.

55. Miller DH, Newton MR, van der Poel JC, et al. Magnetic resonance imaging of the optic nerve in optic neuritis. Neurology 1988;38(2):175–179.

56. Compston A. Brain repair. J Intern Med 1995;237(2):127–134.

57. McDonald WI. Rachelle Fishman-Matthew Moore Lec-ture. The pathological and clinical dynamics of multiple sclerosis. J Neuropathol Exp Neurol 1994;53(4):338–343.

58. Rao SM, Leo GJ, Ellington L, et al. Cognitive dysfunction in multiple sclerosis. II. Impact on employment and social functioning. Neurology 1991;41(5):692–696.

59. Pozzilli C, Fieschi C, Perani D, et al. Relationship between corpus callosum atrophy and cerebral metabolic asymmetries in multiple sclerosis. J Neurol Sci 1992;112(1–2):51–57.

60. Rao SM. Neuropsychology of multiple sclerosis: a critical review. J Clin Exp Neuropsychol 1986;8(5):503–542.

61. Damian MS, Schilling G, Bachmann G, et al. White mat-ter lesions and cognitive deficits: relevance of lesion pat-tern? Acta Neurol Scand 1994;90(6):430–436.

62. The IFNB Multiple Sclerosis Study Group and the Uni-versity of British Columbia MS/MRI Analysis Group. Interferon beta-1b in the treatment of multiple sclerosis: final outcome of the randomized controlled trial. Neurol-ogy 1995;45(7):1277–1285.

63. Grimaud J, Barker GJ, Wang L, et al. Correlation of mag-netic resonance imaging parameters with clinical disabil-ity in multiple sclerosis: a preliminary study. J Neurol 1999;246(10):961–967.

64. O'Riordan JI, Thompson AJ, Kingsley DP, et al. The prognostic value of brain MRI in clinically isolated syn-dromes of the CNS. A 10-year follow-up. Brain 1998; 121(Pt 3):495–503.

65. Lee KH, Hashimoto SA, Hooge JP, et al. Magnetic reso-nance imaging of the head in the diagnosis of multiple sclerosis: a prospective 2-year follow-up with comparison of clinical evaluation, evoked potentials, oligoclonal banding, and CT. Neurology 1991;41(5):657–660.

66. Paty DW, Oger JJ, Kastrukoff LF, et al. MRI in the diag-nosis of MS: a prospective study with comparison of clin-ical evaluation, evoked potentials, oligoclonal banding, and CT. Neurology 1988;38(2):180–185.

67. Optic Neuritis Study Group. The clinical profile of optic neuritis. Experience of the Optic Neuritis Treatment Trial. Arch Ophthalmol 1991;109(12):1673–1678.

68. Optic Neuritis Study Group. The 5-year risk of MS after optic neuritis. Experience of the optic neuritis treatment trial. Optic Neuritis Study Group. Neurology 1997;49(5):1404–1413.

69. Thompson AJ, Kermode AG, MacManus DG, et al. Patterns of disease activity in multiple sclerosis: clinical and magnetic resonance imaging study. BMJ 1990;300(6725):631–634.

70. Thompson AJ, Kermode AG, Wicks D, et al. Major differences in the dynamics of primary and secondary progressive multiple sclerosis. Ann Neurol 1991;29(1):53–62.

71. van Walderveen MA, Barkhof F, Tas MW, et al. Patterns of brain magnetic resonance abnormalities on T2-weighted spin echo images in clinical subgroups of multiple sclerosis: a large cross-sectional study. Eur Neurol 1998;40(2):91–98.

72. Dastidar P, Heinonen T, Lehtimaki T, et al. Volumes of brain atrophy and plaques correlated with neurological disability in secondary progressive multiple sclerosis. J Neurol Sci 1999;165(1):36–42.

73. Stevenson VL, Miller DH, Leary SM, et al. One year follow up study of primary and transitional progressive multiple sclerosis. J Neurol Neurosurg Psychiatry 2000;68(6):713–718.

74. Kidd D, Thorpe JW, Kendall BE, et al. MRI dynamics of brain and spinal cord in progressive multiple sclerosis. J Neurol Neurosurg Psychiatry 1996;60(1):15–19.

75. Kastrukoff LF, Oger JJ, Hashimoto SA, et al. Systemic lymphoblastoid interferon therapy in chronic progressive multiple sclerosis. I. Clinical and MRI evaluation. Neurology 1990;40(3 Pt 1):479–486.

76. Zhao GJ, Li DK, Wolinsky JS, et al. Clinical and magnetic resonance imaging changes correlate in a clinical trial monitoring cyclosporine therapy for multiple sclerosis. The MS Study Group. J Neuroimaging 1997;7(1):1–7.

77. The Once Weekly Interferon for MS Study Group. Evidence of interferon beta-1a dose response in relapsing-remitting MS: the OWIMS Study. Neurology 1999;53(4):679–686.

78. van Oosten BW, Barkhof F, Truyen L, et al. Increased MRI activity and immune activation in two multiple sclerosis patients treated with the monoclonal anti-tumor necrosis factor antibody cA2. Neurology 1996;47(6):1531–1534.

79. The Lenercept Multiple Sclerosis Study Group and the University of British Columbia MS/MRI Analysis Group. TNF neutralization in MS: results of a randomized, placebo-controlled multicenter study. Neurology 1999;53(3):457–465.

80. Coles AJ, Wing MG, Molyneux P, et al. Monoclonal antibody treatment exposes three mechanisms underlying the clinical course of multiple sclerosis. Ann Neurol 1999;46(3):296–304.

81. Rice GP, Filippi M, Comi G. Cladribine and progressive MS: clinical and MRI outcomes of a multicenter controlled trial. Cladribine MRI Study Group. Neurology 2000;54(5):1145–1155.

82. Li DK, Paty DW. Magnetic resonance imaging results of the PRISMS trial: a randomized, double-blind, placebo-controlled study of interferon-beta1a in relapsing-remitting multiple sclerosis. Prevention of Relapses and Disability by Interferon-beta1a Subcutaneously in Multiple Sclerosis. Ann Neurol 1999;46(2):197–206.

83. Jacobs L. Magnetic resonance imaging in clinical therapeutic trials of multiple sclerosis. West J Med 1996;164(6):531–532.

84. Simon JH, Jacobs LD, Campion M, et al. Magnetic resonance studies of intramuscular interferon beta-1a for relapsing multiple sclerosis. The Multiple Sclerosis Collaborative Research Group. Ann Neurol 1998;43(1):79–87.

85. Noseworthy JH, Paty DW, Ebers GC. Neuroimaging in multiple sclerosis. Neurol Clin 1984;2(4):759–777.

86. Cala LA, Mastaglia FL, Black JL. Computerized tomography of brain and optic nerve in multiple sclerosis. Observations in 100 patients, including serial studies in 16. J Neurol Sci 1978;36(3):411–426.

87. Losseff NA, Miller DH. Measures of brain and spinal cord atrophy in multiple sclerosis. J Neurol Neurosurg Psychiatry 1998;64(Suppl 1):S102–S105.

88. Ge Y, Grossman RI, Udupa JK, et al. Brain atrophy in relapsing-remitting multiple sclerosis and secondary progressive multiple sclerosis: longitudinal quantitative analysis. Radiology 2000;214(3):665–670.

89. Fox NC, Jenkins R, Leary SM, et al. Progressive cerebral atrophy in MS: a serial study using registered, volumetric MRI. Neurology 2000;54(4):807–812.

90. Liu C, Edwards S, Gong Q, et al. Three dimensional MRI estimates of brain and spinal cord atrophy in multiple sclerosis. J Neurol Neurosurg Psychiatry 1999;66(3):323–330.

91. Paolillo A, Pozzilli C, Gasperini C, et al. Brain atrophy in relapsing-remitting multiple sclerosis: relationship with 'black holes', disease duration and clinical disability. J Neurol Sci 2000;174(2):85–91.

92. Filippi M, Mastronardo G, Rocca MA, et al. Quantitative volumetric analysis of brain magnetic resonance imaging from patients with multiple sclerosis. J Neurol Sci 1998;158(2):148–153.

93. Brex PA, Jenkins R, Fox NC, et al. Detection of ventricular enlargement in patients at the earliest clinical stage of MS. Neurology 2000;54(8):1689–1691.

94. Filippi M, Campi A, Colombo B, et al. A spinal cord MRI study of benign and secondary progressive multiple sclerosis. J Neurol 1996;243(7):502–505.

95. Losseff NA, Wang L, Lai HM, et al. Progressive cerebral atrophy in multiple sclerosis. A serial MRI study. Brain 1996;119(Pt 6):2009–2019.

96. Rudick RA, Fisher E, Lee JC, et al. Use of the brain parenchymal fraction to measure whole brain atrophy in relapsing-remitting MS. Multiple Sclerosis Collaborative Research Group. Neurology 1999;53(8):1698–1704.

97. Phillips MD, Grossman RI, Miki Y, et al. Comparison of T2 lesion volume and magnetization transfer ratio histogram analysis and of atrophy and measures of lesion burden in patients with multiple sclerosis. AJNR Am J Neuroradiol 1998;19(6):1055–1060.

98. Simon JH, Jacobs LD, Campion MK, et al. A longitudinal study of brain atrophy in relapsing multiple sclerosis. The Multiple Sclerosis Collaborative Research Group (MSCRG). Neurology 1999;53(1):139–148.

99. Losseff NA, Webb SL, O'Riordan JI, et al. Spinal cord atrophy and disability in multiple sclerosis. A new reproducible and sensitive MRI method with potential to monitor disease progression. Brain 1996;119(Pt 3):701–708.

100. Edwards SG, Gong QY, Liu C, et al. Infratentorial atrophy on magnetic resonance imaging and disability in multiple sclerosis. Brain 1999;122(Pt 2):291–301.

101. Good K, Clark CM, Oger J, et al. Cognitive impairment and depression in mild multiple sclerosis. J Nerv Ment Dis 1992;180(11):730–732.

102. van Walderveen MA, Barkhof F, Hommes OR, et al. Correlating MRI and clinical disease activity in multiple sclerosis: relevance of hypointense lesions on short-TR/short-TE (T1-weighted) spin-echo images. Neurology 1995;45(9):1684–1690.

103. van Walderveen MA, Truyen L, van Oosten BW, et al. Development of hypointense lesions on T1-weighted spin-echo magnetic resonance images in multiple sclerosis: relation to inflammatory activity. Arch Neurol 1999;56(3):345–351.

104. Loevner LA, Grossman RI, McGowan JC, et al. Characterization of multiple sclerosis plaques with T1-weighted MR and quantitative magnetization transfer. AJNR Am J Neuroradiol 1995;16(7):1473–1479.

105. van Walderveen MA, Kamphorst W, Scheltens P, et al. Histopathologic correlate of hypointense lesions on T1-weighted spin-echo MRI in multiple sclerosis. Neurology 1998;50(5):1282–1288.

106. Nijeholt GJ, van Walderveen MA, Castelijns JA, et al. Brain and spinal cord abnormalities in multiple sclerosis. Correlation between MRI parameters, clinical subtypes and symptoms. Brain 1998;121(Pt 4):687–697.

107. Brex PA, Parker GJ, Leary SM, et al. Lesion heterogeneity in multiple sclerosis: a study of the relations between appearances on T1 weighted images, T1 relaxation times, and metabolite concentrations. J Neurol Neurosurg Psychiatry 2000;68(5):627–632.

108. Goodkin DE, Rooney WD, Sloan R, et al. A serial study of new MS lesions and the white matter from which they arise. Neurology 1998;51(6):1689–1697.

109. Arnold DL, Matthews PM, Francis G, Antel J. Proton magnetic resonance spectroscopy of human brain in vivo in the evaluation of multiple sclerosis: assessment of the load of disease. Magn Reson Med 1990;14(1):154–159.

110. Moffett JR, Namboodiri MA, Cangro CB, Neale JH. Immunohistochemical localization of N-acetylaspartate in rat brain. Neuroreport 1991;2(3):131–134.

111. Trapp BD, Peterson J, Ransohoff RM, et al. Axonal transection in the lesions of multiple sclerosis. N Engl J Med 1998;338(5):278–285.

112. Wolinsky JS, Narayana PA, Fenstermacher MJ. Proton magnetic resonance spectroscopy in multiple sclerosis. Neurology 1990;40(11):1764–1769.

113. Davie CA, Barker GJ, Webb S, et al. Persistent functional deficit in multiple sclerosis and autosomal dominant cerebellar ataxia is associated with axon loss [published erratum appears in Brain 1996;119(Pt 4):1415]. Brain 1995;118(Pt 6):1583–1592.

114. Bitsch A, Bruhn H, Vougioukas V, et al. Inflammatory CNS demyelination: histopathologic correlation with in vivo quantitative proton MR spectroscopy. AJNR Am J Neuroradiol 1999;20(9):1619–1627.

115. Koopmans RA, Li DK, Zhu G, et al. Magnetic resonance spectroscopy of multiple sclerosis: in-vivo detection of myelin breakdown products. Lancet 1993;341(8845):631–632.

116. Landtblom AM, Sjoqvist L, Soderfeldt B, et al. Proton MR spectroscopy and MR imaging in acute and chronic multiple sclerosis—ringlike appearances in acute plaques. Acta Radiol 1996;37(3 Pt 1):278–287.

117. Narayana PA, Doyle TJ, Lai D, Wolinsky JS. Serial proton magnetic resonance spectroscopic imaging, contrast-enhanced magnetic resonance imaging, and quantitative lesion volumetry in multiple sclerosis. Ann Neurol 1998;43(1):56–71.

118. Falini A, Calabrese G, Filippi M, et al. Benign versus secondary-progressive multiple sclerosis: the potential role of proton MR spectroscopy in defining the nature of disability. AJNR Am J Neuroradiol 1998;19(2):223–229.

119. Davie CA, Barker GJ, Thompson AJ, et al. 1H magnetic resonance spectroscopy of chronic cerebral white matter lesions and normal appearing white matter in multiple sclerosis. J Neurol Neurosurg Psychiatry 1997;63(6):736–742.

120. Davie CA, Silver NC, Barker GJ, et al. Does the extent of axonal loss and demyelination from chronic lesions in multiple sclerosis correlate with the clinical subgroup? J Neurol Neurosurg Psychiatry 1999;67(6):710–715.

121. Evangelou N, Esiri MM, Smith S, et al. Quantitative pathological evidence for axonal loss in normal appearing white matter in multiple sclerosis. Ann Neurol 2000;47(3):391–395.

122. Lee MA, Blamire AM, Pendlebury S, et al. Axonal injury or loss in the internal capsule and motor impairment in multiple sclerosis. Arch Neurol 2000;57(1):65–70.

123. Narayanan S, Fu L, Pioro E, et al. Imaging of axonal damage in multiple sclerosis: spatial distribution of magnetic resonance imaging lesions. Ann Neurol 1997;41(3):385–391.

124. Sarchielli P, Presciutti O, Pelliccioli GP, et al. Absolute quantification of brain metabolites by proton magnetic resonance spectroscopy in normal-appearing white matter of multiple sclerosis patients. Brain 1999;122(Pt 3):513–521.

125. Cucurella MG, Rovira A, Rio J, et al. Proton magnetic resonance spectroscopy in primary and secondary progressive multiple sclerosis. NMR Biomed 2000;13(2):57–63.

126. Leary SM, Davie CA, Parker GJ, et al. 1H magnetic resonance spectroscopy of normal appearing white matter in primary progressive multiple sclerosis. J Neurol 1999;246(11):1023–1026.

127. Brex PA, Gomez-Anson B, Parker GJ, et al. Proton MR spectroscopy in clinically isolated syndromes suggestive of multiple sclerosis. J Neurol Sci 1999;166(1):16–22.

128. Gonen O, Catalaa I, Babb JS, et al. Total brain N-acetylaspartate: a new measure of disease load in MS. Neurology 2000;54(1):15–19.

129. Arnold DL, Riess GT, Matthews PM, et al. Use of proton magnetic resonance spectroscopy for monitoring disease

progression in multiple sclerosis. Ann Neurol 1994; 36(1):76–82.

130. Fu L, Matthews PM, De Stefano N, et al. Imaging axonal damage of normal-appearing white matter in multiple sclerosis. Brain 1998;121(Pt 1):103–113.

131. Davie CA, Hawkins CP, Barker GJ, et al. Serial proton magnetic resonance spectroscopy in acute multiple sclerosis lesions. Brain 1994;117(Pt 1):49–58.

132. Arnold DL. Magnetic resonance spectroscopy: imaging axonal damage in MS. J Neuroimmunol 1999;98(1):2–6.

133. Silber E, Sharief MK. Axonal degeneration in the pathogenesis of multiple sclerosis. J Neurol Sci 1999;170(1): 11–18.

134. Grossman RI, Lenkinski RE, Ramer KN, et al. MR proton spectroscopy in multiple sclerosis. AJNR Am J Neuroradiol 1992;13(6):1535–1543.

135. Edzes HT, Samulski ET. Cross relaxation and spin diffusion in the proton NMR or hydrated collagen. Nature 1977;265(5594):521–523.

136. Gass A, Barker GJ, Kidd D, et al. Correlation of magnetization transfer ratio with clinical disability in multiple sclerosis. Ann Neurol 1994;36(1):62–67.

137. Filippi M, Rocca MA, Horsfield MA, Comi G. A one year study of new lesions in multiple sclerosis using monthly gadolinium enhanced MRI: correlations with changes of T2 and magnetization transfer lesion loads. J Neurol Sci 1998;158(2):203–208.

138. Filippi M, Rocca MA, Martino G, et al. Magnetization transfer changes in the normal appearing white matter precede the appearance of enhancing lesions in patients with multiple sclerosis. Ann Neurol 1998;43(6):809–814.

139. Rovira A, Alonso J, Cucurella G, et al. Evolution of multiple sclerosis lesions on serial contrast-enhanced T1-weighted and magnetization-transfer MR images. AJNR Am J Neuroradiol 1999;20(10):1939–1945.

140. Filippi M, Campi A, Dousset V, et al. A magnetization transfer imaging study of normal-appearing white matter in multiple sclerosis. Neurology 1995;45(3 Pt 1):478–482.

141. Pike GB, de Stefano N, Narayanan S, et al. Combined magnetization transfer and proton spectroscopic imaging in the assessment of pathologic brain lesions in multiple sclerosis. AJNR Am J Neuroradiol 1999;20(5):829–837.

142. Leary SM, Silver NC, Stevenson VL. Magnetisation transfer of normal appearing white matter in primary progressive multiple sclerosis. Mult Scler 1999;5(5):313–316.

143. Rocca MA, Mastronardo G, Rodegher M, et al. Long-term changes of magnetization transfer-derived measures from patients with relapsing-remitting and secondary progressive multiple sclerosis. AJNR Am J Neuroradiol 1999; 20(5):821–827.

144. Patel UJ, Grossman RI, Phillips MD, et al. Serial analysis of magnetization-transfer histograms and Expanded Disability Status Scale scores in patients with relapsing-remitting multiple sclerosis. AJNR Am J Neuroradiol 1999;20(10):1946–1950.

145. Pike GB, De Stefano N, Narayanan S, et al. Multiple sclerosis: magnetization transfer MR imaging of white matter before lesion appearance on T2-weighted images. Radiology 2000;215(3):824–830.

146. van Buchem MA, Grossman RI, Armstrong C, et al. Correlation of volumetric magnetization transfer imaging with clinical data in MS. Neurology 1998;50(6):1609–1617.

147. Lycklama a Nijeholt GJ, Castelijns JA, Lazeron RH, et al. Magnetization transfer ratio of the spinal cord in multiple sclerosis: relationship to atrophy and neurologic disability. J Neuroimaging 2000;10(2):67–72.

148. Filippi M, Bozzali M, Horsfield MA, et al. A conventional and magnetization transfer MRI study of the cervical cord in patients with MS. Neurology 2000;54(1):207–213.

149. Richert ND, Ostuni JL, Bash CN, et al. Serial whole-brain magnetization transfer imaging in patients with relapsing-remitting multiple sclerosis at baseline and during treatment with interferon beta-1b. AJNR Am J Neuroradiol 1998;19(9):1705–1713.

150. Kita M, Goodkin DE, Bacchetti P, et al. Magnetization transfer ratio in new MS lesions before and during therapy with IFNbeta-1a. Neurology 2000;54(9):1741–1745.

151. MacKay A, Whittall K, Adler J, et al. In vivo visualization of myelin water in brain by magnetic resonance. Magn Reson Med 1994;31(6):673–677.

152. Vavasour IM, Whittall KP, MacKay AL, et al. A comparison between magnetization transfer ratios and myelin water percentages in normals and multiple sclerosis patients. Magn Reson Med 1998;40(5):763–768.

153. Armspach JP, Gounot D, Rumbach L, Chambron J. In vivo determination of multiexponential T2 relaxation in the brain of patients with multiple sclerosis. Magn Reson Imaging 1991;9(1):107–113.

154. Hajnal JV, Doran M, Hall AS, et al. MR imaging of anisotropically restricted diffusion of water in the nervous system: technical, anatomic, and pathologic considerations. J Comput Assist Tomogr 1991;15(1):1–18.

155. Horsfield MA, Larsson HB, Jones DK, Gass A. Diffusion magnetic resonance imaging in multiple sclerosis. J Neurol Neurosurg Psychiatry 1998;64(Suppl 1):S80–S84.

156. Droogan AG, Clark CA, Werring DJ, et al. Comparison of multiple sclerosis clinical subgroups using navigated spin echo diffusion-weighted imaging. Magn Reson Imaging 1999;17(5):653–661.

157. Werring DJ, Clark CA, Barker GJ, et al. Diffusion tensor imaging of lesions and normal-appearing white matter in multiple sclerosis. Neurology 1999;52(8):1626–1632.

158. Tievsky AL, Ptak T, Farkas J. Investigation of apparent diffusion coefficient and diffusion tensor anisotrophy in acute and chronic multiple sclerosis lesions. AJNR Am J Neuroradiol 1999;20(8):1491–1499.

159. Filippi M, Iannucci G, Cercignani M, et al. A quantitative study of water diffusion in multiple sclerosis lesions and normal-appearing white matter using echo-planar imaging. Arch Neurol 2000;57(7):1017–1021.

160. Cercignani M, Iannucci G, Rocca MA, et al. Pathologic damage in MS assessed by diffusion-weighted and magnetization transfer MRI. Neurology 2000;54(5):1139–1144.

161. Horsfield MA, Lai M, Webb SL, et al. Apparent diffusion coefficients in benign and secondary progressive multiple sclerosis by nuclear magnetic resonance. Magn Reson Med 1996;36(3):393–400.

162. Nusbaum AO, Tang CY, Wei T, et al. Whole-brain diffusion MR histograms differ between MS subtypes. Neurology 2000;54(7):1421–1427.

163. Castriota SA, Tomaiuolo F, Sabatini U, et al. Demyelinating plaques in relapsing-remitting and secondary-progressive multiple sclerosis: assessment with diffusion MR imaging. AJNR Am J Neuroradiol 2000;21(5):862–868.

164. Werring DJ, Brassat D, Droogan AG, et al. The pathogenesis of lesions and normal-appearing white matter changes in multiple sclerosis: A serial diffusion MRI study. Brain 2000;123(Pt 8):1667–1676.

165. Trapp BD, Ransohoff R, Rudick R. Axonal pathology in multiple sclerosis: relationship to neurologic disability. Curr Opin Neurol 1999;12(3):295–302.

166. Miller DH, Albert PS, Barkhof F, et al. Guidelines for the use of magnetic resonance techniques in monitoring the treatment of multiple sclerosis. US National MS Society Task Force. Ann Neurol 1996;39(1):6–16.

Chapter 9

Management of Multiple Sclerosis: Disease-Modifying Treatments

Michael J. Olek and Howard L. Weiner

Disease-modifying treatment of multiple sclerosis (MS) has come to rely on prospective clinical trials. Yet, the variety of patient disabilities and heterogeneity in the course of the disease render the choice of treatment for the individual patient difficult. The clinical presentation of patients seen in the office may differ markedly from that of those treated in clinical trials. Table 9-1 outlines the treatment paradigm used at our institution.

Acute Attacks

Acute attacks are typically treated with corticosteroids. Indications for treatment of a relapse include functionally disabling symptoms with objective evidence of neurologic impairment, such as loss of vision and motor or cerebellar symptoms, or both. Thus, mild sensory attacks are typically not treated. Treatment with short courses of intravenous (i.v.) methylprednisolone, 500–1,000 mg daily for 3–7 days, with or without a short prednisone taper, is commonly used.[1] Optic neuritis may occur anytime during the course of MS or be one of the initial symptoms. A recent trial of optic neuritis demonstrated that patients treated with oral prednisone alone were more likely to experience recurrent episodes of optic neuritis as compared to those treated with methylprednisolone followed by oral prednisone.[2,3] Furthermore, definite MS developed in 7.5% of the i.v. methylprednisolone group, 14.7% of the oral prednisone group, and 16.7% of

the placebo group over a 2-year period.[4] Recent 5-year follow-up data from the trial showed an overall risk of development of MS to be 30% and did not differ between treatment groups. The 5-year risk of developing clinically definite MS (CDMS) did differ by magnetic resonance imaging (MRI) group such that only 16% of patients with initial normal MRIs developed CDMS, whereas 51% of patients with three or more lesions on MRI developed CDMS.[5] High-dose i.v. methylprednisolone appears to be accompanied by relatively few side effects in most patients, although mental changes, unmasking of infections, gastric disturbances, and an increased incidence of fractures have been reported. Baseline and yearly bone density scans are recommended for patients undergoing repeated steroid therapy. Anaphylactoid reactions and arrhythmias are rare but may also occur. Two recent trials have focused on oral steroid use. A double-blind placebo-controlled trial of oral methylprednisolone use in acute attacks involving 51 patients followed up over 8 weeks showed a statistically significant beneficial effect of oral steroids.[6] Patients received a total of 3,676 mg of oral methylprednisolone over 15 days, with no serious adverse events. A second randomized trial of 80 patients evaluated oral versus i.v. methylprednisolone in acute relapses.[7] The results showed no statistical difference between the treatment groups. The immunologic mechanisms of high-dose corticosteroids include reduction of CD4+ cells, decrease in cytokine release from lymphocytes, and cytokines

Table 9-1. Multiple Sclerosis Treatment Strategies

Disease Course and Stage	Treatment Options
Monosymptomatic (e.g., optic neuritis)	i.v. methylprednisolone, 1,000 mg/day for 5 days
Relapsing-remitting, no disease activity for several years and no MRI activity	i.v. steroids if attacks do occur
Relapsing-remitting, current disease activity or MRI activity (or both)	i.v. steroids for attacks, plus IFN-β-1a (Avonex), 30 μg i.m. weekly or IFN-β-1b (Betaseron), 1 ml s.c. every other day or glatiramer acetate (Copaxone), 20 mg s.c. daily
Relapsing-remitting, disease activity while on IFN or glatiramer acetate	Add monthly bolus of i.v. methylprednisolone or consider increasing IFN dose
Relapsing-remitting, accumulating disability (IFN, glatiramer acetate, steroid nonresponders)	i.v. monthly cyclophosphamide-steroid, i.v. mitoxantrone pulse therapy
Rapidly progressing disability	i.v. cyclophosphamide and steroid 8-day induction, followed by pulse maintenance
Secondary-progressive	i.v. steroid monthly pulses, i.v. monthly cyclophosphamide-steroid or i.v. mitoxantrone pulse therapy, IFN-β, methotrexate, oral or s.c., 7.5–20.0 mg/wk with or without monthly steroid pulses, consider monthly IVIg
Primary-progressive	i.v. steroid monthly pulses, methotrexate, oral or s.c., 7.5–20.0 mg/wk with or without monthly steroid pulses; monthly IVIg; consider i.v. mitoxantrone pulse therapy*
Fulminating disease not responsive to steroid or immunosuppressive therapy	Plasma exchange

IFN = interferon; IVIg = i.v. immunoglobulin; MRI = magnetic resonance imaging.
*Drugs used for secondary-progressive disease may be given for primary-progressive disease, although these patients are not as responsive to immunosuppressive agents.
Source: Modified from HL Weiner, L Stazzone. Multiple Sclerosis. In RE Rakel, R Kersey (eds), Conn's Current Therapy 1999. Philadelphia: WB Saunders Co, 1998;935–942.

(including tumor necrosis factor, interferon gamma [IFN-γ], and decreased class II expression).[1] Corticosteroids have also been shown to decrease immunoglobulin G synthesis in the central nervous system (CNS) and reduce cerebrospinal fluid antibodies to myelin basic protein and oligoclonal bands. i.v. methylprednisolone may also decrease the entry of cells across the blood-brain barrier.

Relapsing-Remitting Disease: Interferons and Glatiramer Acetate

The first medication approved by the U.S. Food and Drug Administration (FDA) for use in MS was recombinant IFN-β-1b (Betaseron). This medication was shown in a double-blind placebo-controlled trial of 372 patients to decrease the frequency of relapses from 1.27 per year to 0.84 per year after 2 years in relapsing-remitting (RR) patients receiving 8 MIU every other day. This is a 34%

reduction in the relapse rate as compared to placebo.[8] Recent 5-year follow-up data report that disease progression was less in the IFN-β-1b group (35%) when compared with the placebo group (46%).[9] Also seen was a 30% decrease in the annual exacerbation rate in the treated group over 5 years. Although this was not statistically significant, the treatment benefit trend was maintained. The MRI data showed no significant increase in the median MRI lesion burden (3.6%) in the IFN-β-1b patients, whereas the placebo patients had an increase in median MRI lesion burden of 30.2% over 5 years. IFN-β-1b is administered every other day under the skin by self-injection. Systemic flu-like symptoms decreased from 52% to 8% by year 1, with most of the decline seen in the first 2 months. Depressive symptoms decreased from 16.9% to 11.1% over 5 years. Injection site reactions occurred in 85% of patients initially and decreased to 47% at 1 year. Elevated liver enzymes were seen in up to 20% of patients over 5 years.

Lymphopenia was seen initially in 35% of patients and after 5 years in 63%. White blood cell counts of less than 3,000/mm^3 were seen in 16% of patients. Serum monitoring every 3 months is suggested. Not all patients respond to the drug and, with time, all patients involved in the original trials have had additional attacks. Also, 34% of patients developed neutralizing antibodies that could reduce the clinical efficacy of the drug. The precise mechanism of action of IFN-β-1b is currently unknown.[10]

Several mechanisms are possible:

1. IFN-β may be counteracting the deleterious effects of IFN-γ, which in turn has been shown to increase MS attacks.[11,12]
2. IFN-β-1b may help to reverse a suppressor cell defect that has been described in MS,[13] although the defect is more common in progressive MS patients.[14]
3. Viral infections have been associated with increased MS attacks,[15] and IFN-β could be preventing viral infections,[10,16] although there is no evidence from the trial that IFN-β-1b worked by affecting viral infections.
4. IFN-β may favor increased secretion of the type 2 T helper (Th2) (anti-inflammatory, promodulatory) cytokine interleukin-4 (IL-4) and decreased IFN-γ secretion.[17]

More recent evidence found that IFN-β-1a increased IL-10, another Th2 cytokine.[18] IFN-β blocks human leukocyte antigen class II expression on antigen-presenting cells and on several CNS cell types.[19,20] IFN-β may also have an inhibitory effect on the permeability of the blood-brain barrier, which would explain the reduced gadolinium enhancement in head MRIs of MS patients with active disease.[21] Studies have also shown that IFN-β inhibits matrix metalloproteinases, which facilitate migration of T cells into the CNS space.[22]

A second double-blind placebo-controlled study of 301 RR patients investigated the efficacy of weekly intramuscular injections of 6 MIU (30 μg) of IFN-β-1a (Avonex), a glycosylated recombinant IFN-β.[23] Over 2 years, the annual exacerbation rate was 0.90 in the placebo group and 0.61 in the IFN-β-1a group. This is a 29% reduction in the relapse rate as compared to placebo. After 2 years, the MRI data revealed a lesion volume of 122.4 (mean) in the placebo group as compared with 74.1 (mean)

in the IFN-β-1a group. The number of enhancing lesions on MRI over 2 years was 1.65 (mean) in the placebo group and 0.80 (mean) in the IFN-β-1a group. The proportion of patients progressing by the end of 104 weeks of the trial was 34.9% in the placebo group and 21.9% in the IFN-β-1a group. Adverse events included mild flu-like symptoms and mild anemia. Skin reactions were seen in 10–15% of both the IFN-β-1a and placebo groups in the pivotal study. Laboratory monitoring is suggested but not mandatory, as no serious liver toxicities occurred. When present, liver function test elevation is usually reversible on discontinuation of the drug. Also, 22% of patients on treatment developed neutralizing antibodies.

The recently completed Controlled High-Risk Subjects Avonex Multiple Sclerosis Prevention Study of 383 patients who experienced a single, isolated neurologic event and had MRI evidence of demyelinating disease were randomly assigned to receive IFN-β-1a (30 μg intramuscular IFN-β-1a weekly) or placebo. The proposed 5-year randomized, double-blind, placebo-controlled trial was stopped early after an independent monitoring committee revealed that the rate of developing CDMS was reduced by 43% in the IFN-β-1a group (p = .002). The IFN-β-1a–treated group also had a reduced accumulation of T$_2$ lesion volume, decreased accumulation of individual new and enlarging T$_2$ lesions, and reduced number and volume of gadolinium-enhancing lesions on MRI at all intervals.[24]

Another 2-year placebo-controlled trial (ETOMS) examined the efficacy of IFN-β-1a (22 μg subcutaneously weekly) in 311 patients with initial signs suggestive of demyelination. There was a 24% relative risk reduction in the time to develop CDMS in the treated group (p = .047). There was also a 23% relative risk reduction in the annual relapse rate in the treated group (p = .045). The MRI analysis showed a 38% overall reduction in the mean of active T$_2$ lesions per scan and a 10% decrease in the T$_2$ lesion load in the treatment group at year 2.

Glatiramer acetate (Copaxone), formerly termed *copolymer 1*, a daily subcutaneous injectable synthetic polymer, showed positive effects in a small double-blind trial of RRMS[25] but not in progressive disease.[26] A large double-blind trial in RR disease involving 251 randomly assigned patients was recently completed.[27] The glatiramer acetate

Table 9-2. Safety in Pregnancy of Drugs Used in the Treatment of Multiple Sclerosis

Category B: Animal data showing no harm to the fetus (no human data available)
Glatiramer acetate (Copaxone)
Pemoline
Oxybutynin
Selective serotonin reuptake inhibitors
Desmopressin
Category C: Animal data showing harm to the fetus (no human data available)
Corticosteroids
IFN-β-1a (Avonex-Rebif)
IFN-β-1b (Betaseron)
Baclofen
Amantidine
Tizanidine
Carbamazepine
Category D: Known to cause fetal harm when administered to pregnant women
Mitoxantrone
Azathioprine
Cyclophosphamide
Methotrexate (category X)

IFN = interferon.
Source: Modified from DM Damek, EA Shuster. Pregnancy and multiple sclerosis. Mayo Clin Proc 1997;72:977–989.

patients had a 2-year relapse rate of 1.19, compared with 1.68 for patients receiving placebo. There was a 29% reduction in the relapse rate over 2 years for those using glatiramer acetate. Recent extension data show that over 140 weeks, 41% of placebo patients experienced worsening of their disability by more than or equal to 1.5 Kurtzke's Expanded Disability Status Scale (EDSS) steps, whereas only 21.6% of glatiramer acetate–treated patients worsened.[28] Preliminary results of glatiramer acetate on MRI outcome show a 35% reduction in the number of new T_2 lesions. This 18-month trial with 239 patients is awaiting publication. Side effects included local injection site reactions and transient systemic postinjection reactions, including chest pain, flushing, dyspnea, palpitations, and anxiety. No laboratory monitoring is necessary. No neutralizing antibodies were detected in the study.

The mechanism by which copolymer 1 may work in humans is unknown. Current evidence sug-

gests that copolymer may (1) induce regulatory T cells that suppress pathogenic immune responses,[29,30] (2) bind to the major histocompatibility complex peptide groove of antigen-presenting cells that may serve to block the presentation of self-antigens to autoreactive T cells,[31–33] and (3) shift the pattern of secreted cytokines from a proinflammatory (Th1) to a promodulatory (Th2) profile.[34]

Oral tolerance using glatiramer acetate simulates myelin basic protein–induced tolerance immunologically by inducing regulatory cells and has been effective in both the rat and mouse experimental autoimmune encephalomyelitis models.[35,36] Suppression of experimental autoimmune encephalomyelitis by oral tolerance with glatiramer acetate can be adoptively transferred and is dose-dependent. Currently, there is a large worldwide study of two daily doses of oral glatiramer acetate in RR patients.

Another factor to consider is that IFN-β-1b and IFN-β-1a are classified as pregnancy category C, and glatiramer acetate is classified as pregnancy category B. With all three agents, when pregnancy occurs, treatment is discontinued, and, if relapses occur during pregnancy, patients are treated with i.v. steroids. In addition, caution should be exercised when prescribing medications for MS-related symptoms, as some of these drugs may have adverse effects on pregnancy or the fetus (Table 9-2).

With the success of the IFN drugs, a trial (PRISMS: Prevention of Relapses and Disability by Interferon-β-1a Subcutaneously in Multiple Sclerosis) of IFN-β-1a in higher doses was conducted in Europe.[37] This randomized double-blind placebo-controlled study involved 560 RR patients given subcutaneous IFN-β-1a (Rebif). Patients were randomly assigned to placebo, 22 μg, or 44 μg of Rebif thrice weekly for 2 years. There was a 27% reduction in the relapse rate in the 22-μg group and a 33% reduction in the 44-μg group. The MRI lesion burden showed a decrease of 1.2% in the 22-μg group, a decrease of 3.8% in the 44-μg group, and an increase of 10.9% in the placebo group. The side effect profile was similar to the other IFNs. Of note, 23.8% of the 22-μg group and 12.5% of the 44-μg group were positive for neutralizing antibodies. The presence of neutralizing antibodies did not affect the mean relapse count. This medication is currently approved in Canada and is awaiting FDA approval in the United States.

A head-to-head trial of Rebif versus IFN-β-1a is currently underway.

Progressive Disease: Interferon and Glatiramer Acetate Nonresponders

Treatment directed at the progressive phase is the most difficult, as the disease may be harder to affect once the progressive stage has been initiated. Immunosuppressive agents, including total lymphoid irradiation, cyclosporine, methotrexate, 2-chlorodeoxyadenosine, cyclophosphamide, mitoxantrone (Novantrone), azathioprine, IFN-β-1b, steroids, i.v. immunoglobulin (IVIg), and plasma exchange, have shown positive clinical effects in progressive disease. The drugs we use for progressive disease include mitoxantrone, cyclophosphamide, pulse steroids, methotrexate, IVIg, and IFN. Because of their toxicity, immunosuppressive agents cannot be used for extended periods.

Our center has the most experience in the treatment of acute or chronic treatment of MS with cyclophosphamide (Cytoxan). An early study by Hauser et al.[38] showed a short induction course of high-dose daily i.v. cyclophosphamide plus i.v. adrenocorticotropic hormone could modify the clinical course of patients with severe MS.[38] During a 1-year follow-up period, 80% of patients treated with this regimen were neurologically stable, as compared with 50% of patients who received plasma exchange and 20% of patients who received i.v. adrenocorticotropic hormone alone. A Canadian study several years later, in which treated patients were compared with placebo controls, showed no effect from an induction course of cyclophosphamide. It now appears that the main differences between the Canadian study and other studies were related to patient population and dosing issues, similar to the differences found between the IFN-β-1b secondary-progressive trials performed in the United States and Europe. A follow-up study to the original regimen in Hauser et al.[38] was undertaken by the Northeast Cooperative Multiple Sclerosis Treatment Group and involved 256 progressive patients.[39] Patients were given the original or modified cyclophosphamide induction, with one group continuing with monthly boosters. After 30 months, 17% of patients without boosters were stable or improved

as compared with 27% on booster therapy. More recent studies have documented that of 84 patients with chronic progressive MS treated with cyclophosphamide over 12 months, 80% were either stable or improved in their EDSS. Major effects were observed in patients younger than age 40 years, especially in those who had been in the progressive phase for less than 1 year.[40] There is also evidence that cyclophosphamide can be used in patients with fulminating disease, with a study showing that 13 of 17 treated patients were stable or improved by more than or equal to 1 point on the EDSS over a mean of 22 months.[41] In addition, cyclophosphamide has been shown to reduce significantly the enhancing lesions on MRI when given to MS patients followed up for a mean of 28 months.[42] Immunologic data reveal that cyclophosphamide therapy induces a Th2-type response as measured by IL-4, IL-10, and IFN-γ production.[17] When used in our center, the drug is now given concomitantly with i.v. methylprednisolone as a monthly bolus in the first year, every 6 weeks in the second year, and every 8 weeks in the third year. Additional years of treatment are considered in patients who respond well or in those who show a decline after discontinuation of the drug. As with most immunosuppressive agents formerly attempted as potential MS treatments, cyclophosphamide may not provide help for primary-progressive MS patients. Duration of treatment is limited by the risk of bladder cancer, which appears to rise with time, and it also depends on total accumulated drug dose.

A trial of mitoxantrone in 42 active MS patients was recently published.[43] Patients were treated monthly with i.v. methylprednisolone plus i.v. mitoxantrone or i.v. methylprednisolone alone over 6 months. Although the numbers were small, there was a statistically significant reduction in the number of relapses and an increase in the number of patients free of attack. Also, 90% of the i.v. methylprednisolone–i.v. mitoxantrone group showed no new enhancing lesions on MRI versus only 31% in the i.v. methylprednisolone group. After these results, a multicenter, placebo-controlled, randomized, observer-blind trial of 194 progressive MS patients was recently completed in Europe. Patients received i.v. treatment every 3 months for 2 years. The results have not been published, but preliminary data are reportedly encouraging. The risk of cardiotoxicity prevents prolonged usage. There is also a concern over the development of leukemia. Mitoxantrone was recently approved by the FDA for reducing neurologic disability or the frequency of clinical relapses in patients with secondary-progressive, progressive-relapsing, or worsening MS.

IFN-β-1b was recently studied in secondary-progressive MS patients in 32 centers in Europe. In this study, 358 patients received placebo, and 360 patients received IFN-β-1b every other day subcutaneously for up to 3 years.[44] In the IFN-β-1b group, there was a relative reduction of 21.7% in the proportion of patients with progression. The time to becoming wheelchair-bound was also significantly delayed, equivalent to 12 months ($p < .01$). The authors assert that the positive effect of the treatment could not be ascribed merely to reduction in disability as the result of relapses. There appeared to be an effect on progression. Whether this is due to suppression of some ongoing low-level inflammatory process could not be answered directly. The mean relapse rate was reduced overall by approximately 30% in the treatment group. In terms of MRI lesion volume, the placebo group showed a mean increase of 8% as compared to the IFN-β-1b group, which showed a mean decrease of 5%. There was, however, a 45% reduction in the development of T_1 MRI hypointensities (T_1 holes) in a subgroup of 95 patients. The side effect profile was similar to the initial IFN-β-1b study, as described previously. Neutralizing antibodies were seen in 27.8% of patients. Approval of the use of IFN-β-1b in progressive MS in the United States is currently under FDA review.

A 3-year, randomized controlled trial of IFN-β-1b in secondary-progressive MS in North America was recently completed. The three-arm study involved 939 patients placed on either 8 MIU IFN-β-1b, 5 MIU/m² IFN-β-1b, or placebo subcutaneous every other day. There was no treatment effect on the primary outcome measure, which was progression of disease. Treatment effects were seen on secondary clinical and MRI endpoints. One reason for the disparity between studies could be that the European study group was younger and had a shorter duration of MS as well as more relapses before study entry.

The Secondary Progressive Efficacy Clinical Trial of Recombinant Interferon beta-1a in Multiple Sclerosis study evaluated IFN-β-1a (22 μg and 44 μg thrice weekly) versus placebo for up to 3 years. Of 571 evaluable patients, there was no significant difference in the time to sustained progression of disability, which was the primary endpoint.

Weekly low-dose oral methotrexate (7.5 mg) was studied in a randomized, double-blinded, placebo-controlled trial of 60 patients with chronic progressive disease and has been reported to affect positively measures of upper extremity function in progressive MS. Upper extremity function was measured using a 9-Hole Peg Test and a Block-in Box Test. These tests are sensitive measures of repeated use of digits. Conversely, lower extremity function as measured by ambulation and disability scales was not affected.[45] An advantage of methotrexate is that it is an immunomodulator used extensively in other conditions, such as rheumatoid arthritis, with a known side effect profile. Safety of methotrexate has also been established in patients receiving 20 mg subcutaneously weekly.[46] Whether higher doses given intravenously or intrathecally would be more effective in MS is unclear.

These studies have major implications for the treatment of MS. The immunomodulatory drugs are now approved only for the treatment of relapsing disease. Again, it was shown that their side effects are manageable. In the European study, 45 patients on IFN-β-1b stopped because of adverse effects, as opposed to 15 on placebo, but twice as many stopped because of inefficacy of treatment in the placebo group. An intention-to-treat analysis was used for the final data. If others replicate the study, IFN will become standard therapy for secondary-progressive MS, regardless of the stage of the illness. This is the largest single category of MS, and the impact on the cost of medical care and the search for other treatments, which may have to be compared to this treatment, are obvious.

Monthly bolus i.v. steroids, typically 1,000 mg of methylprednisolone, are used at many institutions for treatment of primary- or secondary-progressive MS. This usage remains empiric, as no relevant studies have been reported. A phase II study using monthly steroids in chronic progressive patients showed promise.[47] Steroids may expedite recovery from acute attacks but do not necessarily help the degree of recovery.

IVIg may help a number of autoimmune diseases, including chronic relapsing polyneuropathy and dermatomyositis, and has been used in initial

MS trials.[48] Its mechanism of action is unclear but may relate to anti-idiotypic effects and suppression of the prodemyelinating cytokine tumor necrosis factor-α. A recent randomized placebo-controlled trial of monthly IVIg in RRMS was reported.[49] This placebo-controlled trial involved 150 patients over 2 years. Thirty-six percent of patients from the placebo group were relapse-free as compared to 53% from the IVIg group with a significant p value of .03. Only three IVIg patients (4%) experienced side effects, including cutaneous reactions and depression, although these were not unequivocally related to the IVIg. Observations in animal models of MS revealed that IVIg could promote new myelin synthesis.[50] Results from an ongoing U.S. trial with IVIg are pending.

Plasma exchange has recently been investigated in patients who had acute CNS inflammatory demyelinating disease and did not respond to steroid therapy.[51] This randomized, sham-controlled, double-masked study involved 12 patients with MS and 10 with other demyelinating diseases. These patients had a baseline EDSS of 7.5, and, in all of them, i.v. methylprednisolone therapy failed. Eight patients (four with MS, four with other disease) on active treatment were deemed successful. Responders tended to be male and younger. As this study did not concomitantly administer drugs that depress T-lymphocytes, demyelinating diseases may share a common humoral mechanism that could include antibodies, complement or complement components, circulating immune complexes, or cytokines. It has been shown that antibodies directed to a specific epitope of myelin oligodendrocyte glycoprotein are present in MS brains and are associated with degenerating myelin.

Unanswered Questions Related to Multiple Sclerosis Therapy

Many unanswered questions remain since the introduction of the three approved medications for MS. Analysis and comparison of these trials has been difficult, as each trial used slightly different statistical, clinical, laboratory, and MRI measures. To begin, no direct comparison can be made because each drug was tested against placebo and not against the others. The glatiramer acetate trial had limited data on MRI measures. Although the molecular structures of IFN-

β-1a and IFN-β-1b are similar, the total dose of IFN-β-1a used in the trials was only 21.4% of the IFN-β-1b dose. This may explain the similar but milder side effect profile of IFN-β-1a. In terms of preventing the progression of the disease, there are many questions concerning the data analysis. In the IFN-β-1a study, the difference in the proportion of patients worse at 2 years is not significant between treatment and placebo groups ($p = .07$). Also, 53% of patients had not completed treatment when the study was terminated. Treated patients had progression at an even rate throughout the study, whereas 30% of placebo patients had begun progressing at the semiannual evaluation. In addition, recent MRI data were presented showing a decrease in new or enhancing lesions, but no correlation to change in the EDSS could be made. In the U.S. IFN-β-1b trial, 20% of treated patients and 28% of placebo patients met the definition of confirmed disability (a 3-month sustained 1-point EDSS increase) at the end of 3 years. This was not statistically significant. The study was not powered to assess disease progression. In addition, it has not been shown whether preventing attacks truly translates into preventing disease progression. The European trial of IFN-β-1b showed statistical differences between treated and untreated patients in slowing the time to reach a wheelchair. However, a difference must be noted between statistically significant and clinically significant changes. For instance, only a few patients on IFN-β therapy would be able to detect any change in their rate of disease progression while being able to detect the number of clinical relapses. Of interest is that the relapse rate in the European trial was reduced by approximately the same percentage as in the U.S. IFN-β-1b trial.

The neutralizing antibody (NAB) issue is another unresolved issue. IFN-β-1a and IFN-β-1b have identical receptor-binding regions that are responsible for their biological activity. An independent laboratory recently provided preliminary data supporting the claim of cross-reactivity both in the binding and biological assays. Both IFN-β trials have documented that the patients who developed NABs demonstrate reduced clinical efficacy of the drug as indicated by a higher relapse rate and increased activity on MRI. The current commercial NAB test (NABferon, Athena Diagnostics, Worcester, MA) includes low, medium, and high titer ranges.

The challenge in MS therapeutics at this point is to advance beyond the currently available, partially effective treatments. Statistically convincing data derived from large randomized clinical trials may not always translate into reliable treatments in the clinic. Many unanswered questions remain:

- Are there clear responders and nonresponders to immunomodulatory treatments?
- Do all patients receive a modest benefit? If there are responders, how can we identify them?
- Do neutralizing antibodies play an important role in the response to IFNs?
- Can immunomodulatory treatments, such as glatiramer acetate and IFN-β, be used in combination?
- Can the duration of effectiveness of IFN-β in secondary-progressive MS be extended? Few patients will be satisfied with a treatment that delays progression to wheelchair use by 1 year or less. Will combination treatment with immunosuppressive drugs achieve this goal?
- What is the proper dose of parenteral IFN-β? Should this dose be more flexible and individualized?
- When should therapy with any treatment begin?
- When should therapy be terminated? For instance, should the physician discontinue the drug if a patient has no disease activity after 5 years of treatment?
- Should the treatment of progressing monosymptomatic MS differ (e.g., if the patient exhibits bilateral recurrent optic neuropathy or progressive myelopathy)?
- Should there be differences in treatment depending on age and gender?
- Will the issue of primary-progressive MS, totaling 15–20% of all patients, remain unsolved, and will its treatment approach require a totally new direction?
- Assuming that there are genes for MS susceptibility, will there be a role for gene therapy to alter their presence or levels of expression?
- Can we identify a subset of MS patients with benign MS earlier in their course, which may alter our treatment strategy?
- Will we be able to identify an antigen responsible for the MS immune cascade and develop more specific and less toxic treatment alternatives?
- Will newer MRI techniques help the clinician to better direct the timing and type of treatment?
- Will newer MRI techniques, such as MR spectroscopy, aid in the diagnosis and follow-up of patients? Will MR spectroscopy allow us to perform drug evaluations at a faster rate?
- Can we identify immune markers to identify which treatment is ideal for which patient?
- Can these immune markers be used to follow up patients over time to decide when to terminate and when to change therapy?
- Will we be able to test new drugs against standard therapy and eliminate the need for a placebo arm?
- Will nerve growth factors have a role in the treatment of MS? This question—of repair and remyelination—is of great interest to patients with advanced disease and is a fundamental neurobiological issue that must be addressed.

Conclusions

MS is, for the most part, a progressive neurologic disorder that strikes patients in the prime of their life. With the advent of MRI, the differentiation and diagnosis of MS have become easier, and the importance of early treatment has become apparent. Recent advances in immunology have led to the approval of three new medications that decrease the relapse rate and slow the progression of the disease. Future therapies may combine immunomodulatory and immunosuppressive approaches as well as remyelination-inducing treatments. Patients on these therapies will be followed up closely with MRI and immune markers. This comprehensive approach to patient care will allow physicians to treat MS patients in a way that will prevent accumulation of disability.

References

1. Kupersmith MJ, Kaufman D, Paty DW, et al. Megadose corticosteroids in multiple sclerosis. Neurology 1994;44:1–4.
2. Beck RW, Cleary PA, Anderson MM Jr., et al. A randomized, controlled trial of corticosteroids in the treatment of acute optic neuritis. N Engl J Med 1992;326:581–588.
3. Beck RW, Cleary PA. Optic neuritis treatment trial: one-year follow-up results. Arch Ophthalmol 1993;111:773–775.

4. Beck RW, Cleary PA, Trobe JD, et al. The effect of corticosteroids for acute optic neuritis on the subsequent development of multiple sclerosis. N Engl J Med 1993; 239:1764–1769.

5. The Optic Neuritis Study Group. The 5-year risk of MS after optic neuritis: experience of the Optic Neuritis Treatment Trial. Neurology 1997;49:1404–1413.

6. Sellebjerg F, Frederiksen JL, Nielsen PM, Olesen J. Double-blind, randomized, placebo-controlled study of oral, high-dose methylprednisolone in attacks of MS. Neurology 1998;51:529–534.

7. Barnes D, Hughes RA, Morris RW. Randomised trial of oral and intravenous methylprednisolone in acute relapses of multiple sclerosis. Lancet 1997;349(9056):902–906.

8. The Interferon-beta-1b Multiple Sclerosis Study Group. Interferon beta-1b is effective in relapsing-remitting multiple sclerosis: clinical results of a multicenter, randomized, double-blind, placebo-controlled trial. Neurology 1993;43:655–661.

9. The Interferon-beta-1b Multiple Sclerosis Study Group, The University of British Columbia MS/MRI Analysis Group. Interferon beta-1b in the treatment of multiple sclerosis: Final outcome of the randomized controlled trial. Neurology 1995;45:1277–1285.

10. Arnason BGW. Interferon beta in multiple sclerosis. Neurology 1993;43:641–643.

11. Hirsch RL, Panitch HS, Johnson KP. Lymphocytes from multiple sclerosis patients produce elevated levels of gamma interferon in vitro. J Clin Immunol 1985;22:139.

12. Noronha A, Toscas A, Jensen MA. Interferon beta decreases T cell activation and interferon gamma production in multiple sclerosis. J Neuroimmunol 1993;46(1–2):145–153.

13. Antel JP, Brown-Bania M, Reder A, Cashman N. Activated suppressor cell dysfunction in multiple sclerosis. J Immunol 1986;137:137–141.

14. Noronha A, Toscas A, Jensen MA. Interferon beta augments suppressor cell function in multiple sclerosis. Ann Neurol 1990;27:207–210.

15. Sibley WA, Bamford CR, Clark K. Clinical viral infections and multiple sclerosis. Lancet 1985;1:1313–1315.

16. Al-Sabbagh A, Nelson PA, Weiner HL. Beta interferon enhances oral tolerance to MBP and PLP in experimental autoimmune encephalomyelitis. Neurology (abstract) 1994;44(Suppl2):A242.

17. Smith DR, Balachov K, Hafler DA, et al. Immune deviation following pulse cyclophosphamide/methylprednisolone treatment of multiple sclerosis: increased interleukin-4 production and associated eosinophilia. Ann Neurol 1997;42: 313–318.

18. Rudick RA, Ransohoff RM, Lee JC, et al. In vivo effects of interferon-beta-1a on immunosuppressive cytokines in multiple sclerosis. Neurology 1998;50:1294–1300.

19. Ransohoff RM, Devajyothi C, Estes ML, et al. Interferon beta specifically inhibits interferon gamma induced class II major histocompatibility complex gene transcription in a human astrocytoma cell line. J Neuroimmunol 1991; 33(2):103–112.

20. Jiang H, Milo R, Swovenland P, et al. Interferon beta-1b reduces interferon gamma induced antigen presenting capacity of human glial and B cells. J Neuroimmunol 1995;61:17–25.

21. Calabresi PA, Tranguill LR, Dambrosia JM, et al. Increases in soluble VCAM-1 correlate with a decrease in MRI lesions in multiple sclerosis treated with interferon beta-1b. Ann Neurol 1997;41:669–674.

22. Stuve O, Dooley NP, Ulm JH. Interferon beta-1b decreases the migration of T lymphocytes in vitro: effects on matrix metalloproteinase-9. Ann Neurol 1996;40:853–863.

23. Jacobs LD, Cookfair DL, Rudick RA, et al. Intramuscular interferon beta-1a for disease progression in relapsing multiple sclerosis. Ann Neurol 1996;39(3):285–294.

24. Jacobs LD, Beck RW, Simon JH, et al. Intramuscular interferon beta-1a therapy initiated during a first demyelinating event in multiple sclerosis. CHAMPS Study Group. N Engl J Med 2000;343:898–904.

25. Bornstein MB, Miller A, Slagle S, et al. A pilot trial of Cop 1 in exacerbating-remitting multiple sclerosis. N Engl J Med 1987;41:533–539.

26. Bornstein MB, Miller A, Slagle S, et al. A placebo-controlled, double-blind, randomized, two-center, pilot trial of Cop 1 in chronic progressive multiple sclerosis. Neurology 1991;41:533–539.

27. Johnson KP, Brooks BR, Cohen JA, Copolymer 1 reduces relapse rate and improves disability in relapsing-remitting multiple sclerosis: results of a phase III multicenter, double-blind, placebo-controlled trial. The Copolymer 1 Multiple Sclerosis Study Group. Neurology 1995;45:1268–1276.

28. Johnson KP, Brooks BR, Cohen JA, et al. Extended use of glatiramer acetate (Copaxone) is well tolerated and maintains its clinical effect on multiple sclerosis relapse rate and degree of disability. Neurology 1998;50:701–708.

29. Aharoni R, Teitelbaum D, Sela M, Arnon R. Copolymer 1 induces T cells of the T helper type 2 that crossreact with myelin basic protein and suppress experimental autoimmune encephalomyelitis. Proc Natl Acad Sci U S A 1997; 94(20):10821–10826.

30. Fukaura H, Kent S, Pietruesewicz M, et al. Induction of circulating myelin basic protein and proteolipid protein specific transforming growth factor-β1-secreting Th3 T cells by oral administration of myelin in multiple sclerosis patients. J Clin Invest 1996;98:70–75.

31. Fridkis-Hareli M, Strominger JL. Promiscuous binding of synthetic copolymer 1 to purified HLA-D molecules. J Immunol 1998;160:4386–4397.

32. Fridkis-Hareli M, Teitelbaum D, Gurevich E, et al. Direct binding of myelin basic protein and synthetic copolymer 1 to class II major histocompatibility complex molecules on living antigen presenting cell. Proc Natl Acad Sci U S A 1994;91:4872–4876.

33. Fridkis-Hareli M, Rosloniec E, Fugger L, Strominger J. Synthetic amino acid copolymers that bind to HLA-DR proteins and inhibit type II collagen-reactive T cell clones. Proc Natl Acad Sci U S A 1998;95:12528–12531.

34. Duda PW, Schmied MC, Cook SL, et al. Glatiramer acetate (Copaxone) induces degenerate, Th2-polarized immune responses in patients with multiple sclerosis. J Clin Invest 2000;105(7):967–976.

35. Weiner HL. Oral tolerance with Copolymer 1 for the treatment of multiple sclerosis. Proc Natl Acad Sci U S A 1999;96:3333–3335.

36. Teitelbaum D, Arnon R, Sela M. Immunomodulation of experimental autoimmune encephalomyelitis by oral administration of copolymer 1. Proc Natl Acad Sci U S A 1999;96:3842–3847.

37. PRISMS Study Group. Randomised double-blind placebo-controlled study of interferon beta-1a in relapsing/remitting multiple sclerosis. Lancet 1998;352(9139):1498–1504.

38. Hauser SL, Dawson DM, Lehrich JR, et al. Intensive immunosuppression in progressive multiple sclerosis: a randomized, three-arm study of high dose intravenous cyclophosphamide, plasma exchange and ACTH. N Engl J Med 1983;308:173–180.

39. Weiner HL, Mackin GA, Orav EJ, et al. Intermittent cyclophosphamide pulse therapy in progressive multiple sclerosis: final report of the Northeast Cooperative Multiple Sclerosis Treatment Group. Neurology 1993; 43:910–918.

40. Hohol MJ, Olek MJ, Orav EJ, et al. Treatment of progressive multiple sclerosis with pulse cyclophosphamide/methylprednisolone: response to therapy is linked to the duration of progressive disease. Mult Scler 1999;5:403–409.

41. Weinstock-Guttman B, Kinkel RP, Cohen JA. Treatment of fulminating multiple sclerosis with intravenous cyclophosphamide. Neurologist 1997;3:178–185.

42. Gobbini MI, Smith ME, Richert ND, et al. Effect of open label pulse cyclophosphamide therapy on MRI measures of disease activity in five patients with refractory relapsing-remitting multiple sclerosis. J Neuroimmunol 1999; 99:142–149.

43. Edan G, Miller D, Clanet M, et al. Therapeutic effect of mitoxantrone combined with methylprednisolone in multiple sclerosis: a randomised multicentre study of active disease using MRI and clinical criteria. J Neurol Neurosurg Psychiatry 1997;62(2):112–118.

44. European Study Group of Interferon-beta-1b in Secondary Progressive MS. Placebo-controlled multicentre randomised trial of interferon beta-1b in treatment of secondary progressive multiple sclerosis. Lancet 1998; 352(9139):1491–1497.

45. Goodkin DE, Rudick RA, Medendorp SV, et al. Low-dose (7.5mg) oral methotrexate reduces the rate of progression in chronic progressive multiple sclerosis. Ann of Neurol 1995;37:30–40.

46. Olek MJ, Hohol MJ, Weiner HL. Methotrexate in the treatment of multiple sclerosis. Ann Neurol (Letter) 1996; 39(5):684.

47. Goodkin DE, Kinkel RP, Weinstock-Guttman B, et al. A phase II study of IV methylprednisolone in secondary-progressive multiple sclerosis. Neurology 1998;51:239–245.

48. Achiron A, Pras E, Gilad R, et al. Open controlled therapeutic trial of intravenous immune globulin in relapsing-remitting multiple sclerosis. Arch Neurol 1992;49:1233–1236.

49. Fazekas F, Deisenhammer F, Strasser-Fuchs S and Austrian Immunoglobulin in MS Group. Randomised placebo-controlled trial of monthly intravenous immunoglobulin therapy in relapsing-remitting multiple sclerosis. Lancet 1997; 349:589–593.

50. Noseworthy JH, O'Brien PC, van Engelen BG, Rodriguez M. Intravenous immunoglobulin therapy in multiple sclerosis: progress from remyelination in the Theiler's virus model to a randomized, double-blind, placebo-controlled clinical trial. J Neurol Neurosurg Psychiatry 1994;57: (Suppl):11–14.

51. Weinshenker BG, O'Brien PC, Petterson TM, et al. A randomized trial of plasma exchange in acute central nervous system inflammatory demyelinating disease. Ann Neurol 1999;46(6):878–886.

Chapter 10

Disorders That Mimic Multiple Sclerosis

Derek Smith, Allison E. Morgan, Bonnie I. Glanz,
Shahram Khoshbin, Fernando Dangond, and
David Margolin

Clinicians who treat multiple sclerosis (MS) patients frequently would agree that most cases of MS are not difficult to diagnose. A classic presentation would be a young white woman who was raised in the northern United States or Europe and presents with sensory loss and fatigue. The neurologic examination shows hyperreflexia. Her history reveals that she has had three different attacks, including an episode of documented optic neuritis (ON). The symptom of eye blurriness has recurred when the patient takes hot showers. Brain magnetic resonance imaging (MRI) shows multiple high T_2 signal–intensity lesions, several gadolinium-enhancing T_1 hypointense periventricular lesions, and pericallosal radiation of lesions in a "Dawson's fingers" pattern. A cervical spine MRI shows a 5-mm high T_2 signal–intensity lesion at C2 to C3 and no evidence of disk herniation or trauma. Even in the absence of oligoclonal bands in the cerebrospinal fluid (CSF), an experienced clinician would diagnose MS with this clinical presentation, as very few, if any, diseases may exhibit such a complex mix of signs and symptoms.

More challenging are the many patients who may have MS but present with a less classic history and examination. As always in neurology, the quality of the clinical history is crucial. Patients with prominent neuropsychiatric abnormalities may have their diagnoses delayed. This chapter addresses disorders that can mimic MS, espe-cially atypical forms of MS. Features that should alert the clinician to the possibility of other diseases include an atypical MRI picture, a family history of neurologic disease, a spinal level in the absence of cerebral disease, persistent back pain, findings attributable to one anatomic site, patients older than 60 years or younger than 15 years at onset, and progressive disease. None of these can exclude MS but should lead one to seek other etiologies before accepting this diagnosis. Some useful screening studies to consider in a patient with an atypical presentation include complete blood count with differential, coagulation studies, vitamin B_{12}, rapid plasma reagin test (RPR), Lyme titers, antinuclear antibodies (ANA), anti–double-stranded DNA antibodies, anti-cardiolipin antibodies, lupus anticoagulant, serum immunoelectrophoresis, serum protein electrophoresis, rheumatoid factor, erythrocyte sedimentation rate, antineutrophil cytoplasmic antibodies, angiotensin-converting enzyme levels, creatine phosphokinase, lactate, very-long-chain fatty acids (VLCFAs), arylsulfatase A, paraneoplastic antibodies, or heavy metals; these may help to guide further workup.

Infectious and Postinfectious Disorders

Human T-cell lymphotropic virus type I–associated myelopathy/tropical spastic paraparesis and progressive multifocal leukoencephalopathy are discussed in Chapters 11 and 15, respectively.

Acute Disseminated Encephalomyelitis and Acute Hemorrhagic Encephalomyelitis

Acute disseminated encephalomyelitis (ADEM) represents a syndrome characterized by a single episode of acute or subacute demyelination-inflammation in the central nervous system (CNS) of a presumed autoimmune basis. The acronym ADEM can be used interchangeably with post-infectious or post-vaccinial encephalitis or encephalomyelitis. ADEM develops from a few weeks (approximately 1–2) to a few months (approximately 2) after vaccination or infection. The infections most commonly associated with a postinfectious demyelination include mycoplasma, herpes, hepatitis, varicella zoster, and measles. ADEM may on occasion present with saltatory progression, rendering it difficult to differentiate from relapsing-remitting MS. In fact, some neurologists refer to relapsing ADEM as a particular entity but, for the most part, it is safe to assume that most episodes that fulfill the clinical criteria will be isolated. In some patients, especially children, lesions can be focal and may, for example, involve only the brain stem.

Lesions are characterized by extensive confluent or multifocal demyelination and inflammation, with lymphocytes and monocytes infiltrating the perivenular spaces. Sometimes, ADEM can be unifocal, however, and this may confuse the examiner. On occasion, lesions can also present in only one hemisphere, a puzzling presentation for the clinician. The pathology in the most fulminant form, acute hemorrhagic encephalomyelitis, shows demyelination and inflammation accompanied by diffuse extravasation of red blood cells that accumulate in the perivenular space with a "ring" or "ball" hemorrhage appearance and by infiltration of neutrophils into the brain parenchyma and CSF. It is generally believed that acute hemorrhagic encephalomyelitis is a more severe version of ADEM, as both are inflammatory and demyelinative and occur as part of a postinfectious or post-vaccinial autoimmune response. Acute demyelinative lesions of ADEM can progress to a hemorrhagic state, with the appearance of red blood cells and neutrophils in the CSF heralding the conversion.[1] ADEM and acute

hemorrhagic encephalomyelitis may be fatal but, in those patients who survive, the prognosis is often good.

Herpes Simplex Virus–Associated Disorders

The human herpesvirus (HHV) family currently includes eight distinct viruses: herpes simplex virus type 1 (HSV-1) and type 2 (HSV-2); Epstein-Barr virus; cytomegalovirus (CMV); varicella-zoster; and HHV6, -7, and -8. HHV8 was formerly known as *Kaposi sarcoma–associated herpesvirus*. All herpesviruses are double-stranded DNA viruses that have the capacity to remain latent within host cells, as episomes in the cell nucleus. The molecular mechanisms that induce, maintain, or disrupt latency have been intensively studied but remain poorly understood. On reactivation, a productive and typically lytic infection develops. Some of these can cause neurologic symptoms for which the differential diagnosis might include MS.

There are two types of HSVs: HSV-1 and HSV-2. HSV-1 accounts for almost all cases of herpes encephalitis and causes more than 10% of all cases of sporadic viral encephalitis in the United States. HSV-2 is more often associated with genital infections. HSV-1 encephalitis occurs in children and in adults. In adults with HSV encephalitis, there is usually evidence of previous mucocutaneous HSV-1 infection. Also, latent HSV is present in many areas of the brain,[2] so most cases probably result from reactivation, although reinfection has also been reported.

A diagnosis of HSV encephalitis is usually considered in cases presenting with acute onset of fever and either mental status changes or focal neurologic symptoms. In patients whose fevers are rather low grade, a diagnosis of demyelinating disease (particularly ADEM) might be considered. A diagnosis of possible HSV encephalitis should be evaluated by MRI, which classically shows T_2 hyperintensity in one or both temporal lobes, although other brain regions can be involved.[3–7] The CSF usually shows a pleocytosis beyond the range common in MS, with leukocyte counts between 50–150/mm³, and may be hemorrhagic or xanthochromic. Although differentiation of HSV encephalitis from other infections or noninfectious processes can be difficult, the diagnosis can be established with high specificity and sensitivity by the demonstration of HSV DNA in CSF by polymerase chain reaction (PCR). Brain biopsy, at one time frequently performed for diagnosis, is now rarely required.

HSV can also involve the spinal cord, presenting as either acute[8,9] or recurrent[10–12] transverse myelitis (TM) or radiculomyelitis. These conditions are easily mistaken for demyelinating disease. Recognition of the correct diagnosis may require analysis of CSF, as discussed previously.

Effective antiviral therapy is available for HSV encephalomyelitis. Treatment is most effective when begun early, leading to the current standard practice of beginning treatment with intravenous acyclovir in patients presenting with possible HSV encephalitis even before the diagnosis is proven and discontinuing treatment if HSV is ruled out. Acyclovir is usually continued for 10 days for treatment of HSV encephalitis. Acyclovir has low toxicity and is usually well tolerated if adequate hydration is maintained. Even with early treatment, however, neurologic sequelae are frequent.

Cytomegalovirus

The human CMV is endemic in the United States. Approximately 80% of adults have antibodies indicating previous infection. Like other herpesviruses, latent chronic CMV infection occasionally becomes reactivated and causes disease in adults. This is a particular problem among immunosuppressed individuals; CMV is a frequent cause of retinitis and neurologic disease among acquired immunodeficiency syndrome patients.

Like HSV, CMV can cause encephalitis and radiculomyelitis. The latter syndrome is characterized by progressive, ascending weakness, areflexia, and sensory loss in association with bladder- or anal-sphincter dysfunction. Onset may be acute or subacute. The CSF often demonstrates a pleocytosis beyond the range common in MS, and may have a neutrophilic predominance or be hemorrhagic. As with HSV, PCR analysis of the CSF for detection of the viral DNA can establish the diagnosis with high sensitivity and specificity.

CMV is more difficult to treat than HSV; ganciclovir and foscarnet are most often used, but these drugs may be ineffective and can have substantial toxicity.

Human Herpesvirus 6

HHV6 infection occurs commonly during childhood and has been cited as the most common pathogen responsible for febrile illness in infants. It is a frequent cause of febrile convulsions of infants.[13–17] Latent infection is established at that time, as the immune system suppresses viral replication. In recent years, there has been considerable interest in a possible role for HHV6 as a cause of encephalitis in adults, particularly in the context of immunosuppression. Some reported cases have closely resembled HSV encephalitis[18]; when CSF from cases of suspected herpes encephalitis tests negative for HSV DNA, it is reasonable to test also for HHV6.

Rare cases have been reported of HHV6 encephalitis that was misdiagnosed as MS.[19] There have also been investigations into a role for HHV6 in the pathogenesis of MS, although these reports have been received with considerable skepticism. This skepticism is heightened by conflicting results among published reports, both with regard to the presence of anti-HHV6 antibodies and to the detection of HHV6 nucleic acids in blood of MS patients. At present, there is no justification for routine clinical testing for this agent in cases of suspected MS.

Lyme Neuroborreliosis

Lyme disease in the United States was first described in Connecticut in the 1970s, when individuals began presenting with an atypical skin rash consistent with erythema migrans and with arthropathy signs.[20] In Europe, the first recorded case of Lyme disease dates back to the 1800s. Burgdorfer[21] recognized the association of Lyme with tick transmission, and the organism was isolated from patients with the disease in 1983.[22,23] The spirochete can be recovered from the edge of the erythema migrans lesion.[24] Erythema migrans is recognized as a central macule at the site of the tick bite that expands no less than 5 cm, becoming a papule and then an annular erythematous plaque. The lesion may have a "bull's eye pattern" and is a pathognomonic marker of recent infection (i.e., within 1 month, usually days). Acrodermatitis chronica atrophicans is a late skin manifestation that is predominantly seen in Europe and should not be confused with erythema migrans.

Lyme disease is the most common arthropod-borne disease in the United States and Europe. In the United States, the disease is more common in the northeastern and north-central regions.[25] The *Ixodes* tick is the primary vector of *Borrelia* worldwide. In the United States, *Ixodes scapularis* and *Ixodes pacificus* are found to transmit the spirochete. Common reservoirs are the deer, other mammals, rodents, and birds.[26] Lyme disease has been linked to infection with *Borrelia burgdorferi garinii*, *sensu strico*, and *afzelli*.[27] More recently, *B. valaisiana* has been proposed to have a pathogenic potential for humans as well.[28] *B. burgdorferi garinii* outer surface protein A serotype 4 strain is the principal agent associated with Lyme neuroborreliosis in Europe, and this association has been demonstrated by PCR.[29] Close to one-half of *Borrelia*-infected people are asymptomatic. Fewer than one-half of neuroborreliosis patients recall an antecedent tick bite. In high endemic areas, such as the northeastern United States, where MS is also relatively common, occasional difficulties arise in distinguishing Lyme neuroborreliosis from MS.

Personal protective measures for individuals from high endemic areas who cannot avoid tick-infested habitats are the mainstay of Lyme disease prevention. These include wearing protective gear, using repellents, and seeking and removing attached ticks. A safe, highly immunogenic vaccine (LYMErix) based on the outer surface protein A antigen is available in the United States for preventive use since 1998[30-32] and is recommended for use in adults. However, testing for Lyme seroreactivity of these individuals may be complicated by previous vaccinations; using outer surface protein A–free strains to perform antibody capture immunoassays and Western blots solves this problem,[33] as no cross reactivity of the vaccine-elicited antibodies with these strains has been shown.

Dissemination of the Lyme spirochete occurs via the hematogenous, lymphatic, and cutaneous pathways. Significant evidence has accumulated to suggest that Lyme disease can affect the CNS and peripheral nervous system (PNS) (in 20–50% of symptomatic patients); the eye (uveitis, keratitis, periorbital edema)[34,35]; and joints, skin, and heart (atrioventricular block, cardiomyopathy, or arrhythmias).[36,37] Lesions in the brain parenchyma and peripheral nerve have been shown to harbor the spirochete, and proper treatment with antibiotics can reduce the severity and size of these lesions. Direct damage to the brain parenchyma (astroglial and neuronal cells) has been supported by studies demonstrating elevated glial fibrillary acidic protein, neuron-specific enolase, and neurofilament light subunit in the CSF of Lyme neuroborreliosis patients[38] and normalization after treatment. Antibodies against *Borrelia* strains can be shown in the CSF, and PCR can be used in some cases to amplify nucleic acid sequences corresponding to the micro-organism.

Lyme meningoencephalitis usually presents with lower-grade fever and a longer duration of malaise and neck pain symptomatology than viral meningitis. The CSF is typically lymphocytic. In addition, papilledema, erythema migrans, or radiculoneuritis are commonly found in Lyme but not viral meningitis.[39] Cranial neuropathies are common, and demyelinative facial palsies can present bilaterally.[40,41] Other cranial nerves commonly involved include the optic nerve,[42] nerves III, IV, and VI (extraocular movement–related gaze abnormalities),[43] nerve V (trigeminal neuralgia symptoms),[44] and nerve VIII (hearing difficulty or loss and "buzzing" symptoms).[45-48] Cranial nerves IX–XII are less commonly involved.

Peripheral neuropathies (including median neuropathy) and sensorimotor polyradiculoneuropathies (painful, axonal involvement but often less fulminant than acute presentations) typically appear late during the disease course. A mild encephalopathy that presents with a confusional state is common[49] and does not necessarily occur in association with proven CNS invasion by the spirochete. Chronic encephalomyelitis occurs rarely.

Patients with *Borrelia* infection may present rarely with inflammatory demyelinating neuropathies,[50] brachial plexopathy,[51] mononeuritis multiplex,[52] Guillain-Barré syndrome,[53,54] motor neuron disease–like syndrome,[55] TM,[56] diaphragmatic paralysis,[57] or abdominal muscle weakness with increased girth.[58,59] The latter findings arise from denervation of lower thoracic paraspinal and rectus abdominus muscles. Some authors have described atypical presentations of Lyme neuroborreliosis with a relapsing-remitting course,[60] but whether patients with such symptoms coincidentally have MS has not clearly been resolved.

In addition, Lyme neuroborreliosis can present as an intracranial mass,[61] as has been seen with some atypical MS cases as well. Constitutional symptoms, such as weight loss and headaches, fatigue with fibromyalgia-like symptoms,[62–66] or behavioral disturbances may also occur. Patients with normal pressure hydrocephalus[67,68] improving after treatment of Lyme neuroborreliosis have been reported. In addition, the meningovascular involvement by the infection may lead to stroke and hemiparesis.[69] Finally, movement disorders reported in Lyme neuroborreliosis include chorea, dyskinesias,[70] myoclonus, or opsoclonus-myoclonus.[71,72]

Children present typically with lymphocytic meningitis, headaches, or isolated or multiple facial palsies, usually during the summer and fall months. Ipsilateral palsy from the site of a tick bite in the head or neck is common and suggests direct invasion by the spirochete.[73] These patients respond well to intravenous penicillin G or high-dose cephalosporins. A pseudotumor cerebri-like syndrome,[74] seizures, and failure to thrive[75] have also been described in children with Lyme disease. Meningoradiculitis and peripheral neuropathy are rare in children with Lyme infection.

We have encountered cases in our clinic of patients who have been treated for Lyme disease and present for consultation regarding new onset of MS. Serum immunoreactivity against *B. burgdorferi* but absence of CSF antibody titers are helpful hints in clarifying the clinical diagnosis of MS and not neuroborreliosis.[76] These MS patients raise the interesting question of whether MS is indeed a syndrome composed of several different etiologies (or known diseases), with an autoimmune, persistent response triggered by a foreign antigen (which may or may not persist in the organism after infection).

Upregulation of matrix metalloproteinase 9 activity has been demonstrated in the CSF of 84% of Lyme neuroborreliosis patients. This activity seems to originate in the macrophage population,[77] but astrocytes and neuronal cells are also stimulated to produce matrix metalloproteinase 9 by *B. burgdorferi* in vitro.[78] Similarly, a sixfold upregulation of soluble intracellular adhesion molecule 1 intrathecally has been demonstrated in Lyme neuroborreliosis patients.[79] Immunodominant epitopes of *Borrelia* and potential cross-reactive host epitopes that may trigger molecular mimicry are being investigated.[80]

Upregulated interleukin-6 and, to a lesser extent, increased interferon gamma have been shown in the brains of experimentally infected rhesus macaques with Lyme neuroborreliosis.[81] This nonhuman primate model develops erythema migrans at the site of inoculation and CNS infection with Western blot positivity and is considered a model that is highly representative of the human disease.[82]

Evidence is mounting to support an autoimmune component to central or peripheral nerve involvement by *B. burgdorferi*. Strong upregulation of B7-1 costimulatory molecules has been shown in epineurial infiltrates of sural nerve biopsies from patients with acute Lyme neuroborreliosis.[83] It has also been shown that *Borrelia* induces the expression of tumor necrosis factor-α and interleukin-1.[84–86] Whether these molecules are directed solely toward controlling the Lyme spirochete invasion or instead represent an autoimmune response triggered by the infection needs further investigation. Lyme patients demonstrate autoantibodies to neurons, myelin, and cardiolipin and have been also shown to produce rheumatoid factor and cryoglobulins.[87–91] In addition, shared antigenic determinants between *Borrelia* and axons, Schwann's cells, and myelin have been reported.[92] Studies examining the frequency of Lyme seropositivity in MS patients have yielded conflicting results.[92–94]

The initial antibody response to the spirochete appears as an immunoglobulin M (IgM) titer that peaks at 3–6 weeks, followed by IgG. Patients with Lyme may maintain IgG positivity for years, but in some, these titers fall. Therefore, antibody titer testing after treatment is useful only to document reinfection, which should course with a marked rise of titers. Investigators have demonstrated elevated antibodies in the CSF against myelin basic protein (MBP), especially in severe cases, and normalization of these levels in response to treatment. In addition, high levels of anti–*B. burgdorferi* IgG antibodies and an approximately 20-fold elevation of *B. burgdorferi*–reactive, interferon gamma–secreting T cells in the CSF of affected patients has been shown.[95] Others have confirmed complement membrane attack complexes and macrophage infiltrates around epineurial vessels and within the endoneurium.[96] Alternatively, upregulation of proinflammatory molecules and tissue infiltration by immune cells may be directed solely at attacking the spirochete, as nucleic acid from the micro-organism can in some cases be amplified from affected peripheral nerve. The demonstration that early treatment of neuroborreliosis does not abolish intrathecal IgM antibody synthesis by 6 months and that these antibodies are not directed against *B. burdorgferi*[97–100] suggests that host epitopes may be exposed by the acute infection and contribute to eliciting a chronic, ongoing inflammatory response. In summary, it is believed that most of the symptoms of Lyme neuroborreliosis are explained by the local presence of spirochetes in affected tissues; however, to some degree and especially in cases that become chronic despite proper treatment, parainfectious mechanisms (i.e., humoral or cellular autoimmune processes) may play a role.

In CSF studies, patients with Lyme meningitis may have a lymphocytic pleocytosis of 100–180 cells/mm^3, and most represent mononuclear cells. Protein is elevated at approximately 80 mg/dl. Oligoclonal bands are present in fewer than 50% of patients. Serologic testing by enzyme-linked immunosorbent assay is helpful. The most sensitive test to diagnose Lyme neuroborreliosis is the demonstration of antibodies against the spirochete in the CSF (positive in approximately 90% of neuroborreliosis cases). PCR in CSF for *Borrelia* may be useful very early in the disease process (before the production of antibodies), as current PCR methods in the CSF have limited sensitivities ranging from 17%[29,101] to 38%.[102] The antibody index, which detects intrathecal synthesis of specific antibodies against *Borrelia*,[103] is much more meaningful than simple antibody titers. Oligoclonal bands in Lyme neuroborreliosis CSF contain anti–*B. burgdorferi*–specific IgG antibodies,[104] and these may persist despite successful treatment. *Borrelia* can be cultured successfully from nearly one-third of erythema migrans skin biopsies, but PCR is more sensitive in these samples than cultures, as more than two-thirds of affected individuals test positive.[29] In patients with typical symptoms of neuroborreliosis, a negative serologic test with one strain should prompt testing with other strains of *B. burgdorferi*, as there is risk of false-negative results.[98,99]

Electrophysiologic testing often reveals a mild axonal sensorimotor polyradiculoneuropathy.[105,106] Atrioventricular block and intra-atrial conduction disturbances detected by electrocardiogram or by serial electrophysiologic studies signal lymphocytic myocarditis by the spirochete, and a gallium scan or a myocardial biopsy may be required.[36,37] Brain perfusion studies using technetium-99m hexamethylpropyleneamine oxime (^{99}mTc-HMPAO) single-photon emission computed tomography scanning have indicated diffuse decrease of cerebral blood flow sparing the cerebellar cortex in one patient,[107] but these studies are currently performed only for research purposes.

MRI may show gadolinium enhancement of affected cranial nerves,[108] and lesions typically involve the white matter in the brain.[109] Rarely, atrophy has been reported in association with Lyme infection.[110]

The diagnosis of Lyme neuroborreliosis is clinical; understanding the caveats of the confirmatory tests is critical in decision making for prescribing proper treatment. Positive enzyme-linked immunosorbent assay should be followed by a Western blot. Some authors have proposed long-term oral tetracyclines[111] for Lyme neuroborreliosis. Oral doxycycline (200–400 mg/day for 2 weeks) may be sufficient to treat facial palsy associated with Lyme seropositivity, and CSF findings that suggest inflammation (high white blood cell counts, high protein levels) tend to normalize.[112–114] Doxycycline penetrates the CSF at the previously recommended dose. An alternative treatment may be oral amoxicillin, 500–1,000 mg three times a day for 3–4 weeks. Proper, early treatment usually leads to substantial improvement of signs and symptoms, including hemiparesis, and even two rare cases of normal pressure hydrocephalus associated with Lyme disease[67,68] have responded dramatically to treatment. Interference with the outflow of CSF by the spirochete has been implicated in the development of this reversible type of normal pressure hydrocephalus. Intravenous ceftriaxone, 2 g per day, or cefotaxime (6 g/day) for 2–4 weeks leads to rapid recovery if patients are treated early; improvement is slower and may take months if the treatment is delayed until symptoms are advanced.[106] Although Lyme meningitis and some facial nerve palsy cases may be treated with oral doxycycline, intravenous treatment should be used for cases indicating diffuse CNS or PNS involvement (i.e., encephalopathy, meningitis, polyradiculoneuritis, encephalomyelitis, and severe, multifocal cranial neuropathies). The physician should be aware of the risks of overtreating patients; following strict diagnostic criteria and adhering to guidelines should minimize complications. Awareness of the Jarisch-Herxheimer reaction is also important, as 10–20% of patients undergoing treatment manifest it during the first 48 hours.

The prognosis is excellent in most cases of Lyme disease,[115] including those presenting with carditis,[116] if antibiotics are instituted early. In children with Lyme neuroborreliosis, early treatment prevents long-term cognitive sequelae.[117]

Subacute Sclerosing Panencephalitis

Subacute sclerosing panencephalitis is a rare late complication of measles in unimmunized children that is more likely to be confused with ADEM than with MS. It is caused by a persistent nonproductive infection by a defective measles virus and follows acute measles infection by an average of 8 years. CSF studies are generally normal with the exception of elevated anti-measles IgG. Brain MRI demonstrates T_2 hyperintensities in posterior gray and white matter. Periodic slow wave complexes can be seen on electroencephalogram.

Syphilis

Syphilis formerly was widely known as *the great imitator* because its manifestations could involve many organs, often presenting with symptoms or signs suggestive of other disorders. Diagnosis, then as now, depends on serologic testing. Serum RPR and the VDRL test continue to be important (and inexpensive) screening laboratory tests.

Involvement of the CNS by syphilis may lead to signs and symptoms that are common in MS, leading to diagnostic confusion. Pupillary abnormalities (classically, the small, irregular Argyll Robertson pupil that reacts to accommodation but not to light); ON; and myelopathy (tabes dorsalis) cause gait disorder, foot slap, paresthesias, bladder disturbances, impotence, loss of position, deep pain, and temperature sensations. The diagnostic confusion may persist when the MRI shows white-matter abnormalities and diffuse atrophy.[118,119] A favorable response to glucocorticosteroids may occur in neurosyphilis as in MS, further confounding the diagnosis.

Radiographic features that should suggest a diagnosis of secondary neurosyphilis include prominent meningeal enhancement or the presence of gummata. However, gadolinium contrast is not always administered when MRI is performed, and particular radiographic features may be absent in a given case. Laboratory findings that should raise suspicion for neurosyphilis include high levels of protein in CSF, with or without leukocytic pleocytosis.

Confirmatory testing requires a more specific test, such as fluorescent *Treponema pallidum* absorption or a microhemoagglutination assay with *T. pallidum* antigen. It should be recognized that the antibody titers detected by serologic testing can vary, depending on the stage of disease and the immune competence of the infected individual. For example, the RPR is highly sensitive during secondary syphilis but insensitive during primary or tertiary syphilis, with false-negative rates as high as 30%. The *Treponema*-specific tests are more sensitive and are appropriate screening assays when clinical suspicion of syphilis is high, but all the serologic tests can give a false-negative result (reviewed in reference 120). Thus, where the diagnosis is strongly suspected, the full neurosyphilis treatment regimen should be administered.

Therapy for neurosyphilis involves a course of high-dose parenteral penicillin. Regimens differ, but one standard is 20 MIU of intravenous penicillin G daily for 10 days. An alternative is 2.4 MIU of intramuscular penicillin G benzathine injections, supplemented with oral probenecid, 500 mg four times daily for 28 consecutive days. The single-dose penicillin treatment customarily used for primary syphilis is inadequate to achieve treponemicidal levels in CSF and to prevent relapse of neurosyphilis. Indeed, relapses may occur even after completion of the recommended course of neurosyphilis treatment. Individuals infected with human immunodeficiency virus may be at particular risk for relapse after treatment for syphilis.

Whipple's Disease

Whipple's disease is a rare, multiorgan disease that can produce protean manifestations, including neurologic symptoms in 20% of cases.[121] Infection was long suspected as the etiology, but the causative organism has only recently been established as an actinomycetes bacterium and named *Tropheryma whippelii*. Although concurrent small-bowel involvement (e.g., malabsorption, diarrhea) is most common, some cases present with isolated CNS involvement.[122–124] The histopathology is granulomatous, and lesions usually appear on MRI as ring-enhancing lesions mainly in the white matter and at the gray-white-matter junction.[123,125,126] Rarely, ON or cervical myelopathy can be attributed to Whipple's disease.[127] Up to 20% of patients with neurologic involvement[121] develop an abnormality that is considered pathognomonic for CNS Whipple's disease. This is oculomasticatory myorhythmia, characterized by pendular convergent-divergent oscillations of the eyes synchronous with involuntary rhythmic contraction of the muscles of mastication at a rate of approximately one per second. Another form of the disorder is oculo-facial-skeletal myorhythmia, characterized by synchronous movements of muscles of the extremities and face at the one-per-second rate. Whipple's disease can also manifest more limited oculomotor signs, such as supranuclear vertical gaze palsy or internuclear ophthalmoplegia.[128]

However, many cases of CNS Whipple's disease are not diagnosed until after death. Even in the absence of the pathognomonic signs, a diagnosis of CNS Whipple's disease should be considered in the setting of neurologic signs with concomitant malabsorption diarrhea or weight loss, arthralgias, or inflammatory cardiac disease (pericarditis, myocarditis, or valvular endocarditis). A small-bowel biopsy is often diagnostic, although in approximately 30% of patients, no abnormality is present. In patients with only CNS involvement, a stereotactic brain biopsy can be performed under local anesthesia, but PCR of the blood[129] or CSF to detect the 16S ribosomal RNA of *T. whippelii* may be more sensitive.[130]

Whipple's disease is potentially fatal but may respond dramatically to antibiotic treatment. CNS Whipple's disease can be more resistant to therapy and more prone to relapse.[131] Indeed, the CNS is the most common site for post-treatment relapse.[132] Currently, the recommended initial treatment for CNS Whipple's disease is a combination of parenteral penicillin and streptomycin for at least 14 days, followed by either clotrimoxazole orally 3 times a day for 2 years[132,133] or ceftriaxone parenterally for 1 month followed by 2 years of oral

cefixime.[134] It is important that the patient is closely monitored throughout the duration of treatment because of the potential for relapse despite therapy. Serial brain imaging by MRI is an effective modality for monitoring.

Probable Multiple Sclerosis Variants and Other Localized Neurologic Immune-Mediated Syndromes

Baló's Concentric Sclerosis

Certain atypical patterns of demyelination are sufficiently distinctive or have been observed with sufficient regularity to require a moniker. Alternating areas of demyelinated and myelinated white matter in a concentric pattern are the hallmark of Baló's concentric sclerosis. Aside from their striking concentric arrangement, the demyelinating lesions are similar to those associated with MS. The histopathologic findings include perivascular cuffs, demyelinating lesions of apparently varying ages, and remyelination at the fringes of older lesions and in the bands of less-affected white matter within the concentric lesions. The clinical and histopathologic similarities to MS suggest that Baló's sclerosis is best considered a form of atypical MS. Although Baló's sclerosis–type demyelination often behaves as a fulminant disorder, even extending to involve large portions of a cerebral hemisphere, recovery can also occur, particularly if the patient is treated with corticosteroids. Relapses may occur.

Serial imaging studies in cases of Baló's sclerosis have shed light on the formation of the concentric lesions. One study[135] showed that the layering does not form simultaneously but develops step by step in a centrifugal direction. The development of lesions was preceded by an enhancing ring relatively devoid of demyelination and was followed by progressive demyelination occurring mainly at the inner aspect of the enhancement. The same process recurred on the edge of the previous enhanced zone. Conflicting findings were reported in another case,[136] wherein the concentric demyelinated bands were observed to form simultaneously, not centrifugally. In either case, the pathogenetic mechanisms that led to the concentric pattern of demyelination remain obscure.

Cerebellitis

Acute, isolated ataxia may occur after viral illnesses, most frequently with varicella infections. Cerebellar ataxia accounts for one-half of the postvaricella neurologic syndromes, which overall occur in 1 in 1,000 cases of childhood varicella. The prognosis for recovery is excellent. Duration of symptoms varies from a few days up to 3–4 weeks.

Combined Central and Peripheral Demyelinating Disease

Combined central and peripheral demyelinating disease may be a postinfectious disorder or a complication after administration of vaccines not known to contain PNS and CNS tissue. Cases after swine flu vaccination have been reported. Reports of combined central and peripheral demyelination syndromes do exist, in which onion bulb formation in the PNS is demonstrated, indicating recurrent demyelination and remyelination. Some cases have clinical features consistent with MS. It remains uncertain whether combined demyelination represents a chance coincidence or a distinct disease.

Devic's Disease

Neuromyelitis optica (Devic's disease) is a rare clinical syndrome of unilateral or bilateral ON and TM occurring within an 8-week interval. Neuromyelitis optica is often assumed to be a variant of MS, and certainly many cases presenting with concurrent ON and myelitis do appear on long-term follow-up to have typical MS. Nonetheless, evidence in other cases indicates that Devic's disease may be a different disease altogether. Clinical laboratory findings that have been suggested as indicative of Devic's disease in distinction to MS include CSF pleocytosis (more than 50 cells/mm^3), particularly if polymorphonuclear cells are present[137]; CSF protein (more than 500 mg/dl)[138,139]; and absence of oligoclonal bands.[138–140] Imaging findings that should raise suspicion for Devic's disease include T_1 hypointense lesions in the spinal cord[141] and a persistent absence of white-matter abnormalities beyond the spinal cord or optic nerves. Researchers seeking beyond the usual diagnostic tests have reported that MS

patients typically have increased levels of tissue metalloproteinases in the CSF, but this biochemical abnormality was not found in a small series of Devic's disease cases.[142]

Neuromyelitis optica has been reported as a sequela to a variety of infections, including varicella,[143] *Mycobacterium tuberculosis*,[144] and mycoplasma.[145] Cases have also been reported in association with collagen-vascular disorders, including systemic lupus erythematosis (reviewed in references 146–151) and Sjögren's syndrome.[152] The pathogenesis of the disorder is uncertain. Pathologic examination of Devic's disease cases consistently finds necrotizing lesions in white-matter tracts of the spinal cord and optic nerves and finds minimal inflammation without the perivascular lymphocyte cuffing observed in MS. Some investigators have reported thickening of blood vessel walls in affected areas,[153] whereas others report that blood vessels were not affected.[138,154]

Inasmuch as Devic's myelopathy is necrotizing rather than demyelinating, the prognosis of this syndrome is poor. Still, substantial recovery of function may occur in individual cases. The disorder is too rare to permit large-scale drug treatment trials. Treatments that have been reported effective in small series or anecdotal reports include glucocorticoids, glucocorticoids plus azathioprine,[155] and lymphocytoplasmapheresis.[156]

Eales' Disease

Eales' disease is an idiopathic retinal perivasculitis characterized by recurrent retinal and vitreous hemorrhages. Extraocular CNS involvement occurs and may present with symptoms suggestive of MS together with an MRI appearance[157] and abnormal brain stem auditory and somatosensory evoked potentials[158] similar to those of MS. The neurologic symptoms may improve with glucocorticosteroids, further confounding the diagnosis. Any level of the CNS may be involved in Eales' disease, but the most common neurologic picture is an acute or subacute myelopathy occurring at an interval of a few weeks to a few years after the eye episode.[159] The histopathology of CNS lesions in Eales' disease is primarily demyelination after a perivenous distribution,[160] but cerebral infarction also may result from Eales' vasculitis.[161–163]

The diagnosis of Eales' disease should be suggested first by a history or finding of retinal or vitreous hemorrhages in a patient with CNS white-matter abnormalities. Differentiation of Eales' disease and MS is facilitated by analysis of the CSF, which in Eales' disease cases may show substantial elevations in leukocytes and total protein, beyond the range typical of MS.[164–166]

Gluten-Sensitive Ataxia and Related Syndromes

A number of neurologic syndromes have been described in association with the autoimmune gastrointestinal disorder known variously as *celiac disease*, nontropical sprue, or *gluten-sensitive enteropathy*. Celiac disease is precipitated by ingestion of the protein gliadin, a component of wheat gluten, and usually resolves on its withdrawal. Celiac disease–associated villous atrophy is a cause of intestinal malabsorption, but the neurologic syndrome can develop in the absence of apparent malabsorption or, indeed, any gastrointestinal symptoms, so that neurologic disorders may be the presenting symptom. Gluten-sensitive neurologic disorders most commonly include ataxia, memory impairment and neuropathy; internuclear opthalmoplegia, progressive multifocal leukoencephalopathy, dementia, epilepsy, and myoclonus have also been reported.

MRI may reveal isolated cerebellar atrophy affecting the vermis and hemispheres in many cases with gluten-sensitive ataxia[167] but, in other cases, the MRI shows patchy or confluent cerebral white-matter involvement mimicking MS.[168,169] Neuropathologic findings (reviewed in reference 170) may vary with the clinical syndrome. Cerebellar ataxia appears to correlate with Purkinje cell loss, whereas cases with sensory ataxia or pyramidal tract symptoms may have demyelination in the spinal cord and neuropathy. Infiltration of T-lymphocytes in the brain and perivascular cuffing with inflammatory cells are found in only a subset of cases, calling into question the role of cellular immune responses in disease pathogenesis.

Although gluten ingestion precipitates the disorder, the pathogenesis of the intestinal disorder involves an autoimmune reaction to an enzyme—tissue transglutaminase[171]—that avidly binds gliadin protein present in gluten. It is not yet proven that this same enzyme is the target for autoimmunity in the CNS. Detection of serum IgA or IgG antibodies to tissue transglutaminase provides the most sensitive and specific screening test for celiac disease. These antibodies are often detected by their reactivity with endomysium (i.e., anti-endomysial antibodies) in immunofluorescence assays. Small-bowel biopsy and human leukocyte antigen (HLA) typing are useful in establishing the diagnosis.

The genetics of celiac disease is an active area of investigation (reviewed in references 172 and 173). The disorder is strongly linked to the susceptibility locus in the major histocompatibility complex region, with a particular association with DQ2 and DQ8. The HLA-DQ alleles identified by molecular genotyping are DQA1*0501 and DQB1*0201. However, it is clear that non–major histocompatibility complex loci also contribute to susceptibility. A polymorphism of cytotoxic T lymphocyte antigen 4 is associated with increased risk in some populations. Infection with hepatitis C virus may predispose to celiac disease[174] in genetically susceptible individuals.

Treatment of gluten-sensitive disorders involves lifelong dietary restriction to eliminate gluten-containing foods. The response to a gluten-free diet is variable; in some cases, the neurologic symptoms entirely resolve, whereas other cases experience progressive neurologic deterioration. Information regarding the disease and gluten-free diets is available from the Celiac Sprue Association on the World Wide Web: http://www.csaceliacs.org.

Marburg Variant (Acute Fulminant Multiple Sclerosis)

Severe, acute demyelination has been termed the *Marburg variant of MS*. This variant may be suspected with a large acute lesion of one hemisphere or, rarely, the spinal cord. Much of the T_2 lesion volume is edema and usually rapidly responds to corticosteroids. Biopsy is often required to exclude a malignancy. Rapidly developing brain lesions may lead to quadriplegia, blindness, or obtundation or coma and sometimes lead to death. Subsequent to recovery, the disease may follow a more typical relapsing-remitting course.[175]

The pathology in Marburg-type MS is inflammatory and demyelinating.[176] Biochemical investigation in a single case of Marburg-type MS identified an unusual post-translational modification of MBP that might adversely affect its ability to stabilize the myelin sheath and that increases MBP susceptibility to proteolytic degradation and formation of an encephalitogenic peptide.[177–181] Although plausible, a pathogenetic role for this modification of MBP has not yet been proven.

Optic Neuritis

Simultaneous bilateral ON is rare in MS, except in Devic's disease. The estimated incidence of subsequent development of MS after an initial episode of ON varies widely among different series, from less than 20% to more than 70%. T_2 hyperintensities on brain MRI are an important predictor of risk of developing MS after ON.[182]

Progressive Myelopathy

Slowly progressive spinal cord dysfunction can present a diagnostic challenge. If there are no sensory symptoms, primary lateral sclerosis may be the cause. Human T-cell leukemia virus type 1 infection, vitamin B_{12} deficiency, and human immunodeficiency virus infection all can be excluded by appropriate testing. Spinal dural arteriovenous fistula can cause a steadily or stepwise progressive myelopathy, usually in the lower spinal segments and can be difficult to detect without spinal angiography. Adrenomyeloneuropathy should also be considered. Some patients do not fit into these categories, and spinal MRI as well as brain MRI, spinal fluid assessment, and electrophysiology results may be negative. In these cases, no diagnosis is possible. Significant cervical intervertebral disk disease may be difficult to assess in middle-aged patients because most have some disk disease. Progressive myelopathy may represent the primary progressive form of MS, which carries a poor prognosis.

Schilder's Disease (Myelinoclastic Diffuse Sclerosis)

Schilder's disease, a very rare disorder, presents with large, lobar demyelinating lesions with a destructive component, sometimes termed *tumefactive demyelination*. The lobar lesions may be bilateral and symmetric. Histopathologic findings are indistinguishable from those of MS, especially the Marburg variant, and it has been suggested that Schilder's disease is a variant of MS.[183] A diagnosis of Schilder's disease cannot be established unless adrenoleukodystrophy has been ruled out by biochemical analysis. This disorder occurs more often in children or young adolescents but on occasion has been described in adults.[184,185] Schilder's disease causes symptoms appropriate to the site of cerebral involvement, often blindness, limb paralysis, and mental deterioration. The natural history of the disease is variable and may be monophasic, relapsing-remitting, or progressive and fatal. Treatment with glucocorticoids appears to improve recovery in at least some cases.[186]

Transverse Myelitis

TM is an isolated spinal cord dysfunction that evolves over hours or days in patients with no evidence of a compressive lesion. Some patients report a preceding febrile illness. The initial symptoms are paresthesias, back pain, or leg weakness. Patients have the maximal deficit within 1–10 days. The prognosis may be worse in the rapid-onset group of patients. Only approximately 7% of patients with complete TM develop MS by clinical criteria. Acute TM may occur on a background of systemic vasculitis. One must distinguish complete TM from the partial or incomplete syndromes, as the latter predict evolution to MS in 50–90% of patients.

Acquired Metabolic and Hereditary Genetic Disorders

A complete discussion of childhood dysmyelinating disorders is included in Chapter 4.

Adrenoleukodystrophy and Adrenomyeloneuropathy

Although best known as the cause of adrenoleukodystrophy (ALD) in childhood, abnormalities in the metabolism of VLCFAs can also present as neurologic disorders in adults. Classically, young adults with the disorder develop adrenomyeloneuropathy (AMN), but reports of cases with adult-onset cerebral involvement have considerably widened the phenotypic spectrum. These disorders should be considered whenever appropriate neurologic symptoms are accompanied by evidence of adrenal cortical dysfunction, such as Addison's disease or hypergonadotropic hypogonadism.

Although ALD and AMN differ clinically, the underlying genetic and biochemical abnormalities are the same: an elevation in VLCFA that can present with demyelinating spinal cord or cerebral involvement, alone or in combination. Indeed, individual kindreds may include some individuals with ALD and others with AMN. The spinal form usually is manifested as a slowly progressive myelopathy causing spastic paraparesis or spinocerebellar ataxia, sphincter dysfunction, and impotence. The cerebral form manifests as progressive dementia and ataxia. ALD and AMN are inherited as X-linked recessive traits, although carriers (heterozygotes) can also be symptomatic. A form of ALD is seen in up to 20% of women who are carriers of the disorder.[187] In heterozygotes, symptoms usually progress slowly but can become moderately severe and may include spastic paraparesis of the lower limbs, ataxia, mild peripheral neuropathy, and urinary control problems.

The endocrine dysfunction associated with the disorder is highly variable in its severity. The endocrine disturbance may be severe or asymptomatic, although evidence of glandular involvement is always evident when tissues are examined pathologically. The hypogonadism may cause pubertal delay or be sufficiently mild to permit fertility.

The phenotypic variability associated with elevated VLCFA extends even to monozygotic twins.[188] Clearly, nongenetic factors are important determinants of disease pathogenesis. There is circumstantial evidence that immunologic factors contribute to the pathogenesis of the CNS lesions in ALD.

The gene responsible for X-linked ALD/AMN encodes a peroxisomal membrane protein, ALDP, which is a member of the ABC (adenosine triphosphate–binding cassette) transporter superfamily. The defective peroxisomes are unable to metabolize unbranched saturated fatty acids with a chain length from 24 to 30 carbons, particularly the 26-carbon hexacosanoate. The disease results from accumulation of these VLCFAs in the cholesterol esters of

brain white matter and in adrenal cortex. The accumulating long-chain fatty acids are, at least in part, of exogenous origin, lending support to approaches for the dietary control of disease progression, the most famous being "Lorenzo's oil," a combination of oleic and erucic acids.

Lorenzo's oil has been studied as a treatment for ALD and AMN. Consistently, such dietary therapy succeeds in normalizing the serum levels of VLCFAs, but nonetheless has disappointing clinical efficacy[189] and can have substantial toxicity.[189] Similarly, MRI studies have not shown regression of leukodystrophy with treatment.[190,191] Bone marrow transplantation (BMT) can be strikingly effective when performed early in the disease course.[192,193] Inhibitors of 3-hydroxy-3-methylglutaryl coenzyme A reductase (e.g., lovastatin and simvastatin) have recently been shown to normalize plasma VLCFA levels[194]; their efficacy is being studied in clinical trials. Gene therapy aimed at replacing the defective enzymes could theoretically cure the disorder. Adrenoleukodystrophy-related gene transfer can correct VLCFA accumulation in adrenoleukodystrophy fibroblasts in vitro,[195] but no satisfactory methods for somatic cell gene therapy of the brain are currently available.

Adult Polyglucosan Body Disease

Adult polyglucosan body disease (also known as *glycogen-branching enzyme deficiency*) is a rare glycogen storage disease. A more profound deficiency of the same enzyme appears responsible for the fatal early childhood disorder known as *glycogen storage disease type IV*.[196] Inheritance is usually autosomal recessive and usually occurs in patients of Ashkenazi Jewish origin. This clinicopathologic entity is usually manifested as progressive upper and lower motor neuron dysfunction, sensory loss in the lower extremities, neurogenic bladder, and often dementia. As an adult-onset, progressive gait disturbance with urinary incontinence, its presentation may lead to diagnostic confusion with MS. This confusion may be compounded by MRI of the brain revealing extensive leukoencephalopathy. A variant presentation has been reported, with dementia of frontal lobe type and neurogenic bladder but no symptoms of sensory motor peripheral neuropathy or gait disorder.[197]

The histopathologic hallmark of the disease is a profusion of microscopic bodies resembling corpora amylacea or Lafora bodies but restricted to processes of neurons and astrocytes. Similar but especially large bodies are seen within axons of peripheral nerves.

Alcohol-Related Disorders

Some of the clinical manifestations of alcohol-related diseases can mimic MS. Alcoholism has been defined as a disease. Alcohol-related neuropathologic changes seen in the brain vary considerably. They may be the result of direct toxicity to the neurons or related to dietary factors, such as malnutrition and folate-thiamine deficiency. Generalized atrophy as a result of loss of white matter has been noted. More specifically, cortical atrophy secondary to neuronal loss occurs in the superior frontal regions and in cerebellum. Neuronal loss is also seen in the hypothalamus and other regions of the diencephalon. A relationship has been observed between alcohol and increased risk of stroke. Alcohol is thought to increase the friability of the vascular bed. Therefore, at autopsy, there is often evidence of changes consistent with old scars as a result of strokes.[198] White-matter lesions similar to those seen in MS may be present. However, because of the impact on many systems in the body, the manifestations of this disease are multifocal. Three important alcohol-related neurologic disorders are described here.

Marchiafava-Bignami Disease

Marchiafava-Bignami disease is a rare disorder that is seen in cases of chronic alcoholism, but there have been some reported cases in nonalcoholics. The clinical course is varied, and symptoms differ in the acute, subacute, and chronic stages.[199] The clinical features range from a change in mental status with confusional state, rigidity of the extremities to seizures, and death.[200] Dysarthria and apraxia have been reported.[201] Steroid treatment has been successfully used in the treatment of this disease. It is postulated that the presence of early edema may have an impact on the integrity of the blood-brain barrier. Steroid treatment, therefore, may help to restore the blood-brain barrier to its original state.[202]

Treatment with vitamin B supplementation has also been reported to improve the clinical status.[203] Severe global dementia is seen in the late stages of the disease.[204] A syndrome of interhemispheric disconnection is seen in many patients. Signs such as mutism, alexia with agraphia, and impaired language comprehension and constructional ability have been observed.[205]

Pathology consists of extrapontine myelinolysis, atrophy, and demyelinating lesions of the corpus callosum. Myelin sheaths show disseminated, perivascular, spongy degeneration. Sclerosis and perivascular gliosis of blood vessels are also observed.[206]

Imaging studies show hyperintense T_2 lesions located in the corpus callosum on MRI.[202] The lesions are typically large and symmetric and located in the midline in the splenium of the corpus callosum.[207] Swelling of the corpus callosum has been observed. Other reports[201] have made similar observations of symmetric isointense lesions on T_1-weighted images and hyperintense lesions on T_2-weighted and fluid-attenuated inversion recovery (FLAIR) images, located in the body and splenium of the corpus callosum. On diffusion-weighted images, these lesions may be hyperintense. This is not the case in MS; thus, "bright" diffusion-weighted images may be used to differentiate the two diseases. Imaging performed at various stages of the disease show the development of fluidlike layers in the corpus callosum, which eventually become lesions with central hypointense necrotic cores surrounded by a hyperintense rim of demyelination.[208] Atrophy of the corpus callosum eventually occurs. Cortical and subcortical atrophy is also present.

Central Pontine Myelinolysis

The central pontine myelinolysis disorder usually presents with cranial nerve signs related to the brain stem. It may be caused by rapid, aggressive, and excessive correction of hyponatremia, which results in lesions in the central pons evolving over a period of 48 hours. It is also seen in the setting of alcohol toxicity. Because central pontine myelinolysis is often observed in malnourished alcoholics, nutritional deficiency has been proposed as its cause. However, it is now thought that a combination of factors, including metabolic derangements and nutritional factors, may play a role. MRI demonstrates confluent hyperintense lesions on T_2-weighted images, located centrally and bilaterally in the pons.

Wernicke-Korsakoff Syndrome

The Wernicke-Korsakoff syndrome is seen in the later stages of alcoholism. A hallmark finding is atrophy of the opercula. This pathologic abnormality is thought to be the cause of the amnestic syndrome seen in alcoholics with Korsakoff dementia.[209] Wernicke's encephalopathy presents with altered mental status, ataxia, and nystagmus and is associated with thiamine deficiency.

Autosomal Dominant Leukodystrophy

Autosomal dominant leukodystrophy can mimic primary-progressive MS. Autosomal dominant leukodystrophy differs from MS, however, in the strikingly symmetric appearance of white-matter lesions. The autosomal dominant leukodystrophy gene localizes to chromosomal region 5q31.[210]

Cerebral Autosomal Dominant Arteriopathy with Subcortical Infarcts and Leukoencephalopathy

Cerebral autosomal dominant arteriopathy with subcortical infarcts and leukoencephalopathy (CADASIL) was named in 1991.[211] In its prototypic presentation, the episodic pattern of neurologic symptoms in young adults, together with white-matter lesions on MRI, may erroneously suggest a diagnosis of MS. Since its original description, the phenotypic spectrum of CADASIL has broadened considerably. In addition to stroke, the presenting symptom in CADASIL may be migraine,[212–215] seizures,[216] dementia,[217,218] or even a psychiatric illness.[215,219,220] Any of the foregoing may occur in the absence of stroke-like episodes. Although a family history of neurologic disease can usually be elicited, the diverse manifestations of CADASIL may prevent its being recognized as a heritable condition. Moreover, CADASIL can also occur in sporadic cases because of de novo mutations in the causative gene.[221]

Although the various clinical phenomena associated with CADASIL may occur alone or in com-

bination, a progression of symptoms is typically observed.[215] Migraine-like headaches with or without aura are frequently an early symptom of the disease. Recurrent episodes of transient ischemic attack or stroke often occur in individuals with history of migraine. Slowly progressive subcortical dementia often develops at a later stage.

The underlying cause of CADASIL is a characteristic angiopathy of small and medium-sized cerebral arteries. Ultrastructural analysis reveals electron-dense granular deposits in the basal lamina of the vessels. The genetic abnormality causing CADASIL involves a variety of mutations in the *Notch3* gene on chromosome 19p. All known CADASIL mutations are similar in that they increase or decrease the number of cysteines within the epidermal growth factor–like repeats of the Notch3 protein.[222]

Brain MRI and computed tomography typically show scattered white-matter lesions or diffuse leukoencephalopathy, which may easily be mistaken for demyelinating disease. One-third of cases may have white-matter hyperintensities in the absence of small deep infarcts on T_1-weighted images.[223] Radiographic evidence of lesions in gray matter (most commonly in the basal ganglia and thalamus) should provide a clue that a diagnosis of MS may be in error. The diagnosis of CADASIL may be confirmed either by genetic testing of the *Notch3* gene or by electron microscopic examination of skin[214,224] or muscle[225] biopsies to detect the characteristic vasculopathy.

Fabry's Disease

Fabry's disease is an X-linked recessive lysosomal storage disorder caused by a deficiency of alpha-galactosidase A. Intracellular accumulation of globotriaosylceramide, the glycolipid substrate of this enzyme, leads to severe painful small-fiber neuropathy with progressive renal, cardiovascular, and cerebrovascular dysfunction and death by middle age. Neuropathic pain may be an early and presenting symptom and, although the pain may be very severe, routine physical examination and electrophysiology may fail to detect any neurologic abnormality. Moreover, other neurologic manifestations may include progressive sensorineural hearing loss and vertigo. The scattered brain lesions in Fabry's disease, T_2-hyperintense on MRI, may be confined to white matter in up to one-third of cases,[226] leading to misdiagnosis as MS.

Features of Fabry's disease that might provide a clue to the diagnosis include (1) physical stigmata, such as reddish-purple angiokeratomas in skin and mucous membranes, and characteristic benign corneal abnormalities; (2) concomitant renal or cardiac failure or strokes; or (3) autonomic dysfunction,[227] classically manifested as episodic abdominal pain but also including reduced sweating.

Anticonvulsant medications, such as carbamazepine, may alleviate the neuropathic pain, although autonomic dysfunction may be exacerbated.[228] The finding of a marked decreased activity of alpha-galactosidase A in white blood cells or cultured skin fibroblasts confirms the diagnosis.

Familial Ataxias

The familial ataxias are heterogeneous, both clinically and genetically. These varied disorders present with symptoms that are common in MS and, in some cases, also resemble MS in their MRI appearance. Some types of familial ataxia are highly treatable and deserve special consideration in the differential diagnosis of MS presenting with ataxia.

Clinically, the heritable ataxias may present with a bewildering variety of associated neurologic and systemic symptoms. Genetically, subtypes have been described with autosomal recessive, autosomal dominant, X-linked, and mitochondrial inheritance. The nosology of heritable ataxias promulgated by Harding[229] has undergone revision in recent years as the genetic basis for many ataxias has been elucidated (recently reviewed in references 230–232). We do not attempt to review this subject comprehensively or to describe all the subtypes. Instead, we focus here on subtypes that may pose a particular diagnostic challenge in cases of possible MS and on clues that may help to differentiate the heritable ataxias from MS.

Ataxia with vitamin E deficiency (reviewed in reference 233) is an autosomal recessive condition usually associated with a defect in the alpha-tocopherol transfer protein. Symptom onset may be in childhood or adult years. Clinically, it manifests as a progressive ataxia with a phenotype resembling that of Friedreich's ataxia. Diagnosis is established by assay of serum vitamin E level or by genetic assay for mutations in the alpha-tocopherol transfer protein gene. Supplementation with vitamin E is highly effective in arresting or reversing the neurologic symptoms.

The episodic ataxias (EAs) are perhaps misnamed, as cerebellar or oculomotor abnormalities are common even between attacks. At least two subtypes are recognized, EA-1 and EA-2. In both subtypes, peak symptoms during an episode last from one to several hours. EA-1 is an autosomal dominant syndrome characterized by myokymia and periodic ataxia, associated with mutations in the potassium channel gene *KCNA1* on chromosome 12.[234] Phenytoin reportedly produces good control of the symptoms. EA-2 is also an autosomal dominant disorder but has a more complex phenotype. Some of the complexity is introduced by the fact that familial hemiplegic migraine and spinocerebellar ataxia type 6 are associated with mutations in the same calcium channel gene, *CACNA1A*, and have overlapping clinical phenotypes. Spinocerebellar ataxia type 6 results from a CAG-repeat expansion in the gene[235]; EA-2 and familial hemiplegic migraine are more often associated with point mutations in the gene but also occur in patients with small CAG-repeat expansions.[236] Although the disorders are inherited in an autosomal dominant manner, the penetrance is variable; some carriers may not show any clinical symptoms.[237] Family history may be lacking for this reason and also because the point mutations can readily arise de novo.[238] Thus, a diagnosis of EA-2 should be entertained in patients with EA even without a family history, particularly because it is treatable: Acetazolamide can reverse most of or all the symptoms in many cases.[239]

The autosomal dominant spinocerebellar ataxias can mimic progressive MS clinically, causing ataxia, weakness and spasticity affecting the lower extremities, and Babinski's sign; some subtypes are accompanied by vision loss. MRI may be helpful in diagnosing some of the subtypes, particularly those in which the white matter is normal and the cerebellum and perhaps the brain stem show atrophy. Where vision loss occurs, ocular funduscopy may show pigmentary retinopathy. Genetic tests are available to detect the trinucleotide repeat expansions associated with several of the spinocerebellar ataxias.

Friedreich's ataxia typically causes incoordination of limb movements, dysarthria and nystagmus,

Babinski's sign, and impairment of position and vibratory senses. These signs are also common in MS, although in Friedreich's ataxia, the symptoms are progressive and unremitting. An important clue to the diagnosis is diminished or absent tendon reflexes rather than the exaggerated reflexes commonly occurring in MS patients. The triad of hypoactive knee and ankle jerks, signs of progressive cerebellar dysfunction, and preadolescent onset is commonly regarded as sufficient for diagnosis of Friedreich's ataxia, although occasional patients first develop symptoms in adulthood.[240] The disease is caused by mutations in the frataxin gene on chromosome 9. More than 90% of patients are homozygous for GAA trinucleotide repeat expansions in the first intron of the frataxin gene. The trinucleotide repeat expansions generally contain between 100 and several thousand copies; normally, there are fewer than 20 repeats. The remaining cases are compound heterozygotes for a GAA expansion and a frataxin point mutation. In cases with such genetic heterozygosity, the phenotype may vary from that of classic Friedreich's ataxia. For example, the tendon reflexes may be retained, and optic pallor may occur.[241] The pathogenesis of Friedreich's ataxia remains incompletely understood. No treatment has been shown to slow the disease progression.

Hypoxia-Anoxia

Anoxic brain injury produces an encephalopathy. A most frequently reported deficit in cases of anoxia is memory loss. Other sequelae are personality changes, behavioral changes, and visuospatial deficits. An unusual clinical presentation seen in the setting of anoxia is "the man in the barrel" syndrome. This is secondary to bilateral hypoxic border-zone infarcts in the frontal lobe cortex.[242] The phenomenon of Ondine's curse is due to hypoxic events causing an impact on the brain stem and producing disturbances in respiratory function.[243] A frontal lobe-like syndrome described as loss of drive, inertia, and stereotypical activities has also been seen, as well as extrapyramidal signs. Lesions restricted to white matter are uncommonly associated with hypoxic injuries.

Carbon monoxide (CO) poisoning results in a syndrome of delayed post-anoxic encephalopathy.

CO poisoning is the most common accidental poisoning in the United States. It is also associated with suicide attempts. It results in an anoxic-ischemic encephalopathy targeting the gray matter predominantly but with white-matter involvement as well. In the white matter, the periventricular and subcortical areas, corpus callosum, and internal capsule are all affected.[244] In the gray matter, the globus pallidus appears to be the most common site affected.[245] Speech and gait disturbance with pyramidal signs and clumsiness of the hands occurs in individuals with CO poisoning. The sequelae of CO poisoning may include personality changes and cognitive delay.[246] Visual agnosia secondary to lesions in the parieto-occipital regions, parkinsonian signs related to lesions in the basal ganglia, apathy, and memory deficits are observed clinical signs. Tics and obsessive compulsive disorder have been reported.

Cerebral hypoxic-ischemic events occur during episodes of hypotension and result from hypoperfusion of the cerebral tissue. This is particularly noted to occur during surgical intervention, such as cardiac and neurosurgical procedures. Cardiac arrhythmias, episodes of bradycardia, and cardiac ischemia or infarction may result in similar hypoxic episodes or anoxic events involving the basal ganglia. Vascular stenosis or occlusion, particularly in the vertebrobasilar artery territory, may lead to ischemia or infarction of the brain stem with similar results.

In renal disease patients who receive intravenous fluids, care is taken to avoid episodes of acute pulmonary edema that may result in hypoxemia. An overdose of illegal drugs, such as heroin, may produce ischemic lesions in the globus pallidus and cerebral hypoxia. Cocaine is known to produce vasospasm, increasing the risk of stroke. Subclinical or silent anoxic vascular events related to cocaine involving the white and gray matter have been seen on imaging studies. An ischemic-embolic picture has been described for the lesions attributed to heroin. Near-drowning can produce a severe anoxic encephalopathy or hypoxemia. Pulmonary edema aspiration pneumonia or pneumothorax is thought to be the precipitating factor. The duration of submersion is the main factor with regard to severity of symptoms.

Imaging studies in patients with anoxia-hypoxia display demyelinating lesions in the periventricular white matter. However, unlike MS, frequently present are cortical watershed-border zone infarcts that are the result of hypoperfusion in areas that are at the ends of arterial territories. The parieto-occipital and temporal lobes are frequent sites of watershed infarcts. Lesions in the basal ganglia are a hallmark sign of anoxia-hypoxia. The thalamus, hippocampus, pons, and cerebellum are often affected. Medial temporal lobe atrophy involving the hippocampal and parahippocampal regions often develops after anoxia, which is best seen on MRI in the coronal plane.[247] More specific is the pattern seen with CO poisoning, displaying general cerebral atrophy, hippocampal atrophy, and lesions in the globus pallidus. In the acute state, FLAIR images may show the presence of demyelinating lesions in the deep white matter.

Inherited Spastic Paraparesis

Familial spastic paraparesis (FSP) is a genetically heterogeneous group of upper motor neuron syndromes. In its simplest form, the disease is characterized by progressive spasticity of the legs and increased reflexes without other associated neurologic signs. More complicated cases have also been included under this rubric, with such additional features as dementia, visual abnormalities, and ataxia, for example.

FSP can be inherited as an autosomal dominant (Online Mendelian Inheritance in Man 182600 and 182601), autosomal recessive (Online Mendelian Inheritance in Man 270800), or X-linked (Online Mendelian Inheritance in Man 312900) disorder. Four loci for autosomal dominant FSP have been genetically mapped, and two genes have been shown responsible for the X-linked type. In addition, two loci for autosomal recessive types have been reported and mapped to chromosomes 8q and 16q. The gene for the 16q locus has been characterized as a mitochondrial protein. Some cases of apparently "pure" FSP have been shown to have elevated levels of VLCFA, diagnostic of adrenoleukodystrophy-adrenomyeloneuropathy. The mechanism of neurodegeneration has not yet been established.

The radiographic appearance depends on the genetic subtype. In X-linked FSP, MRI of the brain of affected individuals often shows discrete white-matter lesions in the periatrial regions,[248–250] leading to misdiagnosis as MS. By contrast, in autosomal dominant disease, brain and spinal cord MRI may not disclose any significant abnormalities.[251] In advanced cases, MRI may reveal atrophy of the thoracic spinal cord without evidence for white-matter disease in the cerebrum, cerebellum, or brain stem.

Krabbe's Disease (Globoid Cell Leukodystrophy)

Globoid cell leukodystrophy (GLD) is an autosomal recessive inherited disorder caused by the deficiency of a lysosomal enzyme, galactocerebrosidase (GalC). GalC is a beta-galactosidase required for the hydrolysis of the galactosyl moiety from several myelin-associated lipids, including galactosylceramide and psychosine. Infantile- and juvenile-onset forms are far more common, but adult-onset cases are reported. In the adult-onset form, a typical presentation is progressive spastic hemiparesis or tetraparesis, followed by optic atrophy, dementia, and large-fiber demyelinating neuropathy. In some cases, only the pyramidal tracts appear involved, perhaps asymmetrically.[252,253] Cerebellar involvement is more common in early-onset forms[254] but has been described in adults.[255] In some cases, the peripheral nerves are not clinically affected.[256]

In both early- and late-onset forms, galactosphingolipid accumulation in cells of monocytic origin gives these cells a globoid appearance, hence the name globoid cell leukodystrophy. Accumulation of psychosine (beta-galactosyl-sphingosine) is thought to be responsible for the induction of pathologic changes. GLD is characterized by extensive demyelination in both the PNS and the CNS.

The *GalC* gene has been mapped to the 14q31 chromosomal region. More than 60 mutations in the *GalC* gene have been identified in patients with all clinical types of GLD (reviewed in reference 257). The most common involves a deletion,[258] but missense and nonsense mutations are also reported. Severe or homozygous mutations result in the infantile type; late-onset forms more often occur in heterozygous individuals. Among heterozygotes, even patients with the same genotype can have very different clinical presentations and course.

Naturally occurring deficiencies of GalC in a mouse strain (*twitcher*), several breeds of dog, and rhesus monkeys are equivalent to human

GLD at the molecular level and provide useful models for the human disorder, for both pathogenesis and treatment (reviewed in reference 259). Diagnostic clues to the presence of a leukodystrophy usually include a family history, moderate increases in the CSF protein content, and MRI showing confluent white-matter involvement.[253] Definitive diagnosis depends on identification of GalC deficiency in leukocytes. However, as with metachromatic leukodystrophy (MLD), a condition of pseudodeficiency is recognized.[260] Pseudodeficiency is defined as the in vitro measurement of low activity (usually less than 15% of the normal mean for controls) of an enzyme in a healthy person. Therefore, a positive test result should be confirmed using a more specific test, either genetic or biochemical.

Treatment of GLD hinges on replacing the deficient enzyme activity in the marrow-derived CNS cells. BMT has proven effective if performed before irreversible signs of neurologic damage appear.[261] Gene therapy for GLD is under development, but no satisfactory methods for somatic cell gene therapy of the brain are currently available.

Leber's Hereditary Optic Neuropathy

All three primary Leber's hereditary optic neuropathy (LHON) mutations occurring in the European and North American populations have been found to be associated with an MS-like syndrome. Harboring a primary LHON mutation (nucleotide [nt]-3460 and nt-11778 mitochondrial DNA mutations) may be a risk factor for developing MS.[262] At the least, certain mitochondrial DNA variations, when coincidentally associated with MS, likely predispose to ON.[263,264] However, it does not appear that LHON mutations are a common cause for familial MS.[265–271]

The primary neurologic characteristic of MS associated with LHON is severe and bilateral visual symptoms and signs. In other respects, these cases are clinically indistinguishable from those of MS in general. Therefore, it appears most reasonable to select for LHON mutation screening those MS patients with peripapillary telangiectasia typical of LHON, with relatives harboring LHON, or with early severe bilateral optic neuropathy.

Leigh's Syndrome

Originally described in 1951 as an infantile disorder, Leigh's syndrome was later recognized in juvenile- and adult-onset forms. In most cases, the clinical and radiographic features and family history would pose no diagnostic confusion with MS. However, some individuals do not present with typical features, and diagnosis may be challenging in these cases.

The main pathology in Leigh's syndrome involves foci of necrosis in basal ganglia and thalamic gray matter or brain stem. The main biochemical findings are high pyruvate and lactate in the blood. Leigh's syndrome can be caused by defects in a variety of chromosomal and mitochondrial genes. The chromosomal genes implicated to date include *SURF1*, which encodes a factor involved in the biogenesis of cytochrome c oxidase; E1-alpha subunit of pyruvate dehydrogenase (*PDHA1*); *NDUFV1*; and the *NDUFS8* subunits of mitochondrial complex I; however, these forms of Leigh's syndrome have less phenotypic variability. The mitochondrial gene defects, conversely, may present with a baffling variety of phenotypes. A given mitochondrial mutation may manifest as a variety of syndromes, whereas a given syndrome may be caused by mutation in a variety of mitochondrial genes.

The mutations in mitochondrial genes that have been associated with Leigh's syndrome include nt-9176 in the adenosine triphosphatase gene[272]; two differing mutations at nt-8993 in the same gene,[273–276] which also may cause mitochondrial encephalomyopathy, lactic acidosis, and stroke-like episodes (MELAS) or the syndrome of neuropathy, ataxia, and retinitis pigmentosa[277] and cardiomyopathy; nt-3243 in the leucine *transfer RNA* (*tRNA*) gene, which is also a cause of MELAS[278]; nt-1644 in the valine *tRNA* gene[279]; and a thymidine insertion at nt position 5537 in the tryptophan *tRNA* gene.[280] Of the two mutations at nt 8993, the T8993C mutation may lead to less severe disease, compared to the T8993G mutation.[281] Still, even the T8993G mutation may have highly variable manifestations. In an examination of six pedigrees,[276] individuals harboring the mutation manifested a range of symptoms from severe infantile subacute necrotizing encephalomyelopathy (prototypical Leigh's disease) to MELAS to juvenile-onset neuropathy, ataxia, and retinitis pigmentosa and sensory axonal neuropathy. In the most provocative case, a woman with the T8993G mutation developed an MS-like clinical syndrome associated with oligoclonal bands and periventricular white-matter abnormalities. Whether the mitochondrial mutation contributed to the MS-like findings remains an interesting but as yet unproved hypothesis.

Diagnosis of Leigh's syndrome may be made on the basis of combined clinical, laboratory, radiographic, and genetic evidence. In the case of an MS-like presentation, a diagnosis of (and appropriate genetic testing for) Leigh's syndrome should be considered only in the context of an appropriate family history or radiographic picture.

Metachromatic Leukodystrophy

MLD is an autosomal recessive disorder that results from deficiency of the lysosomal enzyme arylsulfatase A. This enzyme is required for the metabolism of cerebroside sulfate. Accumulations of sulfated glycolipid form the metachromatic-staining material found in white matter that gives rise to the name of the disorder. The infantile and juvenile forms are more common, but adult-onset MLD also occurs. In the late-onset forms, the disease progresses slowly. Symptoms, which begin after age 16, may include impaired concentration, psychiatric disturbances, optic atrophy, nystagmus, ataxia, spasticity, urinary incontinence, and dementia. In rare cases, the disease may follow a relapsing-remitting course.[282] The combination of CNS signs and symptoms with white matter abnormalities on MRI may lead to diagnostic confusion with MS.

In the adult form of MLD, initial symptoms are usually psychiatric. Disorders of movement, optic nerve degeneration, and other signs appear late, possibly accompanied by peripheral neuropathy. In mild cases, the diagnosis may even go unsuspected during life. Thus, the disorder should be suspected in individuals with white-matter lesions and prominent psychiatric disorders, particularly if there is a family history of these problems.

Pathologically, the hallmark of MLD is an accumulation of galactosphingosulfatides in the white matter of the CNS, which appear pink with the periodic acid-Schiff stain and doubly refractile in polarized light. The granules stain brown, rather than the usual violet, with acetic acid–cresyl violet, giving rise to the term *metachromatic*. Laboratory findings that help to distinguish MLD from MS include MRI of the brain showing bilateral, fairly symmetric, and confluent white-matter abnormalities rather than the multifocal, asymmetric, ovoid lesions typical of MS; CSF protein concentrations in excess of 100 mg/dl; electrophysiologic evidence of concomitant peripheral neuropathy; and most importantly, assay of arylsulfatase A deficient activity in blood leukocytes.

Normal levels of arylsulfatase activity rules out MLD. However, in the absence of appropriate neurologic signs or symptoms, low arylsulfatase A is not necessarily indicative of this disease. A condition of arylsulfatase A pseudodeficiency is recognized, which is characterized by the in vitro measurement of low enzyme activity using the routine assay in the absence of symptomatic or presymptomatic disease.[260] Therefore, confirmation of a diagnosis of MLD requires additional testing, including radiolabeled-sulfatide loading in cultured skin fibroblasts, examination of urine for excretion of undegraded lipids, and molecular analysis of DNA samples for known mutations.

Treatment of lysosomal storage diseases, such as MLD, requires correction of the underlying enzymatic deficiency. Strategies for enzyme replacement include allogeneic BMT and gene therapy. To be effective, BMT must be performed early in the course of the disease, before the development of irreversible neurologic damage. BMT has been most effective in the later-onset forms of MLD. Donor marrow–derived macrophages or microglia enter the CNS and provide a source of arylsulfatase A activity, although little of the enzyme may be expected to enter host neuronal or glial cells. Thus, these treatments are only partially effective, at best. In a juvenile case with 7 years of follow-up, the disease was stabilized after BMT. In one adult case, modest improvements were seen after transplantation in the electroencephalogram, in peripheral nerve conduction, and in neuropsychological tests.[283] However, in most cases, the damage is not reversed or stabilized in the more severe, infantile-onset form. In principle, gene therapy may correct the metabolic defect within host neuronal and glial cells and prevent MLD. Currently, no satisfactory methods for somatic cell gene therapy of the human brain have been demonstrated. However, impressive results were obtained in a mouse model of MLD using a retroviral vector to deliver a functional human arylsulfatase A gene to the CNS.[284] Even though the mice were treated after the expected onset of neuropathologic changes, the neuropathology appeared almost normal within months, and the treated mice performed as well as wild-type mice in a maze-learning task.

Mitochondrial Encephalomyopathy, Lactic Acidosis, and Stroke-Like Episodes

The syndrome of MELAS[285] in its prototypic form would not be confused with MS. The clinical features originally recognized in MELAS include migraine, episodic vomiting, seizures, and recurrent cerebral insults resembling strokes. However, in some cases, the clinical and MR findings may be indistinguishable from MS.[286] The myopathy may be mild and asymptomatic, the lactic acidemia may be detectable only on vigorous exercise, and some individuals may not develop stroke-like episodes.[287]

The disorder has been associated with a variety of point mutations in the mitochondrial genes encoding tRNAs. The most common mutation is at nt-3243 in the *tRNA[Leu(UUR)]* gene of mitochondrial DNA.[288] Other MELAS-associated mutations in the *tRNA[Leu(UUR)]* gene lie at nt-3271,[289] -3291,[290] -3256,[291] or -3260.[292] Additionally, a mutation at nt-8316 in the mitochondrial DNA *tRNA(Lys)* gene[293] and another at nt-1642 in the mitochondrial *tRNA(Val)* gene have been associated with MELAS.[294,295]

Mitochondrial mutations are typically heteroplasmic, so that mitochondria containing the mutant DNA coexist with mitochondria containing wild-type DNA. The proportion of mutant mitochondrial DNA can vary widely among individuals and among tissues within an individual.[296] The percentage of mutant mitochondrial DNA and its tissue distribution appear to be determinants of disease pathogenesis.[287] The co-occurrence of other mutations that alter mitochondrial function also modifies disease pathogenesis, in particular the risk of stroke.[297]

When an individual does not present the prototypic syndrome, an appropriate family history will sometimes suggest a diagnosis of MELAS. In addition to CNS disorders, MELAS-associated mutations may present with demyelinating polyneuropathy,[298] progressive external ophthalmoplegia,[299] maternally inherited diabetes and sensorineural deafness,[300] or cardiomyopathy.[301] Genetic testing of the mitochondrial DNA (e.g., from blood leukocytes or muscle biopsy) for the associated mutations can establish the diagnosis.

Mercury Toxicity

Mercury poisoning is also termed *acrodynia*, *pink disease*, or *Minamata disease*. Chronic exposure to or ingestion of mercury leads to signs and symptoms that mimic those of MS. Cognitive changes, such as asthenia, behavioral changes, short-term memory loss, and psychological symptoms may result from mercury toxicity. Encephalopathy, a confusional state, headache, and seizures have been seen with exposure to organic mercury absorbed via skin or aspiration. Cerebellar signs, such as tremor and ataxia, are often seen. A sensorimotor axonal polyneuropathy, fasciculations of the muscles of the trunk and extremities, and painful paresthesias have been reported. The phenomenon of delayed neurotoxicity (Minamata disease) was observed in a population around Minamata Bay in Japan in those who had ingested mercury-contaminated marine life[302] and in Zulu mine workers.[303] The symptoms were mainly neurobehavioral and developed as late as 5 years after exposure to mercury in many instances. Attention deficits, memory loss, and delayed motor speed were found. Psychological symptoms, such as anxiety, depression, and phobia, were present. Tremor, motor weakness of the extremities, and profuse sweating were also prevalent. Impairment of color vision and cortical blindness has often been reported.[304] Quadriplegia and mental retardation have been observed in children exposed to mercury at an early age. The cutaneous manifestations of mercury poisoning are termed *pink disease*. They include gingivitis, erythematous peeling of the palmar surface, and a miliary rash. Anorexia, sweating, weight loss, and irritability may accompany these symptoms. Cortical blindness with concentric constriction of the visual fields, decreased proprioception, choreoathetosis, and attention deficits were symptoms observed in a family whose members had ingested mercury-contaminated pork. The diagnosis is made by the appearance of the appropriate clinical features and the measurement of hair, blood, and urinary levels of mercury. The treatment is dimercaprol (British Anti-Lewisite, BAL) for 2 months. This substance increases the urinary excretion of mercury.

Several attempts have been made to link dental amalgams to mercury poisoning. One study showed evidence that the level of mercury released in 24 hours from dental fillings is equal to that ingested in a normal meal, which is significantly below the neurotoxic level.[305] A clustering of MS cases located in close proximity to sites polluted with mercury have led to a heightened suspicion for mercury as a cause of MS.[306] In patients who present with mercury toxicity as their chief symptom, a large percentage have been found to have a significant degree of somatization on psychological testing.[307]

Pathologic signs of cortical atrophy, neuronal loss, and gliosis are found in the parieto-occipital and paracentral areas.[304] On MRI, atrophy is noted in the parietal and cerebellar lobes and in the calcarine area. This latter finding correlates well with the visual symptoms observed in some patients.[308] Cerebellar atrophy is prominent in the middle and inferior vermis.[309] Hypointense T_1 lesions and hyperintense T_2 lesions can be seen in the calcarine area, cerebellum, and posterior central gyri.

Prion Protein Gene Mutation

Familial cases of spongiform encephalopathy typically result from inherited mutations in the cellular genes that encode prion proteins. Although most such disorders do not present clinical or MRI appearances likely to be mistaken for MS, rare cases have been reported that have features in common with MS.[310] The absence of stepwise exacerbations and the severity of the dementia, which eventually culminate in mutism, readily differentiate this disorder from demyelinating disease.

Retinal Vasculopathy with Cerebral Leukodystrophy (Hereditary Cerebroretinal Vasculopathy)

Retinal vasculopathy with cerebral leukodystrophy, a rare disorder, is characterized by progressive CNS degeneration and retinal vasculopathy, inherited in apparent autosomal dominant fashion.[311,312] Onset is in middle adult years. In some individuals, the vasculopathy presents the radiographic picture of a mass lesion simulating tumor, whereas in other cases, the MRI shows periventricular white-matter lesions. The latter cases might be mistaken for MS, particularly because of the accompanying visual symptoms.

Common clinical features include fluctuating or progressive vision loss, weakness and hyperreflexia, and mild cognitive impairment. Elevated erythrocyte sedimentation rate and cutaneous vasculitis are reported.[312] As the visual impairment reflects retinal vasculopathy rather than ON, a careful examination might disclose the presence of retinal exudates or hemorrhages. Fluorescein angiography is useful to confirm the diagnosis of retinal vasculopathy.

Vitamin B_{12} (Cobalamin) Deficiency and Related Disorders

Serum deficiency of cobalamin can have adverse consequences for the nervous system, the bone marrow, and the gastrointestinal system. The neurologic disorder is known as *combined subacute degeneration* and is characterized by progressive demyelination that can involve peripheral nerve, spinal cord or brain. The hematologic disorder is known as *megaloblastic anemia* and is characterized by anemia with macrocytosis and hypersegmented neutrophils. Gastrointestinal symptoms may include changes in the tongue, anorexia, and diarrhea. The neurologic, hematologic, and gastrointestinal disorders may occur alone or in combination.

Combined subacute degeneration may present with posterior column sensory symptoms, progressive spastic and ataxic weakness or, in recent years, with a variety of neurologic symptoms together with radiographic evidence of demyelination in the spinal cord or brain (Figure 10-1). The myelopathy tends to be symmetric. Reflexes may be increased because of corticospinal tract interruption, decreased because of concomitant peripheral neuropathy, or neutral. Optic atrophy and mental changes may occur.

Vitamin B_{12} is actually cyanocobalamin, which must be converted to biologically active forms (methylcobalamin and adenosylcobalamin) before it can be used by tissues. The most common cause for the cobalamin deficiency state is pernicious anemia,

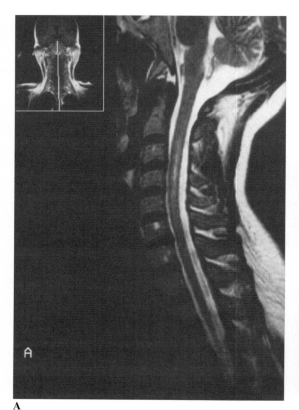

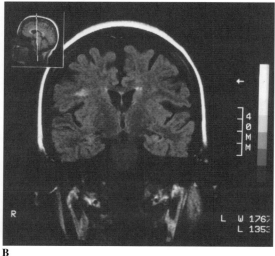

Figure 10-1. A. Magnetic resonance imaging of the spine of a middle-aged woman who presented with bilateral arm numbness and a pseudoataxic gait. Laboratory tests revealed vitamin B_{12} deficiency. A posteriorly localized area of demyelination can be seen in the spinal cord. **B.** Magnetic resonance imaging of the brain of the same patient shows scattered areas of demyelination. The patient's symptoms improved after several weeks of treatment with vitamin B_{12}.

A

B

in which absorption of dietary cobalamin is reduced because autoantibodies reduce the availability of "intrinsic factor," which is necessary for intestinal absorption of vitamin B_{12}. Intestinal absorption of vitamin B_{12} is determined by a Schilling test, in which a patient ingests radiolabeled cobalamin and urinary excretion is measured. Elevated levels of serum methylmalonic acid or homocysteine may help in the diagnosis. Rarely, a dietary inadequacy of vitamin B_{12} (the only natural dietary sources are meat and dairy foods), alteration of gastric parietal cells or the terminal ileum by resection or disease, or an abnormal vitamin B_{12}–binding protein leads to deficiency. Nitrous oxide anesthesia can precipitate an acute neurologic deterioration, particularly in individuals with borderline cobalamin deficiency.[313–315] This is attributable to an effect of the gas on multiple aspects of cobalamin metabolism.[316] Folate deficiency states can present a clinical picture that is highly similar to that of cobalamin deficiency[317–321] but is much less common.

The pathogenesis of combined subacute degeneration is incompletely understood. Methylcobalamin and adenosylcobalamin have differing but important roles in metabolism, so cobalamin deficiency impairs the function of disparate biochemical pathways. Deficiency of both forms of cobalamin could have an impact on the production of myelin, but impairment of methionine synthetase activity from methylcobalamin deficiency is probably the most important factor. Treatment of cobalamin deficiency involves supplementation of vitamin B_{12}. The route of administration depends on the mechanism underlying the deficiency state. A dietary deficiency may be remedied by nutritional supplementation, but malabsorption syndromes may require parenteral therapy. An important caution when initiating replacement therapy is that folate administration may cause neurologic deterioration in vitamin B_{12}–deficient patients. Therefore, if folate therapy is indicated, it should not be given until cobalamin stores have been repleted for 1–2 weeks.

There has been widespread interest in a possible role for cobalamin deficiency states in MS. It has been observed that people with MS have an increased incidence of low serum B_{12} levels,[322,323] although the metabolic significance of these mild deficiencies has been disputed.[324] Although serum B_{12} levels may be reduced by corticosteroid treatments in MS,[325] widespread use of this standard therapy probably does not account for the observed incidence of low serum B_{12}. A correlation of serum B_{12} levels with the age of onset of MS has been reported.[326] Overall, the possibility that coexisting vitamin B_{12} deficiency might aggravate MS or impair recovery from MS provides a strong justification for determining serum B_{12} levels in all patients presenting with demyelinating disease. Other B vitamin deficiencies (folate, biotin) are rare but may also mimic MS.

Wilson's Disease

Wilson's disease results from abnormally increased serum copper, which becomes deposited in the organs and causes primarily neurologic and hepatic dysfunction. The cerebral dysfunction associated with Wilson's disease may have cognitive, motor, and psychiatric manifestations. Although MRI may reveal T_2 hyperintense lesions in white matter, the disease is readily distinguished from MS by the prominent involvement of gray-matter structures, notably the basal ganglia, thalamus, and substantia nigra.

Other Immune-Mediated and Neoplastic Disorders

Behçet's Disease

Behçet's disease is defined by the combination of uveitis and oral or genital ulcers. Aseptic meningitis or meningoencephalitis occurs in some cases. Neurologic findings may localize to the brain or spinal cord. The relapsing-remitting variety of neuro–Behçet's syndrome overlaps in some clinical aspects with MS.[327] The CSF shows a mild pleocytosis and increased protein concentration. MRI findings include a predilection for periventricular areas, extensive brain stem lesions, and involvement of both white and gray matter.[328,329]

Isolated Central Nervous System Angiitis

Isolated CNS angiitis is a rare cause of multifocal CNS disease. Systemic vasculitides can cause similar problems if they involve the CNS.[330] Symptoms may develop suddenly or evolve over days or months. Common findings[331] include ataxia, aphasia, visual symptoms, paraparesis, or quadriparesis. Patients may have fever, night sweats, anorexia, weight loss, mild anemia, or an elevated sedimentation rate, but the diagnosis must be questioned with other evidence of disease outside the CNS. An unexplained, multifocal, severe neurologic illness progressing over weeks or months accompanied by headache merits aggressive workup, which may require cerebral angiography and brain biopsy. Isolated CNS angiitis can present as myelopathy.[332–334] Nearly one-fifth of patients with isolated CNS angiitis have evidence of myelopathy sometime during their illness.[335] Unihemispheric herpes zoster infection–associated vasculitis presenting with contralateral hemiparesis is a distinct syndrome.

Patients frequently have increased CSF IgG levels or oligoclonal bands. Most patients with isolated CNS angiitis have abnormal CSF protein levels or cell counts.[336] The CSF mononuclear cell count may be mildly elevated and is rarely in excess of 300 white blood cells/µl. Spinal cord MRI scans may show intramedullary lesions that are hyperintense on T_2-weighted images or enhance with gadolinium.[333] MRI brain scans often show areas of brightness on T_2-weighted images in both hemispheres, either in a multifocal pattern consistent with cerebral infarctions or in a more diffuse, confluent pattern. Focal lesions may have a mass effect.[337] Lesions may enhance with gadolinium and improve with steroid therapy. Focal brain lesions seen on MRI scans are most frequently visible in cortex or deep white matter but may also occur in subcortical white matter or deep gray matter. MRI abnormalities may match angiographic findings in a given patient; in addition, other areas of focal vasculopathy may not accompany MRI brain abnormalities.[338,339] The angiographic findings of cerebral angiitis are multifocal narrowing of blood vessels, mild post-stenotic dilatations, and focal variations in blood flow.[340] Stenoses usually are seen in multiple vessels asymmetrically.[341] Cerebral angiograms may appear normal. CNS biopsy specimens should include meningeal tissue and brain parenchyma with a longitudinally oriented surface vessel. Biopsy necessarily produces only a limited sample of tissue, and the results may be negative in nearly 30% of cases of isolated CNS angiitis.[336]

Lymphomatoid Granulomatosis

Patients with lymphomatoid granulomatosis typically present with skin manifestations or involvement of other organs (kidneys, lungs) by an angiocentric, vascular infiltrate usually composed of B cells. Lymphomatoid granulomatosis is considered a pre–B-cell lymphoma. Involvement of the brain can be circumscribed to the white matter.[342] Progressive multifocal leukoencephalopathy develops rarely in patients with lymphomatoid granulomatosis.[343] Another unusual complication of lymphomatoid granulomatosis is disseminated necrotizing leukoencephalopathy after brain irradiation and chemotherapy.[344]

Primary Central Nervous System Lymphoma

CNS Lymphoma may present with multiple white-matter lesions that can sometimes be confused with active MS plaques[345,346] because they usually enhance with gadolinium. The physician should be aware that lymphoma lesions may decrease in size and sometimes seem to disappear on treatment with intravenous steroids. Diagnosis often can be established by serial cytologies of the CSF. Flow cytometry to establish clonality may be helpful. In cases presenting with large lesions, a brain biopsy may be indicated. Patients should be tested for human immunodeficiency virus infection.

Paraneoplastic Neurologic Disorders

Several CNS syndromes occur in association with particular non-CNS tumors and without direct malignant cell invasion of the CNS.[347,348] The clinical manifestations of these syndromes such as ataxia, brain stem dysfunction, and blindness may raise suspicion of MS. The symptoms are generally acute or subacute in onset, but, unlike MS, the symptoms rarely remit.

Because these disorders are consistently associated with particular autoantibodies, an immune

pathogenesis has been postulated. At least nine autoantibodies have been associated with particular syndromes, and others are being sought. These autoantibodies appear to be elicited by tumor antigens but cross-react with neuronal antigens. Recently, investigators have begun to identify cytologic and helper T cells that respond to the tumor antigens and that may play an important role in the neuropathogenesis.

Oddly, some of the autoantibodies have been associated with a variety of tumors and with a variety of neurologic syndromes. For example, anti-Hu antibodies may occur in association with limbic encephalitis, cerebellar ataxia, and sensory or autonomic neuronopathy and have been elicited by small cell lung cancer, non-small cell lung cancer, and neuroblastoma. The anti-Ri antibodies that cause opsoclonus/myoclonus may occur with small cell lung cancer, breast cancer, and ovarian or uterine cancers. This diversity can complicate the search for a neoplasm in patients presenting with possible paraneoplastic syndromes. A tumor is not found in all cases but should be sought. Despite the neurologic devastation these disorders can cause, the associated malignancy can be extremely small or occult, further complicating the search for a neoplasm.

It is a curious feature of these disorders that the associated malignancy often has a more benign course than in otherwise similar tumor cases without paraneoplastic symptoms. This suggests that the immune response may contribute to the control of the tumor.

Other Central Nervous System Neoplasms

Neoplasms and other space-occupying lesions of the CNS often produce slowly progressive symptoms. The most common presentation is headache presumably secondary to increased intracranial pressure and edema. Memory loss, attention deficits, confusional state, and focal neurologic signs may develop. In lesions located in the posterior fossa, such as the brain stem and cerebellum, various cranial nerve and cerebellar signs may result. Internuclear opthalmoplegia, facial palsy, dysarthria, dysphagia, hearing loss, ataxia, hemiparesis, and one-and-a-half syndrome are some of the reported signs.

The response to steroid therapy may be similar in tumors of both the CNS and MS. Therefore, this radiographic or clinical responsiveness is not helpful in differentiating these entities, especially if lymphoma is suspected. Similarly, the presence of oligoclonal bands in the CSF was thought to be a strong identifying clue for MS. However, oligoclonal bands may be seen in patients with other structural CNS lesions, such as tumors, arteriovenous malformation, compressive cervical myelopathy, and Arnold-Chiari malformation.[349] Neoplasms that may be particularly difficult to distinguish from MS include oligodendroglial gliomatosis cerebri,[350] brain stem gliomas, and ependymoma of the conus medullaris. Nonexpansile lesions of the cord and brain stem have the greatest likelihood of representing MS. Vascular lesions, such as cavernous angiomas, arteriovenous malformations, and venous angiomas are also often mistaken for lesions of MS. The question of whether MS patients are at increased risk for gliomas remains unresolved.[351,352]

Pathologic changes of necrosis, cystic areas, and edema are associated with both MS and neoplasms. The multiplicity of some tumors may falsely lead to the suspicion for MS. However, the pathologic changes in MS patients for whom a brain biopsy is performed often show areas of demyelination leading to the correct diagnosis. The CSF in patients with neoplasms may reveal a lymphocytic pleocytosis similar to that seen in MS. Dysembryoplastic neuroepithelial tumors reveal histologic changes of oligodendroglia-like cells, astrocytes, and neurons[353] that are present in the white matter of the brain. The presence of multiple nodules is the characteristic that distinguishes this disease from MS. Some of the neoplasms that may mimic MS with lesions apparent in the CNS white matter are metastatic large B-cell lymphoma,[354,355] gliomas, infiltrating-anaplastic astrocytomas, meningiomas, glioblastoma, metastatic lesions, or Langerhans cell histiocytosis. Astrocytomas and gliomas are the tumors most often misdiagnosed as MS.

The histopathology of demyelinating lesions often reveals some preservation of axons, foamy macrophages, and normal or reactive astrocytes.[356] Necrosis is not a distinguishing feature. These characteristics help to separate MS from other entities in the differential of space-occupying lesions.

At times, MS lesions may display imaging characteristics that suggest the presence of a space-occupying lesion, such as a tumor.[357–359] The area of demyelination may be solitary, large, and surrounded by edema with an area of ring enhancement. The use of diffusion-weighted MRI is helpful to differentiate various space-occupying lesions of the CNS. By using imaging characteristics, such as a difference in intensity in diffusion-weighted images, the differential diagnosis could be narrowed considerably. The use of diffusion-weighted images may be helpful in differentiating lymphoma and infectious processes, such as abscess, but may be less effective in differentiating other tumors.[360] Similarly, proton-density MRI can be useful to differentiate tumefactive demyelinating lesions from neoplasms and avoid misdiagnosis.[361] The open-ring imaging sign[362] on MRI is useful for differentiation of demyelination versus other etiology, such as neoplasm or infectious processes. This characteristic is described as an open ring of contrast enhancement surrounding a lesion. If present, this may be indicative of a demyelinating lesion.[363] In some cases, the presence of a malignant or infectious lesion can not be excluded without resorting to biopsy. However, stereotactic biopsy can lead to misdiagnosis because of sampling error.

Rheumatoid Arthritis

Rheumatoid arthritis is the most common connective-tissue disease. Systemic vasculitis occurs in up to 25% of patients and rarely may affect the CNS. The MRI appearance is usually similar to Binswanger's disease. Atlantoaxial dislocation may cause a myelopathy or brain stem deficits from direct medullary compression or vertebral artery involvement.

Sarcoidosis

Sarcoidosis is an idiopathic disorder with multi-organ involvement and many different clinical presentations. Cranial neuropathies from basal meningitis are the most common neurologic manifestation. The facial nerve is often affected, sometimes bilaterally. The optic nerve may appear inflamed or atrophic. Increased intracranial pressure from a large non-caseating granuloma or obstructive hydrocephalus may cause papilledema. Disturbances of the hypothalamic region are associated with diabetes insipidus, abnormal thermoregulation, amenorrhea, hypoglycemia, sleep disturbances, obesity, personality changes, or other evidence of hypopituitarism. Occasionally, sarcoidosis can predominantly involve cerebral or spinal cord white matter and be virtually indistinguishable from MS. Neurosarcoidosis often remits spontaneously, but progressive neurologic disease occurs in approximately 30% of cases. The diagnosis of neurosarcoidosis is difficult in the absence of cutaneous or pulmonary involvement. Histologic diagnosis may require biopsy of apparently normal tissue if lesions are not accessible. The tuberculin skin test and serum concentration of angiotensin-converting enzyme cannot establish a definitive diagnosis.

Sjögren's Syndrome

Sjögren's syndrome is characterized by xerostomia and xerophthalmia. Diagnosis requires a positive rose bengal dye test, evidence of diminished salivary gland flow, abnormal biopsy of a salivary gland, and an abnormal rheumatoid factor or ANA. A subset of ANA called SS-A (Ro) and SS-B (La) are highly prevalent in Sjögren's syndrome. Neurologic complications include psychiatric disturbances, migrainous episodes, aseptic meningitis, and myelopathy. Cranial MRI may show hyperintense, small subcortical lesions.[364,365] It has been suggested that MS patients may be at increased risk for Sjögren's syndrome.[366] Sjögren's syndrome can be controlled by corticosteroids in some cases but may require immunosuppressant therapies such as cyclophosphamide.

Systemic Lupus Erythematosus and Lupoid Sclerosis

Systemic lupus erythematosus (SLE) is a chronic multisystem disease characterized by skin, musculoskeletal, cardiac, pulmonary, renal, hematologic, and neuropsychiatric abnormalities.[367] Nervous system involvement occurs in 25–75% of patients[368] and includes cognitive decline, cerebrovascular disease, seizures, neuropathy, headache, and psychosis. Myelopathy is rare, occurring in fewer than 1% of patients with SLE.

The term *lupoid sclerosis* has been applied to patients with overlapping clinical and laboratory features of SLE and MS. Spastic paraplegia due to transverse myelopathy is the most common neuro-

logic finding in lupoid sclerosis. Other clinical and laboratory features include ON, ANA, and antiphospholipid antibodies (APLAs).

There are several case reports dating back to the 1950s that documented spinal cord involvement in patients with SLE.[369–371] Penn and Rowan[372] described four patients with SLE and myelopathy, including two cases in which the myelopathy was the initial manifestation of SLE. In all patients, LE cell preparations were positive.

In 1972, Fulford et al.[373] described six women with a clinical picture resembling MS and laboratory features suggestive of SLE. Five patients had a slowly progressive spastic paraplegia, and one patient had a poorly defined left-sided movement disorder. All patients showed a moderate elevation of protein in the CSF consistent with MS. Laboratory findings suggestive of SLE included positive LE cell tests, false-positive VDRL test results, and the presence of ANA. None of the patients showed involvement of other organ systems. Fulford et al. argued that these patients had a distinct variant of SLE, and they proposed the term *lupoid sclerosis* to describe the syndrome.

TM occurs in fewer than 1% of patients with SLE. It involves the acute or subacute onset of either paraplegia or hemiplegia. There is also weakness, sensory loss, and impaired bowel and bladder control.[374] Hackett et al.[375] examined three patients with ON as a presenting manifestation of SLE. Within 3 years, two of the patients developed a TM syndrome. In one case, the patient demonstrated severe weakness in both legs, a spastic gait, hyperreflexia, and bilateral Babinski's signs. There was no sensory deficit. In the other case, the patient showed paralysis of the legs, weakness of the trunk and shoulder muscles, hypoactive reflexes, bilateral Babinski's signs, and a sensory level at C5-T2. Smith and Pinals[376] described two patients who presented with myelopathy. Both went on to develop ON, one after 1 year and the other after 6 years. Other features of SLE included malar rash, positive ANA, anti-DNA antibodies, anti-ribonucleoprotein Smith antigen (anti-Sm) antibodies, and low complement. Kovacs et al.[377] presented 14 patients with transverse myelopathy who met American College of Rheumatology criteria for the diagnosis of SLE. In all cases, TM was the initial manifestation of the disease or presented within 5 years of diagnosis. Three patients had ON. Six of 11 patients tested were positive for APLAs.

ON is uncommon in patients with SLE. In a prospective study of 150 patients with SLE, Estes and Christian[378] reported three cases of optic atrophy and blindness. Cinefro and Frenkel[379] described a 57-year-old man with unilateral ON. Laboratory findings were consistent with SLE and included a positive LE cell prep, ANA titer of 1:1280, false-positive VDRL test results, cellular casts, elevated sedimentation rate, and reduced complement. Oppenheimer and Hoffbrand[380] reviewed 14 cases of lupus ON. Seven patients developed a myopathy during their clinical course. High titers of anticardiolipin antibodies were also recorded.

A number of features differentiate ON in patients with lupoid sclerosis from ON in patients with MS. Lupus ON is characterized by a persistent, dense central scotoma with severe vision loss after the first attack. In cases of demyelination, approximately 90% of patients recover normal or nearly normal vision after a single episode. In addition, there is an absent visual-evoked response or a decrease in the amplitude of the response. The conduction delay seen in patients with MS does not occur in lupus ON. Finally, lupus ON is marked by steroid responsiveness and steroid dependence. Kupersmith et al.[381] described 14 patients with progressive or recurrent optic neuropathy and laboratory features of SLE. Megadoses of corticosteroid therapy improved the vision in 11 cases, and continued steroid and immunosuppressive therapies were necessary to maintain vision in nine cases. ON in patients with MS commonly remits without treatment.

Positive ANA is a hallmark of SLE. Estes and Christian[378] found positive ANA in 87% of 150 patients with SLE. The frequency of positive ANA in much lower in patients with MS. Fulford et al.[373] reported positive ANA in 10% of 69 patients with MS. In a retrospective chart review of 433 patients with MS, Barned et al.[382] reported positive ANA in 27% of 150 patients with relapsing-remitting MS and 30% of 23 patients with chronic progressive MS. In general, ANA titers are higher in patients with SLE or lupoid sclerosis than in patients with MS. Dore-Duffy et al.[383] detected ANA titers at or less than 1:32 in 81% of patients with MS.

APLAs, including lupus anticoagulant and anti-cardiolipin antibodies, are common in patients with SLE. Toubi et al.[384] reported APLAs in 53 of 96 (55%) of patients with CNS manifestations of SLE and in 20 of 100 (20%) of patients with SLE who did not have CNS manifestations of the disease. Harris et al.[385] described a patient with transverse myelopathy that resulted in spastic paraparesis. Serologic findings included a positive ANA and a false-positive result on the VDRL test. Raised levels of IgM anti-cardiolipin antibodies were also found. There is a low incidence of APLAs in patients with MS. Even when positive, the titers are much lower than those found in patients with SLE. Harris et al.[385] reported only slightly raised anti-cardiolipin antibody levels in 3 of 91 patients with MS.

Several familial cases of MS and SLE have been reported in the literature. Holmes et al.[386] described female identical twins, one with diagnosed SLE and the other with MS. The diagnosis of SLE was based on acute hemolytic anemia, thrombocytopenia, and positive LE cell preparation. The diagnosis of MS was based on lower extremity weakness, bilateral Babinski's signs, absent abdominal reflexes, mild generalized incoordination, hyperactive jaw jerk, and spinal fluid protein. Buckman et al.[387] interviewed 340 patients meeting American Rheumatology Association criteria for the diagnosis of SLE. Twelve percent had affected relatives: Five had two affected relatives, and 36 had one affected relative each. McCombe et al.[388] described two sisters with clinically definite MS. One sister also had a history of Graves' disease. The other sister had a daughter with SLE. Over the next four generations, additional female family members had histories of hyperthyroidism, Addison's disease, sarcoidosis, and MS. McCombe et al. reasoned that familial cases of MS and SLE were the result of a genetic predisposition to autoimmune disease. Sloan et al.[389] reported the occurrence of MS and SLE in two generations of the same family. In one generation, two siblings were given diagnoses of MS. In the second generation, three children of one of the siblings developed SLE. Sloan et al. hypothesized that MS and SLE were separate expressions of the same autoimmune diathesis.

A number of investigators have tried to associate HLA markers with a predisposition to develop MS or SLE. McCombe et al.[388] described the occurrence of MS, SLE, autoimmune thyroid disease, and sarcoidosis in six generations of a single family. All but one of the affected family members was related to the proband on the maternal side, and all the affected females shared an HLA haplotype. This haplotype, however, was also present in unaffected individuals. Sloan et al.,[389] conversely, did not find any association between HLA inheritance of genes and the subsequent development of MS and SLE in two generations of the same family.

Wegener's Granulomatosis

Neurologic involvement occurs in up to 50% of patients with Wegener's granulomatosis and is manifest usually by a mononeuropathy multiplex or polyneuropathy. The brain may be affected by basal meningitis, temporal lobe dysfunction, cranial neuropathies, cerebral infarction, or venous sinus obstruction. In one study of 109 patients with neurologic complications,[390] eight had multiple cranial neuropathies, and five had cerebritis. White-matter disease is not usually found in patients with Wegener's granulomatosis. An exceptional case report is of a woman with Wegener's granulomatosis who had granulomatous basilar meningitis and also had foci of demyelination in her medulla and spinal cord not easily explicable by her granulomatous lesions.[391]

Other Immune-Mediated Disorders with Multiple Sclerosis–Like Central Nervous System Involvement

Associations between MS and other organ-specific autoimmune disorders have been difficult to demonstrate epidemiologically, but the concurrence of several of these in a patient inevitably raises the question of an underlying common causal factor. There are multiple reports of MS or MS-like CNS involvement in autoimmune thyroiditis and Crohn's disease. Another rare systemic disorder that may demonstrate MS-like CNS involvement is systemic histiocytosis-X.

Vascular and Traumatic Disorders

Irradiation

Radiotherapy for primary and metastatic brain tumors is neurotoxic and may result in structural lesions located diffusely in the cerebral periventricular and subcortical white matter. As a result of the diffuse nature of the lesions, a plethora of symptoms may result. It is sometimes difficult to differentiate between symptoms that are a result of radiotherapy versus those secondary to the tumor itself. In most cases, cognitive impairment has been noted ranging from a confusional state to coma. A subcortical dementia has also been described, the onset of which is reported to be 3–12 months after therapy. A predilection for bilateral corticospinal tracts produces impairment in motor function and movement. A pseudo-parkinsonian syndrome may be seen.[392] Akinesia and tremors are part of the clinical spectrum as well. MRI spectroscopy has been used to demonstrate diffuse chemical changes in the white matter after irradiation.[393] The degree of damage to the white matter was observed to be dose dependent.

Pathology shows pallor or spongiosis of the white matter with a vacuolar appearance, tissue necrosis with demyelination, axonal loss, and reactive astrocytosis with white-matter edema. In a study of children receiving a combination of chemotherapy and radiotherapy, multifocal necrotic lesions in the cerebral white matter were seen on autopsy. There was no significant inflammatory response noted. Macrophages were not present; however, loss of myelin axonal damage and glial cell loss was observed. The white matter demonstrated a spongy appearance.[394] Narrowing of small, penetrating vessels in the CNS may occur several years and sometimes decades after whole-brain radiotherapy for tumors and may lead to focal strokes, mimicking demyelinating lesions.

MRI spectroscopy may be used to show the metabolic changes in white matter which appears grossly affected by radiotherapy (identified by T_2 hyperintense lesions on conventional MRI) versus normal-appearing white matter. Decreased metabolite ratios indicate that damage to the axon and membrane had occurred in the areas where lesions were present on routine MRI studies. In patients with cognitive changes, MRI of the brain revealed a rapid progressive ventriculomegaly and diffuse hyperintense T_2 lesions in the white matter.[392] Necrotic lesions have been well demonstrated on MRI as T_2 cystic lesions with finger-like extensions in the temporal lobe in a patient with nasopharyngeal carcinoma.[395] Spectroscopy has been used successfully to differentiate the effect of radiotherapy versus the effect of tumor load.[396]

Head Trauma

Head trauma presentation is variable and dependent on the cause and consequently the location of the lesions. Early signs may be manifested as an acute confusional state, a comatose state, or a vegetative state, the duration of which may be linked to the location of the lesions produced. Lesions in the corpus callosum, corona radiata, and brain stem were more often found to be the location in patients who showed evidence of a profound change in mental status.[397]

Lesions that are the result of head trauma often produce symptoms of headache, memory deficits, dizziness, and sleep disorders.[398] Cognitive changes correlate well with lesions located in the frontal and temporal lobes. Memory loss is often seen in temporal lobe contusions, and frontal lobe lesions may be manifested as attentional deficits and changes in personality.

A connection between trauma and MS has never been convincingly established. Anecdotal reports have suggested a link between an episode of trauma and the first signs of MS in some patients. It is thought that diligent management and advancements in investigative studies, such as MRIs, may be responsible for the diagnosis of MS in the setting of head trauma in some patients. Some researchers have postulated that trauma leads to the triggering and manifestation of latent disease. Others contend that the emotional stress caused by the trauma may have an impact on pre-existing MS. Regardless of these hypotheses, it is generally accepted that trauma does not play an important role in the pathogenesis of MS.

Imaging studies show that the cerebral lesions that occur as a result of head trauma are best seen on FLAIR and diffusion-weighted MRI.[399] In cases of closed head trauma, the frontal and temporal lobes of the brain and the corpus callosum are the areas most frequently affected. The lesion volumes measured using FLAIR sequences in both the frontal lobes and the corpus callosum were observed to correlate well with disability and cognition scores in the subacute and chronic stages.[400]

The pathology reveals hemorrhagic lesions with the characteristics of contusions in the corpus callosum, subcortical white matter, internal capsule, and pons.[401] These lesions are thought to be the result of diffuse axonal injury (shearing injury).

Ischemic Vascular Disease

The clinical features of the vascular diseases are dependent on the vascular territory supplied by the affected vessel. They may take the form of a stuttering course or an acute and rapidly evident constellation of signs and symptoms. At times, the clinical presentation may resemble that of MS because this disease in itself can be present in any location in the white or gray matter of the cerebral hemisphere. Migraine, Binswanger's disease, embolic strokes, or strokes related to stenotic, occlusive, or hypertensive disease are disorders related to the cerebral vasculature.

The symptoms of migraine are well known and commonly include a severe hemicranial headache with photophobia, nausea, and emesis. Paresthesias involving the extremities and face and motor weakness in a similar distribution are not uncommon. These symptoms at times are mistaken for a transient ischemic attack or stroke. Certain foods and stressors often trigger migraines. Young migraine-prone females who smoke tobacco or use oral contraceptives are known to be at increased risk for strokes. Visual symptoms in migraine include photophobia, phosphenes, teichopsias, and fortification spectra. A phenomenon known as the *Alice in Wonderland syndrome* characterizes some types of migraine (reviewed in reference 402). The clinical features were first described by Lippman in 1952, and the resemblance of symptoms to the variations in size and shape experienced by the main character in the 1865 novel *Alice in Wonderland* prompted Todd to give it this name in 1955.[402] The symptoms are described as distortions of shape, with objects appearing smaller or larger than they are, a sensation of "zooming" of the environment, and an altered sense of time.

The hallmark sign of Binswanger's disease is a subcortical dementia, with signs that are reflective of frontal lobe dysfunction and involvement of the cortex, basal ganglia, thalamus, limbic system and subcortical white matter. This type of dementia is also present in some patients with MS.[403] The dementia is progressive and may be accompanied by incontinence, pseudo-bulbar signs, and motor deficits.[404]

In general, the vasculopathies that produce lesions that clinically mimic MS all ultimately exert their effects by producing ischemic changes in the cortical surface, the subcortical or periventricular white matter, and the brain stem. Cortical territory infarcts, border zone infarcts, or lacunar infarcts may result. The distribution of the lesions usually points to the etiology.[404] The cause may be ischemia secondary to an embolic source from the heart or an established coagulopathy or may be a stenotic-occlusive event attributable to atherosclerotic disease. Other risk factors include use of tobacco, amphetamines, or cocaine or history of hypercholesterolemia, diabetes mellitus, or migraine headaches. Other rare diseases include Susac's syndrome, which is manifested by encephalopathy and visual and hearing deficits and is caused by a microangiopathy that affects the small arteries of the brain, retina, and cochlea.[405]

Patients with CADASIL may present with severe migraine, stroke-like symptoms, psychiatric symptoms, and subcortical dementia. Binswanger's disease is thought to be secondary to a diffuse cerebral arteriosclerosis. Associations have been made in the past with hypertensive disease; however, the presence of dementia does not seem to correlate well with hypertensive disease in these patients. Lacunar infarcts may present as a "multi-infarct state" that manifests as a subcortical dementia; these small strokes have been found to be associated with hypertension, diabetes, and alcohol consumption.

The pathologic changes in Binswanger's disease are described as a periventricular cap of glial accumulations, loss of the ependymal lining, the presence of finely textured myelin as a result of myelin architecture, and a disrupted axonal glial pattern with axonal loss. This pattern is suggestive of fibrosis involving the vascular bed and is seen primarily in the subcortical white matter in Binswanger's disease and in MS. Lacunar lesions were also noted with an increase in fluid content.[406,407] On MRI, Binswanger's disease is characterized by extensive diffuse confluent lesions in the white matter. Focal lesions in the white matter may be present as well.

The vascular lesions mimicking MS on imaging studies have been attributed to hypertensive small-vessel ischemic disease, Binswanger's disease, CADASIL, embolic infarcts secondary to subacute bacterial endocarditis or atrial myxoma, and ischemic lesions that are the result of an underlying coagulopathy. The vascular ischemic lesions that result from migraines tend to be located in the deep or subcortical white matter of the posterior parietal and occipital lobes. Bilateral anterior cerebral artery infarcts are

rare but have been reported.[408] It should be noted that the cerebral vascular lesions of migraine appear to be much less numerous than the demyelinative lesions seen in MS.[409] Cardioembolic events, particularly those associated with subacute bacterial endocarditis, may manifest as multiple lesions distributed diffusely throughout the vascular bed. Embolic events, hypotensive events, and atherosclerosis have been known to produce border zone infarcts that sometimes can be misinterpreted as demyelinative lesions. Furthermore, an association between border zone infarcts and periventricular white-matter changes has been described.[410] Similarly, an association has been recognized between lacunar infarction and severe white-matter changes. In patients with CADASIL, diffuse subcortical infarcts are identified in the basal ganglia and white matter.[411]

The use of MRIs to differentiate lesions in the white matter has proved to be useful. Using a sophisticated technique of three-dimensional tissue segmentation, the differences in the type of lesions becomes evident. Using this technique, the images of patients with MS revealed that gliosis, edema, and demyelination were the prominent findings. In subcortical lesions that produced a vascular dementia, the lesions appeared more homogeneous. In lesions caused by lacunar infarction, a cystic central area of necrosis is found to be encircled by reactive gliosis.[412]

Other Vascular Lesions

Of the various vascular malformation syndromes, cavernous angioma or hemangioma most frequently are misdiagnosed as MS, especially when located in the brain stem or spinal cord.[413,414] Cases involving capillary telangiectasia, dural arteriovenous fistula, venous angioma, epidural angiolipoma, and arteriovenous malformations also have been reported.[415–417] Arteriovenous malformations in particular may be associated with ischemic lesions in the cerebral white matter. Recognition of a single well-circumscribed or multilobulated brightly enhancing lesion leads to the correct diagnosis.

Conclusions

Although most textbooks include long lists of diseases that should be in the differential diagnosis of

MS, a classic presentation of MS can be readily diagnosed by detailed history taking and clinical examination together with a confirmatory MRI. Understanding that some disorders that mimic MS, in particular Lyme disease (in some geographic regions) and vitamin B_{12} deficiency, are relatively common and may respond to treatment justifies routine screening for these disorders. It is the atypical presentations of MS that may require very extensive testing, and clinical knowledge of the usually rare disorders in the differential diagnosis thus helps to direct the investigation. Thus, the following questions gain relevance in the workup of cases that clinically resemble MS:

- Is there a family history of similar episodes?
- Are the lesions symmetric or otherwise atypical on MRI?
- Has the patient had a rash, mucocutaneous ulcer, or trunk angiokeratomas?
- Is there a systemic illness accompanying the symptoms?
- Is there a history of migraines, arthralgias, or venous thrombosis?
- Is there evidence of a peripheral neuropathy?

References

1. Dangond F, Lacomis D, Schwartz RB, et al. Acute disseminated encephalomyelitis progressing to hemorrhagic encephalitis. Neurology 1991;41:1697–1698.
2. Baringer JR, Pisani P. Herpes simplex virus genomes in human nervous system tissue analyzed by polymerase chain reaction. Ann Neurol 1994;36(6):823–829.
3. Kaji M, Kusuhara T, Ayabe M, et al. Survey of herpes simplex virus infections of the central nervous system, including acute disseminated encephalomyelitis, in the Kyushu and Okinawa regions of Japan. Mult Scler 1996;2(2):83–87.
4. Duarte J, Argente J, Gutierrez P, et al. Herpes simplex brainstem encephalitis with a relapsing course. J Neurol 1994;241(6):401–403.
5. Rose JW, Stroop WG, Matsuo F, Henkel J. Atypical herpes simplex encephalitis: clinical, virologic, and neuropathologic evaluation. Neurology 1992;42(9):1809–1812.
6. Tyler KL, Tedder DG, Yamamoto LJ, et al. Recurrent brainstem encephalitis associated with herpes simplex virus type 1 DNA in cerebrospinal fluid. Neurology 1995;45(12):2246–2250.
7. Moulignier A, Baudrimont M, Martin-Negrier ML, et al. Fatal brain stem encephalitis due to herpes simplex virus type 1 in AIDS. J Neurol 1996;243(6):491–493.
8. Folpe A, Lapham LW, Smith HC. Herpes simplex myelitis as a cause of acute necrotizing myelitis syndrome. Neurology 1994;44(10):1955–1957.
9. Ellie E, Rozenberg F, Dousset V, Beylot-Barry M. Herpes simplex virus type 2 ascending myeloradiculitis: MRI findings and rapid diagnosis by the polymerase chain method. J Neurol Neurosurg Psychiatry 1994;57(7):869–870.
10. Nakajima H, Furutama D, Kimura F, et al. Herpes simplex virus myelitis: clinical manifestations and diagnosis by the polymerase chain reaction method. Eur Neurol 1998;39(3):163–167.
11. Shyu WC, Lin JC, Chang BC, et al. Recurrent ascending myelitis: an unusual presentation of herpes simplex virus type 1 infection. Ann Neurol 1993;34(4):625–627.
12. Nakajima H, Furutama D, Kimura F, et al. Herpes simplex virus type 2 infections presenting as brainstem encephalitis and recurrent myelitis. Intern Med 1995;34(9):839–842.
13. Chua KB, Lam SK, AbuBakar S, et al. The incidence of human herpesvirus 6 infection in children with febrile convulsion admitted to the University Hospital, Kuala Lumpur. Med J Malaysia 1997;52(4):335–341.
14. Suga S, Suzuki K, Ihira M, et al. Clinical characteristics of febrile convulsions during primary HHV-6 infection. Arch Dis Child 2000;82(1):62–66.
15. Bland RM, Mackie PL, Shorts T, et al. The rapid diagnosis and clinical features of human herpesvirus 6. J Infect 1998;36(2):161–165.
16. Bertolani MF, Portolani M, Marotti F, et al. A study of childhood febrile convulsions with particular reference to HHV-6 infection: pathogenic considerations. Childs Nerv Syst 1996;12(9):534–539.
17. Barone SR, Kaplan MH, Krilov LR. Human herpesvirus-6 infection in children with first febrile seizures. J Pediatr 1995;127(1):95–97.
18. McCullers JA, Lakeman FD, Whitley RJ. Human herpesvirus 6 is associated with focal encephalitis. Clin Infect Dis 1995;21(3):571–576.
19. Carrigan DR, Harrington D, Knox KK. Subacute leukoencephalitis caused by CNS infection with human herpesvirus-6 manifesting as acute multiple sclerosis. Neurology 1996;47(1):145–148.
20. Steere AC, Malarwista SE, Snydman DR, et al. Lyme arthritis: an epidemic of oligoarticular arthritis in children and adults in three Connecticut communities. Arthritis Rheum 1977;20:7–17.
21. Burgdorfer W, Barbour AG, Hayes SF, et al. Lyme disease—a tick-borne spirochetosis? Science 1982;216:1317–1319.
22. Benach JL, Bosler EM, Hanrahan JP, et al. Spirochetes isolated from the blood of two patients with Lyme disease. N Engl J Med 1983;308:740–742.
23. Steere A. The spirochetal etiology of Lyme disease. N Engl J Med 1983;308:733–740.
24. Berger BW, Johnson RC, Kodner C, Coleman L. Cultivation of *Borrelia burgdorferi* from erythema migrans lesions and perilesional skin. J Clin Microbiol 1992;30:359–361.
25. Orloski KA, Hayes EB, Campbell GL, Dennis DT. Surveillance for Lyme disease—United States, 1992–1998. Mor Mortal Wkly Rep CDC Surveill Summ 2000;49:1–11.

26. Anderson JF. Ecology of Lyme disease. Conn Med 1989; 53:343–346.

27. Evans J. Lyme disease. Curr Opin Rheumatol 2000;12: 311–317.

28. Ryffel K, Peter O, Rutti B, et al. Scored antibody reactivity determined by immunoblotting shows an association between clinical manifestations and presence of *Borrelia burgdorferi* sensu stricto, *B. garinii*, *B. afzelii*, and *B. valaisiana* in humans. J Clin Microbiol 1999;37:4086–4092.

29. Lebech AM, Hansen K, Brandrup F, et al. Diagnostic value of PCR for detection of *Borrelia burgdorferi* DNA in clinical specimens from patients with erythema migrans and lyme neuroborreliosis. Mol Diagn 2000;5: 139–150.

30. Sigal LH, Zahradnik JM, Lavin P, et al. A vaccine consisting of recombinant *Borrelia burgdorferi* outer-surface protein A to prevent Lyme disease. Recombinant Outer-Surface Protein A Lyme Disease Vaccine Study Consortium [published erratum appears in N Engl J Med 1998;339(8):571]. N Engl J Med 1998;339(4):216–222.

31. Steere AC, Sikan VK, Maurice F, et al. Vaccination against Lyme disease with recombinant *Borrelia burgdorferi* outer–surface lipoprotein A with adjuvant. Lyme Disease Vaccine Study Group. N Engl J Med 1998;339:209–215.

32. Rutter T. Lyme disease vaccine given guarded approval in the US [news]. BMJ 1998;316:1695.

33. Molloy PJ, Berardi VP, Persing D, Sigal LH. Detection of multiple reactive protein species by immunoblotting after recombinant outer surface protein A lyme disease vaccination. Clin Infect Dis 2000;31:42–47.

34. Steere A, Duray PH, Kauffmann DJ, Wormser GP. Unilateral blindness caused by infection with the Lyme disease spirochete, *Borrelia burgdorferi*. Ann Intern Med 1985; 103:382–384.

35. Breeveld J, Rothova A, Kuiper H. Intermediate uveitis and Lyme borreliosis. Br J Ophthalmol 1992;76:181–182.

36. Reznick JW, Braunstein DB, Walsh RL, et al. Lyme carditis. Electrophysiologic and histopathologic study. Am J Med 1986;81:923–927.

37. Linde MRVD, Crijns HJ, Lie KI. Transient complete AV block in Lyme disease. Electrophysiologic observations. Chest 1989;96:219–221.

38. Dotevall L, Hagberg L, Karlsson JE, Rosengren LE. Astroglial and neuronal proteins in cerebrospinal fluid as markers of CNS involvement in Lyme neuroborreliosis. Eur J Neurol 1999;6:169–178.

39. Eppes SC, Nelson DK, Lewis LL, Klein JD. Characterization of Lyme meningitis and comparison with viral meningitis in children. Pediatrics 1999;103:957–960.

40. Glasscock M, Pensak ML, Gulya AJ, Baker DC. Lyme disease. A cause of bilateral facial paralysis. Arch Otolaryngol 1985;111:47–49.

41. Eng GD. Lyme disease presenting with bilateral facial nerve palsy. Arch Phys Med Rehabil 1990;71:749–750.

42. Bouat C, Meyer F, Rosier S, et al. [Unusual case of bilateral optic neuritis in Lyme neuroborreliosis.] Med Trop (Mars) 1995;55:462–465.

43. Lesser RL, Kornmehl EW, Pachner AR, et al. Neuro–ophthalmologic manifestations of Lyme disease. Ophthalmology 1990;97:699–706.

44. Fritz C, Rosler A, Heyden B, Braune HJ. Trigeminal neuralgia as a clinical manifestation of Lyme neuroborreliosis [letter]. J Neurol 1996;243:367–368.

45. Hanner P, Rosenhall U, Edstrom S, Kaijser B. Hearing impairment in patients with antibody production against *Borrelia burgdorferi* antigen. Lancet 1989;1:13–15.

46. Hyden D, Roberg M, Odkvist L. Borreliosis as a cause of sudden deafness and vestibular neuritis in Sweden. Acta Otolaryngol Suppl 1995;520:320–322.

47. Quinn S, Boucher BJ, Booth JB. Reversible sensorineural hearing loss in Lyme disease. J Laryngol Otol 1997;111: 562–564.

48. Bertholon P, Damon G, Antoine J, et al. Bilateral sensorineural hearing loss and spastic paraparesis in Lyme disease. Otolaryngol Head Neck Surg 2000;122:458–460.

49. Halperin J, Krupp L, Golightly M, Volkman D. Lyme borreliosis–associated encephalopathy. Neurology 1990;40: 1340–1343.

50. Zifko U, Wondrusch E, Machacek E, Grisold W. [Inflammatory demyelinating neuropathy in neuroborreliosis.] Wien Med Wochenschr 1995;145:188–190.

51. Horowitz HW, Marks SJ, Weintraub M, Dumler JS. Brachial plexopathy associated with human granulocytic ehrlichiosis. Neurology 1996;46:1026–1029.

52. Tezzon F, Corradini C, Huber R, et al. Vasculitic mononeuritis multiplex in patient with Lyme disease. Ital J Neurol Sci 1991;12:229–232.

53. Shapiro EE. Guillain-Barre syndrome in a child with serologic evidence of *Borrelia burgdorferi* infection [published erratum appears in Pediatr Infect Dis J 1998;17(6):481]. Pediatr Infect Dis J 1998;17:264–265.

54. Horneff G, Huppertz HI, Muller K, et al. Demonstration of *Borrelia burgdorferi* infection in a child with Guillain-Barré syndrome. Eur J Pediatr 1993;152:810–812.

55. Hemmer B, Glocker FX, Kaiser R, et al. Generalised motor neuron disease as an unusual manifestation of *Borrelia burgdorferi* infection [letter]. J Neurol Neurosurg Psychiatry 1997;63:257–258.

56. Huisman TA, Wohlrab G, Nadal D, et al. Unusual presentations of neuroborreliosis (Lyme disease) in childhood. J Comput Assist Tomogr 1999;23:39–42.

57. Faul JL, Ruoss S, Doyle RL, Kao PN. Diaphragmatic paralysis due to Lyme disease. Eur Respir J 1999;13:700–702.

58. Daffner KR, Saver JL, Biber MP. Lyme polyradiculoneuropathy presenting as increasing abdominal girth. Neurology 1990;40:373–375.

59. Krishnamurthy KB, Liu GT, Logigan EL. Acute Lyme neuropathy presenting with polyradicular pain, abdominal protrusion, and cranial neuropathy. Muscle Nerve 1993;16:1261–1264.

60. Zamponi N, Cardinali C, Tavoni MA, et al. Chronic neuroborreliosis in infancy. Ital J Neurol Sci 1999;20:303–307.

61. Curless RG, Schatz NJ, Bowen BC, et al. Lyme neuroborreliosis masquerading as a brainstem tumor in a 15-year-old. Pediatr Neurol 1996;15:258–260.

62. Dinerman H, Steere AC. Lyme disease associated with fibromyalgia. Ann Intern Med 1992;117:281–285.

63. Goldenberg DL. Fibromyalgia, chronic fatigue syndrome,

and myofascial pain syndrome. Curr Opin Rheumatol 1994;6:223–233.

64. Goldenberg DL. Fibromyalgia, chronic fatigue syndrome, and myofascial pain syndrome. Curr Opin Rheumatol 1995;7:127–135.

65. Lightfoot RW Jr., Luft BJ, Rahn DW, et al. Empiric parenteral antibiotic treatment of patients with fibromyalgia and fatigue and a positive serologic result for Lyme disease. A cost-effectiveness analysis. Ann Intern Med 1993;119:503–509.

66. Schned ES, Williams DN. Special concerns in Lyme disease. Seropositivity with vague symptoms and development of fibrositis. Postgrad Med 1992;91:65–68, 70.

67. Danek A, Uttner I, Yoursry T, Pfister HW. Lyme neuroborreliosis disguised as normal pressure hydrocephalus. Neurology 1996;46:1743–1745.

68. Druschky K, Stefan H, Grehl H, Neundorfer B. [Secondary normal pressure hydrocephalus. A complication of chronic neuroborreliosis.] Nervenarzt 1999;70:556–559.

69. Reik L Jr. Stroke due to Lyme disease. Neurology 1993;43:2705–2707.

70. Piccolo I, Thiella G, Sterzi R, et al. Chorea as a symptom of neuroborreliosis: a case study. Ital J Neurol Sci 1998;19:235–239.

71. de la Sayette V, Schaeffer S, Queruel C, et al. Lyme neuroborreliosis presenting with propriospinal myoclonus [letter]. J Neurol Neurosurg Psychiatry 1996;61:420.

72. Vukelic D, Bozinovic D, Morovic M, et al. Opsoclonus-myoclonus syndrome in a child with neuroborreliosis. J Infect 2000;40:189–191.

73. Christen HJ, Bartlan N, Hanefield F, et al. Peripheral facial palsy in childhood—Lyme borreliosis to be suspected unless proven otherwise. Acta Paediatr Scand 1990;79:1219–1224.

74. Belman AL, Lyer M, Coyle PK, Dattwyler R. Neurologic manifestations in children with North American Lyme disease. Neurology 1993;43:2609–2614.

75. Wilke M, Eiffert H, Christen HJ, Hanefeld F. Primarily chronic and cerebrovascular course of Lyme neuroborreliosis: case reports and literature review. Arch Dis Child 2000;83:67–71.

76. Halperin JJ, Luft BJ, Anand AK, et al. Lyme neuroborreliosis: central nervous system manifestations. Neurology 1989;39:753–759.

77. Kirchner A, Koedel V, Fingerle V, et al. Upregulation of matrix metalloproteinase-9 in the cerebrospinal fluid of patients with acute Lyme neuroborreliosis. J Neurol Neurosurg Psychiatry 2000;68:368–3671.

78. Perides G. Tanner-Brown LM, Klempner MS. *Borrelia burgdorferi* induces matrix metalloproteinases by neural cultures. J Neurosci Res 1999;58:779–790.

79. Lewczuk P, Reiber H, Korenke GC, et al. Intrathecal release of sICAM-1 into CSF in neuroborreliosis—increased brain-derived fraction. J Neuroimmunol 2000;103:93–96.

80. Hemmer B, Gran B, Zhao Y, et al. Identification of candidate T-cell epitopes and molecular mimics in chronic Lyme disease. Nat Med 1999;5:1375–1382.

81. Pachner AR, Amemiya K, Delaney E, et al. Interleukin-6 is expressed at high levels in the CNS in Lyme neuroborreliosis. Neurology 1997;49:147–152.

82. Pachner AR, Delaney E, O'Neill T, Major E. Inoculation of nonhuman primates with the N40 strain of *Borrelia burgdorferi* leads to a model of Lyme neuroborreliosis faithful to the human disease. Neurology 1995;45:165–172.

83. Kiefer R, Dangond F, Mueller M, et al. Enhanced B7 costimulatory molecule expression in inflammatory human sural nerve biopsies. J Neurol Neurosurg Psychiatry 2000;69:362–368.

84. Defosse DL, Johnson RC. In vitro and in vivo induction of tumor necrosis factor alpha by *Borrelia burgdorferi*. Infect Immun 1992;60:1109–1113.

85. Habicht GS, Beck G, Benach JL, et al. Lyme disease spirochetes induce human and murine interleukin 1 production. J Immunol 1985;134:3147–3154.

86. Radolf JD, Norgard MV, Brandt ME, et al. Lipoproteins of *Borrelia burgdorferi* and *Treponema pallidum* activate cachectin/tumor necrosis factor synthesis. Analysis using a CAT reporter construct. J Immunol 1991;147:1968–1974.

87. Sigal LH, Tatum AH. Lyme disease patients' serum contains IgM antibodies to *Borrelia burgdorferi* that cross-react with neuronal antigens. Neurology 1988;38:1439–1442.

88. Ryberg B, Hindfelt B, Nilsson B, Olsson JE. Antineural antibodies in Guillain-Barré syndrome and lymphocytic meningoradiculitis (Bannwarth's syndrome). Arch Neurol 1984;41:1277–1281.

89. Mackworth-Young CG, Harris EN, Steere AC, et al. Anti-cardiolipin antibodies in Lyme disease. Arthritis Rheum 1988;31:1052–1059.

90. Garcia-Monco JC, Coleman JL, Benach JL. Antibodies to myelin basic protein in Lyme disease [letter]. J Infect Dis 1988;158:667–668.

91. Baig S, Olsson T, Hojeberg B, Link H. Cells secreting antibodies to myelin basic protein in cerebrospinal fluid of patients with Lyme neuroborreliosis. Neurology 1991;41:581–587.

92. Aberer E, Brunner C, Suchanek G, et al. Molecular mimicry and Lyme borreliosis: a shared antigenic determinant between *Borrelia burgdorferi* and human tissue. Ann Neurol 1989;26:732–737.

93. Chmielewska-Badora J, Cisak E, Dutkiewicz J. Lyme borreliosis and multiple sclerosis: any connection? A seroepidemic study. Ann Agric Environ Med 2000;7(2):141–143.

94. Coyle P, Krupp L, Doscher C. Significance of reactive Lyme serology in multiple sclerosis. Ann Neurol 1993;34(5):745–747.

95. Wang WZ, Fredrikson S, Sun JB, Link H. Lyme neuroborreliosis: evidence for persistent up-regulation of *Borrelia burgdorferi*-reactive cells secreting interferon-gamma. Scand J Immunol 1995;42:694–700.

96. Maimone D, Villanova M, Stanta G, et al. Detection of *Borrelia burgdorferi* DNA and complement membrane attack complex deposits in the sural nerve of a patient with chronic polyneuropathy and tertiary Lyme disease. Muscle Nerve 1997;20:969–975.

97. Kaiser R, Lucking CH. Intrathecal synthesis of specific antibodies in neuroborreliosis. Comparison of different ELISA techniques and calculation methods. J Neurol Sci 1993;118:64–72.

98. Kaiser R, Rasiah C, Gassmann G, et al. Intrathecal antibody

synthesis in Lyme neuroborreliosis: use of recombinant p41 and a 14-kDa flagellin fragment in ELISA. J Med Microbiol 1993;39:290–297.

99. Kaiser R. Variable CSF findings in early and late Lyme neuroborreliosis: a follow-up study in 47 patients. J Neurol 1994;242:26–36.

100. Kaiser R. Intrathecal immune response in neuroborreliosis: importance of cross-reactive antibodies. Zentralbl Bakteriol 1995;282:303–314.

101. Lebech AM, Hansen K. Detection of *Borrelia burgdorferi* DNA in urine samples and cerebrospinal fluid samples from patients with early and late Lyme neuroborreliosis by polymerase chain reaction. J Clin Microbiol 1992;30: 1646–1653.

102. Nocton JJ, Bloom BJ, Rutledge BJ, et al. Detection of *Borrelia burgdorferi* DNA by polymerase chain reaction in cerebrospinal fluid in Lyme neuroborreliosis. J Infect Dis 1996;174:623–627.

103. Picha D, Moravcova L, Zdarsky E, Benes J. Clinical comparison of immunoblot and antibody index for detection of intrathecal synthesis of specific antibodies in Lyme neuroborreliosis. Eur J Clin Microbiol Infect Dis 2000; 19:805–806.

104. Hansen K, Cruz M, Link H. Oligoclonal *Borrelia burgdorferi*–specific IgG antibodies in cerebrospinal fluid in Lyme neuroborreliosis. J Infect Dis 1990;161:1194–202.

105. Logigian EL, Steere AC. Clinical and electrophysiologic findings in chronic neuropathy of Lyme disease. Neurology 1992;42:303–311.

106. Logigian EL. Peripheral nervous system Lyme borreliosis. Semin Neurol 1997;17:25–30.

107. Sumiya H, Kobayashi K, Mizukoshi C, et al. Brain perfusion SPECT in Lyme neuroborreliosis. J Nucl Med 1997; 38:1120–1122.

108. Marsot-Dupuch K, Gallouedec G, Bousson V, et al. [Facial palsy, enhancement of cranial nerves and Lyme disease.] J Radiol 2000;81:43–45.

109. Fernandez RE, Rothberg M, Ferncz G, Wujack D. Lyme disease of the CNS: MR imaging findings in 14 cases. AJNR Am J Neuroradiol 1990;11:479–481.

110. Aasly J, Nilsen G. Cerebral atrophy in Lyme disease. Neuroradiology 1990;32:252.

111. De Maria AD, Primavera A. Possibility of the use of oral long-acting tetracyclines in the treatment of Lyme neuroborreliosis. Clin Infect Dis 2000;31:848–849.

112. Dotevall L, Alestig K, Hanner P, et al. The use of doxycycline in nervous system *Borrelia burgdorferi* infection. Scand J Infect Dis Suppl 1988;53:74–79.

113. Dotevall L, Hagberg L. Penetration of doxycycline into cerebrospinal fluid in patients treated for suspected Lyme neuroborreliosis. Antimicrob Agents Chemother 1989;33: 1078–1080.

114. Dotevall L, Hagberg L. Successful oral doxycycline treatment of Lyme disease-associated facial palsy and meningitis. Clin Infect Dis 1999;28:569–574.

115. Seltzer EG, Gerber MA, Cartter ML, et al. Long-term outcomes of persons with Lyme disease. JAMA 2000;283: 609–616.

116. Bateman H, Sigal L. Update on Lyme Carditis. Curr Infect Dis Rep 2000;2:299–301.

117. Adams WV, Rose CD, Eppes SC, Klein JD. Long-term cognitive effects of Lyme disease in children. Appl Neuropsychol 1999;6:39–45.

118. Brightbill TC, Ihmeidan IH, Post MJ, et al. Neurosyphilis in HIV-positive and HIV-negative patients: neuroimaging findings. AJNR Am J Neuroradiol 1995;16(4):703–711.

119. Yamaguchi S, Johkura K, Nagatomo H, et al. A case of Lissauer's general paresis with left hemisphere dominant brain atrophy and leuko-araiosis in the deep white matter on MRI. Rinsho Shinkeigaku 1995;35(8):904–907.

120. Browning DJ. Posterior segment manifestations of active ocular syphilis, their response to a neurosyphilis regimen of penicillin therapy, and the influence of human immunodeficiency virus status on response. Ophthalmology 2000; 107(11):2015–2023.

121. Durand DV, Lecomte C, Cathebras P, et al. Whipple disease. Clinical review of 52 cases. The SNFMI Research Group on Whipple Disease. Societe Nationale Francaise de Medecine Interne. Medicine (Baltimore) 1997;76(3):170–184.

122. Suzer T, Demirkan N, Tahta K, et al. Whipple's disease confined to the central nervous system: case report and review of the literature. Scand J Infect Dis 1999;31(4): 411–414.

123. De Coene B, Gilliard C, Indekeu P, et al. Whipple's disease confined to the central nervous system. Neuroradiology 1996;38(4):325–327.

124. Brown AP, Lane JC, Murayama S, Vollmer DG. Whipple's disease presenting with isolated neurological symptoms. Case report. J Neurosurg 1990;73(4):623–627.

125. Erdem E, Carlier R, Delvalle A, et al. Gadolinium-enhanced MRI in cerebral Whipple's disease. Neuroradiology 1993;35(8):581–583.

126. Schnider P, Trattnig S, Kollegger H, Auff E. MR of cerebral Whipple disease. AJNR Am J Neuroradiol 1995;16(6): 1328–1329.

127. Clarke CE, Falope ZF, Abdelhadi HA, Franks AJ. Cervical myelopathy caused by Whipple's disease. Neurology 1998;50(5):1505–1506.

128. Verhagen WI, Huygen PL, Dalman JE, Schuurmans MM. Whipple's disease and the central nervous system. A case report and a review of the literature. Clin Neurol Neurosurg 1996;98(4):299–304.

129. Coria F, Cuadrado N, Velasco C, et al. Whipple's disease with isolated central nervous system symptomatology diagnosed by molecular identification of *Tropheryma whippelii* in peripheral blood. Neurologia 2000;15(4): 173–176.

130. von Herbay A, Ditton HJ, Schuhmacher F, Maiwald M. Whipple's disease: staging and monitoring by cytology and polymerase chain reaction analysis of cerebrospinal fluid. Gastroenterology 1997;113(2):434–441.

131. Carella F, Valla P, Bernardi G, et al. Cerebral Whipple's disease: clinical and cerebrospinal fluid findings. Ital J Neurol Sci 1998;19(2):101–105.

132. Keinath RD, Merrell DE, Vlietstra R, Dobbins WO. Antibiotic treatment and relapse in Whipple's disease. Long-term follow-up of 88 patients. Gastroenterology 1985;88(6): 1867–1873.

133. Cooper GS, Blades EW, Remler BF, et al. Central nervous system Whipple's disease: relapse during therapy with tri-

methoprim-sulfamethoxazole and remission with cefixime. Gastroenterology 1994;106(3):782–786.

134. Anderson M. Neurology of Whipple's disease. J Neurol Neurosurg Psychiatry 2000;68(1):2–5.

135. Chen CJ, Chu NS, Lu CS, Sung CY. Serial magnetic resonance imaging in patients with Balo's concentric sclerosis: natural history of lesion development. Ann Neurol 1999;46(4):651–656.

136. Sekijima Y, Tokuda T, Hashimoto T, et al. Serial magnetic resonance imaging (MRI) study of a patient with Baló's concentric sclerosis treated with immunoadsorption plasmapheresis. Mult Scler 1997;2(6):291–294.

137. Wingerchuk DM, Hogancamp WF, O'Brien PC, Weinshenker BG. The clinical course of neuromyelitis optica (Devic's syndrome). Neurology 1999;53(5):1107–1114.

138. Katz JD, Ropper AH. Progressive necrotic myelopathy: clinical course in 9 patients. Arch Neurol 2000;57(3):355–361.

139. Carod Artal FJ, Brenner C, Melo M, et al. Devic's neuromyelitis optica. Presentation of 2 new cases and review of the bibliography. Neurologia 2000;15(7):307–312.

140. Piccolo G, Franciotta DM, Camana C, et al. Devic's neuromyelitis optica: long-term follow-up and serial CSF findings in two cases. J Neurol 1990;237(4):262–264.

141. Filippi M, Rocca MA, Moiola L, et al. MRI and magnetization transfer imaging changes in the brain and cervical cord of patients with Devic's neuromyelitis optica. Neurology 1999;53(8):1705–1710.

142. Mandler RN, Dencoff JD, Midani F, et al. Matrix metalloproteinases and tissue inhibitors of metalloproteinases in cerebrospinal fluid differ in multiple sclerosis and Devic's neuromyelitis optica. Brain 2001;124(Pt 3):493–498.

143. Chusid MJ, Williamson SJ, Murphy JV, Ramey LS. Neuromyelitis optica (Devic disease) following varicella infection. J Pediatr 1979;95(5 Pt 1):737–738.

144. Silber MH, Willcox PA, Bowen RM, Unger A. Neuromyelitis optica (Devic's syndrome) and pulmonary tuberculosis. Neurology 1990;40(6):934–938.

145. Perez-Garcia C, Maravi Petri E, Goni Iturralde R, et al. Devic's syndrome complicating a *Mycoplasma pneumoniae* infection. Rev Clin Esp 1987;181(1):29–31.

146. Giorgi D, Balacco Gabrieli C, Bonomo L. The association of optic neuropathy with transverse myelitis in systemic lupus erythematosus. Rheumatology (Oxford) 1999;38(2):191–192.

147. Bonnet F, Mercie P, Morlat P, et al. Devic's neuromyelitis optica during pregnancy in a patient with systemic lupus erythematosus. Lupus 1999;8(3):244–247.

148. Margaux J, Hayem G, Meyer O, Kahn MF. Systemic lupus erythematosus with optical neuromyelitis (Devic's syndrome). A case with a 35-year follow-up. Rev Rhum Engl Ed 1999;66(2):102–105.

149. Inslicht DV, Stein AB, Pomerantz F, Ragnarsson KT. Three women with lupus transverse myelitis: case reports and differential diagnosis. Arch Phys Med Rehabil 1998;79(4):456–459.

150. Kinney EL, Berdoff RL, Rao NS, Fox LM. Devic's syndrome and systemic lupus erythematosus: a case report with necropsy. Arch Neurol 1979;36(10):643–644.

151. April RS, Vansonnenberg E. A case of neuromyelitis optica (Devic's syndrome) in systemic lupus erythemato-

sus. Clinicopathologic report and review of the literature. Neurology 1976;26(11):1066–1070.

152. Mochizuki A, Hayashi A, Hisahara S, Shoji S. Steroid-responsive Devic's variant in Sjögren's syndrome. Neurology 2000;54(6):1391–1392.

153. Mandler RN, Davis LE, Jeffery DR, Kornfeld M. Devic's neuromyelitis optica: a clinicopathological study of 8 patients. Ann Neurol 1993;34(2):162–168.

154. Cartier L, Arellano R, Garcia L, et al. Optic neuromyelitis: a necrotizing disease of the central nervous system. Rev Med Chil, 1998;126(8):981–986.

155. Mandler RN, Ahmed W, Dencoff JE. Devic's neuromyelitis optica: a prospective study of seven patients treated with prednisone and azathioprine. Neurology 1998;51(4):1219–1220.

156. Aguilera AJ, Carlow TJ, Smith KJ, Simon TL. Lymphocytaplasmapheresis in Devic's syndrome. Transfusion 1985;25(1):54–56.

157. Masson C, Denis P, Prier S, et al. Eales' disease with neurologic disorders. Rev Neurol (Paris) 1988;144(12):817–819.

158. Antiguedad A, Zarranz JJ. Eales' disease involving central nervous system white matter. Neurologia 1994;9(7):307–310.

159. Singhal BS, Dastur DK. Eales' disease with neurological involvement Part 1. Clinical features in 9 patients. J Neurol Sci 1976;27(3):313–321.

160. Dastur DK, Singhal BS. Eales' disease with neurological involvement. Part 2. Pathology and pathogenesis. J Neurol Sci 1976;27(3):323–345.

161. Misra UK, Jha S, Kalita J, Sharma K. Stroke—a rare presentation of Eales' disease. A case report. Angiology 1996;47(1):73–76.

162. Gordon MF, Coyle PK, Golub B. Eales' disease presenting as stroke in the young adult. Ann Neurol 1988;24(2):264–266.

163. Katz B, Wheeler D, Weinreb RN, Swenson MR. Eales' disease with central nervous system infarction. Ann Ophthalmol 1991;23(12):460–463.

164. Alfieri G, Barontini F, Brogelli S, Maurri S. Unusual association of Eales disease with multifocal neurological deficit. Ital J Neurol Sci 1984;5(4):461–462.

165. Sawhney IM, Chopra JS, Bansal SK, Gupta AK. Eales' disease with myelopathy. Clin Neurol Neurosurg 1986;88(3):213–215.

166. Pepin B, Goldstein B, Man HX, et al. Eales's disease with neurological involvement. Rev Neurol (Paris) 1978;134(6–7):427–436.

167. Hadjivassiliou M, Grunewald RA, Chattopadhyay AK, et al. Clinical, radiological, neurophysiological, and neuropathological characteristics of gluten ataxia. Lancet 1998;352(9140):1582–1585.

168. Hadjivassiliou M, Grunewald RA, Lawden M, et al. Headache and CNS white matter abnormalities associated with gluten sensitivity. Neurology 2001;56(3):385–388.

169. Ghezzi A, Filippi M, Falini A, Zaffaroni M. Cerebral involvement in celiac disease: a serial MRI study in a patient with brainstem and cerebellar symptoms. Neurology 1997;49(5):1447–1450.

170. Wills AJ. The neurology and neuropathology of coeliac disease. Neuropathol Appl Neurobiol 2000;26(6):493–496.

171. Dieterich W, Ehnis T, Bauer M, et al. Identification of tissue transglutaminase as the autoantigen of celiac disease. Nat Med 1997;3(7):797–801.

172. Clot F, Babron MC. Genetics of celiac disease. Mol Genet Metab 2000;71(1–2):76–80.

173. King AL, Ciclitira PJ. Celiac disease: strongly heritable, oligogenic, but genetically complex. Mol Genet Metab 2000;71(1–2):70–75.

174. Fine KD, Ogunji F, Saloum Y. Celiac sprue: another autoimmune syndrome associated with hepatitis C. Am J Gastroenterol 2001;96(1):138–145.

175. Giubilei F, Sarrantonio A, Tisei P, et al. Four-year follow-up of a case of acute multiple sclerosis of the Marburg type. Ital J Neurol Sci 1997;18(3):163–166.

176. Bitsch A, Wegener C, da Costa C, et al. Lesion development in Marburg's type of acute multiple sclerosis: from inflammation to demyelination. Mult Scler 1999;5(3):138–146.

177. Beniac DR, Wood DD, Palaniyar N, et al. Cryoelectron microscopy of protein-lipid complexes of human myelin basic protein charge isomers differing in degree of citrullination. J Struct Biol 2000;129(1):80–95.

178. Boggs JM, Rangaraj G, Koshy KM, et al. Highly deiminated isoform of myelin basic protein from multiple sclerosis brain causes fragmentation of lipid vesicles. J Neurosci Res 1999;57(4):529–535.

179. Cao L, Goodin R, Wood D, et al. Rapid release and unusual stability of immunodominant peptide 45-89 from citrullinated myelin basic protein. Biochemistry 1999;38(19):6157–6163.

180. Beniac DR, Wood DD, Palaniyar N, et al. Marburg's variant of multiple sclerosis correlates with a less compact structure of myelin basic protein. Mol Cell Biol Res Commun 1999;1(1):48–51.

181. Wood DD, Bilbao JM, O'Connors P, Moscarello MA. Acute multiple sclerosis (Marburg type) is associated with developmentally immature myelin basic protein. Ann Neurol 1996;40(1):18–24.

182. Beck R, Cleary P, Trobe J. The effect of corticosteroids for acute optic neuritis on the subsequent development of multiple sclerosis. N Engl J Med 1993;329:1764–1769.

183. Hainfellner JA, Schmidbauer M, Schmutzhard E, et al. Devic's neuromyelitis optica and Schilder's myelinoclastic diffuse sclerosis. J Neurol Neurosurg Psychiatry 1992;55(12):1194–1196.

184. Dresser LP, Tourian AY, Anthony DC. A case of myelinoclastic diffuse sclerosis in an adult. Neurology 1991;41(2 Pt 1):316–318.

185. Iniguez C, Pascual LF, Ramon y Cajal S, et al. Transitional multiple sclerosis (Schilder's disease): a case report. J Neurol 2000;247(12):974–976.

186. Poser CM, Goutieres F, Carpentier MA, Aicardi J. Schilder's myelinoclastic diffuse sclerosis. Pediatrics 1986;77(1):107–112.

187. Moser HW, Moser AB, Naidu S, Bergin A. Clinical aspects of adrenoleukodystrophy and adrenomyeloneuropathy. Dev Neurosci 1991;13(4–5):254–261.

188. Sobue G, Ueno-Natsukari I, Okamoto H, et al. Phenotypic heterogeneity of an adult form of adrenoleukodystrophy in monozygotic twins. Ann Neurol 1994;36(6):912–915.

189. van Geel BM, Assies J, Haverkort EB, et al. Progression of abnormalities in adrenomyeloneuropathy and neurologically asymptomatic X-linked adrenoleukodystrophy despite treatment with "Lorenzo's oil." J Neurol Neurosurg Psychiatry 1999;67(3):290–299.

190. Restuccia D, Di Lazzaro V, Valeriani M, et al. Neurophysiologic follow-up of long-term dietary treatment in adult-onset adrenoleukodystrophy. Neurology 1999;52(4):810–816.

191. Duchesne N, Dufour M, Bouchard G, et al. Adrenoleukodystrophy: magnetic resonance follow-up after Lorenzo's oil therapy. Can Assoc Radiol J 1995;46(5): 386–391.

192. Shapiro E, Krivit W, Lockman L, et al. Long-term effect of bone-marrow transplantation for childhood-onset cerebral X-linked adrenoleukodystrophy. Lancet 2000;356(9231):713–718.

193. Suzuki Y, Isogai K, Teramoto T, et al. Bone marrow transplantation for the treatment of X-linked adrenoleukodystrophy. J Inherit Metab Dis 2000;23(5):453–458.

194. Pai GS, Khan M, Barbosa E, et al. Lovastatin therapy for X-linked adrenoleukodystrophy: clinical and biochemical observations on 12 patients. Mol Genet Metab 2000;69(4):312–322.

195. Flavigny E, Sanhaj A, Aubourg P, Cartier N. Retroviral-mediated adrenoleukodystrophy-related gene transfer corrects very long chain fatty acid metabolism in adrenoleukodystrophy fibroblasts: implications for therapy. FEBS Lett 1999;448(2–3):261–264.

196. Lossos A, Meiner Z, Barash V, et al. Adult polyglucosan body disease in Ashkenazi Jewish patients carrying the Tyr329Ser mutation in the glycogen-branching enzyme gene. Ann Neurol 1998;44(6):867–872.

197. Boulan-Predseil P, Vital A, Brochet B, et al. Dementia of frontal lobe type due to adult polyglucosan body disease. J Neurol 1995;242(8):512–516.

198. Skullerud K, Andersen SN, Lundevall J. Cerebral lesions and causes of death in male alcoholics. A forensic autopsy study. Int J Legal Med 1991;104(4):209–213.

199. Navarro JF, Noriega S. [Marchiafava-Bignami disease.] Rev Neurol 1999;28(5):519–523.

200. Helenius J, Tatlisumak T, Soinne L, et al. Marchiafava-Bignami disease: two cases with favourable outcome. Eur J Neurol 2001;8(3):269–272.

201. Inagaki T, Saito K. [A case of Marchiafava-Bignami disease demonstrated by MR diffusion-weighted image.] No To Shinkei 2000;52(7):633–637.

202. Kikkawa Y, Takaya Y, Niwa N. [A case of Marchiafava-Bignami disease that responded to high-dose intravenous corticosteroid administration.] Rinsho Shinkeigaku 2000;40(11):1122–1125.

203. Gabriel S, Grossmann A, Hoppner J, et al. [Marchiafava-Bignami syndrome. Extrapontine myelinolysis in chronic alcoholism.] Nervenarzt 1999;70(4):349–356.

204. Kohler CG, Ances BM, Coleman AR, et al. Marchiafava-Bignami disease: literature review and case report. Neuropsychiatry Neuropsychol Behav Neurol 2000;13(1):67–76.

205. Ferracci F, Conte F, Gentile M, et al. Marchiafava-Bignami disease: computed tomographic scan, 99mTc HMPAO-SPECT, and FLAIR MRI findings in a patient

with subcortical aphasia, alexia, bilateral agraphia, and left-handed deficit of constructional ability. Arch Neurol 1999;56(1):107–110.

206. Tarnowska-Dziduszko E, Bertrand E, Szpak GM. Morphological changes in the corpus callosum in chronic alcoholism. Folia Neuropathol 1995;33(1):25–29.

207. Friese SA, Bitzer M, Freudenstein D, et al. Classification of acquired lesions of the corpus callosum with MRI. Neuroradiology 2000;42(11):795–802.

208. Yamamoto T, Ashikaga R, Araki Y, Nishimura Y. A case of Marchiafava-Bignami disease: MRI findings on spin-echo and fluid attenuated inversion recovery (FLAIR) images. Eur J Radiol 2000;34(2):141–143.

209. Blansjaar BA, Vielvoye GJ, van Dijk JG, Rijnders RJ. Similar brain lesions in alcoholics and Korsakoff patients: MRI, psychometric and clinical findings. Clin Neurol Neurosurg 1992;94(3):197–203.

210. Coffeen CM, McKenna CE, Koeppen AH, et al. Genetic localization of an autosomal dominant leukodystrophy mimicking chronic progressive multiple sclerosis to chromosome 5q31. Hum Mol Genet 2000;9(5):787–793.

211. Tournier-Lasserve E, Iba-Zizen MT, Romero N, Bousser MG. Autosomal dominant syndrome with strokelike episodes and leukoencephalopathy. Stroke 1991;22(10):1297–1302.

212. Ceroni M, Poloni TE, Tonietti S, et al. Migraine with aura and white matter abnormalities: Notch3 mutation. Neurology 2000;54(9):1869–1871.

213. Mellies JK, Baumer T, Muller JA, et al. SPECT study of a German CADASIL family: a phenotype with migraine and progressive dementia only. Neurology 1998;50(6):1715–1721.

214. Ebke M, Dichgans M, Bergmann M, et al. CADASIL: skin biopsy allows diagnosis in early stages. Acta Neurol Scand 1997;95(6):351–357.

215. Verin M, Rolland Y, Landgraf F, et al. New phenotype of the cerebral autosomal dominant arteriopathy mapped to chromosome 19: migraine as the prominent clinical feature. J Neurol Neurosurg Psychiatry 1995;59(6):579–585.

216. Malandrini A, Carrera P, Ciacci G, et al. Unusual clinical features and early brain MRI lesions in a family with cerebral autosomal dominant arteriopathy. Neurology 1997;48(5):1200–1203.

217. Hedera P, Friedland RP. Cerebral autosomal dominant arteriopathy with subcortical infarcts and leukoencephalopathy: study of two American families with predominant dementia. J Neurol Sci 1997;146(1):27–33.

218. Filley CM, Thompson LL, Sze CI, et al. White matter dementia in CADASIL. J Neurol Sci 1999;163(2):163–167.

219. Adair JC, Hart BL, Kornfeld M, et al. Autosomal dominant cerebral arteriopathy: neuropsychiatric syndrome in a family. Neuropsychiatry Neuropsychol Behav Neurol 1998;11(1):31–39.

220. Chabriat H, Vahedi K, Iba-Zizen MT, et al. Clinical spectrum of CADASIL: a study of 7 families. Cerebral autosomal dominant arteriopathy with subcortical infarcts and leukoencephalopathy. Lancet 1995;346(8980):934–939.

221. Joutel A, Dodick DD, Parisi JE, et al. De novo mutation in the Notch3 gene causing CADASIL. Ann Neurol 2000;47(3):388–391.

222. Joutel A, Vahedi K, Corpechot C, et al. Strong clustering and stereotyped nature of Notch3 mutations in CADASIL patients. Lancet 1997;350(9090):1511–1515.

223. Chabriat H, Levy C, Taillia H, et al. Patterns of MRI lesions in CADASIL. Neurology 1998;51(2):452–457.

224. Ruchoux MM, Brulin P, Leteurtre E, Maurage CA. Skin biopsy value and leukoaraiosis. Ann N Y Acad Sci 2000;903:285–292.

225. Mayer M, Straube A, Bruening R, et al. Muscle and skin biopsies are a sensitive diagnostic tool in the diagnosis of CADASIL. J Neurol 1999;246(7):526–532.

226. Crutchfield KE, Patronas NJ, Dambrosia JM, et al. Quantitative analysis of cerebral vasculopathy in patients with Fabry disease. Neurology 1998;50(6):1746–1749.

227. Cable WJ, Kolodny EH, Adams RD. Fabry disease: impaired autonomic function. Neurology 1982;32(5):498–502.

228. Filling-Katz MR, Merrick HF, Fink JK, et al. Carbamazepine in Fabry's disease: effective analgesia with dose-dependent exacerbation of autonomic dysfunction. Neurology 1989;39(4):598–600.

229. Harding AE. The inherited ataxias. Adv Neurol 1988;48:37–46.

230. Schelhaas HJ, Ippel PF, Beemer FA, Hageman G. Similarities and differences in the phenotype, genotype and pathogenesis of different spinocerebellar ataxias. Eur J Neurol 2000;7(3):309–314.

231. Klockgether T. Recent advances in degenerative ataxias. Curr Opin Neurol 2000;13(4):451–455.

232. Evidente VG, Gwinn-Hardy KA, Caviness JN, Gilman S. Hereditary ataxias. Mayo Clin Proc 2000;75(5):475–490.

233. Cavalier L, Ouahchi K, Kayden HJ, et al. Ataxia with isolated vitamin E deficiency: heterogeneity of mutations and phenotypic variability in a large number of families. Am J Hum Genet 1998;62(2):301–310.

234. Browne DL, Gancher ST, Nutt JG, et al. Episodic ataxia/myokymia syndrome is associated with point mutations in the human potassium channel gene, KCNA1. Nat Genet 1994;8(2):136–140.

235. Zhuchenko O, Bailey J, Bonnen P, et al. Autosomal dominant cerebellar ataxia (SCA6) associated with small polyglutamine expansions in the alpha 1A-voltage-dependent calcium channel. Nat Genet 1997;15(1):62–69.

236. Jodice C, Mantuano E, Veneziano L, et al. Episodic ataxia type 2 (EA2) and spinocerebellar ataxia type 6 (SCA6) due to CAG repeat expansion in the CACNA1A gene on chromosome 19p. Hum Mol Genet 1997;6(11):1973–1978.

237. Denier C, Ducros A, Vahedi K, et al. High prevalence of CACNA1A truncations and broader clinical spectrum in episodic ataxia type 2. Neurology 1999;52(9):1816–1821.

238. Yue Q, Jen JC, Thwe MM, et al. De novo mutation in CACNA1A caused acetazolamide-responsive episodic ataxia. Am J Med Genet 1998;77(4):298–301.

239. Griggs RC, Moxley RT 3rd, Lafrance RA, McQuillen J. Hereditary paroxysmal ataxia: response to acetazolamide. Neurology 1978;28(12):1259–1264.

240. Pujana MA, Corral J, Gratacos M, et al. Spinocerebellar ataxias in Spanish patients: genetic analysis of familial and sporadic cases. The Ataxia Study Group. Hum Genet 1999;104(6):516–522.

241. Cossee M, Durr A, Schmitt M, et al. Friedreich's ataxia: point mutations and clinical presentation of compound heterozygotes. Ann Neurol 1999;45(2):200–206.

242. Elting JW, Haaxma R, Sulter G, De Keyser J. Predicting outcome from coma: man-in-the-barrel syndrome as potential pitfall. Clin Neurol Neurosurg 2000;102(1):23–25.

243. Kraus J, Heckmann JG, Druschky A, et al. Ondine's curse in association with diabetes insipidus following transient vertebrobasilar ischemia. Clin Neurol Neurosurg 1999;101(3):196–198.

244. Chalela JA, Wolf RL, Maldjian JA, Kasner SE. MRI identification of early white matter injury in anoxic-ischemic encephalopathy. Neurology 2001;56(4):481–485.

245. O'Donnell P, Buxton PJ, Pitkin A, Jarvis LJ. The magnetic resonance imaging appearances of the brain in acute carbon monoxide poisoning. Clin Radiol 2000;55(4):273–280.

246. Priscu VR, Halperin D, Soroker D. [Delayed post-anoxic encephalopathy.] Harefuah 1994;127(10):384–385, 431.

247. Murata T, Itoh S, Koshino Y, et al. Serial cerebral MRI with FLAIR sequences in acute carbon monoxide poisoning. J Comput Assist Tomogr 1995;19(4):631–634.

248. Cambi F, Tartaglino L, Lublin F, McCarren D. X-linked pure familial spastic paraparesis. Characterization of a large kindred with magnetic resonance imaging studies. Arch Neurol 1995;52(7):665–669.

249. Yousem DM, Gutmann DH, Milestone BN, Lenkinski RE. Integrated MR imaging and proton nuclear magnetic resonance spectroscopy in a family with an X-linked spastic paraparesis. AJNR Am J Neuroradiol 1991;12(4):785–789.

250. Gutmann DH, Fischbeck KH, Kamholz J. Complicated hereditary spastic paraparesis with cerebral white matter lesions. Am J Med Genet 1990;36(2):251–257.

251. Nielsen JE, Krabbe K, Jennum P, et al. Autosomal dominant pure spastic paraplegia: a clinical, paraclinical, and genetic study. J Neurol Neurosurg Psychiatry 1998;64(1):61–66.

252. Satoh JI, Tokumoto H, Kurohara K, et al. Adult-onset Krabbe disease with homozygous T1853C mutation in the galactocerebrosidase gene. Unusual MRI findings of corticospinal tract demyelination. Neurology 1997;49(5):1392–1399.

253. Farina L, Bizzi A, Finocchiaro G, et al. MR imaging and proton MR spectroscopy in adult Krabbe disease. AJNR Am J Neuroradiol 2000;21(8):1478–1482.

254. Loes DJ, Peters C, Krivit W. Globoid cell leukodystrophy: distinguishing early-onset from late-onset disease using a brain MR imaging scoring method. AJNR Am J Neuroradiol 1999;20(2):316–323.

255. Inatomi Y, Tomoda H, Itoh Y, et al. An adult patient with Krabbe's disease—the first case reported in Japan. Rinsho Shinkeigaku 1993;33(11):1188–1194.

256. Turazzini M, Beltramello A, Bassi R, et al. Adult onset Krabbe's leukodystrophy: a report of 2 cases. Acta Neurol Scand 1997;96(6):413–415.

257. Wenger DA, Rafi MA, Luzi P, et al. Krabbe disease: genetic aspects and progress toward therapy. Mol Genet Metab 2000;70(1):1–9.

258. Rafi MA, Luzi P, Chen YQ, Wenger DA. A large deletion together with a point mutation in the GALC gene is a common mutant allele in patients with infantile Krabbe disease. Hum Mol Genet 1995;4(8):1285–1289.

259. Wenger DA. Murine, canine and non-human primate models of Krabbe disease. Mol Med Today 2000;6(11):449–451.

260. Wenger DA, Louie E. Pseudodeficiencies of arylsulfatase A and galactocerebrosidase activities. Dev Neurosci 1991;13(4–5):216–221.

261. Krivit W, Shapiro EG, Peters C, et al. Hematopoietic stem-cell transplantation in globoid-cell leukodystrophy. N Engl J Med 1998;338(16):1119–1126.

262. Vanopdenbosch L, Dubois B, D'Hooghe MB, et al. Mitochondrial mutations of Leber's hereditary optic neuropathy: a risk factor for multiple sclerosis. J Neurol 2000;247(7):535–543.

263. Mayr-Wohlfart U, Paulus C, Henneberg A, Rodel G. Mitochondrial DNA mutations in multiple sclerosis patients with severe optic involvement. Acta Neurol Scand 1996;94(3):167–171.

264. Reynier P, Penisson-Besnier I, Moreau C, et al. mtDNA haplogroup J: a contributing factor of optic neuritis. Eur J Hum Genet 1999;7(3):404–406.

265. Mojon DS, Fujihara K, Hirano M, et al. Leber's hereditary optic neuropathy mitochondrial DNA mutations in familial multiple sclerosis. Graefes Arch Clin Exp Ophthalmol 1999;237(4):348–350.

266. Mojon DS, Herbert J, Sadiq SA, et al. Leber's hereditary optic neuropathy mitochondrial DNA mutations at nucleotides 11778 and 3460 in multiple sclerosis. Ophthalmologica 1999;213(3):171–175.

267. Ohlenbusch A, Wilichowski E, Hanefeld F. Characterization of the mitochondrial genome in childhood multiple sclerosis. III. Multiple sclerosis without optic neuritis and the non-LHON–associated genes. Neuropediatrics 1998;29(6):313–319.

268. Wilichowski E, Ohlenbusch A, Hanefeld F. Characterization of the mitochondrial genome in childhood multiple sclerosis. II. Multiple sclerosis without optic neuritis and LHON-associated genes. Neuropediatrics 1998;29(6):307–312.

269. Leuzzi V, Carducci C, Lenza M, et al. LHON mutations in Italian patients affected by multiple sclerosis. Acta Neurol Scand 1997;96(3):145–148.

270. Kalman B, Rodriguez-Valdez JL, Bosch U, Lublin FD. Screening for Leber's hereditary optic neuropathy associated mitochondrial DNA mutations in patients with prominent optic neuritis. Mult Scler 1997;2(6):279–282.

271. Ohlenbusch A, Wilichowski E, Hanefeld F. Characterization of the mitochondrial genome in childhood multiple sclerosis. I. Optic neuritis and LHON mutations. Neuropediatrics 1998;29(4):175–179.

272. Dionisi-Vici C, Seneca S, Zeviani M, et al. Fulminant Leigh syndrome and sudden unexpected death in a family with the T9176C mutation of the mitochondrial ATPase 6 gene. J Inherit Metab Dis 1998;21(1):2–8.

273. Shoffner JM, Fernhoff PM, Krawiecki NS, et al. Subacute necrotizing encephalopathy: oxidative phosphorylation defects and the ATPase 6 point mutation. Neurology 1992;42(11):2168–2174.

274. Tatuch Y, Christodoulou J, Feigenbaum A, et al. Heteroplasmic mtDNA mutation (T----G) at 8993 can cause Leigh disease when the percentage of abnormal mtDNA is high. Am J Hum Genet 1992;50(4):852–858.

275. de Vries DD, van Engelen BG, Gabreels FJ, et al. A second missense mutation in the mitochondrial ATPase 6 gene in Leigh's syndrome. Ann Neurol 1993;34(3):410–412.

276. Uziel G, Moroni I, Lamantea E, et al. Mitochondrial disease associated with the T8993G mutation of the mitochondrial ATPase 6 gene: a clinical, biochemical, and molecular study in six families. J Neurol Neurosurg Psychiatry 1997;63(1):16–22.

277. Holt IJ, Harding AE, Petty RK, Morgan-Hughes JA. A new mitochondrial disease associated with mitochondrial DNA heteroplasmy. Am J Hum Genet 1990;46(3):428–433.

278. Koga Y, Akita Y, Takane N, et al. Heterogeneous presentation in A3243G mutation in the mitochondrial tRNA(Leu(UUR)) gene. Arch Dis Child 2000;82(5):407–411.

279. Chalmers RM, Lamont PJ, Nelson I, et al. A mitochondrial DNA tRNA(Val) point mutation associated with adult-onset Leigh syndrome. Neurology 1997;49(2):589–592.

280. Santorelli FM, Tanji K, Sano M, et al. Maternally inherited encephalopathy associated with a single-base insertion in the mitochondrial tRNATrp gene. Ann Neurol 1997;42(2):256–260.

281. Santorelli FM, Mak SC, Vazquez-Memije E, et al. Clinical heterogeneity associated with the mitochondrial DNA T8993C point mutation. Pediatr Res 1996;39(5):914–917.

282. Sadeh M, Kuritzky A, Ben-David E, Goldhammer Y. Adult metachromatic leukodystrophy with an unusual relapsing-remitting course. Postgrad Med J 1992;68(797):192–195.

283. Solders G, Celsing G, Hagenfeldt L, et al. Improved peripheral nerve conduction, EEG and verbal IQ after bone marrow transplantation for adult metachromatic leukodystrophy. Bone Marrow Transplant 1998;22(11):1119–1122.

284. Consiglio A, Quattrini A, Martino S, et al. In vivo gene therapy of metachromatic leukodystrophy by lentiviral vectors: correction of neuropathology and protection against learning impairments in affected mice. Nat Med 2001;7(3):310–316.

285. Pavlakis SG, Phillips PC, DiMauro S, et al. Mitochondrial myopathy, encephalopathy, lactic acidosis, and strokelike episodes: a distinctive clinical syndrome. Ann Neurol 1984;16(4):481–488.

286. Iniguez C, Arenas J, Montoya J, et al. Mitochondrial respiratory chain deficiency may present as multiple sclerosis. Neurologia 1998;13(4):199–203.

287. Mosewich RK, Donat JR, DiMauro S, et al. The syndrome of mitochondrial encephalomyopathy, lactic acidosis, and strokelike episodes presenting without stroke. Arch Neurol 1993;50(3):275–278.

288. Kobayashi Y, Momoi MY, Tominaga K, et al. A point mutation in the mitochondrial tRNA(Leu(UUR)) gene in MELAS (mitochondrial myopathy, encephalopathy, lactic acidosis and stroke-like episodes). Biochem Biophys Res Commun 1990;173(3):816–822.

289. Goto Y, Nonaka I, Horai S. A new mtDNA mutation associated with mitochondrial myopathy, encephalopathy, lactic acidosis and stroke-like episodes (MELAS). Biochim Biophys Acta 1991;1097(3):238–240.

290. Goto Y, Tsugane K, Tanabe Y, et al. A new point mutation at nucleotide pair 3291 of the mitochondrial tRNA (Leu(UUR)) gene in a patient with mitochondrial myopathy, encephalopathy, lactic acidosis, and stroke-like episodes (MELAS). Biochem Biophys Res Commun 1994;202(3):1624–1630.

291. Sato W, Hayasaka K, Shoji Y, et al. A mitochondrial tRNA(Leu)(UUR) mutation at 3,256 associated with mitochondrial myopathy, encephalopathy, lactic acidosis, and stroke-like episodes (MELAS). Biochem Mol Biol Int 1994;33(6):1055–1061.

292. Nishino I, Komatsu M, Kodama S, et al. The 3260 mutation in mitochondrial DNA can cause mitochondrial myopathy, encephalopathy, lactic acidosis, and strokelike episodes (MELAS). Muscle Nerve 1996;19(12):1603–1604.

293. Campos Y, Lorenzo G, Martin MA, et al. A mitochondrial tRNA(Lys) gene mutation (T8316C) in a patient with mitochondrial myopathy, lactic acidosis, and stroke–like episodes. Neuromuscul Disord 2000;10(7):493–496.

294. de Coo IF, Sistermans EA, de Wijs IJ, et al. A mitochondrial tRNA(Val) gene mutation (G1642A) in a patient with mitochondrial myopathy, lactic acidosis, and stroke-like episodes. Neurology 1998;50(1):293–295.

295. Taylor RW, Chinnery PF, Haldane F, et al. MELAS associated with a mutation in the valine transfer RNA gene of mitochondrial DNA. Ann Neurol 1996;40(3):459–462.

296. Ciafaloni E, Ricci E, Shanske S, et al. MELAS: clinical features, biochemistry, and molecular genetics. Ann Neurol 1992;31(4):391–398.

297. Pulkes T, Sweeney MG, Hanna MG. Increased risk of stroke in patients with the A12308G polymorphism in mitochondria. Lancet 2000;356(9247):2068–2069.

298. Rusanen H, Majamaa K, Tolonen U, et al. Demyelinating polyneuropathy in a patient with the tRNA(Leu(UUR)) mutation at base pair 3243 of the mitochondrial DNA. Neurology 1995;45(6):1188–1192.

299. Lertrit P, Kapsa RM, Jean-Francois MJ, et al. Mitochondrial DNA polymorphism in disease: a possible contributor to respiratory dysfunction. Hum Mol Genet 1994;3(11):1973–1981.

300. van den Ouweland JM, Lemkes HH, Trembath RC, et al. Maternally inherited diabetes and deafness is a distinct subtype of diabetes and associates with a single point mutation in the mitochondrial tRNA(Leu(UUR)) gene. Diabetes 1994;43(6):746–751.

301. Vilarinho L, Santorelli FM, Rosas MJ, et al. The mitochondrial A3243G mutation presenting as severe cardiomyopathy. J Med Genet 1997;34(7):607–609.

302. Harada M. Minamata disease: methylmercury poisoning in Japan caused by environmental pollution. Crit Rev Toxicol 1995;25(1):1–24.

303. Powell TJ. Chronic neurobehavioural effects of mercury

poisoning on a group of Zulu chemical workers. Brain Inj 2000;14(9):797–814.

304. Davis LE, Kornfeld M, Mooney HS, et al. Methylmercury poisoning: long-term clinical, radiological, toxicological, and pathological studies of an affected family. Ann Neurol 1994;35(6):680–688.

305. Moreau T, Loudenot V. [Dental amalgam and multiple sclerosis: what is the connection?]. Presse Med 1999; 28(25):1378–1380.

306. Ingalls TH. Endemic clustering of multiple sclerosis in time and place, 1934–1984. Confirmation of a hypothesis. Am J Forensic Med Pathol 1986;7(1):3–8.

307. Langauer-Lewowicka H, Zajac-Nedza M. [Changes in the nervous system due to occupational metallic mercury poisoning.] Neurol Neurochir Pol 1997;31(5):905–913.

308. Korogi Y, Takahashi M, Hirai T, et al. Representation of the visual field in the striate cortex: comparison of MR findings with visual field deficits in organic mercury poisoning (Minamata disease). AJNR Am J Neuroradiol 1997;18(6):1127–1130.

309. Ikeda O, Okajima T, Korogi Y, et al. [Cerebellar atrophy in Minamata disease: comparison with spino-cerebellar degeneration on MR images.] Nippon Igaku Hoshasen Gakkai Zasshi 1997;57(3):99–103.

310. Mallucci GR, Campbell TA, Dickinson A, et al. Inherited prion disease with an alanine to valine mutation at codon 117 in the prion protein gene. brain 1999;122:1823–1837.

311. Grand MG, Kaine J, Fulling K, et al. Cerebroretinal vasculopathy. A new hereditary syndrome. Ophthalmology 1988;95(5):649–659.

312. Gutmann DH, Fischbeck KH, Sergott RC. Hereditary retinal vasculopathy with cerebral white matter lesions. Am J Med Genet 1989;34(2):217–220.

313. Alarcia R, Ara JR, Serrano M, et al. Severe polyneuropathy after using nitrous oxide as an anesthetic. A preventable disease? Rev Neurol 1999;29(1):36–38.

314. Schilling RF. Is nitrous oxide a dangerous anesthetic for vitamin B_{12}-deficient subjects? JAMA 1986;255(12): 1605–1606.

315. Marie RM, Le Biez E, Busson P, et al. Nitrous oxide anesthesia-associated myelopathy. Arch Neurol 2000; 57(3):380–382.

316. Kondo H, Osborne ML, Kolhouse JF, et al. Nitrous oxide has multiple deleterious effects on cobalamin metabolism and causes decreases in activities of both mammalian cobalamin–dependent enzymes in rats. J Clin Invest 1981;67(5):1270–1283.

317. Ravakhah K, West BC. Case report: subacute combined degeneration of the spinal cord from folate deficiency. Am J Med Sci 1995;310(5):214–216.

318. Lever EG, Elwes RD, Williams A, Reynolds EH. Subacute combined degeneration of the cord due to folate deficiency: response to methyl folate treatment. J Neurol Neurosurg Psychiatry 1986;49(10):1203–1207.

319. Guard O, Dumas R, Audry D, et al. Clinical and pathological study of a case of subacute combined degeneration of the cord with folic acid deficiency. Rev Neurol (Paris) 1981;137(6–7):435–446.

320. Raphael JC, Choutet P, Barois A, et al. Myelopathy and macrocytic anemia associated with a folate deficiency.

Cure by folic acid. Ann Med Interne (Paris) 1975; 126(5):339–348.

321. Le Prise PY, Boutin J, Menault F, Richier JL. Folic acid deficiency and combined sclerosis of the spinal cord. Sem Hop 1974;50(37–38):2325–2326.

322. Reynolds EH, Bottiglieri T, Laundy M, et al. Vitamin B12 metabolism in multiple sclerosis. Arch Neurol 1992; 49(6):649–652.

323. Nijst TQ, Wevers RA, Schoonderwaldt HC, et al. Vitamin B12 and folate concentrations in serum and cerebrospinal fluid of neurological patients with special reference to multiple sclerosis and dementia. J Neurol Neurosurg Psychiatry 1990;53(11):951–954.

324. Goodkin DE, Jacobsen DW, Galvez N, et al. Serum cobalamin deficiency is uncommon in multiple sclerosis. Arch Neurol 1994;51(11):1110–1114.

325. Frequin ST, Wevers RA, Braam M, et al. Decreased vitamin B12 and folate levels in cerebrospinal fluid and serum of multiple sclerosis patients after high-dose intravenous methylprednisolone. J Neurol 1993;240(5):305–308.

326. Sandyk R, Awerbuch GI. Vitamin B_{12} and its relationship to age of onset of multiple sclerosis. Int J Neurosci 1993;71(1–4):93–99.

327. Motomura S, Tabira T, Kurosawa Y. A clinical comparative study of multiple sclerosis and neuro-Behçet's syndrome. J Neurol Neurosurg Psychiatry 1980;43:210–213.

328. Banna M, El-Ramahi K. Neurologic involvement in Behçet disease: imaging findings in 16 patients. AJNR Am J Neuroradiol 1991;12:791–796.

329. Wechsler B, Dellilsola B, Vidailhet M. MRI in 31 patients with Behçet's disease and neurological involvement: prospective study with clinical correlation. J Neurol Neurosurg Psychiatry 1993;56:793–798.

330. Case records of the Massachusetts General Hospital (Case 14-1967). N Engl J Med 1967;276:741.

331. Younger D, Hays A, Brust J. Granulomatous angiitis of the brain. An inflammatory reaction of diverse etiology. Arch Neurol 1988;45:514–518.

332. Feasby T, Ferguson G, Kaufmann J. Isolated spinal cord arteritis. Can J Neurol Sci 1975;2:143–146.

333. Giovanini M, Eskin T, Mukherji S. Granulomatous angiitis of the spinal cord: a case report. Neurosurgery 1994; 34:540–543.

334. Kattah J, Cupps T, DiChiro G. An unusual case of central nervous system vasculitis. J Neurol 1987;234:344–347.

335. Calabrese L, Furlan A, Gragg L. Primary angiitis of the central nervous system: diagnostic criteria and clinical approach. Cleve Clin J Med 1992;59:293–306.

336. Calabrese L, Mallek J. Primary angiitis of the central nervous system: report of 8 new cases, review of the literature, and proposal for diagnostic criteria. Medicine (Baltimore MD) 1987;67:20.

337. Johnson M, Maciunas R, Dutt P. Granulomatous angiitis masquerading as a mass lesion. Magnetic resonance imaging and stereotactic biopsy findings in a patient with occult Hodgkin's disease. Surg Neurol 1989;31:49–53.

338. Greenan T, Grossman R, Goldberg H. Cerebral vasculitis: MR imaging and angiographic correlation. Radiology 1992;182:65–72.

339. Harris K, Tran D, Sickels W, et al. Diagnosing intracranial vasculitis: the roles of MRI and angiography. AJNR Am J Neurodiol 1994;15:317–330.

340. Ferris E, Levine H. Cerebral arteritis: classification. Radiology 1973;109:327–341.

341. Alhalabi M, Moore P. Serial angiography in isolated angiitis of the central nervous system. Neurology 1994;44:1221–1226.

342. Smith A, Huang T, Weinstein M. Periventricular involvement in CNS lymphomatoid granulomatosis: MR demonstration. J Comput Assist Tomogr 1990;14(2):291–293.

343. Warner T. Lymphomatoid granulomatosis, progressive multifocal leucoencephalopathy and recurrent staphylococcal infections of childhood: report of a case. J Irish Med Assoc 1975;68:61–68.

344. Verity M, Wolfson W. Cerebral lymphomatoid granulomatosis: a report of two cases, with disseminated necrotizing leukoencephalopathy in one. Acta Neuropathol (Berl) 1976;36:117–124.

345. Brecher K, Hochberg F, Louis D, et al. Case report of unusual leukoencephalopathy preceding primary CNS lymphoma. J Neurol Neurosurg Psychiatry 1998;65(6):917–920.

346. DeAngelis L. Primary central nervous system lymphoma imitates multiple sclerosis. J Neurooncol 1990;9(2):177–181.

347. Furneaux H, Reich L, Posner J. Autoantibody synthesis in the CNS of patients with paraneoplastic syndromes. Neurology 1990;7:1085–1091.

348. Gultekin S, Rosenfeld M, Voltz R, et al. Paraneoplastic limbic encephalitis: neurological symptoms, immunological findings and tumour association in 50 patients. Brain 2000;123(7):1481–1494.

349. Cohen O, Biran I, Steiner I Cerebrospinal fluid oligoclonal IgG bands in patients with spinal arteriovenous malformation and structural central nervous system lesions. Arch Neurol 2000;57(4):553–557.

350. Balko MG, Blisard KS, Samaha FJ. Oligodendroglial gliomatosis cerebri. Hum Pathol 1992;23(6):706–707.

351. Malmgren R, Detels R, Verity M. Co-occurrence of multiple sclerosis and glioma—case report and neuropathologic and epidemiologic review. Clin Neuropathol 1984;3(1):1–9.

352. Nahser H, Vieregge P, Nau H, Reinhardt V. Coincidence of multiple sclerosis and glioma. Clinical and radiological remarks on two cases. Surg Neurol 1986;26(1):45–51.

353. Fujimoto K, Ohnishi H, Tsujimoto M, et al. Dysembryoplastic neuroepithelial tumor of the cerebellum and brainstem. Case report. J Neurosurg 2000;93(3):487–489.

354. Heckmann JG, Druschky A, Kern PM, et al. ["Ghost and mimicry-tumor"—primary CNS lymphoma.] Nervenarzt 2000;71(4):305–310.

355. Pels H, Deckert-Schluter M, Glasmacher A, et al. Primary central nervous system lymphoma: a clinicopathological study of 28 cases. Hematol Oncol 2000;18(1):21–32.

356. Raisanen J, Goodman HS, Ghougassian DF, Harper CG. Role of cytology in the intraoperative diagnosis of central demyelinating disease. Acta Cytol 1998;42(4):907–912.

357. Giang DW, Poduri KR, Eskin TA, et al. Multiple sclerosis masquerading as a mass lesion. Neuroradiology 1992;34(2):150–154.

358. Dagher AP, Smirniotopoulos J. Tumefactive demyelinating lesions. Neuroradiology 1996;38(6):560–565.

359. Kepes JJ. Large focal tumor-like demyelinating lesions of the brain: intermediate entity between multiple sclerosis and acute disseminated encephalomyelitis? A study of 31 patients. Ann Neurol 1993;33(1):18–27.

360. Stadnik TW, Chaskis C, Michotte A, et al. Diffusion-weighted mr imaging of intracerebral masses: comparison with conventional mr imaging and histologic findings. AJNR Am J Neuroradiol 2001;22(5):969–976.

361. DeStefano N, Caramanos Z, Preul M, et al. In vivo differentiation of astrocytic brain tumors and isolated demyelinating lesions of the type seen in multiple sclerosis using 1H magnetic resonance spectroscopic imaging. Ann Neurol 1998;44(2):273–278.

362. Cha S, Pierce S, Knopp EA, et al. Dynamic contrast-enhanced t2*-weighted mr imaging of tumefactive demyelinating lesions. AJNR Am J Neuroradiol 2001;22(6):1109–1116.

363. Masdeu JC, Quinto C, Olivera C, et al. Open-ring imaging sign: highly specific for atypical brain demyelination. Neurology 2000;54(7):1427–1433.

364. Escudero D, Latorre P, Codina M. Central nervous system disease in Sjögren's syndrome. Ann Med Intern 1995;146:239–242.

365. Coates T, Slavotinek J, Rischmueller M, et al. Cerebral white matter lesions in primary Sjögren's syndrome: a controlled study. J Rheumatol 1999;26(6):1301–1305.

366. Ellemann K, Krogh E, Arlien-Soeborg P, Halberg P. Sjögren's syndrome in patients with multiple sclerosis. Acta Neurologica Scandinavica 1991;84(1):68–69.

367. Schur P (ed). General symptomatology: The Clinical Management of Systemic Lupus Erythematosus (2nd ed). Philadelphia: Lippincott–Raven, 1996;9–16.

368. Kovacs J, Urowitz M, Gladman D. Dilemmas in neuropsychiatric lupus. Rheum Dis Clin North Am 1993;19:795–814.

369. Granger D. Transverse myelitis with recovery; the only manifestation of systemic lupus erythematosus. Neurology Minneap 1960;42:325–329.

370. Piper P. Disseminated lupus erythematosus with involvement of the spinal cord. JAMA 1953;153:215–217.

371. Siekert R, Clark E. Neurologic signs and symptoms as early manifestations of systemic lupus erythematosus. Neurology Minneap 1955;5:84–88.

372. Penn A, Rowan A. Myelopathy in systemic lupus erythematosus. Arch Neurol 1968;18:337–349.

373. Fulford K, Catterall R, Delhanty J, et al. A collagen disorder of the nervous system presenting as multiple sclerosis. Brain 1972;95:373–386.

374. Inslicht D, Stein A, Ragnarsson FP. Three women with lupus transverse myelitis: Case reports and differential diagnosis. Arch Phys Med Rehabil 1998;79:456–459.

375. Hackett E, Martinez R, Larson P, Paddison R. Optic neuritis in systemic lupus erythematosus. Arch Neurol 1974;31:9–11.

376. Smith C, Pinals R. Optic neuritis in systemic lupus erythematosus. J Rheumatol 1982;9:963–966.

377. Kovacs B, Lafferty T, Brent L, DeHoratius R. Transverse

myelopathy in systemic lupus erythematosus: an analysis of 14 cases and review of the literature. Ann Rheum Dis 2000;59:120–124.

378. Estes D, Christian C. The natural history of systemic lupus erythematosus by prospective analysis. Medicine 1971;50:85–95.

379. Cinefro R, Frenkel M. Systemic lupus erythematosus presenting as optic neuritis. Ann Ophthal 1978;10:559–563.

380. Oppenheimer S, Hoffbrand B. Optic neuritis and myelopathy in systemic lupus erythematosus. Can J Neurol Sci 1986;13:129–132.

381. Kupersmith M, Burde R, Warren F, et al. Autoimmune optic neuropathy: evaluation and treatment. J Neurol Neurosurg Psychiat 1988;51:1381–1386.

382. Barned S, Goodman A, Mattson D. Frequency of antinuclear antibodies in multiple sclerosis. Neurology 1995;45:384–385.

383. Dore-Duffy P, Donaldson J, Rothman B, Zurier R. Antinuclear antibodies in multiple sclerosis. Arch Neurol 1982;39:504–506.

384. Toubi E, Khamashta M, Panarra A, Hughes G. Association of antiphospholipid antibodies with central nervous system disease in systemic lupus erythematosus. Am J Med 1995;99:397–401.

385. Harris E, Gharavi A, Mackworth-Young C, et al. Lupoid sclerosis: a possible pathogenetic role for antiphospholipid antibodies. Ann Rheum Dis 1985;44:281–283.

386. Holmes F, Stubbs D, Larsen W. Systemic lupus erythematosus and multiple sclerosis in identical twins. Arch Intern Med 1967;119:302–304.

387. Buchman K, Moore S, Ebbin A, et al. Familial systemic lupus erythematosus. Arch Intern Med 1978;138:1674–1676.

388. McCombe P, Chalk J, Pender M. Familial occurrence of multiple sclerosis with thyroid disease and systemic lupus erythematosus. J Neurol 1990;97:163–171.

389. Sloan J, Berk M, Gebel H, Fretzin D. Multiple sclerosis and systemic lupus erythematosus. Occurrence in two generations of the same family. Arch Intern Med 1987;147:1317–1320.

390. Nishino H, Rubino F, DeRemee R. Neurological involvement in Wegener's granulomatosis: an analysis of 324 consecutive patients at the Mayo Clinic. Ann Neurol 1993;33:4–9.

391. Feola R, Matakis F, Rafii M. Cerebral manifestations of Wegenerís granulomatosis with funicular demyelination. Virchows Arch 1971;354:169.

392. Vigliani MC, Duyckaerts C, Hauw JJ, et al. Dementia following treatment of brain tumors with radiotherapy administered alone or in combination with nitrosourea-based chemotherapy: a clinical and pathological study. J Neurooncol 1999;41(2):137–149.

393. Virta A, Patronas N, Raman R, et al. Spectroscopic imaging of radiation-induced effects in the white matter of glioma patients. Magn Reson Imaging 2000;18(7):851–857.

394. Rubinstein LJ, Herman MM, Long TF, Wilbur JR. Disseminated necrotizing leukoencephalopathy: a complication of treated central nervous system leukemia and lymphoma. Cancer 1975;35(2):291–305.

395. Tsui EY, Chan JH, Leung TW, et al. Radionecrosis of the temporal lobe: dynamic susceptibility contrast MRI. Neuroradiology 2000;42(2):149–152.

396. Arai M, Hayakawa K, Takahashi T, et al. The study of 201Tl, 123I-IMP-SPECT before and after radiation therapy of brain tumor. Kaku Igaku 1990;27(3):279–283.

397. Kampfl A, Franz G, Aichner F, et al. The persistent vegetative state after closed head injury: clinical and magnetic resonance imaging findings in 42 patients. J Neurosurg 1998;88(5):809–816.

398. Abu-Judeh HH, Parker R, Singh M, et al. SPET brain perfusion imaging in mild traumatic brain injury without loss of consciousness and normal computed tomography. Nucl Med Commun 1999;20(6):505–510.

399. Liu AY, Maldjian JA, Bagley LJ, et al. Traumatic brain injury: diffusion-weighted MR imaging findings. AJNR Am J Neuroradiol 1999;20(9):1636–1641.

400. Pierallini A, Pantano P, Fantozzi LM, et al. Correlation between MRI findings and long-term outcome in patients with severe brain trauma. Neuroradiology 2000;42(12): 860–867.

401. Toupalik P, Klir P, Bouska I, Chadova L. [Immunohistochemical methods in the differential diagnosis of primary traumatic and subsequent secondary cerebral changes.] Soud Lek 2000;45(2):18–2.1

402. Cau C. [The Alice in Wonderland syndrome.] Minerva Med 1999;90(10):397–401.

403. Nadeau SE. Multi-infarct dementia, subcortical dementia, and hydrocephalus. South Med J 1991;84(5 Suppl 1):S41–S52.

404. McQuinn BA, O'Leary DH. White matter lucencies on computed tomography, subacute arteriosclerotic encephalopathy (Binswanger's disease), and blood pressure. Stroke 1987;18(5):900–905.

405. Meca-Lallana JE, Martin JJ, Lucas C, et al. [Susac syndrome: clinical and diagnostic approach. A new case report.] Rev Neurol 1999;29(11):1027–1032.

406. Leifer D, Buonanno FS, Richardson EP Jr. Clinicopathologic correlations of cranial magnetic resonance imaging of periventricular white matter. Neurology 1990;40(6): 911–918.

407. Revesz T, Hawkins CP, du Boulay EP, et al. Pathological findings correlated with magnetic resonance imaging in subcortical arteriosclerotic encephalopathy (Binswanger's disease). J Neurol Neurosurg Psychiatry 1989;52(12): 1337–1344.

408. Demirkaya S, Odabasi Z, Gokcil Z, et al. Migrainous stroke causing bilateral anterior cerebral artery territory infarction. Headache 1999;39(7):513–516.

409. Rocca MA, Colombo B, Pratesi A, et al. A magnetization transfer imaging study of the brain in patients with migraine. Neurology 2000;54(2):507–509.

410. Mantyla R, Aronen HJ, Salonen O, et al. Magnetic resonance imaging white matter hyperintensities and mechanism of ischemic stroke. Stroke 1999;30(10):2053–2058.

411. Davous P. CADASIL: a review with proposed diagnostic criteria. Eur J Neurol 1998;5(3):219–233.

412. Mahmoud-Ahmed AS, Suh JH, Barnett GH, et al. Tumor distribution and survival in six patients with brain

metastases from cervical carcinoma. Gynecol Oncol 2001;81(2):196–200.

413. Cader M, Winer J. Lesson of the week: cavernous haemangioma mimicking multiple sclerosis. BMJ 1999;318: 1604–1605.

414. Vrethem M, Thuomas K, Hillman J. Cavernous angioma of the brain stem mimicking multiple sclerosis. N Engl J Med 1997;336(12):875–876.

415. Stahl S, Johnson K, Malamud N. The clinical and pathological spectrum of brain-stem vascular malformations.

Long-term course simulates multiple sclerosis. Arch Neurol 1980;37(1):25–29.

416. Sadeh M, Shacked I. Rappaport Z, Tadmor R. Surgical extirpation of a venous angioma of the medulla oblongata simulating multiple sclerosis. Surg Neurol 1982;17(5): 334–337.

417. Akhaddar A, Gazzaz M, Derraz S, et al. Spinal epidural angiolipomas: a rare cause of spinal cord compression. A report of 8 cases and review of the literature. Neuro-Chirurgie 2000;46(6):523–533.

Chapter 11

Immunologic and Clinical Aspects of Human T-Cell Lymphotropic Virus Type I–Associated Myelopathy/Tropical Spastic Paraparesis

Fernando Dangond and David A. Hafler

Many different human brain and spinal cord disorders have been found to be triggered by infectious agents, including viruses. How these viruses affect the nervous system has been a subject of great interest to biomedical researchers. Demyelinative disorders in humans associated with viral infection range from those associated with a hyporesponsive immune system (e.g., human immunodeficiency virus–associated myelopathy and progressive multifocal leukoencephalopathy; see Chapters 14 and 15, respectively) to those associated with an activated, hyperresponsive immune system (e.g., human T-cell lymphotropic virus type I [HTLV-I]–associated myelopathy/tropical spastic paraparesis [HAM/TSP]).

Zaninovic and colleagues[1] described a syndrome of endemic spastic paraparesis in the Tumaco island of the Pacific coast of Colombia in 1981 and named it *spastic paraparesis of the Pacific*. A similar syndrome named *Jamaican neuropathy* had been described earlier by Cruickshank in Jamaica. In South India, Mani and colleagues[2] described a similar disorder and gave it the term *South Indian paraplegia* in 1966. By 1985, Gessain et al.[3] had described the association of tropical paraparesis in the Caribbean (in Martinique) with infection by HTLV-I. This virus had been described in 1980 by Poiesz and collaborators as a type C retrovirus.[4] A few years later, Osame et al.[5] and Roman et al.[6] realized that these disorders represented a disease identi-

cal to one that had been described in Japan by Osame and collaborators in 1987 and in the Seychelles Islands. Roman had coined the name *TSP*[7] but, in an effort to avoid confusion and to categorize these disorders as a single disease entity, the term *HAM/TSP* was coined and promptly gained widespread acceptance. Endemic cases of spastic paraparesis from different parts of the world soon became associated with HTLV-I, including cases from Melanesia, equatorial Africa, Japan, the Middle East, South America,[8] and the Caribbean basin.[9]

It has now become clear that HTLV-I–associated disease not only involves the spinal cord (i.e., as a myelopathy) but also, to a lesser degree, other regions of the central nervous system (CNS) and the peripheral nervous system. In addition, HTLV-I infection is associated with uveitis,[10] bronchoalveolitis,[11] autoimmune thyroiditis,[12] arthritis,[13] polymyositis,[14] Sjögren's syndrome,[15] and cutaneous manifestations. Besides the occurrence of infective dermatitis in HTLV-I carrier children,[16] it is now known that a small percentage (less than 1–2%) of infected individuals may develop adult T-cell leukemia-lymphoma (ATLL).[17] ATLL is classified among the skin-involving lymphomas in the same class as mycosis fungoides, Sézary syndrome, lymphomatoid papulosis, and CD30+ large-cell lymphoma.

It is still unclear whether the spinal cord specificity is determined by the activation state of specific viral-reactive T cells or by particular predisposing genetic factors. Although we still do not know the answer, one possible explanation would be that the organ specificity is the reflection of the high frequency of organ-specific reactive T cells in the peripheral circulation. Although CNS or ocular antigens may be sequestered and this may not impede a negative deletion of reactive T cells in the thymus, it is also possible that other antigens commonly encountered in the environment, such as viral or bacterial antigens, may be responsible for triggering autoimmune responses. In addition, the random infection of potentially autoreactive T cells by a retrovirus with a high transactivating capability may eliminate their state of tolerance or immune ignorance and result in a spinal cord–specific immune response. Furthermore, there is no evidence that different strains of the virus account for the different syndromes; rather, different host susceptibility and immune response factors are believed to influence the development of HTLV-I–associated disease. HTLV-I from human carriers has been shown to lead to HAM/TSP in recipients of blood transfusions,[18] demonstrating that specific host factors or else a degree of proviral load at onset can play a key role in disease transmission.

Immunology of Human T-Cell Lymphotropic Virus Type I

HTLV-I can induce T-cell transformation or activation. The HTLV-I–associated diseases described earlier are thought to be immune-mediated. The immune cell type most frequently infected by HTLV-I in vivo expresses the CD4+CD45RO memory phenotype,[19] but CD8+ T cells can also be infected. CD4+ T-cell infection by HTLV-I may result in either a latent or a productive infection. It is unclear whether a latent infection can be reactivated in vivo and converted to a productive infection. However, in vitro studies have shown that the levels of expression of HTLV-I proteins can be enhanced with agents, such as phytohemagglutinin and phorbol 12-myristate 13-acetate; combinations of cytokines; and use of the histone deacetylase inhibitors sodium butyrate[20] and trichostatin A (F. Dangond, unpublished data, 2001). It has been shown that the majority of infected T cells from HAM/TSP patients is latently infected and remains

so during in vitro culture. The phenotype of HTLV-I–infected T cells seems to progress in at least two phases: the initial phase characterized by a dependence on interleukin-2 (IL-2) and the second phase characterized by a downregulation of the T-cell receptor (TCR) and growth that is IL-2–independent.[21] In the second phase, T cells are transformed and immortalized, and the exact mechanisms behind this immortalization are not as yet defined.

Humoral Response

HTLV-I infection is followed by an antibody response against viral structural proteins. The most important proteins recognized by antibodies are env and gag (p19 and p24). In some cases, the antibody response is detected against gag p19 or against p24 but not against env by Western blotting. This "indeterminate" pattern presents a diagnostic dilemma because it remains questionable whether this is associated with HTLV-I infection. In patients with HAM/TSP, the synthesis of intrathecal antibodies may manifest as cerebrospinal fluid (CSF) oligoclonal bands, and a fraction of this humoral response is specific against HTLV-I proteins. Recently, it has been shown that immunoglobulin G isolated from HAM/TSP patients binds to uninfected human neuronal cells and that this binding can be blocked by preincubating the immunoglobulin G with the HTLV-I tax protein.[22] These results suggest that an antiviral antibody response directed against the viral tax protein can cross react, in a process known as *molecular mimicry*, with uninfected neurons and possibly contribute to CNS degeneration.

Cellular Response

Role of Antigen Presentation by Human Leukocyte Antigen

Antigenic protein fragments of HTLV-I can be presented by human leukocyte antigen (HLA) class I or by class II molecules. The presentation of viral protein fragments by HLA class I induces a response mediated by CD8+ T cells, whereas the presentation of viral antigen by class II molecules induces an antiviral response mediated by CD4+ T cells.

Although a CD4+ T-cell response has been reported in HAM/TSP,[23,24] the dominant response is mediated by CD8+ T cells that are specifically reactive against the HTLV-I tax fragment.[25] In patients who express class I HLA-A2, the immunodominant response is directed against the 11-19 tax peptide fragment, whereas in patients with class I HLA-B14, the dominant response is directed against amino acids 186-194 from tax. The frequency of CD8+ T cells had been reported to be high, with approximately 1 in 500 cells that were specific against the virus.[26] Paradoxically, the high CD8+ T-cell response occurs concomitantly with a high viral load,[27] indicating that the antiviral immune response is compensatory but still inefficient in eliminating the virus. CD4+ viral-reactive T cells specifically directed against HTLV-I env protein epitopes in the context of HLA DRB1*0101 presentation have also been demonstrated,[24] but their in vivo significance remains unknown.

Role of the B7 Family of Molecules

The activation of T cells requires two signals, one derived from the contact of the TCR with the antigenic peptide (e.g., an HTLV-I antigen) bound to the HLA molecule; the second is a costimulatory signal in which the CD28 molecule on the surface of the T cell binds the B7 molecule on the surface of the antigen-presenting cell. The modulation of levels of expression of the B7 costimulatory molecules has been associated with autoimmunity, which suggests that these are important molecules regulating autoreactive immune responses. Recent observations have suggested that the infection of antigen-specific T cells by HTLV-I results in activation of these cells, by a mechanism that does not depend on costimulatory signals via B7.[28] This suggests the possibility that a random infection of autoreactive T cells by HTLV-I may result in lymphoproliferative responses against CNS tissue despite the absence of proinflammatory B7 molecule expression in the peripheral blood or in the target tissue.

Role of Adhesion Molecules

Cell adhesion molecules are responsible for cell-cell interactions and tissue infiltration. Infection of immune cells by HTLV-I results in the expression of cell-surface adhesion molecules that may mediate migration into CNS tissues.[29] The upregulated expression of intercellular cell adhesion molecule I with an increase in the adherence of T cells to endothelial cells has been described in HAM/TSP,[30] and this phenomenon is enhanced by interferon gamma (IFN-γ), a proinflammatory cytokine. Besides intercellular cell adhesion molecule I, tax transactivates the promoter for E-selectin in HTLV-I–transformed T cells, possibly promoting the entry of these malignant cells into tissues. L-selectin has also been shown to be upregulated by tax in transformed cells.[31] In addition, the lymphocyte-functional–associated antigen 3-CD2 pathway is used by HTLV-I–infected T cells to activate noninfected T cells[32] and may account for the phenomenon of spontaneous proliferation (see Mechanisms That Mediate Proliferation or Transformation Induced by Human T-Cell Lymphotropic Virus Type I) observed in peripheral blood mononuclear cells from HAM/TSP patients.

Hypotheses Regarding Human T-Cell Lymphotropic Virus Type I–Associated Myelopathy/Tropical Spastic Paraparesis Immunopathogenesis

Several hypotheses have been suggested to explain the immunopathogenesis of HAM/TSP. The cytotoxic hypothesis predicts that CD8+ T cells develop a cytotoxic (i.e., cell-destructive) response against infected cells in the CNS. Cytotoxicity of CD8+ T cells might be preceded by initial entry into the CNS by infected CD4+ T cells, a process that may contribute to dissemination of infection within the CNS. The bystander hypothesis predicts that the migration of IFN-γ–secreting infected CD4+ T cells from the peripheral blood to the CNS would be in part determined by hemodynamic conditions in the thoracic spinal cord and would induce the secretion of prodemyelinating and proinflammatory factors by microglia and the recruitment of an antiviral CD8+ T-cell response in the CNS (Figure 11-1). Invading T cells may also secrete cytokines with demyelinating properties, such as tumor necrosis factor-α, resulting in an amplification of the immune response. Finally, the autoimmune hypothesis predicts that an autoreactive T cell is infected by HTLV-I, becomes activated, and results in the destruction of a specific tissue.[17]

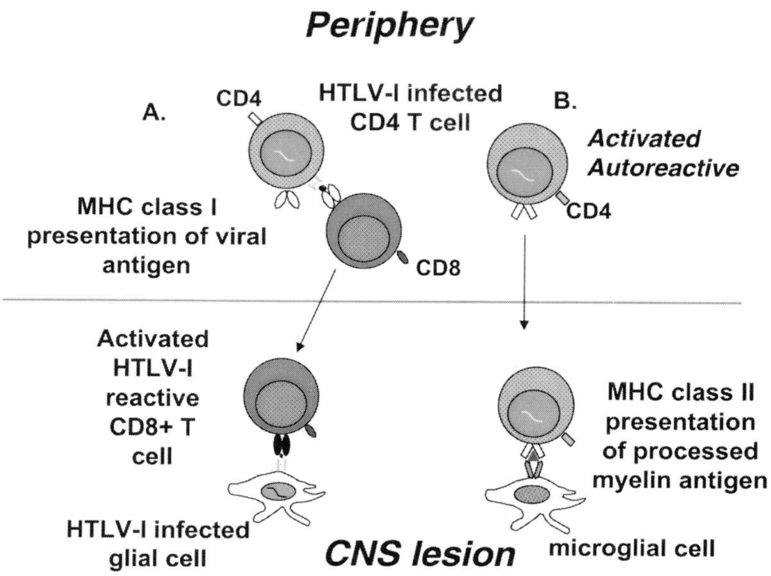

Figure 11-1. Mechanisms of T-cell activation induced by human T-cell lymphotropic virus type I (HTLV-I). The two major hypotheses regarding the pathogenesis of HTLV-I–associated myelopathy/tropical spastic paraparesis are as follows. In hypothesis A, the HTLV-I–infected CD4 T cell presents antigen to CD8 antigen–reactive T cells, leading to their activation. The activated HTLV-I–reactive CD8 T cell then migrates into the central nervous system (CNS), where it recognizes infected glial cells, leading to tissue destruction. In hypothesis B, the random infection of CD4 T cells (approximately 10% of CD4 cells) occurs in an autoreactive T cell. As the activation of an autoreactive T cell is all that is required to induce chronic inflammation in the CNS in this scenario, activated autoreactive T cells migrate into the CNS, leading to tissue destruction. (MHC = major histocompatibility complex.) (Reprinted with permission from F Dangond, DA Hafler. Neuroimmunology. In R Ransohoff [ed], Continuum Series, Vol. 7. St. Paul, Minnesota: American Academy of Neurology, 2001.)

Organ Specificity of Human T-Cell Lymphotropic Virus Type I Infection

Evidence documenting the presence of HTLV-I virions and nucleic acids in the spinal cord has accumulated. Particles similar to HTLV-I have been observed by electron microscopy in postmortem tissues of spinal cord, and specific HTLV-I sequences have been amplified by polymerase chain reaction (PCR) in spinal cord samples. Other investigators have reported the presence of viral antigens in areas of demyelination by immunohistochemistry, whereas in situ hybridization has detected HTLV-I RNA in astrocytes even in noninflamed spinal cord regions. HTLV-I–infected T cells have been demonstrated in the perivascular space of inflammatory lesions by PCR in situ hybridization.[33] In HTLV-I–induced arthropathy, clones of HTLV-I–infected non-T synovial cells

have been isolated. These clones proliferate, in contrast to uninfected synovial cells. In addition, transfection of these synovial cells with tax alone leads to the same phenotype of augmented proliferation, indicating that tax may mediate the altered phenotype. Clones of HTLV-I–infected T cells have also been generated from the intraocular fluid in patients with HTLV-I–associated uveitis.

Mechanisms That Mediate Proliferation or Transformation Induced by Human T-Cell Lymphotropic Virus Type I

Circulating blood cells from HAM/TSP patients and carriers exhibit the phenomenon of "spontaneous proliferation," meaning that freshly isolated peripheral blood lymphocytes divide and expand continuously for 4–6 days after being placed in vitro, in the absence of growth factors. This is in striking contrast to peripheral blood lymphocytes from normal, noninfected individuals, which require exogenous IL-2 added to the culture plate to expand. The phenomenon of spontaneous proliferation is thought to reflect a level of activation that is induced exclusively by HTLV-I infection. As stated earlier, the HTLV-I tax transactivator protein is thought to mediate the expression of various proinflammatory molecules, including IFN-α. An interesting phenomenon seen in in vitro T cells infected by HTLV-I is the prolonged state of activation after initial restimulation of the clone. This type of T-cell activation correlates with the expression of tax and is sensitive to rapamycin, a p70 S6 kinase blocker that also arrests cells in G_1 but is resistant to cyclosporin A or FK506, which inhibits IL-2 production.[34]

Transformation and immortalization of T cells by HTLV-I is characterized by downregulation of the TCR and IL-2–independent growth.[35] The mechanisms responsible for the transformation are largely unknown, but tax has been clearly implicated.[36] Recent reports have demonstrated constitutive activation of the janus kinase 3–signal transducer and activator of transcription 5 (JAK3/STAT5) pathway in HTLV-I–transformed T cells.[37,38] However, it is unclear whether this is related to the HTLV-I infection because tax-transfected T cells show no activation of the JAK3/STAT5 pathway and tax is sufficient for transforming T cells in vitro. Tax also binds proteins involved directly or indirectly in cell cycle progression, signal transduction, or transcriptional activation, promoting the deregulation of these pathways. For instance, Tax binds the P/CAF-interacting and DNA-binding protein NF-Y[39] and also binds CBP/P300,[40] a transcriptional activator protein with histone acetyltransferase function. In fact, tax interacts directly with DNA [41,42] and with the ATF/CREB family of transcription factors, which bind to cyclic adenosine monophosphate–responsive elements in the HTLV-I long terminal repeats region, leading to activation of HTLV-I as well. Tax also binds MEKK1, a protein kinase that, when activated, results in NFκB nuclear translocation[43] and binds the cell cycle–related proteins cyclin D3,[44] P16[INK4a],[45] and MAD1.[46] It has recently been reported that tax may bind internexin-α, a neuronal protein involved in neurofilament assembly,[47] raising the intriguing question of whether some of the neuropathogenetic

mechanisms of HTLV-I lie in its ability to disrupt neuronal architecture.

Role of T Cells and Antigen-Presenting Cells in Immunopathogenesis

HTLV-I infection has been associated with clonal expansion of the CD4+ and CD8+ T-cell populations.[23] Involvement of the spinal cord, brain stem, brain, and even meninges by lymphocytic cuffs with loss of myelin is observed in neuropathologic specimens (see Chapter 12). Anterior horns and lateral and posterior columns may reveal these lymphocytic cuffs. Pycnosis and chromatolysis of motor neurons can be rarely seen. Fibroblasts from thickened adventitia exhibit large nuclei. However, adventitial thickening does not lead to a decrease in luminal caliber. Although the pyramidal tract is most commonly involved, most pathologic reports describe variable levels of posterior column involvement. Infiltration of the pia arachnoid by lymphocytic cuffs and along the folds where the dorsal roots join the spinal cord has been described. In addition, an axomyelinic loss and fibrillar gliosis that primarily involve the lateral columns have been described.[48] CNS resident antigen-presenting cells, such as astrocytes, are known to harbor the virus, and it is believed that an antiviral CD8+ T-cell response is, at least in part, responsible for the secondary inflammation. Jacobson and colleagues[25] first demonstrated high frequencies of HTLV-I-tax–reactive CD8+ T cells in the blood and CSF of HAM/TSP patients, and these cells have also been successfully cloned from spinal cord tissue of one postmortem specimen. As stated earlier, the frequency of these anti-tax–specific CD8+ T cells by limiting dilution analysis had been shown to be high, with approximately 1 in 500 cells or more exhibiting viral specificity. Remarkably, the use of *major histocompatibility complex class I tetramers*, loaded with viral peptides, a new technique, has recently revealed significantly higher frequencies of tax-reactive T cells, approaching 10% of the circulating CD8 T cells.[49] This anti–HTLV-I cellular response can be manipulated in vitro using altered peptide ligands.[50]

Breakdown of the brain-blood barrier has also been suggested at the molecular level, with the finding of enhanced expression of matrix metalloproteinase 2 and 9 in the blood and CSF, as well as in inflammatory lesions of HAM/TSP.[51] Matrix metalloproteinases may help to mediate the migration of inflammatory cells within the perivascular spaces. Activated HTLV-I–reactive CD8+ T cells isolated from HAM/TSP patients have been shown to secrete IFN-γ, tumor necrosis factor-α, macrophage inflammatory proteins 1-α and -β, IL-16, and matrix metalloproteinase 9.[52] In addition, when compared to cells from asymptomatic HTLV-I carriers, nearly 50% of CD8+ T lymphocytes from HAM/TSP patients with high proviral loads and longer disease chronicity express high levels of fas ligand,[53] a proapoptotic surface molecule. Fas ligand on the surface of a T cell binds to fas on the target cell and triggers cell death, suggesting a potential mechanism for CNS tissue damage in HAM/TSP. Whether other factors (i.e., CNS self-antigens as targets) participate in the immune response to HTLV-I has been suspected but not yet demonstrated. In the peripheral circulation, dendritic cells can become infected with HTLV-I and are capable of stimulating clonal expansion of lymphocytes.[54,55] The finding of massive latent HTLV-I infection in bone marrow cells of HAM/TSP patients[56] suggests that this site may be an important reservoir for the virus.

Our studies have shown that HTLV-I is capable of inducing a proinflammatory phenotype in organ-specific CD4+ T cells, suggesting that HTLV-I–induced autoreactive T-cell activation and clonal expansion may play an important role in autoimmunity (i.e., random infection of a myelin-reactive T-cell clone would lead to inflammation of the spinal cord). Tax is thought to play an important role in disturbing the cellular machinery in a process that results in prolonged T-cell activation and in serving as a target antigen for cytotoxic CD8+ T cells, as seen in HAM/TSP. Whether immunopathogenetic factors in different organs are triggered by cytotoxicity against organ-specific virally infected cells, by bystander activation, or by direct HTLV-I–induced T-cell activation and clonal expansion remains to be shown.

What Have We Learned from Human T-Cell Lymphotropic Virus Type I Infection in Animal Models?

The generation of animal models of HAM/TSP has not resulted in an exact replica, with infected WKA rats as the strain most closely resembling human disease. However, HTLV-I–associated, rheumatoid factor–positive arthropathy can be modeled in mice that are transgenic for tax env-pX and in rats that are transgenic for env-pX (the viral envelope determinant along with the tax-containing pX region), suggesting a triggering role for tax in inducing autoimmune arthropathy. WKA rats infected with HTLV-I have prominent involvement of cervical, thoracic, and lumbar spinal cord levels, the peripheral nervous system, predominant macrophage infiltration, and severe vacuolization of the spinal cord,[57] features that differ from the human disease. In WKA rats, HTLV-I sequences can be detected by reverse transcriptase PCR in the spinal cord and peripheral nerves. Schwann cells from the peripheral nerves of these rats have been shown to undergo apoptosis. In addition, WKA rats exhibit some degree of weakness of hind limbs 16–26 months after the infection.[58] Investigators have also shown oligodendrocyte apoptosis in thoracic cords of WKA rats and increased CSF production of tumor necrosis factor-α. Of interest, the congenitally transmitted retrovirus murine leukemia virus Lake Casitas strain has been associated with both lymphoma and a motor neuron paralysis in mice, thus resembling the pathogenesis of HAM/TSP and ATLL by HTLV-I.[59]

Need for Predictive Biomarkers

HTLV-I antibody titers by enzyme-linked immunoabsorbent assay (ELISA) are necessary for confirmation; however, occasional false-positive results may be found, and a Western analysis may be required to reveal characteristic HTLV-I antigen bands. Positive antibody titers to HTLV-I are found in CSF and serum of both carriers and HAM/TSP patients. Recently, quantification of proviral load by PCR has shown that HTLV-I proviral load is highest at the onset of the infection and tends to decrease with time. Antibody titers, however, are generally higher in HAM/TSP patients than in asymptomatic carriers. In addition, it is possible that a higher proviral load at the time of seroconversion in a patient infected with HTLV-I via transfusion may correlate with the development of HAM/TSP later on. Quantification of proviral load, which reflects degree of integrated viral genome in host cells and can serve as a surrogate marker of HTLV-I production, may play an important role as a future biomarker for predicting disease onset and for clinical studies assessing early treatment approaches for HAM/TSP.[18,27] However, there is a need for more precise biomarkers that reflect the triggering of proinflammatory pathways by HTLV-I. There is also a need for clinical markers for the HTLV-I carrier status, and it is of interest that infective dermatitis has been proposed as a clinical marker for HTLV-I carrier children.[16] *Strongyloides stercoralis* gastrointestinal tract hyperinfection has also been suggested as a potential clinical marker of HTLV-I infection in Latin America.[8]

Clinical Features of Human T-Cell Lymphotropic Virus Type I–Associated Myelopathy/Tropical Spastic Paraparesis

HAM/TSP develops in approximately 1–2% of individuals carrying HTLV-I. HAM/TSP rarely presents in patients who have already developed T-cell lymphoma or vice versa. The onset of HAM/TSP occurs after several (5 or more) years of harboring the HTLV-I virus and, for this reason, the peak of median age of onset occurs in the fifth decade. However, cases in children have been reported. HAM/TSP initially manifests as leg stiffness (Figure 11-2) and occasional urinary hesitancy and rarely presents with paresthesias and dysesthesias of legs. Decreased vibration sense may be found on examination. In addition, approximately one-third of patients exhibit abnormal perception of light touch, pain, and cold temperature. Position sense is impaired in only approximately 20% of patients with HAM/TSP. The most frequently reported subjective pain symptoms are those due to spasticity-associated muscle spasms. Hip flexor weakness tends to be asymmetric in the initial stage, but gradually symptoms of symmetric leg weakness and spasticity progress, so that assistance is required a few years later for ambulation. The disorder thus clinically resembles the spinal form of primary progressive multiple sclerosis. Some patients may have associated uveitis, arthritis, or respiratory problems. By the time patients reach the wheelchair-bound stage, most have urinary or bowel symptoms of a neurogenic origin, such as urgency, frequency, or incontinence. Impotence is a frequent manifestation. Arm strength and reflexes can be compromised to a much lesser degree and frequency, and the examination more consistently shows distinct and remark-

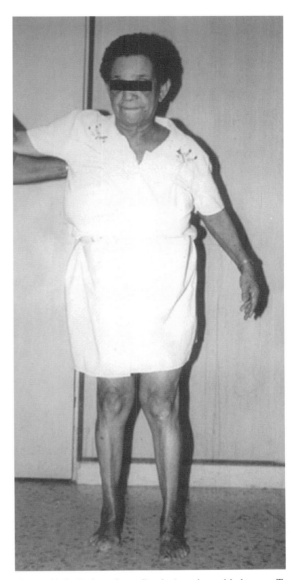

Figure 11-2. Patient from South America with human T-cell lymphotropic virus type I–associated myelopathy/tropical spastic paraparesis. She had a history of arthritis and uveitis and was found to have a progressive spastic paraparesis. She required constant assistance with ambulation. Presence of human T-cell lymphotropic virus type I infection–related antibodies was confirmed by enzyme-linked immunosorbent assay and Western blots. (Reprinted with permission from F Dangond, DA Hafler. Neuroimmunology. In R Ransohoff [ed], Continuum Series, Vol. 7. St. Paul, Minnesota: American Academy of Neurology, 2001.)

able lower extremity hyperreflexia, clonus, and Babinski signs. Cognitive decline, ocular movement abnormalities, visual dysfunction, and sensory level findings on examination are exceptionally rare but can occur. In fact, a subcortical dementia related to HTLV-I infection has been described, but more cases are needed to establish a true association. In addition, highly sensitive tests, such as visual-evoked potentials, have detected bilateral abnormalities (prolongation of P100) in as high as 50% of HAM/TSP patients, reflecting the subclinical involvement of brain regions.

At the time of diagnosis, most patients walk only with support. This might be an explanation for the variable and generally transient and poor response to treatment with most agents, including intravenous steroids.[60–62] Perhaps early intervention during the first 2 years of symptoms helps to change the clinical outcome of the disease.

Diagnostic and Confirmatory Tests

Viral Confirmation

Positive antibody titers to HTLV-I by ELISA are found in serum and CSF of both carriers and HAM/TSP patients. ELISA titers are necessary for confirmation; however, a Western blot may be required to reveal characteristic bands for HTLV-I when false-positive results are suspected.

Magnetic Resonance Imaging in Human T-Cell Lymphotropic Virus Type I–Associated Myelopathy/Tropical Spastic Paraparesis

The most common diagnosis carried by HAM/TSP patients before laboratory confirmation of HTLV-I myelopathy is that of multiple sclerosis. Not surprisingly, MRI may be helpful in diagnosis. However, due to the chronic nature of HAM/TSP, demyelinative lesions rarely enhance with gadolinium on T_1-weighted images unless the study is performed in the early years. These lesions predominantly appear in the lower levels of the thoracic spinal cord and sometimes can be difficult to ascertain due to the minimal involvement in some cases. Chronic findings in head and spine MRIs in some cases include multiple bihemi-

spheric white matter or brain stem lesions and cord atrophy.

Evoked Potentials

Recent studies using motor- and somatosensory-evoked potentials in HAM/TSP[63] showed a clear correlation with the pathologic findings. These studies show that 73.8% of HAM/TSP patients have abnormal lower extremity central motor conduction time as measured using the transcranial magnetic stimulation technique, whereas only 17.6% exhibit involvement of upper extremities, reflecting a predominant involvement of the descending corticospinal pathways at the thoracic level. Somatosensory-evoked potentials may also be abnormal, reflecting prominent subclinical involvement of large-fiber afferent pathways, including the dorsal columns, medial lemniscus, and thalamocortical pathways. However, involvement of these ascending pathways is seen in only 31.3% of HAM/TSP patients as assessed by central sensory conduction time of all limbs.[64] Visual-evoked responses can be altered in as many as 50% of patients, despite the absence of visual symptoms. Auditory-evoked responses are less helpful, with most studies reporting little or no involvement of auditory pathways.

Cerebrospinal Fluid Examination

The presence of HTLV-I can be ascertained by PCR. Intrathecal production of antibodies against HTLV-I may also be demonstrated by ELISA or Western blot. Some cases present with oligoclonal bands, and there is a mononuclear pleocytosis (less than 20 cells) but no significant increases in protein (less than 50 mg/dl) or glucose are demonstrated. The immunoglobulin G index may be elevated. Microscopic analysis of CSF or peripheral blood may reveal characteristic nuclear hyperlobulation in HTLV-I–infected T cells (see Color Plate 12), a finding that may suggest ATLL or a preleukemic (pre-ATLL) stage.[65]

Transmission

The virus is transmitted by blood transfusion, sexual intercourse, or needle sharing or from mother to offspring via placenta or breast-feeding. As compared to human immunodeficiency virus infection, wherein transmission can occur by contact with the virus itself, HTLV-I infection requires direct exposure to infected cells. The recent detection of the HTLV-I provirus in salivary lymphocytes of HTLV-I carriers and HAM/TSP patients by in situ PCR[66] suggests that these lymphocytes could transmit the infection.

Treatment

Antiviral Therapy

At present, there is no curative or standard treatment for HAM/TSP. Most studies have examined the short-term effects of therapies with few patients, and some reports are anecdotal. IFN-α is an immunomodulatory and antiviral compound that has been used for the treatment of hepatitis B and C, Kaposi sarcoma in acquired immune deficiency syndrome, and ATLL. Treatment with IFN-α stands out as a potentially useful treatment for HAM/TSP, as this medication has been shown to decrease HTLV-I viral titers and T-cell proliferation, with some studies claiming both short- and long-term improvement in motor performance.[67,68] However, these reports do not describe striking results. A combination of IFN-α and -β results in a partial inhibition of early infection by HTLV-I in in vitro mononuclear cells derived from umbilical blood. The human recombinant IFN-α and -β also seem to inhibit the HTLV-I–induced transformation of peripheral blood lymphocytes in vitro. Glucocorticoids are widely used and may have transient beneficial effects in some patients with HAM/TSP, but their long-term impact on disease course is questionable. Perhaps a combination treatment with antiretroviral compounds (i.e., protease inhibitors) and IFN-α may yield better clinical responses.

Immunotherapy

Immunotherapeutic interventions in HAM/TSP could be directed against specific T cells activated by CD4+ or against the generalized immune activation mediated by HTLV-I. The high frequency of viral-responsive CD8+ T cells could also be a target of immunotherapy. However, it is as yet unclear whether the high-frequency CD8+ T-cell response is inefficient in eliminating the virus and thus should be strengthened or whether it mediates the damage in the CNS by increasing the size of the lesions, in which case the objective would be to downregulate this T-cell population. It has been determined that the restricted use of the TCR by these cells in HAM/TSP and the number, also limited, of immunodominant epitopes that are responsible for the antiviral response can make it possible to design a CD8+ T-cell–specific immune therapy. For example, we have demonstrated that if we alter key amino acids in the immunodominant tax_{11-19} protein fragment of HTLV-I, the response of the CD8+ T cells can be manipulated in a selective manner toward proliferation, cytotoxicity, or anergy.[50] In addition, the demonstrated ability of monoclonal antibodies against IL-15 or IL-2 or their receptors[69] to inhibit spontaneous proliferation of HTLV-I–infected cells suggests that immunotherapy with cytokine or cytokine receptor–specific antibodies may be beneficial in HAM/TSP. Finally, our growing knowledge of adhesion molecules that participate in CNS migration of lymphocytes will help to establish likely targets of immunomodulation therapies.

Symptomatic Therapy

Medical care in HAM/TSP is primarily palliative, and treatment is fairly similar to the symptomatic management of multiple sclerosis patients (see Chapter 5). There is no activity restriction. Patients should maintain a regular exercise regimen, if the degree of weakness allows it. There is no dietary restriction specific for HAM/TSP, and patients are encouraged to eat a balanced diet. HAM/TSP patients have multiple needs, including neuropsychological counseling, physical therapy, and access to orthotic equipment. End-stage HAM/TSP patients may develop impaired arm strength resulting in inability to perform activities of daily living, including handling utensils for self-feeding. Home health aides can be helpful in feeding the patient in whom upper limb involvement has become significant. Physical therapy should be aimed at enhancing muscle function and relieving spasticity. In addition, these patients commonly develop decubitus ulcers, skin infections, atelectasis, pneumonia, or aspiration. Urinary tract infections are commonly secondary to neurogenic bladder dysfunction.

Medications, such as baclofen (Lioresal), tizanidine (Zanaflex), dantrolene, and diazepam, may be used to relieve severe spasticity. A combination of these drugs is allowed in cases in which maximum doses are not achieving the desired effect. Finally, surgical procedures to alleviate contractures perceived as painful spasms or neuropathic pain include adductor leg muscle tendon release and rhizotomy, respectively.

Baclofen is a γ-aminobutyric acid agonist drug that is metabolized in the liver and primarily excreted in the urine. The medication can be started at 5 mg by mouth three times a day and may be gradually advanced as needed to a maximum of 80 mg by mouth every day. Hypersensitivity to the drug or its components is the only major contraindication for its use. Caution should be exercised when using antipsychotics, monoamine oxidase inhibitors, narcotics, tricyclic antidepressants, oral hypoglycemics, or insulin or when used concomitantly with alcohol intake. Baclofen should be used with caution in patients with seizures or impaired kidney function. Serious reactions include stupor, cardiovascular collapse, tachypnea, and seizures. Common side effects include headaches, dizziness, light-headedness, blurred vision, slurred speech, rash, weight gain, pruritus, constipation, and increased perspiration. Excessive dosing of baclofen may lead to flaccidity and significant worsening of weakness. The safety of baclofen in pregnancy has not been established.

Tizanidine is a central α-adrenergic agonist that is metabolized in the liver and primarily excreted in the feces and urine. A starting dose of 4–8 mg by mouth every 8 hours as needed is advanced gradually to a maximum of 36 mg per day. It is contraindicated in patients with known hypersensitivity to the drug or its components and should be used with caution in elderly patients or in patients with impaired kidney function. Tizanidine may interact with alcohol, resulting in drowsiness or stupor. Its safety in pregnancy has not yet been established. Serious reactions of tizanidine include hallucinations, severe bradycardia, and liver damage. More common side effects include dryness of the mouth, somnolence and sedation, dizziness, light-headedness, malaise, constipation, increased spasms, and hypotension.

Urologic consultation may be necessary to assess better the degree and type of incontinence. Drugs commonly used for incontinence in HAM/TSP patients include tolterodine tartrate (Detrol), propantheline bromide (Pro-Banthine), oxybutynin (Ditropan), and imipramine (Tofranil). The use of self-catheterization intermittently is important in avoiding recurrent infections.

High-fiber diets, over-the-counter laxatives, and stool softeners are advised for patients with severe constipation. No effective medications are listed for the long-term control of recurrent bowel incontinence.

Sildenafil (Viagra) has been shown to be effective in spinal cord disorders of diverse etiologies and should be of first choice in HAM/TSP. Other approaches include the use of intracorporeal papaverine (not U.S. Food and Drug Administration approved) and penile prostheses. Several newer medications for the treatment of erectile dysfunction are currently under development, and the physician should be aware of alternative new options for patients with HAM/TSP.

Painful tonic spasms are a frequent symptom and can become incapacitating to the patient, who may be awakened at night by their severity. These symptoms may respond to medications such as carbamazepine, baclofen, gabapentin, or phenytoin.

Although not as prominent as that described by multiple sclerosis patients, fatigue and exhaustion also occur in HAM/TSP. Medications commonly used to treat fatigue include amantadine, pemoline, fluoxetine (Prozac), methylphenidate (Ritalin), or selegiline and more recently, modafinil (Provigil).

Conclusions

HTLV-I is a human retrovirus that leads, in a minority of infected patients, to a neurologic disease termed *HAM/TSP* or to a malignant disease, termed *ATLL*. The neurologic aspects of HAM/TSP are interesting to neuroscientists and neuroimmunologists, as there is clearly an inflammatory and probably autoimmune component to the spinal cord injury in this disease. HAM/TSP clinically resembles the spinal form of primary progressive multiple sclerosis, a disorder for which a viral hypothesis has been entertained. HTLV-I can be transmitted by sexual intercourse, blood transfusion, or needle sharing or from mother to offspring via placenta or breastfeeding. Despite the wealth of literature regarding modes of transmission and HTLV-I proviral expression, little is known regarding the molecular mechanisms behind the pathogenesis, including the signal transduction and transcriptional activation pathways responsible for mediating the CNS manifestations in HAM/TSP. Treatment of HAM/TSP and ATLL is difficult, as most studies have examined the short-term effects of therapies with few patients, and some reports are anecdotal. Recent approaches have included attempts at decreasing proviral loads. Efforts to treat HAM/TSP patients with plasmapheresis have resulted in only slight to modest improvement.[70] Studies of safety and possible efficacy of therapy with zidovudine have been performed.[71] Treatments with IFN-α or anti–IL-2 receptor antibody[69] or other anticytokine antibodies stand out as potentially useful treatments for HAM/TSP disease or even lymphoma. Antagonism of a proinflammatory phenotype may explain the response to these treatments. Elucidation of the molecular pathways triggering this phenotype is a first step toward our better understanding of HTLV-I–induced diseases and their potential treatments.

References

1. Zaninovic V, Biojo R, Barreto P. Paraparesia Espastica del Pacifico. Colombia Medica 1981;111–117.
2. Mani KS, Punekar BD, Rao KT, Nair DS. South Indian paraplegia: a spastic paraplegic syndrome of obscure etiology. Neurol India 1966;14:19–24.
3. Gessain A, Barin F, Vernant JC, et al. Antibodies to human T-lymphotropic virus type-I in patients with tropical spastic paraparesis. Lancet 1985;2:407–410.
4. Poiesz BJ, Ruscetti FW, Gazdar AF, et al. Detection and isolation of type C retrovirus particles from fresh and cultured lymphocytes of a patient with cutaneous T-cell lymphoma. Proc Natl Acad Sci U S A 1980;77:7415–7419.
5. Osame M, Matsumoto M, Usuku K, et al. Chronic progressive myelopathy associated with elevated antibodies to human T-lymphotropic virus type I and adult T-cell leukemialike cells. Ann Neurol 1987;21:117–122.
6. Roman GC, Schoenberg BS, Madden DL, et al. Human T-lymphotropic virus type I antibodies in the serum of patients with tropical spastic paraparesis in the Seychelles. Arch Neurol 1987;44:605–607.
7. Roman GC, Roman LN, Spencer PS, Schoenberg BS. Tropical spastic paraparesis: a neuroepidemiological study in Colombia. Ann Neurol 1985;17:361–365.
8. Gotuzzo E, Arango C, de Queiroz-Campos A, Isturiz RE. Human T-cell lymphotropic virus-I in Latin America. Infect Dis Clin North Am 2000;14(1):211–239, x–xi.
9. Dangond F, Daza JS, Rosania A, et al. Tropical spastic paraparesis on the Caribbean coast of Colombia. Am J Trop Med Hyg 1995;52:155–158.
10. Mochizuki M, Watanabe T, Yamaguchi K, et al. HTLV-I uveitis: a distinct clinical entity caused by HTLV-I. Jpn J Cancer Res 1992;83:236–239.
11. Mita S, Sugimoto M, Nakamura M, et al. Increased human T lymphotropic virus type-1 (HTLV-1) proviral DNA in peripheral blood mononuclear cells and bronchoalveolar lavage cells from Japanese patients with HTLV-1-associated myelopathy. Am J Trop Med Hyg 1993;48:170–177.
12. Kawai H, Inui T, Kashiwagi S, et al. HTLV-I infection in patients with autoimmune thyroiditis (Hashimoto's thyroiditis). J Med Virol 1992;38:138–141.
13. Nishioka K, Maruyama I, Sato K, et al. Chronic inflammatory arthropathy associated with HTLV-I. Lancet 1989;1:441.
14. Sowa JM. Human T lymphotropic virus I, myelopathy, polymyositis and synovitis: an expanding rheumatic spectrum. J Rheumatol 1992;19:316–318.
15. Terada K, Katamine S, Eguchi K, et al. Prevalence of serum and salivary antibodies to HTLV-1 in Sjögren's syndrome. Lancet 1994;344:1116–1119.
16. LaGrenade L, Hanchard B, Fletcher V, et al. Infective dermatitis of Jamaican children: a marker for HTLV-I infection. Lancet 1990;336:1345–1347.
17. Höllsberg P, Hafler DA. Seminars in medicine of the Beth Israel Hospital, Boston. Pathogenesis of diseases induced by human lymphotropic virus type I infection. N Engl J Med 1993;328:1173–1182.
18. Manns A, Miley WJ, Wilks RJ, et al. Quantitative proviral DNA and antibody levels in the natural history of HTLV-I infection. J Infect Dis 1999;180:1487–1493.
19. Richardson JH, Edwards AJ, Cruickshank JK, et al. In vivo cellular tropism of human T-cell leukemia virus type 1. J Virol 1990;64:5682–5687.
20. Lin HC, Dezzutti CS, Lal RB, Rabson AB. Activation of human T-cell leukemia virus type 1 tax gene expression in chronically infected T cells. J Virol 1998;72:6264–6270.
21. Yssel H, de Waal Malefyt R, Duc Dodon MD, et al. Human T cell leukemia/lymphoma virus type I infection of a CD4+ proliferative/cytotoxic T cell clone progresses in at least two distinct phases based on changes in function and phenotype of the infected cells. J Immunol 1989;142:2279–2289.
22. Levin MC, Krichavsky M, Berk J, et al. Neuronal molecular mimicry in immune-mediated neurologic disease. Ann Neurol 1998;44:87–98.
23. Eiraku N, Hingorani R, Ijichi S, et al. Clonal expansion within CD4+ and CD8+ T cell subsets in human T lymphotropic virus type I-infected individuals. J Immunol 1998;161:6674–6680.
24. Kitze B, Usuku K, Yamano Y, et al. Human CD4+ T lymphocytes recognize a highly conserved epitope of human T lymphotropic virus type 1 (HTLV-1) env gp21 restricted by HLA DRB1*0101. Clin Exp Immunol 1998;111:278–285.
25. Jacobson S, Shida H, McFarlin DE, et al. Circulating CD8+ cytotoxic T lymphocytes specific for HTLV-I pX in patients with HTLV-I associated neurological disease. Nature 1990;348:245–248.

26. Elovaara I, Koenig S, Brewah AY, et al. High human T cell lymphotropic virus type 1 (HTLV-1)-specific precursor cytotoxic T lymphocyte frequencies in patients with HTLV-1-associated neurological disease. J Exp Med 1993;177:1567–1573.

27. Nagai M, Usuku K, Matsumoto W, et al. Analysis of HTLV-I proviral load in 202 HAM/TSP patients and 243 asymptomatic HTLV-I carriers: high proviral load strongly predisposes to HAM/TSP. J Neurovirol 1998; 4:586–593.

28. Scholz C, Freeman GJ, Greenfield EA, et al. Activation of human T cell lymphotropic virus type I-infected T cells is independent of B7 costimulation. J Immunol 1996; 157:2932–2938.

29. Ichinose K, Nakamura T, Kawakami A, et al. Increased adherence of T cells to human endothelial cells in patients with human T-cell lymphotropic virus type I-associated myelopathy. Arch Neurol 1992;49:74–76.

30. Tanaka Y, Fukudome K, Hayashi M, et al. Induction of ICAM-1 and LFA-3 by Tax1 of human T-cell leukemia virus type 1 and mechanism of down-regulation of ICAM-1 or LFA-1 in adult-T-cell-leukemia cell lines. Int J Cancer 1995;60:554–561.

31. Tatewaki M, Yamaguchi K, Matsuoka M, et al. Constitutive overexpression of the L-selectin gene in fresh leukemic cells of adult T-cell leukemia that can be transactivated by human T-cell lymphotropic virus type 1 Tax. Blood 1995;86:3109–3117.

32. Wucherpfennig KW, Höllsberg P, Richardson JH, et al. T-cell activation by autologous human T-cell leukemia virus type I-infected T-cell clones. Proc Natl Acad Sci U S A 1992;89:2110–2114.

33. Matsuoka E, Takenouchi N, Hashimoto K, et al. Perivascular T cells are infected with HTLV-I in the spinal cord lesions with HTLV-I-associated myelopathy/tropical spastic paraparesis: double staining of immunohistochemistry and polymerase chain reaction in situ hybridization. Acta Neuropathol (Berl) 1998;96:340–346.

34. Höllsberg P, Wucherpfennig KW, Ausubel LJ, et al. Characterization of HTLV-I in vivo infected T cell clones. IL-2-independent growth of nontransformed T cells. J Immunol 1992;148:3256–3263.

35. de Waal Malefyt R, Yssel H, Spits H, et al. Human T cell leukemia virus type I prevents cell surface expression of the T cell receptor through down-regulation of the CD3-gamma, -delta, -epsilon, and -zeta genes. J Immunol 1990;145:2297–2303.

36. Grassmann R, Berchtold S, Radant I, et al. Role of human T-cell leukemia virus type 1 X region proteins in immortalization of primary human lymphocytes in culture. J Virol 1992;66:4570–4575.

37. Xu X, Kang SH, Heidenreich O, et al. Constitutive activation of different Jak tyrosine kinases in human T cell leukemia virus type 1 (HTLV-1) tax protein or virus-transformed cells. J Clin Invest 1995;96:1548–1555.

38. Migone TS, Lin JX, Cereseto A, et al. Constitutively activated Jak-STAT pathway in T cells transformed with HTLV-I. Science 1995;269:79–81.

39. Pise-Masison CA, Dittmer J, Clemens KE, Brady JN. Physical and functional interaction between the human T-cell lymphotropic virus type 1 Tax1 protein and the CCAAT binding protein NF-Y. Mol Cell Biol 1997;17: 1236–1243.

40. Bex F, Yin MJ, Burny A, Gaynor RB. Differential transcriptional activation by human T-cell leukemia virus type 1 Tax mutants is mediated by distinct interactions with CREB binding protein and p300. Mol Cell Biol 1998;18:2392–2405.

41. Lundblad JR, Kwok RP, Laurance ME, et al. The human T-cell leukemia virus-1 transcriptional activator Tax enhances cAMP-responsive element-binding protein (CREB) binding activity through interactions with the DNA minor groove. J Biol Chem 1998;273(30):19251–19259.

42. Lenzmeier BA, Giebler HA, Nyborg JK. Human T-cell leukemia virus type 1 Tax requires direct access to DNA for recruitment of CREB binding protein to the viral promoter. Mol Cell Biol 1998;18(2):721–731.

43. Nicot C, Tie F, Giam CZ. Cytoplasmic forms of human T-cell leukemia virus type 1 Tax induce NF-kappaB activation. J Virol 1998;72:6777–6784.

44. Neuveut C, Low KG, Maldarelli F, et al. Human T-cell leukemia virus type 1 Tax and cell cycle progression: role of cyclin D-cdk and p110Rb. Mol Cell Biol 1998;18:3620–3632.

45. Low KG, Dorner LF, Fernando DB, et al. Human T-cell leukemia virus type 1 Tax releases cell cycle arrest induced by p16INK4a. J Virol 1997;71:1956–1962.

46. Jin DY, Spencer F, Jeang KT. Human T cell leukemia virus type 1 oncoprotein Tax targets the human mitotic checkpoint protein MAD1. Cell 1998;93:81–91.

47. Reddy TR, Li X, Jones Y, et al. Specific interaction of HTLV tax protein and a human type IV neuronal intermediate filament protein. Proc Natl Acad Sci U S A 1998;95:702–707.

48. Cartier LM, Cea JG, Vergara C, et al. Clinical and neuropathological study of six patients with spastic paraparesis associated with HTLV-I: an axomyelinic degeneration of the central nervous system. J Neuropathol Exp Neurol 1997;56:403–413.

49. Bieganowska K, Höllsberg P, Buckle GJ, et al. Direct analysis of viral-specific CD8+ T cells with soluble HLA-A2/Tax11-19 tetramer complexes in patients with human T cell lymphotropic virus-associated myelopathy. J Immunol 1999;162:1765–1671.

50. Höllsberg P, Weber WE, Dangond F, et al. Differential activation of proliferation and cytotoxicity in human T-cell lymphotropic virus type I Tax-specific CD8 T cells by an altered peptide ligand. Proc Natl Acad Sci U S A 1995;92:4036–4040.

51. Umehara F, Okada Y, Fujimoto N, et al. Expression of matrix metalloproteinases and tissue inhibitors of metalloproteinases in HTLV-I-associated myelopathy. J Neuropathol Exp Neurol 1998;57:839–849.

52. Biddison WE, Kubota R, Kawanishi T, et al. Human T cell leukemia virus type I (HTLV-I)-specific CD8+ CTL clones from patients with HTLV-I-associated neurologic disease secrete proinflammatory cytokines, chemokines, and matrix metalloproteinase. J Immunol 1997;159:2018–2025.

53. Kawahigashi N, Furukawa Y, Saito M, et al. Predominant expression of Fas ligand mRNA in CD8+ T lymphocytes

in patients with HTLV-1 associated myelopathy. J Neuroimmunol 1998;90:199–206.

54. Macatonia SE, Cruickshank JK, Rudge P, Knight SC. Dendritic cells from patients with tropical spastic paraparesis are infected with HTLV-1 and stimulate autologous lymphocyte proliferation. AIDS Res Hum Retroviruses 1992;8:1699–1706.

55. Makino M, Shimokubo S, Wakamatsu SI, et al. The role of human T-lymphotropic virus type 1 (HTLV-1)-infected dendritic cells in the development of HTLV-1-associated myelopathy/tropical spastic paraparesis. J Virol 1999;73:4575–4581.

56. Jacobson S, Krichavsky M, Flerlage N, Levin M. Immunopathogenesis of HTLV-I associated neurologic disease: massive latent HTLV-I infection in bone marrow of HAM/TSP patients. Leukemia 1997;11(Suppl 3):73–75.

57. Kushida S, Mizusawa H, Matsumura M, et al. High incidence of HAM/TSP-like symptoms in WKA rats after administration of human T-cell leukemia virus type 1-producing cells. J Virol 1994;68:7221–7226.

58. Sun B, Fang J, Yagami K, et al. Age-dependent paraparesis in WKA rats: evaluation of MHC κ-haplotype and HTLV-1 infection. J Neurol Sci 1999;167:16–21.

59. Gardner MB, Chiri A, Dougherty MF, et al. Congenital transmission of murine leukemia virus from wild mice prone to the development of lymphoma and paralysis. J Natl Cancer Inst 1979;62:63–70.

60. Honig LS, Lipka JJ, Young KY, et al. HTLV-I-associated myelopathy in a Californian: diagnosis by reactivity to a viral recombinant antigen. Neurology 1991;41:448–450.

61. Kira J, Fujihara K, Itoyama Y, et al. Leukoencephalopathy in HTLV-I-associated myelopathy/tropical spastic paraparesis: MRI analysis and a two year follow-up study after corticosteroid therapy. J Neurol Sci 1991;106:41–49.

62. McKendall RR, Oas J, Lairmore MD. HTLV-I-associated myelopathy endemic in Texas-born residents and isolation of virus from CSF cells. Neurology 1991;41:831–836.

63. Suga R, Tobimatsu S, Kira J, Kato M. Motor and somatosensory evoked potential findings in HTLV-I associated myelopathy. J Neurol Sci 1999;167:102–106.

64. Castillo JL, Cea JG, Verdugo RJ, Cartier L. Sensory dysfunction in HTLV-I-associated myelopathy/tropical spastic paraparesis. A comprehensive neurophysiological study. Eur Neurol 1999;42:17–22.

65. Kinoshita K, Amagasaki T, Ikeda S, et al. Preleukemic state of adult T cell leukemia: abnormal T lymphocytosis induced by human adult T cell leukemia-lymphoma virus. Blood 1985;66:120–127.

66. Achiron A, Higuchi I, Takenouchi N, et al. Detection of HTLV type I provirus by in situ polymerase chain reaction in mouthwash mononuclear cells of HAM/TSP patients and HTLV type I carriers. AIDS Res Hum Retroviruses 1997;13:1067–1070.

67. Izumo S, Goto I, Itoyama Y, et al. Interferon-alpha is effective in HTLV-I-associated myelopathy: a multicenter, randomized, double-blind, controlled trial. Neurology 1996;46:1016–1021.

68. Yamasaki K, Kira J, Koyanagi Y, et al. Long-term, high dose interferon-alpha treatment in HTLV-I-associated myelopathy/tropical spastic paraparesis: a combined clinical, virological and immunological study. J Neurol Sci 1997;147:35–44.

69. Azimi N, Jacobson S, Leist T, Waldmann TA. Involvement of IL-15 in the pathogenesis of human T lymphotropic virus type I-associated myelopathy/tropical spastic paraparesis: implications for therapy with a monoclonal antibody directed to the IL-2/15R beta receptor. J Immunol 1999;163:4064–4072.

70. Matsuo H, Nakamura T, Tsujihata M, et al. Plasmapheresis in treatment of human T-lymphotropic virus type-I associated myelopathy. Lancet 1988;2:1109–1113.

71. Sheremata WA, Benedict D, Squilacote DC, et al. High-dose zidovudine induction in HTLV-I-associated myelopathy: safety and possible efficacy. Neurology 1993;43:2125–2129.

Chapter 12

Virologic and Neuroimmunopathologic Aspects of Human T-Cell Lymphotropic Virus Type I–Associated Myelopathy/Tropical Spastic Paraparesis

Carlos A. Pardo and Suzanne Gartner

Human T-cell lymphotropic virus type I (HTLV-I) is a human oncogenic retrovirus associated with development of T-cell lymphomas and a variety of disorders, including forms of uveitis, polymyositis, arthritis, Sjögren's syndrome, and infective dermatitis.[1–4] In the central nervous system (CNS), infection by HTLV-I leads to a progressive and chronic neurologic disorder characterized by spastic paraparesis, sensory symptoms, and sphincter dysfunction known as *HTLV-I–associated myelopathy* (HAM) or *tropical spastic paraparesis* (TSP).[5–12] In HAM/TSP, the involvement of the white-matter tracts of the spinal cord appears to be the main factor responsible for the clinical symptoms,[13] but other white-matter areas of the CNS may be involved as well. Geographic clusters of HAM/TSP were initially described in Jamaica and other Caribbean islands and later in Japan, Colombia, and other regions of South America and Africa.[14–19]

The prevalence of HTLV-I infection is variable worldwide but is endemic in many regions, particularly in the Caribbean, South America, Japan, and some equatorial regions of Africa, where the HTLV-I seroprevalence ranges from 3% to 30%.[20–25] In the United States and Europe, the seroprevalence of HTLV-I infection among low-risk populations is lower than 1% but is particularly high among intravenous drug users, homosexual men, prostitutes,

and patients infected with human immunodeficiency virus.[26–30] The seroprevalence increases with age and is higher among females in reproductive age. HTLV-I infection is linked mostly to three forms of transmission: sexual contact, vertical transmission from HTLV-I–infected mother to child through prolonged breast-feeding, or transfusion of blood components. Sexual transmission and maternal passage of the virus through breast-feeding appear to be the most common forms of infection.[2,31–35] The risk of sexual transmission increases if the sexual partner has high antibody titer or proviral load. Infection by HTLV-I through sexual contact appears to be more efficient from males to females, as the rate of infection is four times higher as compared with the female-to-male route in sexually active age groups.[36] However, among risk factors, transfusion of blood components such as packed red blood cells, whole blood, and platelets (but not fresh frozen plasma) appears to be the most effective route of HTLV-I transmission.[37,38] In recent years, co-infection of HTLV-I with human immunodeficiency virus is a source of concern in some regions of the world, as the course of disease in co-infected patients appears to be one of rapid progression of disability.[39,40]

The prevalence of HAM/TSP parallels the seroprevalence of HTLV-I infection. In regions of high

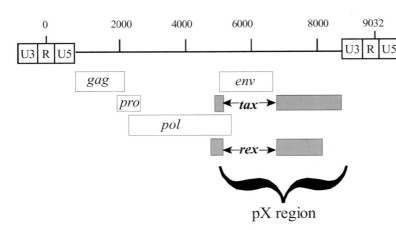

Figure 12-1. Diagrammatic representation of the human T-cell lymphotropic virus type I genome.

pX region

seroprevalence, approximately 2% of the infected population develops HTLV-I–associated disease, either HAM/TSP[41] or a distinct form of adult T-cell leukemia-lymphoma (ATLL).[21] However, HAM/TSP and ATLL rarely coincide in the same patient. The lifetime risk for developing HAM/TSP is lower than that of ATLL, with an age-standardized incidence in endemic areas of 2 per 100,000 person-years.[21,31] The factors that determine the risk of HAM/TSP among HTLV-I carriers remain unknown, but they appear to be associated with differences in host genetic factors and immune responses rather than the virus itself. No specific strains of HTLV-I have been demonstrated to be associated with the outcome of infection or development of HAM/TSP.[3] However, the mode of transmission and cultural factors have been also invoked as determinants of susceptibility. The incubation period from time of infection to the development of disease is variable, and it may take months to years before the onset of first symptoms. In some cases in which blood transfusion was the risk factor, the incubation period appears to be particularly short, with a rapid evolution of the disease.[42] The clinical, immunologic, and treatment issues of HAM/TSP are discussed extensively in this book (see Chapter 11).

Human T-Cell Lymphotropic Virus Type I Virology

Viral Genome: Structure and Function

Based primarily on phylogenetic relatedness, retroviruses are now commonly grouped into seven gen-

era.[43] HTLV-I is a member of the HTLV-BLV group, which also includes HTLV-II and bovine leukemia virus. The HTLV-I particles, which consist of the typical retroviral envelope and core structures, are spherical, and measure 110–140 nm in diameter. The envelope is composed of a host cell–derived lipid bilayer studded with the viral envelope protein. Ultrastructurally, the viral core is reminiscent of the mammalian C-type retroviruses, the mature particle appearing with an electron-dense central core surrounded by an electron-lucent halo.[44] The dense central core contains two copies of the viral RNA genome packaged together with certain of the viral proteins.

HTLV-I displays the genomic organization characteristic of all retroviruses: *gag*, *pol*, and *env* genes (ordered 5' to 3') bound by identical long-terminal repeat (LTR) regions at either end of the coding regions (Figure 12-1). The *group-specific antigen* (*gag*) gene encodes a 48-kD polyprotein that is cleaved by the viral protease[45] to form the three major core proteins: the 19-kD matrix protein, the 24-kD capsid protein, and the 15-kD nucleocapsid protein. The *polymerase* (*pol*) gene encodes a 99-kD polyprotein that includes the reverse transcriptase, integrase, and RNase H enzymes. The HTLV-I protease is encoded by an open reading frame that overlaps with the 3' end of the *gag* gene and the 5' end of *pol*; ribosomal frame-shifting is required for production of this protein.[45] The *envelope* (*env*) gene encodes a 54-kD product that includes a 46-kD external surface glycoprotein and a 21-kD transmembrane portion. The LTRs contain transcription factors and other regulatory elements (see Regulation of Virus Expression). There appears to be little genetic variability among HTLV-I strains recovered from different geographic regions,[46] and no specific strains have been linked to the development of HAM/TSP versus ATLL.[47]

Like other so-called complex retroviruses, HTLV-I encodes additional nonstructural gene products unique to this virus. These genes, designated collectively as pX (see Figure 12-1), are located at the 3' end of the viral genome.[48] Four open reading frames have been identified, termed X-I, X-II, X-III, and X-IV. The X-III and X-IV domains encode the 27-kD Rex and 40-kD tax proteins, respectively. These proteins are produced from double-spliced messenger RNAs (mRNAs), and the AUG initiation codons for both are located in the second exon of the double-spliced message. Rex and tax are both nuclear phosphoproteins required for the viral life cycle, and they play key roles in the regulation of viral gene expression. Another protein, designated p21[rex] because it can be precipitated by anti-rex antibodies, is produced from the X-III and X-IV open reading frames by means of an internal AUG codon[49]; p21[rex] may function as a rex antagonist. Three proteins derived from the X-I and X-II domains have been identified[48,50]: p12, p13, and p30; they arise via alternative splicing. A few studies have examined the subcellular localization of these, but little is known about their functional activities.

Regulation of Virus Expression

The U3 region of the LTR contains three 21-bp tandem repeats that, along with intervening sequences, constitute the tax-responsive element (TRE-1).[51] tax can greatly upregulate or "transactivate" HTLV-I transcription by interacting with TRE-1. The binding of tax to the TRE-1 within the 5' LTR leads to increased production of the full-length (genomic) viral mRNA.[52] Tax can also interact with a number of cellular transcription factors and signaling molecules,[10,53,54] and it may play a critical role in the early steps leading to HTLV-I–mediated transformation of T-lymphocytes.[55] Rex can also upregulate viral expression but does so at the post-transcriptional level. Rex promotes export of the unspliced genomic and single-spliced env

mRNAs from the host cell nucleus, which, in turn, results in decreased levels of tax and rex and increased levels of the *gag*, *pol*, and *env* gene products.[56] Rex-mediated regulation is complex. A cis-acting repressive sequence (CRS) is located within the U5 region of the 5' LTR, whereas a rex-responsive element is present within the 3' LTR.[57,58] Rex binding to the responsive element appears to outcompete the cis-acting repressive sequence–mediated suppression.

Tax can also promote or enhance the expression of a number of cellular genes, including genes encoding cytokines and chemokines; receptors; enzymes; and various regulatory proteins.[59,60] Included among the cytokines and growth factors are interleukin-2 (IL-2), IL-3, granulocyte-macrophage colony stimulating factor, tumor necrosis factor-α (TNF-α), transforming growth factor-1 beta, c-sis, c-fos, and nerve growth factor. It has also been suggested that tax can be secreted from infected cells and then taken up by others, with pathologic consequences. For example, exposure of cultured primary human adult microglial cells to extracellular tax results in the production of TNF-α and IL-6.[61] Also, in infected T cells, tax is sufficient to induce expression of certain chemokines, among them RANTES (*r*egulated upon *a*ctivation *n*ormal *T* cell *e*xpressed and *s*ecreted), macrophage inflammatory protein 1-α, macrophage inflammatory protein 1-β, and stromal cell–derived factor-1.[62,63] Tax-mediated transactivation of some other cellular genes is clearly important to the process of T-cell transformation during the development of ATLL. Whether this is also the case in HAM/TSP remains to be established.

Viral Life Cycle

The life cycle of HTLV-I is similar to that of other retroviruses. Viral entry is mediated by binding of the virion to an as-yet unidentified receptor on the surface of the target cell, followed by membrane fusion and internalization of the viral core. In vitro studies suggest that HTLV-I has properties of a cell-associated virus, meaning that efficient transmission requires cell-to-cell contact. In vivo, it is likely that transmission occurs via the transfer of infected cells. After internalization, reverse transcription is initiated, and the newly synthesized double-stranded DNA is transported to the nucleus, where it becomes integrated into the host cell genome. Integration appears to occur at random sites.[64] All these initial steps are performed by virus-encoded products packaged into the virion along with the genomic RNA. As a consequence of undefined conditions, the integrated provirus can remain silent or become transcriptionally active. Transcriptional activation leads to the production of various viral mRNAs that become translated and further processed. Essentially, three kinds of viral mRNA are produced: the unspliced, full-length genomic RNA; a single-spliced 4.2-kb species that produces the envelope protein; and a double-spliced 2.1-kb species that gives rise to the pX products.[48,50] The life cycle is completed with packaging of the viral structural proteins and enzymes into particle cores, transporting of the viral envelope protein to the cell surface, and subsequent budding of the structures from the cell surface. Budding results in envelopment of the viral core with the host cell membrane.

Host Cells for Infection in Human T-Cell Lymphotropic Virus Type I–Associated Myelopathy/Tropical Spastic Paraparesis

HTLV-I can infect a number of different types of cells in vitro, including astrocytes, microglia, and neuroblastoma cells.[65,66] Controversy exists, however, as to the in vivo relevance of these observations, particularly with respect to the pathogenesis of HAM/TSP. Several investigators have detected HTLV-I DNA in nervous tissue specimens from patients with HAM/TSP, particularly in specimens taken from the spinal cord.[67–71] In most cases, however, the identity of the infected cells was not established. Even less clear is whether a significant number of these viral genomes become transcriptionally active within the CNS. Bhigjee and colleagues[70] were unable to detect HTLV-I particles, proteins, or mRNA in spinal cord tissues that clearly harbored viral DNA. In contrast, Matsuoka et al.[69] combined in situ DNA polymerase chain reaction with immunostaining for cell markers and found that most of the virus-expressing cells were of T-lympho-

cyte origin and were located within the perivascular areas. Using a probe for *Tax*, Lehky and coworkers[72] detected HTLV-I RNA in the spinal cord and cerebellum of HAM/TSP patients. Interestingly, however, although the typical perivascular infiltrates were present, the virus-positive cells did not localize to these regions but rather were deeper within the parenchyma. Colocalization techniques demonstrated that some of the virus-expressing cells were astrocytes. Some investigators have suggested that this variability in findings may be attributable, in some cases, to the presence of replication-defective viral genomes.[71] However, infectious HTLV-I has been isolated from cerebrospinal fluid (CSF) cells of HAM/TSP patients using phytohemagglutinin stimulation and cocultivation.[73] Clearly, a more definitive identification of the virus-infected cells within the CNS is needed, along with a better understanding of the conditions that initiate and control virus expression.

Two additional observations bear relevance to the issue of HTLV-I host cells in HAM/TSP. First, Sueyoshi et al.[68] detected approximately 1 copy of HTLV-I DNA per 10 cells in tissue recovered from the spinal cord, sciatic nerve, and liver of a patient with HAM/TSP. No viral DNA was recovered from the kidney, cerebellum, or multiple regions of the cerebrum, and only minimal numbers of copies were present within the lungs and the T-cell–rich lymph nodes. Similar findings were obtained by Kuroda et al.[74] Second, Levin and colleagues[75] found extensive latent infection of HTLV-I in the bone marrow of HAM/TSP patients (i.e., high levels of viral DNA were detected in the absence of significant HTLV-I expression). Although the cells harboring the viral genomes were not identified in any of these studies, it is conceivable that macrophages may represent a significant target population in some of these tissues, particularly given their numbers as compared to T cells, as seen for example within the liver sinusoids. They may also represent an important target within the nervous system wherein increased numbers of macrophages and activated microglia have been observed in spinal cord tissues in situ.[69] Latent infection in macrophages could reflect their nonproliferative status or their state of activation or differentiation.

Neuropathologic Features of Human T-Cell Lymphotropic Virus Type I–Associated Myelopathy

Human T-Cell Lymphotropic Virus Type I–Associated Myelopathy/Tropical Spastic Paraparesis Neuropathology

Autopsy and histopathologic studies in patients with HAM/TSP were described for the first time in the late 1980s when there was clear evidence that cases of TSP and myelopathies described in Jamaica and Japan were associated with HTLV-I infection.[76–78] These pathologic studies showed similar features to those of the Jamaican myelo-neuropathies described years before the discovery of the association of HTLV-I with HAM/TSP.[79,80] Although the neuropathologic studies in HAM/TSP have focused on few small case-series, all of them demonstrate[76] that specific segments of the spinal cord, particularly the thoracic region, are the main sites of lesions. In the spinal cord of HAM/TSP patients, both gray- and white-matter structures are involved by pathologic processes characterized by extensive loss of myelin and axons in anterolateral and posterior tracts (see Color Plate 13A) and by inflammatory reactions in the perivascular and leptomeningeal compartments (see Color Plate 14D).[81,82] The extent and severity of histopathologic features of HAM/TSP correlate with duration of the disease. Autopsies and biopsies performed in patients who died early during the course of disease (less than 3 years' duration) have shown mostly inflammatory reactions affecting the leptomeninges, perivascular spaces, white-matter tracts, and anterior horn of the spinal cord.[77,78,82,83] At this early stage, damage to the myelin sheaths and axonal injury appear to be prominent.[83] Infiltration by phagocytic and perivascular macrophages (see Color Plates 14B and 14C), many of them loaded with myelin debris, may be also observed.[76] Marked astroglial reaction is present in areas undergoing spinal cord inflammation (see Color Plate 14A). Similar histologic changes have also been described in regions other than the spinal cord, such as the white matter and gray nuclei of supratentorial and infratentorial structures.[76,82–85] During the intermediate stage of disease (4–9 years' duration), the most important feature is the degeneration of lateral and posterior white-matter tracts of the spinal cord with minimal inflammatory reaction.[81,85] In late or chronic stages of disease (more than 10 years' duration), marked degeneration of white-matter tracts and of the anterior horn of the spinal cord (with notable absence of inflammation) are the most prominent features.[81,86] Thickening and fibrosis of the adventitia of small blood vessels (see Color Plate 13B) in both the gray and white matter represent a common histologic change, particularly in cases in the intermediate to chronic stages of the disease.[76,81]

Multiple neuropathologic studies have shown that, despite the presence of extensive myelin loss in the spinal cord superficially resembling the changes seen in cases of multiple sclerosis, the classic features of demyelinating plaques were absent. In HAM/TSP, the infiltration by inflammatory cells and macrophages in the lateral tracts of the spinal cord appears to have a symmetric distribution in contrast to the patchy involvement typical of multiple sclerosis. The magnitude and symmetry of the anterior and posterior tract involvement are less conspicuous than the lateral tract involvement. Additionally, although the inflammatory foci are observed throughout the spinal cord, the lower thoracic segments appear to be affected the most.[9,81,82] The factors that contribute to the almost selective involvement of the thoracic cord in HAM/TSP remain unclear. In areas of the spinal cord affected by inflammation, an active process of axonal injury has been demonstrated by immunocytochemical studies that showed the intra-axonal accumulation of β-amyloid precursor protein.[87] This finding suggests that during early stages of disease, inflammatory factors likely contribute to defective axonal transport and subsequent neuronal dysfunction. This hypothesis is also supported by the observation of neuroaxonal dystrophy changes and intra-axonal accumulation of cytoskeletal proteins in intermediate or chronic stages of HAM/TSP.[88–90] In addition to the axonal injury present during early phases of inflammation, electron microscopy has shown an active process of demyelination and remyelination within myelinated axons of the lateral tracts of the spinal cord.[91,92] Thus, HAM/TSP is a disorder that exhibits both demyelination-remyelination processes and axonal injury as the main neuropathologic features.

Immunopathologic Features of Human T-Cell Lymphotropic Virus Type I–Associated Myelopathy/Tropical Spastic Paraparesis

Immunocytochemical characterization of the inflammatory reactions present in the spinal cord of HAM/TSP patients demonstrates the presence of a mixture of CD4[+] and CD8[+] lymphocytes.[93] Few perivascular B cells are seen in areas of inflammation. However, in the majority of inflammatory lesions, predominantly CD8[+] lymphocytes appear to be present.[83,85,90,94] Reactive astrogliosis, microglial activation, and macrophages are also prominent.[81,85,95] The presence of T-cell infiltration and monocyte-macrophage activation is directly correlated with the stage of activity of the spinal cord lesions. In early stages of disease or active-chronic inflammation, CD4[+] and CD8[+] lymphocytes appear to be equally present in areas of perivascular and parenchymal infiltration along with activated monocytes, macrophages, and microglia.[93,95]

In addition to the immunotypification of inflammatory reactions in the CNS of patients affected by HAM/TSP, other studies have examined the profile of cytokine expression in spinal cord lesions. A marked increase in the expression of TNF-α, IL-1β, and interferon gamma (IFN-γ) was found in immunocytochemical studies of spinal cords from patients with HAM/TSP. Macrophages, microglia, and perivascular astrocytes were found to express this particular set of cytokines in active-chronic lesions. Other cytokines, such as IFN-α, IFN-β, IL-6, and transforming growth factor beta were less common.[96] The presence of TNF-α, IL-1β, and IFN-γ appears to be correlated with duration of disease and suggests that an active process of immune reaction likely facilitates the perpetuation of inflammatory responses and activation of other immune mechanisms in lesion sites. Other immune mediators and soluble factors produced within areas of lesion have been documented in HAM/TSP. Macrophage and monocyte production of matrix metalloproteinases (MMPs), such as MMP-2 and MMP-9, has been shown in immunocytochemical studies complemented by zymography in CSF from patients with HAM/TSP.[97] These MMPs have important roles in the blood-brain barrier breakdown and remodeling of tissue after injury.

Human T-Cell Lymphotropic Virus Type I Expression in the Central Nervous System

Although the inflammatory and immunopathologic profile of HTLV-I infection is relatively well described, details regarding the presence of HTLV-I itself in the CNS are more elusive. The presence of HTLV-I infection within the CNS neuronal or neuroglial cell population has been explored by different morphologic and molecular techniques. HTLV-I–like particles were initially reported by Liberski et al.[88,89] in an electron microscopy study of autopsy tissue obtained from a Jamaican patient. The morphologic identification of the virus in these types of study is, however, difficult to interpret due to postmortem deterioration or suboptimal fixation. However, molecular biological analysis using polymerase chain reaction has demonstrated the presence of HTLV-I DNA in different segments of the spinal cord of patients affected by HAM/TSP.[67,68,70,71,98] Some of these studies found the highest concentration of HTLV-I proviral DNA within the thoracic spinal cord,[70] but the correlation with the magnitude of inflammatory infiltration has been contradictory. One study showed a lack of correlation between the magnitude of inflammatory infiltration and presence of HTLV-I proviral DNA.[71,99,100] In situ hybridization studies and in situ polymerase chain reaction techniques showed that perivascular lymphocytes within areas of spinal cord inflammation are the main group of cells harboring the HTLV-I genome.[69,71,72,74,98] Some studies showed that the CD4[+] T cell population in the perivascular infiltrates appears to be the main reservoir for the virus.[74,98,100] The potential infection of astrocytes has been suggested by one study.[72] The lack of the HTLV-I genome in microglia or macrophages as suggested by in situ hybridization studies[69,99] suggests that the reactions by these cells are driven by the activation of specific T-cell populations rather than primary or direct effect of infection of this particular cell population. Thus, the presence of CD8[+] lymphocytes, activated microglia, and macrophages in the absence of viral infection of neuronal populations suggests that immunologic reactions rather than direct viral neurocytopathic effects are part of the pathogenic mechanisms in HAM/TSP.

Pathogenic Mechanisms of Human T-Cell Lymphotropic Virus Type I Infection in the Central Nervous System

Different immunopathogenic mechanisms have been proposed to explain the role of HTLV-I in the development of HAM/TSP. These mechanisms are based on the concept that immunopathogenic reactions triggered by HTLV-I infection of T-lymphocytes lead to extensive damage to myelin and axons in the spinal cord. At least three different mechanistic hypotheses have been proposed. The first mechanism proposes that HTLV-I–specific CD8[+] cytotoxic T-lymphocytes (CTLs) target glial populations and induce glial lysis and secretion of cytokines.[101,102] This CTL response appear to be directed to the viral transactivator protein tax. This reaction would facilitate persistent inflammatory activation and destruction of myelin and axons at lesion sites. This hypothesis is supported by the demonstration of a high frequency of CTLs in peripheral blood and CSF, accumulation of CD8[+] T cells in areas of spinal cord lesions,[102–104] and the presence of HTLV-I tax mRNA in astrocytes.[72] A second mechanism invokes the development of autoimmunity by activation of autoreactive T-lymphocytes that migrate into the CNS and initiate immune responses that target CNS antigens.[105] The factors that facilitate the entry of infected lymphocytes into the CNS are unknown. Some studies showed evidence that HTLV-I–infected lymphocytes crossed the blood-brain barrier and that the presence of HTLV-I in the CSF was associated with clonal expansion of these infected lymphocytes.[106,107] In addition, other studies have shown an increase in the adhesion and permeability properties of HTLV-I–infected lymphocytes in an in vitro model of endothelial cell–lymphocyte interaction.[108] These autoreactive T-lymphocytes would induce the local production of proinflammatory cytokines that produce tissue damage. A third mechanism proposes that HTLV-I infected CD4[+] T cells penetrate into the CNS, where significant expression of viral antigen promotes immunologic responses, both cellular and humoral, and production of neurotoxic cytokines cause bystander neuroglial injury. The bystander hypothesis may be complementary also to the autoimmune or cytolytic hypotheses.

The production of cytokines, chemokines, and other soluble factors by lymphocytes, macrophages, activated microglia, and astroglia may also contribute to further CNS injury. The increased production of TNF-α and other soluble factors secreted by lymphocytes and macrophages in areas of spinal cord lesions has been well documented in HAM/TSP.[96,97] TNF-α modifies the metabolism of glutamate and can contribute to further neuronal and neuroglial injury.[109] In vitro experiments with human and rat astrocytes exposed to HTLV-I–infected lymphocytes resulted in significant reduction of glutamate uptake and downregulation of the glutamate transporters GLAST and GLT-1. This effect appeared to be modulated by the viral protein tax and mediated by TNF-α.[11,110] Other soluble factors, such as MMPs, may also contribute to the pathogenesis of HAM/TSP. MMP-2 and MMP-9 are found in areas of active lesion in macrophages, monocytes, and lymphocytes,[97] and in vitro studies showed that astrocytes exposed to HTLV-I–infected lymphocytes increased the production of MMP-3 and MMP-9 despite the expression of the tissue inhibitors of MMP-3 and MMP-9.[111] In lymphocytes, production of MMP-2 appears to be increased by vascular cell adhesion molecule-1, an adhesion molecule frequently present in areas of inflammation and leukocyte recruitment.[112] These finding are relevant to the pathogenesis of HAM/TSP because of the potential disruptive effect of the MMPs on the integrity of the blood-brain barrier and tissue damage.

Although it is clear that patients with HAM/TSP develop a strong and persistent class I–restricted CTL response to HTLV-I infection, there continues to be controversy over whether the role of CTLs is pathogenic or protective. Arguments that favor the potential role of CTLs in tissue damage[101] are counterbalanced by evidence that the persistent CTL response benefits the host by reducing the viral load.[103,113,114] In patients with HAM/TSP, virus-specific CTLs are positively correlated with the proviral loads in peripheral blood cells.[104,115,116] These patients have 10- to 100-fold greater proviral loads and a higher frequency of circulating CTLs in the peripheral blood than do asymptomatic HTLV-I carriers. The CTL response is specifically directed at the viral transactivator protein tax and eventually contributes to the reduction of viral load.[113,117]

Finally, in addition to the pathogenic factors determined by HTLV-I and immune responses, host genetic factors appear to play important roles in determining susceptibility to HAM/TSP. The presence of host genetic factors that favor the pathogenesis of HAM/TSP comes from studies demonstrating associations between various human leukocyte antigen (HLA) class I or class II alleles and the risk of HAM/TSP.[113,118,119] In Japanese patients, the most consistent association between HLA alleles and susceptibility to HAM/TSP has been found with the allele HLA-DRB1*0101. However, this pattern of susceptibility is found only in the absence of the protective effect of the *HLA-A*02* gene. The presence of HLA-A*02 subtypes facilitates the presentation of an immunodominant peptide from HTLV-I tax (tax_{11-19}) to CTLs and confers protection from HAM/TSP.[113,119]

Conclusions

The neuropathologic changes in HAM/TSP are determined by immunopathogenic mechanisms derived from a strong CTL response and the effects of multiple soluble factors such as TNF-α and MMPs produced by infiltrating inflammatory cells and neuroglia. The effect of these mechanisms results in an almost selective injury of the spinal cord that degenerates the white-matter tracts and other CNS structures.

Acknowledgments

Carlos A. Pardo is supported by the Passano Foundation. Suzanne Gartner receives support from the National Institutes of Health Grants NS-39800 and MH63039.

References

1. Bangham CR. HTLV-I infections. J Clin Pathol 2000; 53:581–586.
2. Manns A, Hisada M, La Grenade L. Human T-lymphotropic virus type I infection. Lancet 1999;353:1951–1958.
3. Uchiyama T. Human T cell leukemia virus type I (HTLV-I) and human diseases. Annu Rev Immunol 1997;15:15–37.
4. Höllsberg P, Hafler DA. Seminars in medicine of the Beth Israel Hospital, Boston. Pathogenesis of diseases induced by human lymphotropic virus type I infection. N Engl J Med 1993;328:1173–1182.
5. Rodgers-Johnson PE, Ono SG, Asher DM, Gibbs CJ Jr. Tropical spastic paraparesis and HTLV-I myelopathy: clinical features and pathogenesis. Res Publ Assoc Res Nerv Ment Dis 1990;68:117–130.
6. Rodgers-Johnson PE. Tropical spastic paraparesis/HTLV-I associated myelopathy. Etiology and clinical spectrum. Mol Neurobiol 1994;8:175–179.
7. Roman GC, Roman LN. Tropical spastic paraparesis. A clinical study of 50 patients from Tumaco (Colombia) and review of the worldwide features of the syndrome. J Neurol Sci 1988;87:121–138.
8. Vernant JC, Maurs L, Gout O, et al. HTLV-I-associated tropical spastic paraparesis in Martinique: a reappraisal. Ann Neurol 1988;23(Suppl):S133–S135.
9. Osame M, Nakagawa M, Umehara F, et al. Recent studies on the epidemiology, clinical features and pathogenic mechanisms of HTLV-I associated myelopathy (HAM/TSP) and other diseases associated to HTLV. J Neurovirol 1997; 3(Suppl 1):S50–S51.
10. Fujii M, Sassone-Corsi P, Verma IM. c-fos promoter transactivation by the tax1 protein of human T-cell leukemia virus type I. Proc Natl Acad Sci U S A 1988;85:8526–8530.
11. Szymocha R, Akaoka H, Brisson C, et al. Astrocytic alterations induced by HTLV type 1-infected T lymphocytes: a role for Tax-1 and tumor necrosis factor alpha. AIDS Res Hum Retroviruses 2000;16:1723–1729.
12. Izumo S, Umehara F, Osame M. HTLV-I-associated myelopathy. Neuropathology 2000;20(Suppl):S65–S68.
13. Izumo S, Umehara F, Kashio N, et al. Neuropathology of HTLV-I-associated myelopathy (HAM/TSP). Leukemia 1997;11(Suppl 3):82–84.
14. Morgan OS, Montgomery RD, Rodgers-Johnson P. The myeloneuropathies of Jamaica: an unfolding story. QJM 1988;67:273–281.
15. Arango C, Concha M, Zaninovic V, et al. Epidemiology of tropical spastic paraparesis in Columbia and associated HTLV-I infection. Ann Neurol 1988;23(Suppl):S161–S165.
16. Zaninovic V, Arango C, Biojo R, et al. Tropical spastic paraparesis in Colombia. Ann Neurol 1988;23(Suppl):S127–S132.
17. St Clair MO. The myeloneuropathies of Jamaica. Mol Neurobiol 1994;8:149–153.
18. Osame M, Usuku K, Izumo S, et al. HTLV-I associated myelopathy, a new clinical entity. Lancet 1986;1:1031–1032.
19. Gessain A, Francis H, Sonan T, et al. HTLV-I and tropical spastic paraparesis in Africa. Lancet 1986;2:698.
20. Murphy EL, Figueroa JP, Gibbs WN, et al. Human T-lymphotropic virus type I (HTLV-I) seroprevalence in Jamaica. I. Demographic determinants. Am J Epidemiol 1991;133:1114–1124.
21. Manns A, Blattner WA. The epidemiology of the human T-cell lymphotrophic virus type I and type II: etiologic role in human disease. Transfusion 1991;31:67–75.
22. Yamaguchi K. Human T-lymphotropic virus type I in Japan. Lancet 1994;343:213–216.
23. Edlich RF, Arnette JA, Williams FM. Global epidemic of human T-cell lymphotropic virus type-I (HTLV-I). J Emerg Med 2000;18:109–119.
24. Osame M, Janssen R, Kubota H, et al. Nationwide survey of HTLV-I-associated myelopathy in Japan: association with blood transfusion. Ann Neurol 1990;28:50–56.

25. Etoh K, Tamiya S, Yamaguchi K, et al. Persistent clonal proliferation of human T-lymphotropic virus type I-infected cells in vivo. Cancer Res 1997;57:4862–4867.

26. Poiesz BJ, Papsidero LD, Ehrlich G, et al. Prevalence of HTLV-I-associated T-cell lymphoma. Am J Hematol 2001;66:32–38.

27. Dosik H, Goldstein MF, Poiesz BJ, et al. Seroprevalence of human T-lymphotropic virus in blacks from a selected central Brooklyn population. Cancer Invest 1994;12:289–295.

28. Zucker-Franklin D, Pancake BA. Human T-cell lymphotropic virus type 1 tax among American blood donors. Clin Diagn Lab Immunol 1998;5:831–835.

29. Henrard DR, Soriano V, Robertson E, et al. Prevalence of human T-cell lymphotropic virus type 1 (HTLV-I) and HTLV-2 infection among Spanish drug users measured by HTLV-I assay and HTLV-1 and -2 assay. HTLV-I and HTLV-2 Spanish Study Group. J Clin Microbiol 1995; 33:1735–1738.

30. Marinucci G, Di Giacomo C, Dato A, et al. Seropositivity for HTLV-I among Italian prisoners. AIDS 1990;4:930–932.

31. Kramer A, Maloney EM, Morgan OS, et al. Risk factors and cofactors for human T-cell lymphotropic virus type I (HTLV-I)-associated myelopathy/tropical spastic paraparesis (HAM/TSP) in Jamaica. Am J Epidemiol 1995; 142:1212–1220.

32. Furnia A, Lal R, Maloney E, et al. Estimating the time of HTLV-I infection following mother-to-child transmission in a breast-feeding population in Jamaica. J Med Virol 1999;59:541–546.

33. Wilks R, Hanchard B, Morgan O, et al. Patterns of HTLV-I infection among family members of patients with adult T-cell leukemia/lymphoma and HTLV-I associated myelopathy/tropical spastic paraparesis. Int J Cancer 1996; 65:272–273.

34. Sadamori N, Ikeda S, Yamaguchi K, et al. Serum deoxythymidine kinase in adult T-cell leukemia-lymphoma and its related disorders. Leuk Res 1991;15:99–103.

35. Kusuhara K, Sonoda S, Takahashi K, et al. Mother-to-child transmission of human T-cell leukemia virus type I (HTLV-I): a fifteen-year follow-up study in Okinawa, Japan. Int J Cancer 1987;40:755–757.

36. Murphy EL, Figueroa JP, Gibbs WN, et al. Sexual transmission of human T-lymphotropic virus type I (HTLV-I). Ann Intern Med 1989;111:555–560.

37. Kaplan JE, Litchfield B, Rouault C, et al. HTLV-I-associated myelopathy associated with blood transfusion in the United States: epidemiologic and molecular evidence linking donor and recipient. Neurology 1991;41:192–197.

38. Manns A, Wilks RJ, Murphy EL, et al. A prospective study of transmission by transfusion of HTLV-I and risk factors associated with seroconversion. Int J Cancer 1992;51:886–891.

39. Daisley H, Charles WP, Swanston W. Role of HTLV-I co-infection in the AIDS epidemic in the Caribbean: a cause for concern. Int J STD AIDS 1999;10:487–489.

40. Daisley H, Charles WP. Fatal metastatic calcification in a patient with HTLV-I-associated lymphoma. West Indian Med J 1993;42:37–39.

41. Maloney EM, Cleghorn FR, Morgan OS, et al. Incidence of HTLV-I-associated myelopathy/tropical spastic para-paresis (HAM/TSP) in Jamaica and Trinidad. J Acquir Immune Defic Syndr Hum Retrovirol 1998;17:167–170.

42. Gout O, Baulac M, Gessain A, et al. Rapid development of myelopathy after HTLV-I infection acquired by transfusion during cardiac transplantation. N Engl J Med 1990;322:383–388.

43. Coffin J. Retroviridae: The Viruses and Their Replication. In B Fields, D Knip, P Howley, et al. (eds), Fields Virology. Philapdelphia: Lippincott–Raven Publishers, 1996; 1767–1847.

44. Poiesz BJ, Ruscetti FW, Gazdar AF, et al. Detection and isolation of type C retrovirus particles from fresh and cultured lymphocytes of a patient with cutaneous T-cell lymphoma. Proc Natl Acad Sci U S A 1980;77:7415–7419.

45. Nam SH, Kidokoro M, Shida H, Hatanaka M. Processing of gag precursor polyprotein of human T-cell leukemia virus type I by virus-encoded protease. J Virol 1988;62: 3718–3728.

46. Paine E, Garcia J, Philpott TC, et al. Limited sequence variation in human T-lymphotropic virus type 1 isolates from North American and African patients. Virology 1991;182:111–123.

47. Gessain A, Saal F, Morozov V, et al. Characterization of HTLV-I isolates and T lymphoid cell lines derived from French West Indian patients with tropical spastic para-paresis. Int J Cancer 1989;43:327–333.

48. Ciminale V, Pavlakis GN, Derse D, et al. Complex splicing in the human T-cell leukemia virus (HTLV) family of retroviruses: novel mRNAs and proteins produced by HTLV type I. J Virol 1992;66:1737–1745.

49. Nagashima K, Yoshida M, Seiki M. A single species of pX mRNA of human T-cell leukemia virus type I encodes trans-activator p40x and two other phosphoproteins. J Virol 1986;60:394–399.

50. Berneman ZN, Gartenhaus RB, Reitz MS, et al. Expression of alternatively spliced human T-lymphotropic virus type I pX mRNA in infected cell lines and in primary uncultured cells from patients with adult T-cell leukemia/ lymphoma and healthy carriers. Proc Natl Acad Sci U S A 1992;89:3005–3009.

51. Montagne J, Beraud C, Crenon I, et al. Tax1 induction of the HTLV-I 21 bp enhancer requires cooperation between two cellular DNA-binding proteins. EMBO J 1990;9:957–964.

52. Felber BK, Paskalis H, Kleinman-Ewing C, et al. The pX protein of HTLV-I is a transcriptional activator of its long terminal repeats. Science 1985;229:675–679.

53. Leung K, Nabel GJ. HTLV-I transactivator induces interleukin-2 receptor expression through an NF-kappa B-like factor. Nature 1988;333:776–778.

54. Kim SJ, Kehrl JH, Burton J, et al. Transactivation of the transforming growth factor beta 1 (TGF-beta 1) gene by human T lymphotropic virus type 1 tax: a potential mechanism for the increased production of TGF-beta 1 in adult T cell leukemia. J Exp Med 1990;172:121–129.

55. Yoshida M, Inoue J, Fujisawa J, Seiki M. Molecular mechanisms of regulation of HTLV-I gene expression and its association with leukemogenesis. Genome 1989;31: 662–667.

56. Hidaka M, Inoue J, Yoshida M, Seiki M. Post-transcriptional regulator (rex) of HTLV-I initiates expression of

viral structural proteins but suppresses expression of regulatory proteins. EMBO J 1988;7:519–523.

57. Unge T, Solomin L, Mellini M, et al. The Rex regulatory protein of human T-cell lymphotropic virus type I binds specifically to its target site within the viral RNA. Proc Natl Acad Sci U S A 1991;88:7145–7149.

58. Grassmann R, Berchtold S, Aepinus C, et al. In vitro binding of human T-cell leukemia virus rex proteins to the rex-response element of viral transcripts. J Virol 1991;65:3721–3727.

59. Yoshida M. Multiple viral strategies of HTLV-I for dysregulation of cell growth control. Annu Rev Immunol 2001;19:475–496.

60. Yao J, Wigdahl B. Human T cell lymphotropic virus type I genomic expression and impact on intracellular signaling pathways during neurodegenerative disease and leukemia. Front Biosci 2000;5:D138–D168.

61. Dhib-Jalbut S, Hoffman PM, Yamabe T, et al. Extracellular human T-cell lymphotropic virus type I Tax protein induces cytokine production in adult human microglial cells. Ann Neurol 1994;36:787–790.

62. Baba M, Imai T, Yoshida T, Yoshie O. Constitutive expression of various chemokine genes in human T-cell lines infected with human T-cell leukemia virus type 1: role of the viral transactivator Tax. Int J Cancer 1996;66:124–129.

63. Arai M, Ohashi T, Tsukahara T, et al. Human T-cell leukemia virus type 1 Tax protein induces the expression of lymphocyte chemoattractant SDF-1/PBSF. Virology 1998;241:298–303.

64. Seiki M, Eddy R, Shows TB, Yoshida M. Nonspecific integration of the HTLV provirus genome into adult T-cell leukaemia cells. Nature 1984;309:640–642.

65. Hirayama M, Miyadai T, Yokochi T, et al. Infection of human T-lymphotropic virus type I to astrocytes in vitro with induction of the class II major histocompatibility complex. Neurosci Lett 1988;92:34–39.

66. Koyanagi Y, Itoyama Y, Nakamura N, et al. In vivo infection of human T-cell leukemia virus type I in non-T cells. Virology 1993;196:25–33.

67. Namba Y, Oka S, Shimada K, et al. Post-mortem diagnosis of human T lymphotrophic virus type-1 (HTLV-I) associated myelopathy by detection of HTLV-I DNA in the spinal cord of a patient with post-transfusional myelopathy. Mol Cell Probes 1991;5:381–384.

68. Sueyoshi K, Goto M, Johnosono M, et al. Anatomical distribution of HTLV-I proviral sequence in an autopsy case of HTLV-I associated myelopathy: a polymerase chain reaction study. Pathol Int 1994;44:27–33.

69. Matsuoka E, Takenouchi N, Hashimoto K, et al. Perivascular T cells are infected with HTLV-I in the spinal cord lesions with HTLV-I-associated myelopathy/tropical spastic paraparesis: double staining of immunohistochemistry and polymerase chain reaction in situ hybridization. Acta Neuropathol (Berl) 1998;96:340–346.

70. Bhigjee AI, Wiley CA, Wachsman W, et al. HTLV-I-associated myelopathy: clinicopathologic correlation with localization of provirus to spinal cord. Neurology 1991;41:1990–1992.

71. Kira J, Itoyama Y, Koyanagi Y, et al. Presence of HTLV-I proviral DNA in central nervous system of patients with HTLV-I-associated myelopathy. Ann Neurol 1992;31:39–45.

72. Lehky TJ, Fox CH, Koenig S, et al. Detection of human T-lymphotropic virus type I (HTLV-I) tax RNA in the central nervous system of HTLV-I-associated myelopathy/tropical spastic paraparesis patients by in situ hybridization. Ann Neurol 1995;37:167–175.

73. McKendall RR, Oas J, Lairmore MD. HTLV-I-associated myelopathy endemic in Texas-born residents and isolation of virus from CSF cells. Neurology 1991;41:831–836.

74. Kuroda Y, Matsui M, Kikuchi M, et al. In situ demonstration of the HTLV-I genome in the spinal cord of a patient with HTLV-I-associated myelopathy. Neurology 1994;44:2295–2299.

75. Levin MC, Krichavsky M, Fox RJ, et al. Extensive latent retroviral infection in bone marrow of patients with HTLV-I-associated neurologic disease. Blood 1997;89:346–348.

76. Akizuki S, Setoguchi M, Nakazato O, et al. An autopsy case of human T-lymphotropic virus type I-associated myelopathy. Hum Pathol 1988;19:988–990.

77. Johnson RT, Griffin DE, Arregui A, et al. Spastic paraparesis and HTLV-I infection in Peru. Ann Neurol 1988;23(Suppl):S151–S155.

78. Piccardo P, Ceroni M, Rodgers-Johnson P, et al. Pathological and immunological observations on tropical spastic paraparesis in patients from Jamaica. Ann Neurol 1988;23(Suppl):S156–S160.

79. Robertson WB, Cruickshank EK. Jamaican (Tropical) Myeloneuropathy. In J Minkler (ed), Pathology of the Nervous System. New York: McGraw-Hill, 1972;2466–2476.

80. Montgomery RD, Cruickshank EK. Clinical and pathological observations on Jamaican neuropathy, a report on 206 cases. Brain 1964;87:425–462.

81. Iwasaki Y. Pathology of chronic myelopathy associated with HTLV-I infection (HAM/TSP). J Neurol Sci 1990;96:103–123.

82. Cartier LM, Cea JG, Vergara C, et al. Clinical and neuropathological study of six patients with spastic paraparesis associated with HTLV-I: an axomyelinic degeneration of the central nervous system. J Neuropathol Exp Neurol 1997;56:403–413.

83. Yoshioka A, Hirose G, Ueda Y, et al. Neuropathological studies of the spinal cord in early stage HTLV-I-associated myelopathy (HAM). J Neurol Neurosurg Psychiatry 1993;56:1004–1007.

84. Kuroda Y, Sugihara H. Autopsy report of HTLV-I-associated myelopathy presenting with ALS-like manifestations. J Neurol Sci 1991;106:199–205.

85. Aye MM, Matsuoka E, Moritoyo T, et al. Histopathological analysis of four autopsy cases of HTLV-I-associated myelopathy/tropical spastic paraparesis: inflammatory changes occur simultaneously in the entire central nervous system. Acta Neuropathol (Berl) 2000;100:245–252.

86. Sasaki S, Komori T, Maruyama S, et al. An autopsy case of human T lymphotropic virus type I-associated myelopathy (HAM) with a duration of 28 years. Acta Neuropathol (Berl) 1990;81:219–222.

87. Umehara F, Abe M, Koreeda Y, et al. Axonal damage revealed by accumulation of beta-amyloid precursor pro-

tein in HTLV-I-associated myelopathy. J Neurol Sci 2000;176:95–101.

88. Liberski PP, Rodgers-Johnson P, Char G, et al. HTLV-I-like viral particles in spinal cord cells in Jamaican tropical spastic paraparesis. Ann Neurol 1988;23(Suppl):S185–S187.

89. Liberski PP, Rodgers-Johnson P, Yanagihara R, et al. Ultrastructural pathology of human T-cell lymphotropic virus type I encephalomyelopathy in a white patient with adult T-cell leukemia/lymphoma. Ultrastruct Pathol 1994;18:511–518.

90. Wu E, Dickson DW, Jacobson S, Raine CS. Neuroaxonal dystrophy in HTLV-I-associated myelopathy/tropical spastic paraparesis: neuropathologic and neuroimmunologic correlations. Acta Neuropathol (Berl) 1993;86:224–235.

91. Ohama E, Horikawa Y, Shimizu T, et al. Demyelination and remyelination in spinal cord lesions of human lymphotropic virus type I-associated myelopathy. Acta Neuropathol (Berl) 1990;81:78–83.

92. Moore GR, Traugott U, Scheinberg LC, Raine CS. Tropical spastic paraparesis: a model of virus-induced, cytotoxic T-cell-mediated demyelination? Ann Neurol 1989;26:523–530.

93. Umehara F, Izumo S, Nakagawa M, et al. Immunocytochemical analysis of the cellular infiltrate in the spinal cord lesions in HTLV-I-associated myelopathy. J Neuropathol Exp Neurol 1993;52:424–430.

94. Levin MC, Lehky TJ, Flerlage AN, et al. Immunologic analysis of a spinal cord-biopsy specimen from a patient with human T-cell lymphotropic virus type I-associated neurologic disease. N Engl J Med 1997;336:839–845.

95. Abe M, Umehara F, Kubota R, et al. Activation of macrophages/microglia with the calcium-binding proteins MRP14 and MRP8 is related to the lesional activities in the spinal cord of HTLV-I associated myelopathy. J Neurol 1999; 246:358–364.

96. Umehara F, Izumo S, Ronquillo AT, et al. Cytokine expression in the spinal cord lesions in HTLV-I-associated myelopathy. J Neuropathol Exp Neurol 1994;53:72–77.

97. Umehara F, Okada Y, Fujimoto N, et al. Expression of matrix metalloproteinases and tissue inhibitors of metalloproteinases in HTLV-I-associated myelopathy. J Neuropathol Exp Neurol 1998;57:839–849.

98. Hara H, Morita M, Iwaki T, et al. Detection of human T lymphotrophic virus type I (HTLV-I) proviral DNA and analysis of T cell receptor V beta CDR3 sequences in spinal cord lesions of HTLV-I-associated myelopathy/tropical spastic paraparesis. J Exp Med 1994;180:831–839.

99. Moritoyo T, Reinhart TA, Moritoyo H, et al. Human T-lymphotropic virus type I-associated myelopathy and tax gene expression in CD4+ T lymphocytes. Ann Neurol 1996;40:84–90.

100. Kubota R, Umehara F, Izumo S, et al. HTLV-I proviral DNA amount correlates with infiltrating CD4+ lymphocytes in the spinal cord from patients with HTLV-I-associated myelopathy. J Neuroimmunol 1994;53:23–29.

101. Jacobson S, Shida H, McFarlin DE, et al. Circulating CD8+ cytotoxic T lymphocytes specific for HTLV-I pX in patients with HTLV-I associated neurological disease. Nature 1990;348:245–248.

102. Greten TF, Slansky JE, Kubota R, et al. Direct visualiza-

tion of antigen-specific T cells: HTLV-I Tax11-19-specific CD8(+) T cells are activated in peripheral blood and accumulate in cerebrospinal fluid from HAM/TSP patients. Proc Natl Acad Sci U S A 1998;95:7568–7573.

103. Elovaara I, Koenig S, Brewah AY, et al. High human T cell lymphotropic virus type 1 (HTLV-I)-specific precursor cytotoxic T lymphocyte frequencies in patients with HTLV-I-associated neurological disease. J Exp Med 1993;177:1567–1573.

104. Kubota R, Nagai M, Kawanishi T, et al. Increased HTLV type 1 tax specific CD8+ cells in HTLV type 1-aociated myelopathy/tropical spastic paraparesis: correlation with HTLV type 1 proviral load. AIDS Res Hum Retroviruses 2000;16:1705–1709.

105. Hollsberg P, Hafler DA. What is the pathogenesis of human T-cell lymphotropic virus type I-associated myelopathy/tropical spastic paraparesis? Ann Neurol 1995;37:143–145.

106. Cavrois M, Gessain A, Gout O, et al. Common human T cell leukemia virus type 1 (HTLV-I) integration sites in cerebrospinal fluid and blood lymphocytes of patients with HTLV-I-associated myelopathy/tropical spastic paraparesis indicate that HTLV-I crosses the blood-brain barrier via clonal HTLV-I-infected cells. J Infect Dis 2000; 182:1044–1050.

107. Cavrois M, Leclercq I, Gout O, et al. Persistent oligoclonal expansion of human T-cell leukemia virus type 1-infected circulating cells in patients with Tropical spastic paraparesis/HTLV-I associated myelopathy. Oncogene 1998;17:77–82.

108. Romero IA, Prevost MC, Perret E, et al. Interactions between brain endothelial cells and human T-cell leukemia virus type 1-infected lymphocytes: mechanisms of viral entry into the central nervous system. J Virol 2000;74:6021–6030.

109. Fine SM, Angel RA, Perry SW, et al. Tumor necrosis factor alpha inhibits glutamate uptake by primary human astrocytes. Implications for pathogenesis of HIV-1 dementia. J Biol Chem 1996;271:15303–15306.

110. Szymocha R, Akaoka H, Dutuit M, et al. Human T-cell lymphotropic virus type 1-infected T lymphocytes impair catabolism and uptake of glutamate by astrocytes via Tax-1 and tumor necrosis factor alpha. J Virol 2000;74:6433–6441.

111. Giraudon P, Szymocha R, Buart S, et al. T lymphocytes activated by persistent viral infection differentially modify the expression of metalloproteinases and their endogenous inhibitors, TIMPs, in human astrocytes: relevance to HTLV-I-induced neurological disease. J Immunol 2000; 164:2718–2727.

112. Kambara C, Nakamura T, Furuya T, et al. Vascular cell adhesion molecule-1-mediated matrix metalloproteinase-2 induction in peripheral blood T cells is up-regulated in patients with HTLV-I-associated myelopathy. J Neuroimmunol 1999;99:242–247.

113. Bangham CR, Hall SE, Jeffery KJ, et al. Genetic control and dynamics of the cellular immune response to the human T-cell leukaemia virus, HTLV-I. Philos Trans R Soc Lond B Biol Sci 1999;354:691–700.

114. Daenke S, Kermode AG, Hall SE, et al. High activated and

memory cytotoxic T-cell responses to HTLV-I in healthy carriers and patients with tropical spastic paraparesis. Virology 1996;217:139–146.

115. Nagai M, Kubota R, Greten TF, et al. Increased activated human T cell lymphotropic virus type I (HTLV-I) Tax11-19-specific memory and effector CD8+ cells in patients with HTLV-I-associated myelopathy/tropical spastic paraparesis: correlation with HTLV-I provirus load. J Infect Dis 2001;183:197–205.

116. Nagai M, Usuku K, Matsumoto W, et al. Analysis of HTLV-I proviral load in 202 HAM/TSP patients and 243 asymptomatic HTLV-I carriers: high proviral load strongly predisposes to HAM/TSP. J Neurovirol 1998;4:586–593.

117. Bieganowska K, Hollsberg P, Buckle GJ, et al. Direct analysis of viral-specific CD8+ T cells with soluble HLA-A2/Tax11-19 tetramer complexes in patients with human T cell lymphotropic virus-associated myelopathy. J Immunol 1999;162:1765–1771.

118. Usuku K, Nishizawa M, Matsuki K, et al. Association of a particular amino acid sequence of the HLA-DR beta 1 chain with HTLV-I-associated myelopathy. Eur J Immunol 1990;20:1603–1606.

119. Jeffery KJ, Usuku K, Hall SE, et al. HLA alleles determine human T-lymphotropic virus-I (HTLV-I) proviral load and the risk of HTLV-I-associated myelopathy. Proc Natl Acad Sci U S A 1999;96:3848–3853.

Chapter 13

Neuroepidemiology of Human T-Cell Lymphotropic Virus Type I–Associated Myelopathy/Tropical Spastic Paraparesis

Gustavo C. Román

History

In 1904, Vallée and Carré[1] demonstrated that equine infectious anemia could be transmitted by injecting filtered serum from anemic horses into healthy animals. The etiologic agent—equine infectious anemia virus, a retrovirus of the lentivirus family—is the first known example of a retroviral infection with dual hematologic and neurologic involvement. Maedi-visna, the prototypic lentivirus, is the cause of a pulmonary disease of sheep called *maedi,* and it also causes visna, a demyelinating inflammatory encephalopathy.[2] In 1973, Gardner and colleagues[3] discovered in wild mice *(Mus musculus)* in the vicinity of Lake Casitas in California a strain of murine leukemia virus with lymphotropic and neurotropic manifestations. The Casitas strain of murine leukemia virus is exogenously acquired early in life via maternal milk; it discloses geographic and familial clustering, and infected aging mice develop either lymphoma or a progressive paralysis of the hind limbs. A dozen years later, an equivalent human retroviral disease was finally recognized.

Beginning in the 1930s, high-prevalence clusters of spastic paraplegia of unknown etiology were described in the Congo,[4,5] in south India[6,7] (where it was called *tropical spastic paraplegia),*[8] in South Africa,[9,10] in Jamaica,[11–14] and in the Seychelles Islands.[15] In 1981, Zaninovic and colleagues[16] described the first cluster of spastic paraplegia in South America in the island of Tumaco in the Pacific lowlands of Colombia; Román et al.[17–19] called this condition *tropical spastic paraparesis* or TSP. Excluding chronic cyanide intoxication from consumption of cassava (*Manihot esculenta* Crantz) in Africa[20] and neurotoxicity from *Lathyrus sativus* in India,[20] no cause for TSP had been found until 1985, when the association with human T-cell lymphotropic virus type I (HTLV-I), the first human retrovirus, was first reported in Martinique.[21–23] This etiology was promptly confirmed in patients from Jamaica and Colombia,[24] the Seychelles Islands,[25] and Japan.[26] Because Japanese patients were living in nontropical regions, the name *HTLV-I–associated myelopathy* (HAM) was coined for this condition, but the identity of HAM and HTLV-I–associated TSP was rapidly concluded.[27] Neuroepidemiologic studies of TSP by Román et al.[17–19,25] in widely separated populations—Tumaco, Colombia and Mahé, Seychelles—demonstrated that despite geographic distances, TSP presents around the world with common epidemiologic and clinical features.[28]

Clinically similar cases of chronic myelopathy associated with HTLV-II infection have been rarely reported.[29,30] Currently, chronic HTLV-I myelopathy is the most common form of nontraumatic spastic paraparesis and paraplegia in several parts of the world (Table 13-1).

Table 13-1. Geographic Clusters of Human T-Cell Lymphotropic Virus Type I Infection

Region	Locale
Japan	Okinawa, Kyushu, Shikoku
Caribbean region	All the islands except Cuba
South America	Colombia, Ecuador, Peru, Brazil, Chile, French Guyana
Africa	West and Central Africa, South Africa, Seychelles Islands
Middle East	Iran (Mashad region)
Melanesia	—

Human T-Lymphotropic Virus Types I and II

The human retroviruses (family Retroviridae) constitute a group of type-C RNA viruses characterized by the presence in the viral genome of reverse transcriptase, a protein that initiates the translation of viral RNA into DNA after invading host cells. The first human retrovirus to be identified was HTLV-I, isolated from patients with cutaneous T-cell lymphoma[31] and adult T-cell leukemia[32,33]; this was followed by HTLV-II in a T-cell variant of hairy-cell leukemia[34] and finally by the identification of the causative agent of the acquired immune deficiency syndrome, the human immunodeficiency virus (HIV) initially called *HTLV-III*.[35,36] Animal and human retroviruses are currently classified in three subfamilies: Oncovirinae or oncogenic retroviruses (formerly called *animal RNA tumor viruses*); Lentivirinae or "slow viruses" (including visna-maedi and HIV); and Spumavirinae or foamy viruses.[37]

Human T-Cell Lymphotropic Virus Type I (Subfamily Oncovirinae)

HTLV-I is considered the etiologic agent of both adult T-cell leukemia-lymphoma (ATLL) and HAM.[38] ATLL is a malignant form of leukemia with geographic clustering in the southeastern islands of Kyushu and Shikoku in Japan and in the Caribbean. ATLL is characterized by late age of onset, with a median age of 52 years, proliferation of T-lymphocytes with typical segmentation of the nucleus ("flower" lymphocytes; see Color Plate

12), lymphadenopathy, hepatomegaly and splenomegaly, infiltrating skin lesions (Sézary syndrome or mycosis fungoides), hypercalcemia, lytic bone lesions, and immunosuppression. ATLL has been classified into five types: acute, chronic, smoldering, crisis, and lymphoma; it usually follows an aggressive course with a mean survival of 10 months.

As mentioned earlier, HTLV-I causes a chronic myelitis currently denominated HAM in Japan[39] and HTLV-I–associated TSP elsewhere.[40] HTLV-I myelitis is prevalent in southwestern Japan, Africa, the Seychelles islands, South America, the Caribbean islands,[41–45] Papua New Guinea, and Australia (see Table 13-1). HTLV-I myelitis predominates in women, with onset after age 40 years; it is found mainly in blacks and the Japanese, but other racial groups are affected, such as Chileans in South America,[44] the Inuit from Alaska and Greenland, northern Amerindians from British Columbia,[46,47] and Iranian-born Mashhadi Jews.[48]

HTLV-I myelitis presents as a chronic and slowly progressive spastic paraparesis with back pain, spastic bladder, and minimal sensory symptoms.[49] Pyramidal signs, including bilaterally symmetric lower limb brisk reflexes, crossed adductor responses, ankle clonus, and Babinski's sign, are present, along with a mild decrease of vibratory perception in the toes and feet. Spasticity is moderate and predominates in thigh adductors and, to a lesser extent, on the extensors of the thighs and on gastrocnemius muscles. Leg weakness affects proximal muscle groups, mainly glutei and iliopsoas, resulting in a typical slow scissoring gait, with dragging and shuffling of the feet. The severe spasticity of lathyrism with lurching gait is not seen. Severe, usually rapidly progressive cases of HTLV-I myelitis may result in complete paraplegia.[50]

Human T-Cell Lymphotropic Virus Type II

HTLV-II infection has been reported in association with rare cases of hairy-cell leukemia and large-cell lymphoma and in a few instances of chronic myelopathy resembling either TSP[30] or tropical ataxic neuropathy.[51] A familial form of olivopontocerebellar atrophy has been associated with HTLV-II infection in Amerindians from New Mexico.[52] Recently, spinocerebellar involvement in patients with HTLV-I and II infections, a syndrome first noticed by Kira et al.,[53] has been reported.[54,55] HTLV-II is endemic in Amerindian tribes,[56] in isolated populations in Mongolia and North Africa, and in intravenous drug users in Europe and the United States.

Transmission of Human T-Cell Lymphotropic Virus Types I and II

HTLV-I and -II transmission is cell-mediated, involving mainly CD4 lymphocytes. In closed communities, such as those inhabiting islands, the virus is transmitted mainly through breast-feeding and sexual contact.[57] This may also explain the preponderance of TSP in geographically and culturally isolated populations with a high index of consanguinity, such as Amerindian tribes.[40]

Breast-Feeding

It is generally assumed that in endemic areas of Japan, most patients with HTLV-I infection have been infected during the newborn period via breast-feeding, as placental transmission appears to be exceptional. Cell-rich colostrum from infected mothers transmits the infection with 15–25% efficiency. Approximately 22% of children from ages 3 to 10 years who had been breast-fed by HTLV-I–positive mothers seroconverted to HTLV-I[58]; in Martinique, this percentage increased to 33% when polymerase chain reaction was used to detect children who were seronegative carriers of the virus.[59] Measures to prevent breast-feeding during the first trimester of life are effective in decreasing seroconversion of offspring.[60]

Sexual Contact

HTLV-I is present in semen and cervical secretions of infected subjects, but horizontal transmission occurs more effectively from infected male to female. In population studies in Japan, Tajima et al.[61] found that after 10 years of marital life, 60% of women were infected when the husband was HTLV-I positive, but when the wife was HTLV-I positive, only 0.1–1.0% of the men were positive. In some populations with de facto polygamy (such as those in Seychelles and Tumaco, Colombia), one infected man will infect women in several households; this may explain, in part, the preponderance of seropositive women in endemic populations.

Also, in Latin America, the Caribbean, and probably in Africa, HTLV-I should be considered a sexually transmitted disease. Infection occurs in female sex workers and in homosexual men, often associated with syphilis, herpes simplex virus type 2, genital ulcers, and other sexually transmitted diseases.[62,63] Other risk factors include number of sexual partners, promiscuity, and length of time in prostitution.[63,64] Sexual transmission can be reduced by condom use. Dual infection with HIV and HTLV-I is not uncommon among subjects with high-risk sexual behaviors.[65,66]

Blood Transfusion

Seroconversion after blood transfusion with HTLV-I–infected blood occurs in 48–82% of recipients. In contrast with HIV, cell-free cryoprecipitates and fresh frozen plasma have not been associated with HTLV-I transmission.[67,68] Approximately 20% of patients with HAM in Japan and 15–40% of patients in Latin America have a history of previous blood transfusion, with a short incubation period of 2.5 years in Japan and 6 months to 8 years in Martinique.[69] According to Osame et al.,[70] after compulsory testing of all blood for transfusion in Japan,[9] the incident number of cases of HAM dropped substantially. Acute myelitis developing after transfusion of blood infected with HTLV-I during cardiac transplantation has been demonstrated.[50]

Intravenous Drug Abuse

HTLV-II is more prevalent than HTLV-I among needle-sharing intravenous drug users in the United States and Europe and is often associated with HIV infection.[71–73] The likelihood of developing HTLV-I myelopathy is extremely high in countries with high seropositivity rates in blood banks,[69] such as those observed in Kagoshima, Japan (8%); Martinique, French West Indies (4%); and Trinidad and Tobago (1.6%). In the United States, France,

Table 13-2. Geographic Genotypes of Human T-Cell Lymphotropic Virus Type I Based on Molecular Epidemiology

Type	Geographic Locale
Cosmopolitan	Patients with adult T-cell leukemia and HAM/TSP and healthy carriers in West African countries (Mauritania, Guinea-Bissau, Ivory Coast), South Africa (West African subtype), the Americas, the Caribbean, Iran, and Japan (Japanese subtype)
Central African	Zaire, Gabon, Cameroon, and Central African Republic
Australo-Melanesian*	Papua New Guinea, Solomon Islands, and Australia[86,87]

HAM/TSP = human T-cell lymphotropic virus type I–associated myelopathy/tropical spastic paraparesis.
*This last HTLV-I genotype is the most distant one from the Cosmopolitan prototype.
Source: Adapted from A Gessain, G de Thé. Geographic and molecular epidemiology of primate lymphotropic retroviruses: HTLV-I, HTLV-II, STLV-I, STLV-PP, and PTLV-L. Adv Virus Res 1996;47:377–426.

and the United Kingdom, rates are low, ranging from 0.005% to 0.0046%.[69] In Latin America, blood bank seropositivity for HTLV-I ranges from 0.32% in Buenos Aires, Argentina to 0.15% in Sao Paulo, Brazil.[43] Population studies of HTLV-I seroprevalence in Japan and the Caribbean have shown that seropositivity increases with age, female gender, low socioeconomic status, and history of multiple blood transfusions.[74]

Molecular Epidemiology of Human T-Cell Lymphotropic Virus Type I

Seiki et al.[75] first published the complete nucleotide sequence of the provirus genome of HTLV-I isolated from a Japanese patient with adult T-cell leukemia. Numerous other isolates have been sequenced, including viruses obtained from patients with HAM/TSP[76] and from asymptomatic carriers

(reviewed in reference 77). The study of the molecular epidemiology of HTLV-I has been possible by the development of polymerase chain reaction and other molecular biology techniques, such as restriction fragment length polymorphism of amplified polymerase chain reaction fragments. Several subtypes of HTLV-I were identified by sequence analyses of several viral gene fragments, including the *env* gene fragment coding for the transmembrane protein gp 21, the noncoding long-terminal repeat region, and portions of the *pol* gene.

The cosmopolitan, central African, and Australo-Melanesian geographic genotypes of HTLV-I have been recognized (Table 13-2). Despite the variation of the HTLV-I genotypes and subtypes, no specific mutations have been found to explain the preponderant development of either hematopoietic malignancies or neurotropic involvement.[28]

According to Yanagihara et al.,[78] the origin of HTLV-I infection in human groups may be traced to a probable early infection with an African or Indonesian simian T-lymphotropic virus type I. The dissemination of these early human retroviruses to Amerindian populations along the American continent probably occurred from primitive Ahinu populations in Okkaido that migrated through the Bering Strait. HTLV-I infection has been documented in the Inuit from Alaska and Greenland, in northern Amerindians from British Columbia,[46,47] and in a number of native American tribes (reviewed in reference 43). Of interest, HTLV-II has been demonstrated to be endemic also among several Amerindian tribes (reviewed in reference 43), including the Guaymi in Panama.[79] the Seminoles in Florida,[80] the Navajo and Pueblo in New Mexico,[52] the Wayu in northern Colombia,[81] and the Kraho Indians[82]; we have also shown HTLV-II infection among other tribes of Amazonian Indians in the eastern Amazon basin in the state of Para, Brazil.[56]

The black slave trade from Africa (fifteenth to nineteenth centuries) explains the presence of endemic infection with high seroprevalence rates found among the black and mixed-blood populations in the Caribbean basin, Brazil, Tumaco (Colombia), Esmeraldas (Ecuador), Peru, Panama, and North America.[43] Small foci linked to Japanese migration can be found in Brazil,[83] Bolivia,[84] and Hawaii.[85] The Australo-Melanesian is the most distant of the HTLV-I strains.[86,87]

Public Health Measures for Human T-Cell Lymphotropic Virus Types I and II

Public health programs for the control of HTLV-I and II infection in endemic populations should be undertaken to prevent the high morbidity and mortality associated with ATLL and HAM/TSP. It should be noted that even in highly endemic populations, large variations in seroprevalence are found from one village to the next or among closely related population groups. This should not be taken as a reason to discontinue universal testing of all blood donations in blood banks from endemic areas. Control programs require several measures: (1) prenatal control of pregnant women to discourage breast-feeding among women positive for HTLV-I and -II, (2) blood bank screening of all donors, (3) clean-needle programs for intravenous drug users, and (4) safe-sex programs to encourage condom use. All these measures should be implemented along with HIV control programs.

References

1. Vallée M, Carré M. Sur la nature infectieuse de l'anémie du cheval. CR Acad Sci (Paris) 1904;139:331–333.
2. Pétursson G, Pálsson PA, Georgsson G. Maedi-visna in sheep. Host-virus intreractions and utilization as a model. Intervirology 1989;30(Suppl):36–44.
3. Gardner MB, Henderson BE, Officer JE, et al. A spontaneous motor neuron disease apparently caused by indigenous type-C virus in wild mice. J Natl Cancer Inst 1973; 51:1243–1249.
4. Trolli G. Paraplègie spastique épidemique. Konzo, Brussels: Fonds Reine Elisabeth pour l'Assistance Médicale aux Indigènes du Conge Belge, 1938. Trop Dis Bull 1939;36:501–502(abst).
5. Lucasse C. Le Kitondji: une paralysie spastique. Ann Soc Belge Med Trop 1952;32:391–394.
6. Minchin RLH. Primary lateral sclerosis of South India: lathyrism without lathyrus. BMJ 1940;1:253–255.
7. Gopalan C. The lathyrism syndrome. Trans R Soc Trop Med Hyg 1950;44:333–338.
8. Mani KS, Mani AJ, Montgomery RD. A spastic paraplegic syndrome in South India. J Neurol Sci 1969;9:179–199.
9. Cosnett JE. Unexplained spastic myelopathy: 41 cases in a non-European hospital. South Afr Med J 1965;39:592–595.
10. Wallace ID, Cosnett JE. Unexplained spastic paraplegia. South Afr Med J 1983;63:689–691.
11. Cruickshank EK. A neuropathic syndrome of uncertain origin. West Indian Med J 1956;5:147–158.
12. Cruickshank EK, Montgomery RD, Spillane JD. Obscure neurologic disorders in Jamaica. World Neurol 1961;2: 199–211.
13. Montgomery RD, Cruickshank EK, Robertson WB, McMenemey WH. Clinical and pathological observations on Jamaican neuropathy: a report on 206 cases. Brain 1964;87:425–462.
14. Rodgers PEB. The clinical features and aetiology of the neuropathic syndrome in Jamaica. West Indian Med J 1965;14:36–47.
15. Kelly R, De Mol B. Paraplegia in the islands of the Indian Ocean. Afr J Neurol Sci 1982;1:5–7.
16. Zaninovic V, Biojó R, Barreto P. Paraparesia espástica del Pacífico. Colombia Méd 1981;17:361–365.
17. Román GC, Román LN, Spencer PS, Schoenberg BS. An outbreak of spastic paraparesis along the southern Pacific coast of Colombia: Clinical and epidemiological features. Ann Neurol 1983;14:152A.
18. Román GC, Román LN, Schoenberg BS, Spencer PS. Tropical spastic paraparesis. A neuroepidemiological study in Colombia. Ann Neurol 1985;17:361–365.
19. Román GC, Román LN. Tropical spastic paraparesis. A clinical study of 50 patients from Tumaco (Colombia) and review of the worldwide features of the syndrome. J Neurol Sci 1988;87:121–138.
20. Román GC, Spencer PS, Schoenberg BS. Tropical myelo-neuropathies: the hidden endemias. Neurology 1985;35: 1158–1170.
21. Gessain A, Barin F, Vernant JC, et al. Antibodies to human T-lymphotropic virus type 1 in patients with tropical spastic paraparesis. Lancet 1985;2:407–409.
22. Vernant J-C, Gessain A, Gout O, et al. Paraparésies spastiques tropicales en Martinique: Haute prévalence d'anticorps HTLV-1. Presse Med 1986;15:419–422.
23. Vernant J-C, Maurs L, Gessain A, et al. Endemic tropical spastic paraparesis associated with HTLV-I: a clinical and seroepidemiological study of 25 cases. Ann Neurol 1987; 21:123–130.
24. Rodgers-Johnson P, Gajdusek DC, Morgan OSC, et al. HTLV-I and HTLV-III antibodies and tropical spastic paraparesis. Lancet 1985;2:1247–1248.
25. Román GC, Schoenberg BS, Madden DL, et al. Human T-lymphotropic virus I antibodies in the serum of patients with tropical spastic paraparesis in the Seychelles. Arch Neurol 1987;44:605–607.
26. Osame M, Usuku K, Izumo S, et al. HTLV-I-associated myelopathy, a new clinical entity. Lancet 1986;2:104–105.
27. Román GC, Osame M. Identity of HTLV-I-associated tropical spastic paraparesis and HTLV-I-associated myelopathy. Lancet 1988;1:651.
28. Román GC, Román LN, Osame M. Human T lymphotropic virus type I neurotropism. Prog Med Virol 1990;37:190–210.
29. Kira JL, Koyanagi Y, Hamakado T. HTLV-II in patients with HTLV-I-associated myelopathy. Lancet 1991;338:64–65.
30. Jacobson S, Lehky T, Nishimura M, et al. Isolation of HTLV-II from a patient with chronic progressive neurological disease clinically indistinguishable from HTLV-I-associated myelopathy/tropical spastic paraparesis. Ann Neurol 1993;33:392–396.
31. Poiesz BJ, Ruscetti FW, Gadzar AF, et al. Detection and isolation of type C retrovirus particles from fresh and cultured lymphocytes of a patient with cutaneous T-cell lymphoma. Proc Natl Acad Sci U S A 1980;77:7415–7419.

32. Miyoshi I, Kubonishi I, Yoshimoto S, et al. Detection of type C virus particles in a cord T-cell line derived by cocultivation of normal human cord leukocytes and human leukemic T-cells. Nature 1981;294:770–771.

33. Yoshida M, Miyoshi I, Hinuma Y. Isolation and characterization of human adult T-cell leukemia virus and its implication in the disease. Proc Natl Acad Sci U S A 1982;79: 2031–2035.

34. Kalyanaraman V, Sarngadharan M, Robert-Guroff M, et al. A new subtype of human T-cell leukemia virus (HTLV-II) associated with a T-cell variant of hairy cell leukemia. Science 1982;218:571–573.

35. Barré-Sinoussi F, Chermann C, Rey F, et al. Isolation of a T-lymphotropic retrovirus from a patient at risk for acquired immune deficiency syndrome (AIDS). Science 1983;220:868–871.

36. Gallo RC, Salahuddin SZ, Popovic M, et al. Frequent detection and isolation of cytopathic retroviruses (HTLV-III) from patients with AIDS and at risk for AIDS. Science 1984;224:500–503.

37. Román GC. Retrovirus associated myelopathies. Arch Neurol 1987;44:659–663.

38. Román GC. The Enlarging Spectrum of HTLV-I Infection: an Epidemiological and Public Health Perspective. In GC Román, J-C Vernant, M Osame (eds), HTLV-I and the Nervous System. New York: Alan R. Liss, 1989;485–487.

39. Osame M, Igata A, Matsumoto M. HTLV-I-Associated Myelopathy (HAM) Revisited. In GC Román, J-C Vernant, M Osame (eds), HTLV-I and the Nervous System. New York: Alan R. Liss, 1989;213–223.

40. Román GC. The neuroepidemiology of tropical spastic paraparesis. Ann Neurol 1988;23(Suppl):S113–S130.

41. Arango C, Concha M, Zaninovic V, et al. Epidemiology of tropical spastic paraparesis in Colombia and associated HTLV-I infections. Ann Neurol 1988;238:161–165.

42. Gotuzzo E, De las Casas C, Deza L, et al. Tropical spastic paraparesis and HTLV-I infection: Clinical and epidemiological study in Lima, Peru. J Neurol Sci 1996;143:114–117.

43. Gotuzzo E, Arango C, Araujo de Queiroz-Campos A, et al. Human T-cell lymphotropic virus-I in Latin America. Infect Dis Clin N Am 2000;14:211–239.

44. Cartier L, Araya F, Castillo JL, et al. Progressive spastic paraparesis associated with human T-cell leukemia virus type I (HTLV-I). Intern Med 1992;31:1257–1261.

45. Vernant J-C. HTLV-I. In RA Shakir, PK Newman, CM Poser (eds), Tropical Neurology. London: Saunders, 1996; 19–35.

46. Oger J, Werker D, Foti D, Dekaban G. HTLV-I-associated myelopathy: an endemic disease of Canadian aboriginals of the North-West Pacific coast. Canadian J Neurol Sci 1993;20:302–306.

47. Debakan GA, Ward R, Waters, et al. Low level endemic infection of HTLV-I and HTLV-II in an Amerindian tribe of Vancouver Island, British Columbia, Canada (abst). J Acquir Immune Defic Syndr Hum Retrovirol 1995;10:216.

48. Achiron A, Pinhas-Hamiel O, Doll L, et al. Spastic paraparesis associated with HTLV-I: a clinical, serological and genomic study of Iranian-born Mashhadi Jews. Ann Neurol 1993;34:670–675.

49. Vernant J-C, Román GC. Les paraplégies associées au virus HTLV-1. Rev Neurol (Paris) 1989;145:260–266.

50. Gout O, Baulac M, Gessain A, et al. Rapid development of myelopathy after HTLV-I infection acquired by transfusion during cardiac transplantation. N Engl J Med 1990;322:383–388.

51. Harrington WJ Jr., Sheremata W, Hjelle B, et al. Spastic ataxia associated with human T-cell lymphotropic virus type II infection. Ann Neurol 1993;33:411–414.

52. Hjelle B, Appenzeller O, Mills R. Chronic neurodegenerative disease associated with HTLV-II infection. Lancet 1992;339:645–646.

53. Kira J, Goto I, Otsuka M, et al. Chronic progressive spinocerebellar syndrome associated with antibodies to human T-lymphotropic virus type I: Clinico-virological and magnetic resonance imaging studies. J Neurol Sci 1993;115:111–115.

54. Castillo LC, Gracia F, Román GC, et al. Spinocerebellar syndrome in patients infected with Human T-Lymphotropic virus types I and II (HTLV-I/HTLV-II): Report of 3 cases from Panama. Acta Neurol Scand 2000;101:405–412.

55. Carod-Artal FJ, Melo M, Pereira R, et al. Formas subagudas de infección por el virus HTLV-I potencialmente tratables. Rev Neurol (Barcelona) 2000;31:32–35.

56. Gabbai AA, Bordin JO, Vieira-filho PB, et al. Selectivity of human T-lymphotropic virus type-1 (HTLV-1) and HTLV-2 infection among different populations in Brazil. Am J Trop Med Hyg 1993;49:664–671.

57. Nakano S, Ando Y, Ichijo M, et al. Search for possible routes of vertical and horizontal transmission of adult T-cell leukemia virus. Jap J Cancer Res (Gann) 1984;75: 1044–1045.

58. Hino S, Doi H. Mechanisms of HTLV-I Transmission. In G Román, J-C Vernant, M Osame (eds), HTLV-I and the Nervous System. New York: Alan R Liss, 1989;459–501.

59. Monplaisir N, Neisson-Vernant C, Bouillot M, et al. HTLV-I maternal transmission in Martinique, using serology and polymerase chain reaction. AIDS Research Human Retroviruses 1993;9:869–874.

60. Ando Y, Nakano S, Saito K, et al. Transmission of HTLV-I from mother to child: comaprison of bottle- with breast-fed babies. Jap J Cancer Res (Gann) 1987;78:322–324.

61. Tajima K, Tominaga S, Suchi, et al. Epidemiological analysis of the distribution of antibody to adult T-cell leukemia-virus-associated antigen: Possible horizontal transmission of adult T-cell leukemia virus. Jap J Cancer Res (Gann) 1982;73:893–901.

62. Bartholomew C, Saxinger C, Clark JW, et al. Transmission of HTLV-I and HIV among homosexual men in Trinidad. JAMA 1987;257:2604–2608.

63. Murphy E, Figueroa O, Gibbs W, et al. Sexual transmission of human T-lymphocyte virus type I (HTLV-I). Ann Intern Med 1995;111:555–560.

64. Murphy EL, Wilks K, Hanchard B, et al. A case-control study of risk factor for seropositivity to HTLV-I in Jamaica. Int J Epidemiol 1996;25:1083–1089.

65. Schechter M, Harrison LH, Neal AH, et al. Coinfection with human T-cell lymphotropic virus type I and HIV in Brazil. JAMA 1994;271:353.

66. Gotuzzo E, Escamilla J, Phillips I, et al. The impact of human T lymphotropic virus type I/II infection on the prognosis of sexually acquired cases of acquired immunodeficiency syndrome. Arch Intern Med 1992;152:1429–1432.

67. Okochi K, Sata H, Hinuma Y. A retrospective study on transmission of adult T-cell leukemia virus via blood transfusion: seroconversion in recipients. Vox Sang 1984;46:245–253.

68. Sato H, Okochi K. Transmission of human T-cell leukemia virus (HTLV-I) by blood transfusion: demonstration of proviral DNA in recipients' blood lymphocytes. Int J Cancer 1986;37:395–400.

69. Larson C, Taswell H. Human T-cell leukemia virus type I (HTLV-I) and blood transfusion. Mayo Clin Proc 1988;63:869–875.

70. Osame M, Janssen R, Kubota H, et al. Nationwide survey of HTLV-I associated myelopathy in Japan: association with blood transfusion. Ann Neurol 1990;28:50–56.

71. Lee H, Swanson P, Shorty VS, et al. High rate of HTLV-II infection in seropositive IV drug abusers in New Orleans. Science 1989;244:471–475.

72. Grandilone A, Zani M, Barillari G, et al. HTLV-I and HIV infection in drug addicts in Italy. Lancet 1986;2:753–754.

73. Page JB, Shengham L, Chitwood DD, et al. HTLV-I/II seropositivity and death from AIDS among HIV-1 seropositive intravenous drug users. Lancet 1990;335:1439–1441.

74. Dailey H, Charles W, Landeau P, et al. HTLV-I in multiply transfused patients in Trinidad and Tobago, West Indies. Vox Sang 1993;64:189–190.

75. Seiki M, Hattori S, Hiroyama Y, et al. Human adult T-cell leukemia virus: complete nucleotide sequence of the provirus genome integrated in leukemia cell DNA. Proc Natl Acad Sci U S A 1983;80:3618–3622.

76. Bazarbachi A, Huang M, Gessain A, et al. Human T-cell-leukemia virus type I in post-transfusional spastic paraparesis: complete proviral sequence from uncultured blood cells. Int J Cancer 1995;63:494–499.

77. Gessain A, de Thé G. Geographic and molecular epidemiology of primate lymphotropic retroviruses: HTLV-I, HTLV-II, STLV-I, STLV-PP, and PTLV-L. Adv Virus Res 1996;47:377–426.

78. Yanagihara R, Saitou N, Nerurkar VR, et al. Molecular phylogeny and dissemination of human T-cell lymphotropic virus type I viewed within the context of primate evolution and human migration. Cell Mol Biol (Noisy-le-grand Suppl) 1995;41:S145–S161.

79. Lairmore MD, Jacobson S, Gracia F, et al. Isolation of human T-cell lymphotropic virus type 2 from Guaymi indians in Panama. Proc Natl Acad Sci U S A 1990;87:8840–8844.

80. Levine PH, Jacobson S, Elliott R, et al. HTLV-II infection in Florida indians. AIDS Res Hum Retroviruses 1993;90:123–127.

81. Zamora T, Zaninovic V, Kajiwara M, et al. Antibody to HTLV-I in indigenous inhabitants of the Andes and Amazon regions in Colombia. Jap J Cancer Res (Gann) 1990;81:715–719.

82. Maloney EM, Biggar RJ, Neel JV, et al. Endemic human T cell lymphotropic virus type II infection among isolated Brazilian Amerindians. J Infect Dis 1992;166:100–107.

83. Kitagawa T, Fujishita M, Tagushi H, Miyoshi I. Antibodies to HTLV-I in Japanese immigrants in Brazil. JAMA 1986;256:2342.

84. Ohtsu T, Tsugane S, Tobinai K, et al. Prevalence of antibodies to HTLV-I and HIV in Japanese immigrant colonies in Bolivia and Bolivian natives. Jap J Cancer Res (Gann) 1987;78:1347–1353.

85. Blattner WA, Nomura A, Clark JW, et al. Modes of transmission and evidence for viral latency from studies of HTLV-I in Japanese migrant populations to Hawaii. Proc Natl Acad Sci U S A 1986;83:4895–4898.

86. Garruto RM, Slover M, Yanagihara R, et al. High prevalence of HTLV-I infection in isolated populations of the Western Pacific region confirmed by Western immunoblot. Am J Hum Biol 1990;2:439–447.

87. Yanagihara R, Nerukar VR, Ajdukiewicz AB. Comparison between strains of human T lymphotropic virus type I isolated from inhabitants of the Solomon Islands and Papua New Guinea. J Infect Dis 1991;164:443.

Chapter 14

Neuropathologic Aspects of Disorders of Central Nervous System Myelin in Patients with Human Immunodeficiency Virus Type 1 Infection

Umberto De Girolami

Twenty years ago, a new disorder of cell-mediated immunity was described in previously healthy homosexual men[1,2] and was named *acquired immunodeficiency syndrome* (AIDS). The retrovirus human immunodeficiency virus type 1 (HIV-1) was thereafter demonstrated to be the cause of the new disease,[3,4] and the mechanisms of virus injury slowly began to be understood.[5–7]

By several accounts, it was soon discovered that as many as 20–40% of patients infected with HIV-1 develop neurologic dysfunction at some stage of their illness and that HIV-1 can be isolated from the cerebrospinal fluid (CSF) and neural tissues of patients with neurologic syndromes.[8] The spectrum of neurologic dysfunction includes higher cortical intellectual and mood disorders, central sensorimotor deficits, and peripheral neuromuscular disturbances.[9–12] Although recent studies have shown a remarkable decline in the morbidity and mortality among patients with advanced AIDS,[13] neurologic disability is predicted to continue to be a major component of the illness.[14]

Postmortem neuropathologic studies have demonstrated abnormalities in up to 80% of AIDS cases (reviewed in references 15–20), although in the author's recent experience with cases coming to postmortem examination in Boston-area hospitals, this percentage seems to be progressively diminishing. These neuropathologic abnormalities can be subdivided into four principal categories: (1) direct and indirect effects of HIV-1 on the central nervous system (CNS), including HIV-1 encephalitis and vacuolar myelopathy; (2) opportunistic infections; (3) neoplasms (including primary CNS lymphoma and metastatic Kaposi sarcoma); and (4) neuromuscular disorders.

This chapter considers those neuropathologic aspects of HIV-1 infection that relate to myelin injury in the brain and spinal cord of adults and children. Opportunistic infections that damage myelin-forming cells (e.g., the JC virus of progressive multifocal leukoencephalopathy) are addressed in Chapter 15.

Human Immunodeficiency Virus Type 1 Encephalitis in Adults

The possibility that HIV-1 could infect CNS cells was suspected on clinical grounds since the earliest descriptions of AIDS as a distinct clinical syndrome. Numerous autopsy studies of patients with AIDS, including those with thorough examination of the CNS, have been conducted in this continent and in Europe.[9,15,17,20–31] Reviewing this large body of work indicates that the neuropathologic aspects of HIV encephalitis in adult patients differ considerably, depending on the stage of evolution of the disease. These stages can be grouped for convenience of discussion into three phases of the illness: acute HIV-1 encephalitis, subacute HIV-1 encephalitis, and late manifestations of HIV-1 encephalitis.

Acute Human Immunodeficiency Virus Type 1 Encephalitis

Within 1 week of seroconversion, patients may develop symptoms of meningitis and encephalopathy lasting several days or weeks (see Color Plate 15). In these patients, antibodies to HIV-1 are detectable in the CSF, and virus can be isolated from the CSF.[8,32–34] Individuals who have come to postmortem examination at the time of this early phase of HIV-1 invasion, or shortly thereafter, having died of unrelated causes (e.g., accidental death, suicide, homicide), have been found to have mild to moderate meningeal lymphocytosis, focal cerebral white-matter myelin damage, perivascular gliosis, and chronic inflammatory lesions in and around small blood vessels, principally in the white matter.[18,19,35–39]

Subacute Human Immunodeficiency Virus Type 1 Encephalitis

Many of the large postmortem studies of patients dying of AIDS months or years after the onset of the disease, as reported from this country and Europe in the first 10 years of the epidemic, described a distinctive neuropathologic picture.[8,15,17,21–31] This picture was called *subacute encephalitis* by Nielsen and coworkers[23] and, although the term has fallen into disfavor in recent years, it retains validity inasmuch as it emphasizes the cellular response of the inflammatory reaction in this phase of the disease.

In the majority of cases of acute or subacute HIV-1 encephalitis, *macroscopical* external examination of the brain shows that the meninges are clear, and there is no evidence of cortical atrophy. Brain weight is also normal,[15,17] although there has not yet been a large, systematic study of brain weights at different stages of HIV-1 encephalitis. Progressive loss of cerebral volume in AIDS patients has been reported in studies using magnetic resonance imaging methods.[40] On sectioning

of the formalin-fixed brain, a minority of cases show some ventricular dilatation and widening of the Sylvian fissures and adjacent cortical sulci (see Color Plate 16). The cortical mantle is of normal thickness as established by quantitative measurements.[41] Posterior fossa structures and the spinal cord are not remarkable.

By far, the most careful neuropathologic *microscopical* studies of patients with AIDS have been carried out in individuals who have died within several months or a few years of the onset of the illness. The full range of abnormalities that characterize subacute HIV-1 encephalitis has been defined in these cases. This distinctive spectrum of microscopical findings that has been found to affect both the white matter and gray matter are described in detail.

Inflammatory Lesions in White and Gray Matter

The earliest neuropathologic studies described the microglial nodule as a cardinal feature of subacute HIV-1 encephalitis (see Color Plates 17 and 18; Figure 14-1). These are aggregates of nuclei of elongated or bean-shaped microglial glial cells that cluster around regions of tissue disruption (sometimes with clear evidence of micronecrosis). The surrounding tissue shows reactive astrocytosis and slight pallor of myelin staining. The nodules can occur diffusely throughout the brain, although the extent and density of lesions varies considerably, apparently irrespective of the clinical severity of neurologic manifestations; this paradoxical situation is discussed further later. In the experience of Petito and coworkers[25] and Kure and collaborators[42] and in our observations,[17] microglial nodules occur most often in the subcortical white matter, although they may also be seen in the diencephalon–basal ganglia and brain stem–cerebellum, but are extremely rare in the cerebral cortex.

Infiltrates of macrophages, characterized by abundant foamy (sometimes pigment-laden) cytoplasm, are often found in association with the microglial nodules or occur in sizable collections perivascularly, especially in the white matter of the cerebral hemispheres and cerebellum.

Third, an important component of the inflammatory lesion is the multinucleated giant cells. These are macrophage-derived cells with several nuclei either haphazardly arranged or aggregated within a brightly homogeneous, eosinophilic, irregularly shaped cytoplasm. They can occur admixed with other cells in microglial nodules or appear in isolated clusters in the parenchyma and perivascular spaces. They tend to occur in the same distribution as the microglial nodules and macrophages. Studies have shown that multinucleated cells result from fusion of macrophages; they also have the same immunohistochemical properties as macrophages. Special attention to the importance of the multinucleated giant cells was first drawn by the studies of Sharer and collaborators,[43] and other investigators have interpreted their presence as an essential component of the histopathologic picture.[18,44,45] It is now apparent that their occurrence is characteristic of the subacute HIV-1 encephalitis, as they are not seen at either extreme of the illness.[17,18,20]

Many subsequent studies using light-electron microscopy, anti–HIV-1 antibody immunocytochemistry, in situ hybridization, and polymerase chain reaction methods conclusively demonstrated the presence of HIV-1 in tissue sections of brain and spinal cord.[15,20,46–55] HIV-1 was found principally within the macrophages, multinucleated giant cells, and microglial cells that characterize the lesion of subacute HIV-1 encephalitis as described earlier. These affected intracerebral cells have been shown to be CD4+, as are the helper T cells that HIV uses as a binding site.[56,57] Although there had been early speculation that the microglial nodules and multinucleated giant cells might be the result of non-HIV–related opportunistic viral infections, there seems to be no evidence of immunoreactivity to herpes simplex virus, cytomegalovirus, and papovavirus antigens within microglial nodules containing HIV-positive mononuclear cells when these agents are searched with immunohistochemical and electron microscopical methods.[46,48,58–60]

In spite of assiduous search, there has been no morphologic evidence of HIV-1 infection of neurons or oligodendrocytes in human tissue. Recent evidence suggests limited infection of astrocytes,[55,61,62] particularly in the early stages of the disease. Endothelial cell infection is discussed later.

Lesions of the Microcirculation

The second striking abnormality seen in subacute HIV-1 encephalitis is evident in the intracerebral capillaries and venules (i.e., microcirculation) (see

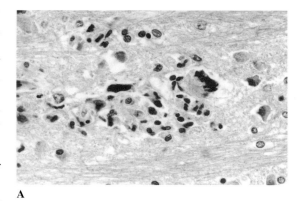

A

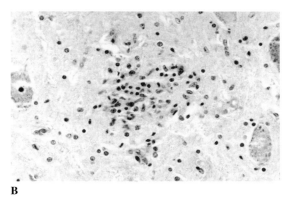

B

Figure 14-1. A. Multinucleated giant cell. Note aggregate of nuclei next to swath of cytoplasm (hematoxylin and eosin). **B.** Neuronophagia. Note presence of mononuclear cells and microglia in the midst of necrotic neuron. Viable neurons are seen at the periphery of the field (hematoxylin and eosin). (Reprinted with permission from U De Girolami, TW Smith, D Hénin, J-J Hauw. Neuropathology and Ophthalmologic Pathology of the Acquired Immunodeficiency Syndrome: A Color Atlas. Boston: Butterworth–Heinemann, 1992.)

Color Plate 19; Figure 14-2). As mentioned previously, an important manifestation of acute HIV-1 encephalitis consists of foci of perivascular and intravascular inflammation[19,39]; recent evidence indicates HIV-1 infection of endothelial cells in this early phase of asymptomatic involvement of the CNS.[62] In the subacute phase of the illness, the inflammatory component subsides, and the microcirculatory changes consist of thickening of the wall of the blood vessels and increased cellularity, with enlargement and pleomorphism of endothelial cells.[63] These vascular abnormalities are usually associated with prominent perivascular aggregates

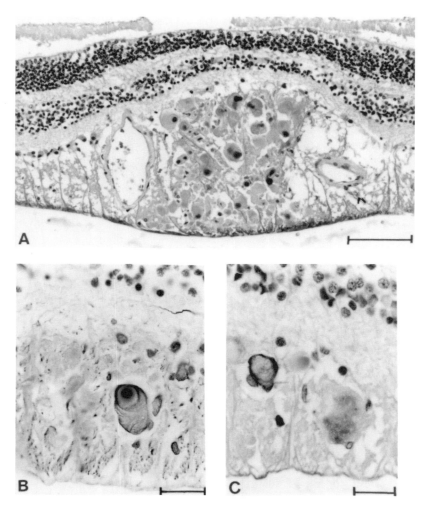

Figure 14-2. Cotton-wool spots in nerve fiber layer of retina (vitreous at bottom of all panels). **A.** Note expanded nerve fiber layer next to blood vessel showing axonal swellings (hematoxylin and eosin). **B.** High magnification showing multiple concentric cores within axonal swelling (hematoxylin and eosin). **C.** High magnification to demonstrate neurofilaments in axonal swelling (immunoperoxidase stain for neurofilaments). (Reprinted with permission from U De Girolami, TW Smith, D Hénin, J-J Hauw. Neuropathology and Ophthalmologic Pathology of the Acquired Immunodeficiency Syndrome: A Color Atlas. Boston: Butterworth–Heinemann, 1992.)

of HIV-1–positive monocytes and multinucleated cells. Microcirculatory abnormalities are most commonly observed in the white matter of the centrum semiovale and in posterior fossa structures. A particularly interesting aspect of both the acute and subacute vascular lesions is that they are sometimes related to microinfarcts. The microinfarcts are characterized by small regions of white-matter necrosis and prominent axonal swelling with little inflammatory reaction. The brain microinfarcts are histologically identical to those seen in the nerve fiber layer of the retina, recognized clinically as cotton-wool spots. Cotton-wool spots are an important and characteristic funduscopic abnormality in patients with AIDS and have an established relationship with the retinal microcirculation.[64]

The pathogenesis of these lesions of the microcirculation could well be related to infection of cerebral endothelial cells by HIV-1, as reported by some investigators[48,55,62]; there are also reports demonstrating infection of retinal endothelial cells.[65,66] These abnormalities of the microcirculation were at first postulated to give rise to altered vascular permeability.[63] Leakage of fluid and plasma proteins around the perivascular extracellular spaces was subsequently demonstrated by Rhodes,[67] Petito and Cash,[68] Power et al.,[69] and Dallasta et al.[70] There has been no systematic neuropathologic study of the topographic distribution of these sites of increased vascular permeability over the course of the disease, although neuroradiologic studies indicate the basal ganglia have increased early enhancement, suggesting disruption of the blood-brain barrier (BBB) in these regions over other areas of the brain.[71] The potential injurious effect of this BBB breakdown on the surrounding white and gray matter is discussed later. Incidentally, lesions of large blood vessels (macrocirculation) are known to occur in patients with AIDS; these may or may not be associated with HIV encephalitis and include instances of embolic cerebral infarction, hemorrhages at various sites of the gray and white matter, and vasculitis.[9,72–77]

Demyelinating Lesions

One of the truly remarkable aspects of the disease, which was especially evident to us on examination of whole-brain sections embedded in celloidin or in paraffin and stained with conventional myelin stains, is the presence of a multifocal, poorly circumscribed, or diffuse faint pallor of myelin staining that involves primarily the centrum semiovale but also less often affects the white matter of the cerebellum and the brain stem (see Color Plate 20). At high magnification, the typical white-matter lesions consist of poorly defined regions of tissue rarefaction wherein there is a moderate reduction in the number of myelinated fibers, scattered macrophages–microglial cells, few reactive astrocytes, relative sparing of axons, and virtual absence of any other inflammatory cell. Microglial nodules or multinucleated giant cells (or both) are sparse or absent within these lesions. Less severe forms of this process (perhaps early lesions) are characterized by focal, often angiocentric regions of myelin loss often around microcirculatory abnormalities, as described earlier. Transitions between the focal and more diffuse white-matter lesions are frequent. Very severe examples (late lesions) show extensive destruction of myelinated fibers, conspicuous axonal damage with axonal spheroids in the centrum semiovale, and secondary degeneration. In these patients with long-standing disease, on macroscopical examination, the white matter of the centrum semiovale appears unusually firm.[15,78] Giometto et al.[79] and Raja and coauthors[80] have documented axonal injury within areas of demyelination using an antibody to β-amyloid precursor protein. This leukoencephalopathy has been studied in detail by several workers.[24,25,45,63,69,80–82]

The pathogenesis of these white-matter abnormalities is uncertain. Some investigators[26,83] have noted alterations in the number and size of oligodendrocytic nuclei within areas of myelin pallor, whereas others have not.[84] Thus far, conclusive evidence of HIV infection of oligodendroglial cells in human tissue has been lacking. Alterations in BBB permeability as discussed earlier could cause accumulation of edema fluid within the extracellular space as well as allow various circulating macromolecules to enter the cerebral parenchyma, which could cause injury to myelinated fibers. Other, as yet, hypothetical causes for the white-matter degeneration include destruction of myelin and axons by soluble substances elaborated by HIV-infected monocytes or autoimmune-associated demyelination.

Clinicopathologic Considerations and Pathogenesis of the Acquired Immunodeficiency Syndrome Dementia Complex in Relation to Lesions of White Matter

Approximately one-fourth to one-half of patients with AIDS develop a neurologic syndrome sometime during the course of their disease, characterized by a variably progressive, subacutely evolving dementia (including principally slowness of thought, loss of retentive memory, apathy, and language disturbances) and associated with motor dysfunction (incoordination of limbs, ataxia of gait, and eye movement abnormalities) and sphincteric disturbances.[85,86] This syndrome has been termed *HIV-associated AIDS dementia complex* (ADC).[12] It is believed by most workers in this field that the neuropathologic substrate of this clinical syndrome is subacute HIV-1 encephalitis as described earlier,[87] albeit with imperfect clinicopathologic correlation as regards severity of the disease.[88] Still inexplicable is why some patients with well-documented, severe ADC show relatively little postmortem morphologic evidence of brain damage.

As indicated earlier, there is good evidence to document that early HIV invasion of the CNS occurs in asymptomatic seropositive individuals, but the sequence of events that leads to penetration of HIV-1 into the human brain and the mechanisms of injury that underlie the ensuing neurologic dementing syndrome are unknown.[16,89–92] At the time of initial viremia, it is speculated that the endothelial cells of the cerebral microcirculation may well become transiently infected; indeed, there is now evidence of infection of the brain endothelial cells of HIV-1–positive asymptomatic patients who died of unrelated causes.[62] The considerable numbers of circulating, latently HIV-infected monocytes[93] may then adhere to the damaged endothelial cells and perivascular astrocytes and be transported across the BBB.[94,95] The mechanisms of HIV-1–infected monocyte migration through the BBB described in experimental models lend credence to these speculations,[96–98] and recent work by Dallasta and coworkers[70] has provided structural evidence that BBB tight-junction proteins are affected in HIV-1 encephalitis. Viral replication within the transformed macrophages might then follow, with a release of virions and subsequently infection of other cells that express CD4 receptors on their surface (i.e., macrophages and microglial cells) through the binding of the HIV envelope glycoprotein gp120 to the CD4 receptor.

Pathogenetic schemes to explain ADC have tried to take into account the following neuropathologic observations:

1. Topography of lesions: Many studies have indicated that there is relatively little evidence of cortical gray-matter tissue destruction in the vast majority of patients with ADC. Indeed, what damage there is (myelin pallor and axonal injury) is in the white matter.
2. Distribution of inflammation: The inflammatory response consisting of macrophages–multinucleated giant cells and microglial cells has largely been a phenomenon of the supratentorial white matter (the brain stem and basal ganglia are affected to a lesser extent).
3. Infected cells: The predominant cells demonstrated to be infected with HIV-1 are not the neurons or oligodendroglial cells, as might be expected, but the macrophage and microglial cells (astrocytes and endothelial cells are also infected at some stage of the disease, as mentioned earlier).

There is considerable evidence that the brain serves as a reservoir of large quantities of proviral (integrated) DNA that apparently is predominantly localized to selective regions, including basal ganglia and hippocampus.[99,100] Some quantitative studies suggest that brain viral burden correlates with the severity of mental dysfunction,[101,102] whereas others

reach the opposite conclusion.[103] A number of workers have suggested that the neuronal dysfunction in ADC is due not to direct infection of neurons (or glia) but to the indirect neurotoxic effects of cytokines liberated by the inflammatory cells (largely macrophages and microglial cells) that permeate the brain in subacute HIV-1 encephalitis; these substances include tumor necrosis factor and other soluble factors or proteolytic enzymes that can be toxic to neurons and their processes or to glia, including astrocytes and oligodendrocytes[104–108] (reviewed in reference 92). Interestingly, the work of Glass et al.[109] has shown that the severity of the dementia in the patients analyzed correlated best with postmortem brain tissue density of macrophages and microglial cells, as identified by immunohistochemical methods, rather than with the viral burden within the infected macrophages and microglial cells. This fact has led to the speculation that control of systemic HIV replication might limit the development of dementia.[110] However, according to the in vitro studies of Lipton,[111,112] a specific mechanism of impairment of neuronal function does involve the HIV envelope glycoprotein gp120, or a fragment of this protein, which was shown to be toxic to rodent neurons by inducing an influx of intraneuronal free calcium. This toxicity was later shown to be mediated through the participation of macrophage-microglial cell–derived factors that acted via the N-methyl-D-aspartate receptors.[113,114] Further evidence of the participation of infected inflammatory cells in mediating neuronal toxicity comes from the experimental study of Tardieu and collaborators,[115] who have demonstrated neuronal cell injury only after adhesion between HIV-infected monocytes and neurons. Cell-to-cell interactions have also been shown to exist between HIV-infected macrophages and astrocytes.[89,95] Finally, Dallasta and collaborators[70] have shown that the disruption in the BBB that occurs in the brains of patients with HIV-1 encephalitis and ADC is associated with HIV-infected macrophages.

The relationship between these neurotoxic factors and the development of neuronal and glial injury are currently under active investigation (reviewed in references 20, 95, and 116). Morphologic evidence of neuronal injury, possibly caused by the release of macrophage-derived neurotoxic factors or other mechanisms, has been presented by several laboratories in an attempt to explain the clinical syndrome of ADC. This evidence rests on the demonstration of quantitative neuronal loss in the cerebral cortex, reduction in cell size, or dendritic injury in cortical neurons.[117–124] Conversely, in a prospective study of six patients with HIV-associated dementia compared with six controls (nondemented, non-AIDS), there was no statistically significant difference in the number of cortical neurons (Brodmann areas 4, 9, 40) in the two groups.[41] Other methods of determining cell death using the terminal deoxytransferase–mediated deoxyuridine triphosphate nick-end labeling technique to detect apoptosis have documented both neuronal and astrocytic injury in HIV encephalitis, although careful quantitation of this phenomenon correlated with morphometric cell counting has not yet been accomplished.[61,125–128]

Still, in spite of all the quoted studies, a plausible pathogenesis for the ADC has remained elusive. It remains a complete mystery how the putative neurotoxic substances could be acting on neurons of the cerebral cortex and elsewhere when systematic neuropathologic examinations in a number of laboratories have shown relatively few microglial nodules, multinucleated giant cells, and macrophages-microglia in patients with clinical evidence of severe dementia. Quantitative assessments of neuronal injury or death have not uncovered damage of such magnitude that would easily explain the clinical syndrome. The abnormalities of the microcirculation described previously are rare in the cortex. Possibly the white-matter injury caused by a breakdown of the BBB might be giving rise to a subcortical dementia, although often enough the neuropathologic changes do not appear to be so severe to afford a reasonable explanation for the dementia in most cases.

Human Immunodeficiency Virus Encephalitis in Children

The neuropathologic abnormalities encountered in children with AIDS, although considerably different from those in adults, also include a disorder of myelin and are therefore mentioned briefly here. Neurologic disease is common in children with AIDS.[129–131] Clinical manifestations of neurologic dysfunction are evident by the first years of life and include microcephaly with mental retardation and motor developmental delay with long-

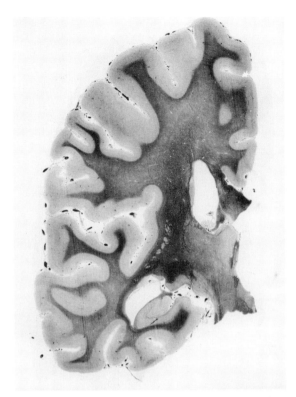

Figure 14-3. Pediatric human immunodeficiency virus type 1 encephalitis. Horizontal myelin-stained section showing extensive myelin pallor in centrum semiovale and cerebral atrophy (Loyez stain for myelin). (Reprinted with permission from U De Girolami, TW Smith, D Hénin, J-J Hauw. Neuropathology and Ophthalmologic Pathology of the Acquired Immunodeficiency Syndrome: A Color Atlas. Boston: Butterworth–Heinemann, 1992.)

tract signs. The neuropathologic features of AIDS in children have been discussed in a few comprehensive reports and reviews.[16,24,78,83,132–139] The most frequently reported macroscopic abnormalities are calcific deposits within the basal ganglia and deep cerebral white matter, microencephaly, and diffuse firmness of the supratentorial white matter (Figure 14-3). These findings are demonstrable with radiologic studies.[131,140] Histopathologically, the characteristic findings include lesions of the medium-sized and small blood vessels of the basal ganglia and subcortical white matter characterized by mineralization of the vessel wall and narrowing of its lumen without associated inflammatory changes of any great severity (see

Color Plate 21A). Calcific deposits may also be found scattered throughout the white matter and in association with destructive lesions. Many patients have also shown the histopathologic findings of subacute encephalitis as described earlier, although the extent and severity of the lesions seems, in general, to be less than that observed in adults (see Color Plate 21B). Immunocytochemical and ultrastructural studies of children with HIV encephalitis have demonstrated the same abnormalities as noted in adults.[139] There has been no detailed quantitative study of neuronal injury; neuronal apoptosis has also been recorded.[141] Also remarkable has been the extent of white-matter damage in the brain and cerebellum, which often shows extensive pallor of myelin staining and evidence of axonal injury. Many more studies are needed to begin to understand the pathogenesis of these findings.

Vacuolar Myelopathy

In early 1985, two separate groups of investigators[142,143] described the clinical and pathologic aspects of a previously unrecognized disorder of the spinal cord in AIDS patients late in the course of their disease. The disease, named *vacuolar myelopathy* by Petito and collaborators,[126] was characterized neuropathologically by multiple 10- to 100-μm vacuoles within the white matter of the posterior and lateral columns of the lower thoracic cord (see Color Plates 22 and 23). They also stressed the importance of finding foamy macrophages in association with these vacuolar lesions so as to be certain to rule out artifactual changes. In the 20 cases recorded, the severity of the lesions was graded (I, mild; II, moderate; III, severe), and transition forms among the prototypes were frequent. In subsequent large studies,[25,60,144–147] the disorder has been estimated to be demonstrable at postmortem in 20–30% of unselected patients with AIDS in this hemisphere and less often in Europe. It has also been noted that, although extensive reactive gliosis is rare, microglial nodules and multinucleated giant cells are not uncommon in the regions of the cord away from the vacuolar myelopathy. Ultrastructural studies indicate both axonal and myelin injury.[148,149]

The etiology and pathogenesis of vacuolar myelopathy are unknown.[150] The early reports pointed out the striking resemblance of the cord lesions to those of vitamin B_{12} deficiency (subacute combined degeneration), but this possibility was negated by appropriate serum assays.[143] The pathogenetic role of HIV-1 in vacuolar myelopathy has been controversial. Ho et al.[8] were able to isolate the virus from the CSF and postmortem spinal cord tissue in a patient with clinical manifestations indicative of a myelopathy. Budka et al.,[151] Maier et al.,[152] and Eilbott et al.[153] have demonstrated by immunohistochemistry and in situ hybridization that the macrophages and multinucleated giant cells in the vicinity of the vacuoles are HIV positive, suggesting that the cause of vacuolar myelopathy is HIV. Conversely, strong evidence has been adduced to demonstrate just the opposite viewpoint. Kamin and Petito[154] reported 12 cases of vacuolar myelopathy in an immunosuppressed patient without AIDS. Rosenblum et al.[155] demonstrated in a comprehensive study combining immunohistochemistry (p24), in situ hybridization (DNA), and HIV isolation, that the presence of the virus correlated not with the presence of vacuolar myelopathy but with an inflammatory myelitis that was in every way similar to subacute HIV-1 encephalitis, as described earlier. Grafe and Wiley[145] also showed a complete lack of association between immunocytologic localization of HIV antigens and vacuolar myelopathy. Shepherd and colleagues[147] studied the spinal cords of 90 patients with AIDS and found no evidence that proximity of productive HIV-1 (quantitative polymerase chain reaction) infection is implicated in the pathogenesis of vacuolar myelopathy. Our own experience with a series of cases from Paris and Boston agrees with these findings.[60] Similarly, the reports of neuropathologic observations of the spinal cords of children with AIDS again dispute the assertion that vacuolar myelopathy is caused by HIV-1.[156–158] Similar lesions have been described in the cerebrum (multifocal vacuolar leukoencephalopathy)[159] and basis pontis (multifocal pontine leukoencephalopathy; see Color Plate 24).[160]

It can now be concluded that AIDS-associated vacuolar myelopathy is probably not related directly to HIV-1 infection of the spinal cord. Available evidence suggests that it may be the result of a yet-unidentified indirect effect, possibly a myelinolytic cytokine.[161] The report by Goudreau et al.,[162] in which transgenic animals expressing HIV genome in oligodendroglia were found to develop vacuolar changes in the white matter of the spinal cord, lends credence to the speculation that there is some indirect role for HIV in the pathogenesis of vacuolar myelopathy.

The spinal cord has also been reported to be the site of "degenerative" changes with limited effects on the corticospinal tracts or the posterior columns. Such changes have been attributed to secondary wallerian degeneration consequent to proximal injury in the pyramidal system or dorsal root ganglia, respectively.[81,163]

Other Acquired Immunodeficiency Syndrome–Associated Disorders of Myelin

Rare instances of fulminating multiple sclerosis–like leukoencephalopathy occurring at almost any stage of AIDS have been described in several clinicopathologic studies. The neuropathology of these lesions closely approximates acute disseminated encephalomyelitis or multiple sclerosis–like syndromes.[164–167] In this context, some cases showing plaque-like demyelinating lesions have been found to be due to opportunistic infection with herpes viruses.[168–171]

References

1. Gottlieb MS, Schroff R, Schanker HM, et al. *Pneumocystis carinii* pneumonia and mucosal candidiasis in previously healthy homosexual men: evidence of a new acquired cellular immunodeficiency. N Engl J Med 1981; 305:1425–1431.
2. Masur H, Michelis MA, Greene JB, et al. An outbreak of community-acquired *Pneumocystis carinii* pneumonia: initial manifestation of cellular immune dysfunction. N Engl J Med 1981;305:1431–1438.
3. Barré-Sinoussi F, Chermann JC, Rey F, et al. Isolation of a T-lymphotropic retrovirus from a patient at risk for acquired immune deficiency syndrome (AIDS). Science 1983;220:868–871.
4. Gallo RC, Salahuddin SZ, Popovic M, et al. Frequent detection and isolation of cytopathic retroviruses (HTLV-III) from patients with AIDS and at risk for AIDS. Science 1984;224:500–503.
5. Ho DD, Pomerantz RJ, Kaplan JC. Pathogenesis of infection with human immunodeficiency virus. N Engl J Med 1987;317(5):278–286.
6. Fauci AS. Multifactorial nature of human immunodeficiency virus disease: Implications for therapy. Science 1993;262:1011–1018.
7. Fauci AS. The AIDS epidemic. Considerations of the 21st century. N Engl J Med 1999;341:1046–1050.
8. Ho DD, Rota TR, Schooley RT, et al. Isolation of HTLV-III from cerebrospinal fluid and neural tissues of patients with neurologic syndromes related to the acquired immunodeficiency syndrome. N Engl J Med 1985;313(24):1493–1497.
9. Snider WD, Simpson DM, Nielsen S, et al. Neurological complications of acquired immune deficiency syndrome: analysis of 50 patients. Ann Neurol 1983;14:403–418.
10. Gabuzda DH, Hirsch MS. Neurologic manifestations of infection with human immunodeficiency virus. Ann Intern Med 1987;107:383–391.
11. de Gans J, Portegies P. Neurological complications of infection with human immunodeficiency virus type 1. Clin Neurol Neurosurg 1989;91(3):199–219.
12. Report of a Working Group of the American Academy of Neurology AIDS Task Force. Nomenclature and research case definitions for neurologic manifestations of human immunodeficiency virus-type 1 (HIV-1) infection. Neurology 1991;41:778–785.
13. Palella FJ, Delaney KM, Moorman AC, et al. Declining morbidity and mortality among patients with advanced human immunodeficiency virus infection. N Engl J Med 1998; 338:853–860.
14. Bacellar H, Muñoz A, Miller EN, et al. Temporal trends in the incidence of HIV-1-related neurologic diseases: multicenter AIDS cohort study, 1985–1992. Neurology 1994; 44:1892–1900.
15. De Girolami U, Smith TW, Hénin D, Hauw J-J. Neuropathology of the acquired immunodeficiency syndrome. Arch Pathol Lab Med 1990;114:643–655.
16. Sharer LR. Pathology of HIV-1 infection of the central nervous system. A review. J Neuropathol Exp Neurol 1992;51(1):3–11.
17. Seilhean D, De Girolami U, Hénin D, Hauw J-J. The Neuropathology of AIDS: the Salpêtrière Experience and Review of the Literature 1983–1993. In RS Weinstein, AR Graham, RE Anderson (eds), Advances in Pathology and Laboratory Medicine. Chicago: Mosby, 1994;221–257.
18. Kibayashi K, Mastri AR, Hirsch CS. Neuropathology of human immunodeficiency virus infection at different disease stages. Hum Pathol 1996;27:637–642.
19. Gray F. Les lésions du système nerveux central aux stades précoces de l'infection par le virus de l'immunodéficience humaine. Revue Neurologique 1997;153:629–640.
20. Bell JE. The neuropathology of adult HIV infection. Revue Neurologique 1998;154:816–829.
21. Moskowitz LB, Hensley GT, Chan JC, et al. The neuropathology of acquired immune deficiency syndrome. Arch Pathol Lab Med 1984;108:867–872.
22. Welch K, Finkbeiner W, Alpers CE, et al. Autopsy findings in the acquired immune deficiency syndrome. JAMA 1984;252(9):1152–1159.
23. Nielsen SL, Petito CK, Urmacher CD, Posner JB. Subacute encephalitis in acquired immune deficiency syndrome: a postmortem study. Am J Clin Pathol 1984;82:678–682.
24. Anders KH, Guerra WF, Tomiyasu U, et al. The neuropathology of AIDS: UCLA experience and review. Am J Pathol 1986;124:537–558.

25. Petito CK, Cho E-S, Lemann W, et al. Neuropathology of acquired immunodeficiency syndrome (AIDS): an autopsy review. J Neuropathol Exp Neurol 1986;45:635–646.

26. de la Monte SM, Schooley RT, Hirsch MS, Richardson EP Jr. Subacute encephalomyelitis of AIDS and its relation to HTLV-III infection. Neurology 1987;37:562–569.

27. Hénin D, Duyckaerts C, Chaunu M-P, et al. Étude neuropathologique de 31 cas de syndrome d'immuno-depression acquise. Revue Neurologique 1987;143:631–642.

28. Kato T, Hirano A, Llena JF, Dembitzer HM. Neuropathology of acquired immune deficiency syndrome (AIDS) in 53 autopsy cases with particular emphasis on microglial nodules and multinucleated giant cells. Acta Neuropathol 1987;73:287–294.

29. Rhodes RH. Histopathology of the central nervous system in the acquired immunodeficiency syndrome. Hum Pathol 1987;18(6):636–643.

30. Lantos PL, McLaughlin JE, Scholtz CL, et al. Neuropathology of the brain in HIV infection. Lancet 1989;1:309–310.

31. Burns DK, Risser RC, White CL 3rd. The neuropathology of human immunodeficiency virus infection. Arch Pathol Lab Med 1991;115:1112–1124.

32. Carne CA, Smith A, Elkington SG, et al. Acute encephalopathy coincident with seroconversion for anti-HTLV-III. Lancet 1985;2:1206.

33. Levy JA, Shimabukuro J, Hollander H, et al. Isolation of AIDS-associated retroviruses from cerebrospinal fluid and brain of patients with neurological symptoms. Lancet 1985;2:586–588.

34. Hollander H, Levy JA. Neurologic abnormalities and recovery of human immunodeficiency virus from cerebrospinal fluid. Ann Intern Med 1987;106:692–696.

35. Lenhardt TM, Super MA, Wiley CA. Neuropathological changes in asymptomatic HIV seropositive man. Ann Neurol 1988;23:210.

36. McArthur JC, Becker PS, Parisi JE, et al. Neuropathological changes in early HIV-1 dementia. Ann Neurol 1989;26:681–684.

37. Davis LE, Hjelle BL, Miller VE, et al. Early viral brain invasion in iatrogenic human immunodeficiency virus infection. Neurology 1992;42:1736–1739.

38. Gray F, Lescs M-C, Keohane C, et al. Early brain changes in HIV infection: neuropathological study of 11 HIV seropositive, non-AIDS cases. J Neuropathol Exp Neurol 1992;51:177–185.

39. Gray F, Scaravilli F, Everall I, et al. Neuropathology of early HIV-1 infection. Brain Pathol 1996;6:1–15.

40. Stout J, Ellis R, Jernigan T, et al. Progressive cerebral volume loss in human immunodeficiency virus infection. Arch Neurol 1998;55:161–168.

41. Seilhean D, Duyckaerts C, Vazeux R, et al. HIV-1-associated cognitive/motor complex: absence of neuronal loss in the cerebral neocortex. Neurology 1993;43(8):1492–1499.

42. Kure K, Weidenheim KM, Lyman WD, Dickson DW. Morphology and distribution of HIV-1 gp41-positive microglia in subacute AIDS encephalitis: pattern of involvement resembling a multisystem degeneration. Acta Neuropathol 1990;80:393–400.

43. Sharer LR, Cho E-S, Epstein LG. Multinucleated giant cells and HTLV-III in AIDS encephalopathy. Hum Pathol 1985;16(8):760.

44. Budka H. Multinucleated giant cells in brain: a hallmark of the acquired immune deficiency syndrome (AIDS). Acta Neuropathol 1986;69:253–258.

45. Navia BA, Cho E-S, Petito CK, Price RW. The AIDS dementia complex: II. Neuropathology. Ann Neurol 1986;19:525–535.

46. Gabuzda DH, Ho DD, de la Monte SM, et al. Immunohistochemical identification of HTLV-III antigen in brains of patients with AIDS. Ann Neurol 1986;20:289–295.

47. Koenig S, Gendelman HE, Orenstein JM, et al. Detection of AIDS virus in macrophages in brain tissue from AIDS patients with encephalopathy. Science 1986;233:1089–1093.

48. Wiley CA, Schrier RD, Nelson JA, et al. Cellular localization of human immunodeficiency virus infection within the brains of acquired immune deficiency syndrome patients. Proc Natl Acad Sci U S A 1986;83:7089–7093.

49. Pumarola-Sune T, Navia BA, Gordon-Cardo C, et al. HIV antigen in the brains of patients with the AIDS dementia complex. Ann Neurol 1987;21:490–496.

50. Vazeux R, Brousse N, Jarry A, et al. AIDS subacute encephalitis: Identification of HIV-infected cells. Am J Pathol 1987;126(3):403–410.

51. Budka H, Wiley CA, Kleihues P, et al. HIV-associated disease of the nervous system: Review of nomenclature and proposal for neuropathology-based terminology. Brain Pathol 1991;1:143–152.

52. Weidenheim KM, Epshteyn I, Lyman WD. Immunocytochemical identification of T-cell in HIV-1 encephalitis; implications for pathogenesis of CNS disease. Mod Pathol 1993;6:167–174.

53. Böni J, Emmerich BS, Leib SL, et al. PCR identification of HIV-1 DNA sequences in brain tissue of patients with AIDS encephalopathy. Neurology 1993;43:1813–1817.

54. Achim CL, Wang R, Miners DK, A WC. Brain viral burden in HIV infection. J Neuropathol Exp Neurol 1994;53:284–294.

55. Takahashi K, Wesselingh S, Griffin D, et al. Localization of HIV-1 in human brain using polymerase chain reaction/in situ hybridization and immunohistochemistry. Ann Neurol 1996;39:705–711.

56. Jameson BA, Rao PE, Kong LI. Location and chemical synthesis of a binding site for HIV-1 on the CD4 protein. Science 1988;240:1335–1341.

57. Jordan CA, Watkins BA, Kufta C, Dubois-Dalcq M. Infection of brain microglial cells by human immunodeficiency virus type 1 is CD4 dependent. J Virol 1991;65:736–742.

58. Wiley CA, Schrier RD, Denaro FJ, et al. Localization of cytomegalovirus proteins and genome during fulminant central nervous system infection in an AIDS patient. J Neuropathol Exp Neurol 1986;45(2):127–139.

59. Meyenhofer MF, Epstein LG, Cho E-S, Sharer LR. Ultrastructural morphology and intracellular production of human immunodeficiency virus (HIV) in brain. J Neuropathol Exp Neurol 1987;46(4):474–484.

60. Hénin D, Smith TW, De Girolami K, et al. Neuropathology of the spinal cord in the acquired immunodeficiency syndrome. Hum Pathol 1992;23:1106–1114.

61. Shi B, De Girolami U, He J, et al. Apoptosis induced HIV-1 infection of the central nervous system. J Clin Invest 1996;98:1979–1990.

62. An SF, Groves M, Gray F, Scaravilli F. Early entry and widespread cellular involvement of HIV-1 in brains of HIV-1 positive asymptomatic individuals. J Neuropathol Exp Neurol 1999;58:1156–1162.

63. Smith TW, De Girolami U, Hénin D, et al. Human immunodeficiency virus (HIV) leukoencephalopathy and the microcirculation. J Neuropathol Exp Neurol 1990;49:357–370.

64. Cunningham ET, Margolis TP. Ocular manifestations of HIV infection. N Engl J Med 1998;339:236–244.

65. Pomerantz RJ, Kuritzkes DR, de la Monte SM. Infection of the retina by human immunodeficiency virus type I. N Engl J Med 1987;317:1643–1647.

66. Reux I, Fillet AM, Fournier J-G, et al. In situ hybridization of HIV-1 RNA in retinal vascular wall. Am J Pathol 1993; 143:1–5.

67. Rhodes RH. Evidence of serum-protein leakage across the blood-brain barrier in acquired immunodeficiency syndrome. J Neuropathol Exp Neurol 1991;50:171–183.

68. Petito CK, Cash KS. Blood-brain barrier abnormalities in the acquired immunodeficiency syndrome: immunohistochemical localization of serum proteins in postmortem brain. Ann Neurol 1992;32:658–666.

69. Power C, Kong P-A, Crawford TO, et al. Cerebral white matter changes in acquired immunodeficiency syndrome dementia: alterations of the blood-brain barrier. Ann Neurol 1993;34:339–350.

70. Dallasta LM, Pisarov LA, Esplen JE, et al. Blood-brain barrier tight junction disruption in human immunodeficiency virus-1 encephalitis. Am J Pathol 1999;155:1915–1927.

71. Berger JR, Nath A, Greenberg RN, et al. Cerebrovascular changes in the basal ganglia with HIV dementia. Neurology 2000;54:921–926.

72. Yankner BA, Skolnik PR, Shoukimas GM, et al. Cerebral granulomatous angiitis associated with isolation of human T-lymphotropic virus type III from the central nervous system. Ann Neurol 1986;20:362–364.

73. Mizusawa H, Hirano A, Llena JF, Shintaku M. Cerebrovascular lesions in acquired immune deficiency syndrome (AIDS). Acta Neuropathol 1988;76:451–457.

74. Vinters HV, Guerra WF, Eppolito L, Keith PE III. Necrotizing vasculitis of the nervous system in a patient with AIDS-related complex. Neuropathol Appl Neurobiol 1988;14:417–424.

75. Scaravilli F, Ellis DS, Tovey G, et al. Unusual development of polyoma virus in the brains of two patients with the acquired immune deficiency syndrome (AIDS). Neuropathol Appl Neurobiol 1989;15:407–418.

76. Berger JR, Harris JO, Gregorios J, Norenberg M. Cerebrovascular disease in AIDS: a case-control study. AIDS 1990;4:239–244.

77. Nogueira Pinto A. AIDS and cerebrovascular disease. Stroke 1996;27:538–543.

78. De Girolami U, Smith TW, Hénin D, Hauw J-J. Neuropathology and Ophthalmologic Pathology of the Acquired Immunodeficiency Syndrome: A Color Atlas. Boston: Butterworth–Heinemann, 1992.

79. Giometto B, An SF, Groves M, et al. Accumulation of β-amyloid precursor protein in HIV encephalitis: relationship with neuropsychological abnormalities. Ann Neurol 1997;42:34–40.

80. Raja F, Sherriff FE, Morris CS, et al. Cerebral white matter damage in HIV infection demonstrated using β-amyloid precursor protein immunoreactivity. Acta Neuropathol 1997;93:184–189.

81. Horoupian DS, Pick P, Spigland I, et al. Acquired immune deficiency syndrome and multiple tract degeneration in a homosexual man. Ann Neurol 1984;15:502–505.

82. Kleihues P, Lang W, Burger PC, et al. Progressive diffuse leukoencephalopathy in patients with acquired immune deficiency syndrome (AIDS). Acta Neuropathol 1985; 68:333–339.

83. Sotrel A. The Nervous System. In SJ Harawi, CJ O'Hara (eds), Pathology and Pathophysiology of AIDS and HIV-Related Diseases. St. Louis: Mosby, 1989;201–268.

84. Morris CS, Esiri MM, Millard PR. The fate of oligodendrocytes in HIV-1 infection. AIDS 1991;5:1081–1088.

85. Brew BJ, Sidtis JJ, Petito CK, Price RW. The Neurologic Complications of AIDS and Human Immunodeficiency Virus Infection. In FD Plum (ed), Advances in Contemporary Neurology. Philadelphia: F. A. Davis, 1988;1–49.

86. Bouwman FH, Skolasky RL, Hes D, et al. Variable progression of HIV-associated dementia. Neurology 1998;50: 1814–1820.

87. Wiley CA, Achim CL. Human immunodeficiency virus encephalitis is the pathological correlate of dementia in the acquired immunodeficiency syndrome. Ann Neurol 1994;36:673–676.

88. Gray F. Démence et infection par le virus de l'immunodéficience humaine. Revue Neurologique 1998;154(Suppl 2):S91–S98.

89. Epstein LG, Gendelman HE. Human immunodeficiency virus type 1 infection of the nervous system: pathogenetic mechanisms. Ann Neurol 1993;33(5):429–436.

90. Lipton SA. Neuropathogenesis of acquired immunodeficiency syndrome dementia. Curr Opin Neurol 1997; 10:247–253.

91. Price RW. Measuring the "viral load" in cerebrospinal fluid in human immunodeficiency virus infection: window into brain infection? Ann Neurol 1997;42:675–678.

92. Seilhean D, Michaud J, Duyckaerts C, Hauw J-J. Physiopathologie de l'infection du système nerveux par le VIH-1 et de la démence du SIDA. Revue Neurologique 1998;154:830–842.

93. Bagasra O, Hauptman SP, Harold DO, et al. Detection of human immunodeficiency virus type 1 provirus in mononuclear cells by in situ polymerase chain reaction. N Engl J Med 1992;326(21):1385–1391.

94. McKelvie PA, De Girolami U, Nasser I. Expression of endothelial adhesion molecules in HIV encephalopathy (Abst). J Neuropathol Exp Neurol 1992;51:354.

95. Seilhean D, Dzia-Lepfoundzou A, Sazdovitch V, et al. Astrocytic adhesion molecules are increased in HIV-1-associated cognitive/motor complex. Neuropathol Appl Neurobiol 1997;23:83–92.

96. Nottet HSLM, Persidsky Y, Sasseville VG, et al. Mechanisms for the transendothelial migration of HIV-1-infected monocytes into brain. J Immunol 1996;156:1284–1295.

97. Persidsky Y, Stins M, Way D, et al. A model for monocyte migration through the blood-brain barrier during HIV-1 encephalitis. J Immunol 1997;158:3499–3510.

98. Persidsky Y, Ghorpade A, Rasmussen J, et al. Microglial and astrocyte chemokines regulate monocyte migration through the blood-brain barrier in human immune deficiency virus-1 encephalitis. Am J Pathol 1999;155:1599–1611.

99. Brew BJ, Rosemblum M, Cronin K, Price RW. AIDS dementia complex and HIV-1 brain infection: clinical-virological correlations. Ann Neurol 1995;38:563–570.

100. Wiley CA, Soontornniyinjuj V, Radhakrishnan L, et al. Distribution of brain HIV load in AIDS. Brain Pathol 1998;8:277–284.

101. McArthur JC, McClernon DR, Cronin MF, et al. Relationship between human immunodeficiency virus-associated dementia and viral load in cerebrospinal fluid and brain. Ann Neurol 1997;42:689–698.

102. Bell JE, Brettle RP, Chiswick A, Simmonds P. HIV encephalitis, proviral load and dementia in drug users and homosexuals with AIDS. Brain 1998;121:2043–2052.

103. Johnson R, Glass J, McArthur J, Chesebro B. Quantitation of human immunodeficiency virus in brains of demented and nondemented patients with acquired immunodeficiency syndrome. Ann Neurol 1996;39:392–395.

104. Giulian D, Vaca K, Noonan CA. Secretion of neurotoxins by mononuclear phagocytes infected with HIV-1. Science 1990;250:1593–1596.

105. Pulliam L, Hendrier BG, Tang NM, McGrath MS. Human immunodeficiency virus-infected macrophages produce soluble factors that cause histological and neurochemical alterations in cultured human brains. J Clin Invest 1991;87:503–512.

106. Wilt SG, Milward E, Zhou JM, et al. In vitro evidence for dual role of tumor necrosis factor-α in human immunodeficiency virus type 1 encephalopathy. Ann Neurol 1995;37:381–394.

107. Adamson D, Wildemann B, Sasaki M, et al. Immunologic NO synthase: elevation in severe AIDS dementia and induction by HIV-1 gp41. Science 1996;274:1917–1921.

108. Rostay K, Monti L, Yiannoutsos C, et al. Human immunodeficiency virus infection, inducible nitric oxide synthase expression, and microglial activation: pathogenetic relationship to the acquired immunodeficiency syndrome dementia complex. Ann Neurol 1999;46:207–216.

109. Glass JD, Fedor H, Wesselingh SL, McArthur JC. Immunocytochemical quantitation of human immunodeficiency virus in the brain: correlations with dementia. Ann Neurol 1995;38:755–762.

110. Gartner S, Markovits P, Markovits DM, et al. Virus isolation from and identification of HTLV-III/LAV-producing cells in brain tissue from a patient with AIDS. JAMA 1986;256(17):2365–2371.

111. Lipton SA. Calcium channel antagonists and human immunodeficiency virus coat protein-mediated neuronal injury. Ann Neurol 1991;30:110–114.

112. Lipton SA. Models of neuronal injury in AIDS: another role for the NMDA receptor? Trends Neurosci 1992;15:75–79.

113. Lipton SA. Human immunodeficiency virus-infected macrophages, gp120 and N-methyl-D-aspartate neurotoxicity. Ann Neurol 1993;33:227–228.

114. Magnuson DSK, Knudsen BE, Geiger JD, et al. Human immunodeficiency virus type 1 Tat activates non-N-methyl-D-aspartate excitatory amino acid receptors and causes neurotoxicity. Ann Neurol 1995;37:373–380.

115. Tardieu M, Héry C, Peudenier S, et al. Human immunodeficiency virus type 1-infected monocytic cells can destroy human neural cells after cell-to-cell adhesion. Ann Neurol 1992;32(1):11–17.

116. Everall I, Luthert P, Lantos P. A review of neuronal damage in human immunodeficiency virus infection: its assessment, possible mechanism and relationship to dementia. J Neuropathol Exp Neurol 1993;52:561–566.

117. Ketzler S, Weis S, Haug H, Budka H. Loss of neurons in the frontal cortex in AIDS brains. Acta Neuropathol 1990;80:92–94.

118. Everall IP, Luthert PJ, Lantos PL. Neuronal loss in the frontal cortex in HIV infection. Lancet 1991;337:1119–1121.

119. Wiley CA, Masliah E, Morey M, et al. Necortical damage during HIV infection. Ann Neurol 1991;29:651–657.

120. Masliah E, Ge N, Achim CL, Hansen LA, Wiley CA. Selective neuronal vulnerability in HIV encephalitis. J Neuropathol Exp Neurol 1992;51(6):585–593.

121. Weis S, Haug H, Budka H. Neuronal damage in the cerebral cortex of AIDS brains: a morphometric study. Acta Neuropathol 1993;85:185–189.

122. Masliah E, Heaton R, Marcotte TD, et al. Dendritic injury is a pathological substrate for human immunodeficiency virus-related cognitive disorders. Ann Neurol 1997;42:963–972.

123. Everall IP, Heaton RK, Marcotte TD, et al. Cortical synaptic density is reduced in mild to moderate human immunodeficiency virus neurocognitive disorder. Brain Pathol 1999;9:209–217.

124. Sá MJ, Madeira MD, Rueda C, et al. AIDS does not alter the total number of neurons in the hippocampal formation but induces cell atrophy: a stereological study. Acta Neuropathol 2000;99:643–653.

125. Adle-Biassette H, Levy Y, Colombei M, et al. Neuronal apoptosis in HIV infection in adults. Neuropathol Appl Neurobiol 1995;21:218–227.

126. Petito CK, Roberts B. Evidence of apoptotic cell death in HIV encephalitis. Am J Pathol 1995;146:1121–1130.

127. An SF, Giometto B, Scaravilli T, et al. Programmed cell death in brains of HIV-1-positive AIDS and pre-AIDS patients. Acta Neuropathol 1996;91:169–173.

128. Kruman II, Nath A, Maragos WF, et al. Evidence that Par-4 participates in the pathogenesis of HIV encephalitis. Am J Pathol 1999;155:39–46.

129. Belman AL, Ultmann MH, Horoupian D, et al. Neurological complications in infants and children with acquired immune deficiency syndrome. Ann Neurol 1985;18:560–566.

130. Belman AL, Diamond G, Dickson D, et al. Pediatric acquired immunodeficiency syndrome. Am J Dis Child 1988;142:29–35.

131. Kozlowski PB, Snider DA, Vietze PM, Wisienwski HM. Brain in Pediatric AIDS. Basel: Karger, 1990.

132. Sharer LR, Epstein LG, Cho E-S, et al. Pathologic features of AIDS encephalopathy in children: evidence for LAV/HTLV-III infection of brain. Hum Pathol 1986; 17(3):271–284.

133. Dickson DW, Belman AL, Park YD, et al. Central nervous system pathology in pediatric AIDS: an autopsy study. APMIS 1989;(8 Suppl):40–57.

134. Cho E-S, Sharer LR. HIV Encephalopathy in Children. In PB Kozlowski, DA Snider, PM Vietze, HM Wisniewski (eds), Pathology of HIV Infection in Children. Basel: Krager, 1990.

135. Joshi VV. Pathology of HIV Infection in Children. In PB Kozlowski, DA Snider, PM Vietze, HM Wisniewski (eds), Brain in Pediatric AIDS. New York: Karger, 1990;122–131.

136. Keohane C, Jousselin CL, Dickson DW. Central Nervous System Pathology in Paediatric AIDS. In F Gray (ed), Atlas of the Neuropathology of HIV Infection. Oxford: Oxford University Press, 1993.

137. Vazeux R, Lacroix-Ciaudo C, Blanche S, et al. Low levels of human immunodeficiency virus replication in the brain tissue of children with severe acquired immunodeficiency syndrome encephalopathy. Am J Pathol 1992;140(1):137–144.

138. Lacroix C, Vazeux R, Brousse N, et al. Étude neuropathologique de 10 enfants infectés par le VIH. Revue Neurologique 1993;149:37–45.

139. Sharer L, Saito Y, Ca Cunha A, et al. In situ amplification and detection of HIV-1 DNA in fixed pediatric AIDS brain tissue. Hum Pathol 1996;27:614–617.

140. Brouwers P, DeCarli C, Civitello L, et al. Correlation between computed tomographic brain scan abnormalities and neuropsychological function in children with symptomatic human immunodeficiency virus disease. Arch Neurol 1995;52:39–44.

141. Gerhard HA, Sharer L, James H, et al. Apoptotic neurons are present in brains from children with HIV-encephalitis (abst). Neurology 1995;45(Suppl):507.

142. Goldstick L, Mandybur TI, Bode R. Spinal cord degeneration in AIDS. Neurology 1985;35:103–106.

143. Petito CK, Navia BA, Cho E-S, et al. Vacuolar myelopathy pathologically resembling subacute combined degeneration in patients with the acquired immunodeficiency syndrome. N Engl J Med 1985;312(14):874–879.

144. Tan SV, Guiloff RJ, Scaravilli S. AIDS-associated vacuolar myelopathy. A morphometric study. Brain 1995;118: 1247–1261.

145. Grafe MR, Wiley CA. Spinal cord and peripheral nerve pathology in AIDS: the roles of cytomegalovirus and human immunodeficiency virus. Ann Neurol 1989;25: 561–566.

146. Dal Pan GJ, Glass JD, McArthur JC. Clinicopathologic correlations of HIV-1-associated vacuolar myelopathy: an autopsy-based case control study. Neurology 1994;44: 2159–2164.

147. Shepherd EJ, Brettle RP, Liberski PP, et al. Spinal cord pathology and viral burden in homosexuals and drug abusers with AIDS. Neuropathol Appl Neurobiol 1999; 25:2–10.

148. Artigas J, Grosse G, Habedank S, et al. Zur Morphologie Vakuolärer Veränderungen des Rückenmarks bei AIDS-patienten (vakuoläre Myelopathie). Der Pathologe 1990; 11:260–267.

149. Artigas J, Grosse G, Niedobitek F. Vacuolar myelopathy in AIDS: a morphological analysis. Pathol Res Pract 1990;186:228–237.

150. Tan SV, Guiloff RJ. Hypothesis on the pathogenesis of vacuolar myelopathy, dementia, and peripheral neuropathy in AIDS. J Neurol Neurosurg Psychiatry 1998;65:23–28.

151. Budka H, Maier H, Pohl P. Human immunodeficiency virus in vacuolar myelopathy of the acquired immunodeficiency syndrome. N Engl J Med 1988;319:1667–1668.

152. Maier H, Budka H, Lassmann H, Pohl P. Vacuolar myelopathy with multinucleated giant cells in the acquired immune deficiency syndrome (AIDS): light and electron microscopic distribution of human immunodeficiency virus (HIV) antigens. Acta Neuropathol 1989;78:497–503.

153. Eilbott DJ, Peress N, Burger H, et al. Human immunodeficiency virus type 1 in spinal cords of acquired immunodeficiency syndrome patients with myelopathy: expression and replication in macrophages. Proc Natl Acad Sci U S A 1989;86:3337–3341.

154. Kamin SS, Petito CK. Vacuolar myelopathy in immunocompromised AIDS patients (abst). J Neuropathol Exp Neurol 1988;47:385.

155. Rosenblum M, Scheck A, Cronin K, et al. Dissociation of vacuolar myelopathy and detectable HIV-I infection of the spinal cord (abst). Lab Invest 1989;60:80A.

156. Sharer L, Epstein LG, Blumberg BM, et al. Histological and molecular probe analysis of spinal cords from children with HIV infection and AIDS. J Neuropathol Exp Neurol 1988;47.

157. Sharer LR, Dowling PC, Michaels J, et al. Spinal cord disease in children with HIV-1 infection: a combined molecular biological and neuropathological study. Neuropathol Appl Neurobiol 1990;16:317–331.

158. Dickson DW, Belman AL, Kim TS, et al. Spinal cord pathology in pediatric acquired immunodeficiency syndrome. Neurology 1989;39:227–235.

159. Schmidbauer M, Budka H, Okeda R, et al. Multifocal vacuolar leucoencephalopathy: a distinct HIV-associated lesion of the brain. Neuropathol Appl Neurobiol 1990;16: 437–443.

160. Vinters HV, Anders KH, Barach P. Focal pontine leukoencephalopathy in immunosuppressed patients. Arch Pathol Lab Med 1987;111:192–196.

161. Tan S, Guiloff R, Henderson D, et al. Aids-associated vacuolar myelopathy and tumor necrosis factor-alpha (TNFα). J Neurol Sci 1996;138:134–144.

162. Goudreau G, Carpenter S, Beaulieu N, Jolicoeur P. Vacuolar myelopathy in transgenic mice expressing human immunodeficiency virus type 1 proteins under the regulation of the myelin basic protein gene promoter. Nat Med 1996;2:655–661.

163. Rance NE, McArthur JC, Cornblatt DR, et al. Gracile tract degeneration in patients with sensory neuropathy and AIDS. Neurology 1988;38:265–271.

164. Jones HR, Ho DD, Forgacs P, et al. Acute fulminating fatal leukoencephalopathy as the only manifestation of

human immunodeficiency virus infection. Ann Neurol 1988;23:519–522.

165. Berger JR, Sheremata WA, Resnick L, et al. Multiple-sclerosis-like illness occurring with human immunodeficiency virus infection. Neurology 1989;39:324–329.

166. Gray F, Chimelli L, Mohr M, et al. Fulminating multiple sclerosis-like leukoencephalopathy revealing human immunodeficiency virus infection. Neurology 1991;41:105–109.

167. Silver B, McAvoy k, Mikesell S, Smith TW. Fulminating encephalopathy with perivenular demyelination and vacuolar myelopathy as the initial presentation of human immunodeficiency virus infection. Arch Neurol 1997;54:647–650.

168. Morgello S, Block GA, Price RW, Petito CK. Varicella-zoster virus leukoencephalitis and cerebral vasculopathy. Arch Pathol Lab Med 1988;112:173.

169. Gray F, Mohr M, Rozenberg F, et al. Varicella-zoster virus encephalitis in acquired immunodeficiency syndrome: report of four cases. Neuropathol Appl Neurobiol 1992;18:502–514.

170. Gray F, Bélec L, Lesce MC, et al. Varicella-zoster virus infection of the central nervous system in the acquired immune deficiency syndrome. Brain 1994;117:987–999.

171. Carrigan DR, Harrington DR, Knox KK. Subacute leukoencephalitis caused by CNS infection with herpesvirus-6 manifesting as acute multiple sclerosis. Neurology 1996;47:145–148.

Chapter 15

Polyomavirus-Induced Demyelination

Igor J. Koralnik

Historical Aspects

Progressive multifocal leukoencephalopathy (PML) is a myelin disorder caused by a lytic viral infection of oligodendrocytes. This disease was originally named in 1958 to describe a demyelinating condition of the central nervous system (CNS) occurring in patients with chronic lymphocytic leukemia and Hodgkin's lymphoma.[1] However, a similar clinical entity associating dementia and leukoencephalopathy had been described already in as early as 1930 by Hallervorden.[2] The histologic hallmarks of this disease are the presence of oligodendrocytes with enlarged nuclei and intranuclear inclusions located at the margins of areas of demyelination, associated with bizarre astrocytes and lipid-laden macrophages.

In 1959, the first clue of a possible viral etiology stemmed from the detection of inclusion bodies in the nuclei of damaged oligodendrocytes.[3] This finding was confirmed 6 years later, when intranuclear inclusions consisting of a dense array of viral particles resembling human polyomaviruses was detected by electron microscopy in oligodendrocytes.[4,5] A human polyomavirus now termed JC virus (JCV) was successfully isolated from the brain of a patient with PML after inoculation of human fetal glial cell cultures.[6] This virus was named according to the patient's initials, which subsequently caused some confusion with another disease of the brain initially thought to be caused by a virus, the prion protein–associated Jakob-Creutzfeldt disease.

Another similar virus was isolated around the same time from the urine of a renal transplant recipient and was named *BK virus*, again according to the patient's initials.[7] This virus, however, has never convincingly been linked to CNS disease. A simian polyomavirus, closely related to JCV and BK virus, was discovered in 1968 as a contaminant of polio vaccines grown in monkey kidney cells and was named *simian vacuolating virus 40* (SV40).[8] A PML-like disease caused by SV40 has been described in a few animals with advanced immunosuppression caused by the simian immunodeficiency virus.[9]

Epidemiology

Seroconversion for JCV occurs in childhood. The primary infection is asymptomatic and may be contracted via respiratory route or through urine-oral contamination. By mid-adulthood, 80–90% of patients have immunoglobulin G (IgG) antibodies against JCV.[10,11] PML was initially a rare condition, affecting a limited number of patients with lymphoproliferative diseases, such as Hodgkin's disease, chronic lymphocytic leukemia, and lymphosarcoma. PML was also described in patients with cancer or granulomatous and inflammatory diseases or in organ transplant recipients. Immune suppression was common among these patients. Therefore, it came as no surprise that at the beginning of the acquired immunodeficiency syndrome (AIDS) epidemic, PML quickly emerged as a major opportunistic infection of the brain, occurring in up to 4% of patients with AIDS.[12] In this population, PML occurs in patients between the ages of 20–50 years.[13] Interestingly, the proportion of PML cases among human immunodeficiency virus (HIV)–related focal brain lesions has increased from 16% before the availability of highly active antiretroviral therapy (HAART) to 28% in 1998.[14] Immunosuppressed children rarely develop PML, perhaps because of the lower percentages who have been exposed to JCV.

Clinical Presentation

PML occurs in patients with severe cellular immunosuppression. In patients with AIDS, PML is seen mainly when the CD4+ T-lymphocyte count drops to less than 200/μl. The clinical presentation is subacute, and, often, neurologic signs and symptoms indicate multiple localizations within the brain. Focal motor deficits, visual defects, and cognitive dysfunction are the most frequent manifestations of this disease. However, speech dysfunction and sensory and coordination deficit occur as well. Indeed, the clinical manifestations of PML are fairly variable, as JCV can infect oligodendrocytes anywhere in the CNS.

Unlike multiple sclerosis (MS), lesions of PML have the tendency to grow unremittingly, due to diffusion of infectious viral particles within the brain parenchyma, and they do not show relapsing-remitting features. A PML lesion can occupy the white matter of an entire hemisphere. However, the lesions are typically not associated with edema and mass effect, and death usually occurs by extension to the respiratory centers of the brain stem or due to other superimposed infectious complications. The clinical features of PML are similar among HIV-infected or HIV-negative immunosuppressed patients.

Diagnostic Procedures

Brain Imaging

Computed tomography of the brain shows hypodense areas in the affected white matter, which are usually devoid of mass effect and do not enhance with contrast. Magnetic resonance imaging is a more sensi-

tive test and shows hyperintense signals in T_2-weighted images in the affected white matter (Figure 15-1). As with computed tomography scan, contrast enhancement is rare. The lesions of PML can occur virtually anywhere in the CNS white matter and, although a predilection for the parieto-occipital lobes has been described, lesions are also found in the basal ganglia, the posterior fossa, the brain stem, and the spinal cord.[15] Other opportunistic infections of the brain, such as toxoplasmosis, cytomegalovirus encephalitis, or CNS lymphoma, also affect the white matter of immunosuppressed patients. However, these diseases are usually associated with edema, mass effect, and contrast enhancement. HIV encephalopathy can be easily mistaken for PML on brain imaging studies. As in PML, white-matter lesions without mass effect and contrast enhancement are the radiologic hallmarks of this disease. However, these lesions tend to be symmetric and less clearly demarcated than the lesions of PML, and they are not associated with focal neurologic deficits. In some cases, lesions of PML can be difficult to distinguish in a background of HIV encephalopathy. Recently, proton magnetic resonance spectroscopy and magnetization transfer studies have shown a promising potential in differentiating PML lesions from HIV encephalopathy.[16]

Cerebrospinal Fluid Analysis

Usual cerebrospinal fluid (CSF) studies are nondiagnostic for PML. CSF abnormalities include moderate mononuclear pleocytosis (fewer than 20 cells/μl) and elevation of proteins (less than 65 mg/dl), which is frequent in HIV infection.[17] Until a few years ago, confirmation of the diagnosis of PML required a brain biopsy. Polymerase chain reaction (PCR) detection of JCV DNA in the CSF has been evaluated in a number of studies and was shown to have a sensitivity of 74–93% and specificity of 92–100% for the diagnosis of PML, respectively.[18–20] CSF PCR has, therefore, been validated as an accurate diagnostic test for PML.

Histologic Studies

If JCV PCR in the CSF is negative or not readily available, a brain biopsy should be performed. His-

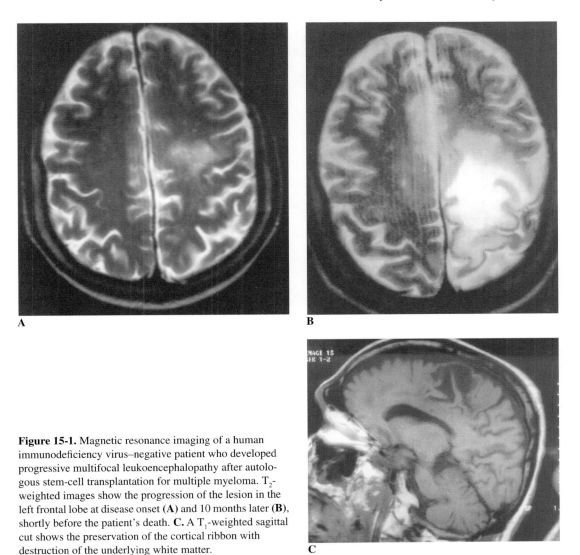

Figure 15-1. Magnetic resonance imaging of a human immunodeficiency virus–negative patient who developed progressive multifocal leukoencephalopathy after autologous stem-cell transplantation for multiple myeloma. T_2-weighted images show the progression of the lesion in the left frontal lobe at disease onset (**A**) and 10 months later (**B**), shortly before the patient's death. **C.** A T_1-weighted sagittal cut shows the preservation of the cortical ribbon with destruction of the underlying white matter.

tologic examination shows that the PML lesions consist of multiple areas of demyelination. They are variable in size, and the large ones appear often to be the result of coalescence of multiple expanding lesions. In some cases, lesions may become necrotic and form cavities. Whereas there is conspicuous loss of oligodendrocytes in the middle of the lesions, these cells display pathognomonic features in the periphery. The nuclei of JCV-infected oligodendrocytes are enlarged two to three times their normal diameter, and the chromatin pattern is altered, such that it appears amphophilic and

denser than normal. Other nuclei stain less densely but display marginated chromatin. Finally, some nuclei harbor irregularly outlined inclusion bodies.

In the center of PML lesions, lipid-laden macrophages are frequently found scavenging myelin and other cellular debris. In addition, reactive gliosis is present. Giant, bizarre astrocytes may be fairly prominent. These cells have pleomorphic, hyperchromatic nuclei, and they resemble the malignant astrocytes of pleomorphic glioblastomas.[5] This transformation is caused by a nonlytic restricted infection of astrocytes by JCV. Axons

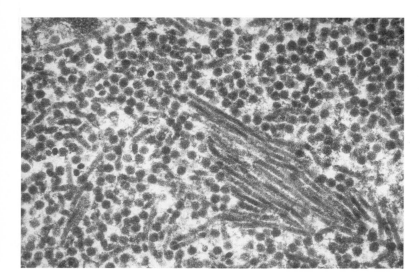

Figure 15-2. Electron microscopy in progressive multifocal leukoencephalopathy. A multitude of JC virions measuring 40 nm in diameter can be seen in the nuclei of infected oligodendrocytes.

going through the areas of demyelination are relatively spared unless necrosis is present. This is also true for neuronal cell bodies in lesions located at the gray-white junction.

The patient reported in Color Plate 25 (giant section and histology) had brain edema and mass effect, which have been described only in rare instances in patients with PML.[21,22] This is the first report of a postmortem analysis of such a form of PML, which indicated that PML alone was responsible for the swelling. This patient had a high CSF JCV DNA load (4.84×10^7 copies/ml). In addition, he had extremely high JCV DNA load in the brain (2.83×10^{10} copies/μg DNA). Although each copy of viral DNA might not correspond to the presence of one infectious viral particle, this finding suggests that a remarkably large number of JC virions were present within the necrotic PML lesions.

Despite the abundance of virions in the lesions of PML, a cellular inflammatory infiltrate is either sparse or absent. When they are present, perivascular mononucleated cell collections are usually small. This phenomenon has been attributed to the profound cellular immunosuppression found in patients who develop PML. Immunohistochemistry, immunoperoxidase, or in situ hybridization reveals the presence of JCV proteins or nucleic acid in infected oligodendrocytes. In situ PCR was also used to detect JCV DNA directly on histologic brain sections of patients with PML.[23,24] This technique was found to be two- to threefold more sensitive than in situ hybridization and confirmed the presence of JCV genome in infected oligodendrocytes and bizarre astrocytes. In addition, significant myelin staining was observed in the neuropil consistent with extracellular virus, suggesting that cell-to-cell contact might not be the only way for the virus to spread but that virus released after cell lysis could possibly also infect new cells.[23]

Electron microscopic studies (Figure 15-2) demonstrate that the enlarged nuclei of oligodendrocytes contain myriad polyomavirus virions that are sometimes densely packed in a crystal-like array. Particles measure approximately 40 nm in diameter. Only small numbers of virions can be found infrequently in the nuclei of astrocytes and in the cytoplasm of macrophages, presumably secondary to phagocytosis of myelin debris. Polyomaviruses are not found in neuronal cells.

Treatment

Despite the fact that the etiology of PML has been known for 30 years, there is still no specific treatment for this disease. There are several reasons for this. First, JCV is tedious to culture in vitro and grows only in primary human fetal glial cells or in few transformed astroglial cell lines. Testing of anti-JCV drugs in vitro is, therefore, difficult. Second, PML is a relatively rare disease, and large groups of patients can be gathered only in multicenter studies. Third, there is a large variability in the natural history of PML. Whereas some patients have a fulminant progression leading to death in few weeks, approximately 9% have a protracted course and a survival exceeding 1 year.[25] Therefore, claims of therapeutic success based on single case reports are often misleading, as they might occur in this population of long-term survivors regardless of their medications.

Over the years, several treatment regimens have been proposed for PML. Nucleoside analogs that act by interfering with the synthesis of viral DNA have been tried for the treatment of PML. Cytosine arabinoside (ARA-C), a drug usually used in the treatment of myeloproliferative disorders, was associated with anecdotal success[26,27] and failures.[28,29] The rationale for this drug was later confirmed after the demonstration that it inhibited JCV replication in vitro.[30] However, the first prospective randomized multicenter treatment study exploring the administration of ARA-C to HIV-positive patients with PML, intravenous or intrathecal, showed no benefit over placebo.[31] In HIV-negative patients with PML, treatment with intravenous ARA-C was associated with disease stabilization in 36% of cases in 1 year, but it was also associated with significant bone marrow toxicity.[32] Other nucleoside analogs, such as adenosine arabinoside and intrathecal idoxuridine in combination with prednisone, were unsuccessful.[33,34] JCV has a double-stranded circular DNA that needs to unwind to allow viral transcription and replication, a task performed by the enzyme topoisomerase. Therefore, camptothecin, a topoisomerase I inhibitor, has been tested in vitro and found to be efficient in blocking JCV replication in doses that were nontoxic to cells.[35] However, its use in patients with PML has been limited.[36,37] To our knowledge, there is no published report of a treatment trial using this medication in patients with PML.

Immunomodulatory agents, such as interferons, have been shown to have antiviral activity, presumably through activation of natural killer cells.[38] Interferon alpha-2A failed to show any promising results in a pilot study.[39] However, a retrospective study showed prolonged survival in one-third of patients treated with interferon alpha-2B as compared to historical controls.[40] However, the long-term follow-up of this patient population showed that interferon alpha-2B did not provide additional benefit when added to HAART.[41] A combined treatment using intravenous ARA-C and interferon beta was unsuccessful in one patient, but intrathecal infusion of interferon beta produced modest clinical and radiologic improvement.[42]

Cidofovir [(S)-1-(3-hydroxy-2-phosphonylmethoxypropyl)cytosine] is an antiviral nucleotide (nt) analog that has been shown to be effective in the treatment of cytomegalovirus retinitis,[43] papillomavirus-induced condilomata,[44,45] and molluscum contagiosum.[46] Cidofovir has recently been shown to be active in vitro in inhibiting the replication of mouse polyomavirus and SV40 in monkey kidney cells.[47] Preliminary reports indicate that cidofovir may be beneficial in the treatment of PML in patients with AIDS.[48–56] Our experience in six patients with AIDS and PML resulted in stabilization and moderate improvement in two and progressive disease with rapid fatal outcome in the other four patients.[57] A recent prospective study showed no additional benefit of cidofovir over HAART alone in HIV-positive patients with PML.[58] The mechanisms by which cidofovir affects JCV replication and spread in the CNS are still unclear. A recent report failed to confirm earlier in vitro studies carried out with animal polyomaviruses and showed that cidofovir had minimal activity against JCV replication in a human neuroglial cell line.[47] Indeed, cidofovir was less efficient than ARA-C in containing JCV replication in vitro.[30] New systems of drug delivery to the brain[59] or combination therapy including HAART, ARA-C, and cidofovir[49] or interferon alpha might be necessary to improve specific treatment in patients with AIDS and PML.

Treatment of PML in HIV-negative patients is even less standardized than in HIV-positive patients, because of the very small number of reported cases and the diversity of underlying diseases. Measures aiming to restore the patient's immune response or to reduce the dosage of immunosuppressant therapies should be favored in these cases. One patient with bone marrow transplantation improved after treatment with low doses of interleukin-2.[60]

Prognosis

The prognosis of PML is poor, both in HIV-infected patients and in patients affected with other immunosuppressive conditions. The median survival is approximately 6 months.[12,61,62] Since the availability of HAART, the survival of HIV-infected patients with PML has increased to 10.5 months.[63] However, approximately 9% of patients have prolonged survival exceeding 1 year. Predictive factors for longer survival include CD4[+] T-lymphocyte counts beyond 300/µl at disease onset, contrast enhancement on brain imaging studies, presence of a mononucleated perivascular inflammatory infiltrate in the PML lesions, absence of brain stem involvement, and PML heralding AIDS.[25]

The development of PML as first manifestation of AIDS is associated with a good prognosis as anti-HIV treatment can be initiated, with subsequent increase in CD4[+] T-lymphocyte counts and improvement of the patient's immune response. The outlook seems even better if the CD4[+] counts are not profoundly depressed at the onset of the disease. An intact brain stem is associated with a better survival because of the preservation of the respiratory centers. Lesions restricted to the cerebral hemispheres cause death only after extensive and bilateral involvement, leading to paralysis, coma, and secondary infectious complications. Contrast enhancement seen on imaging studies is a rare feature of PML and likely corresponds to a minor breakdown of the blood-brain barrier. This in turn might be associated with the presence of the perivascular inflammatory infiltrate that has independently been associated with a better prognosis.[64]

Virologic studies have also shed some light on the pathogenesis of JCV in PML. Measures of the CSF JC viral load at disease onset have shown that a high JC viral load in the CSF correlates with poor clinical outcome in HIV-infected patients with PML.[18] Analyses of JCV regulatory region (JCV RR) from kidney isolates show a very conserved sequence, which has therefore been called *the archetype*. Rearrangements, such as deletions and duplications of the RR, are usually observed in isolates from the CSF and brain of patients with PML. These changes occur in the setting of immunosuppression and might be implicated in neurotropism and neurovirulence. It is likely that JCV reaches the brain via the hematogenous route, but the events that trigger JC viremia are poorly understood. Sequence analysis from blood isolates of JCV suggests that the presence of a rearranged JCV RR in the plasma is associated with a poor

clinical outcome, whereas detection of archetype sequences in the blood is found in survivors of PML. It therefore appears that both the amount of virus present in CNS and the molecular structure of JCV RR are implicated in the patient's prognosis. (JCV sequence variation will be discussed further in JC Virus Genome.)

The host's immune response against JCV is also a crucial determinant for disease outcome. As the presence of antibodies against JCV does not protect against PML, the cellular immune response is likely instrumental in keeping JCV in check and preventing viral spread and the onset of PML. Indeed, PML occurs almost exclusively in patients with depressed cellular immunity. Study of the cellular immune response against JCV showed that detection of JCV-specific cytotoxic T-lymphocytes (CTLs) in the peripheral blood mononuclear cells (PBMCs) of HIV-infected patients with PML was associated with long-term survival, whereas those with an undetectable cellular immune response against the virus had a progressive neurologic disease and a fatal outcome.[57,65] (The cellular immune response against JCV will be discussed further in Immune Response Against JC Virus.)

In light of all these data, it appears that PML patients with good prognosis are less immunosuppressed at disease onset or benefit from anti-HIV drugs that improve their immune system. This in turn leads to a better control of JCV replication and prevents the development of mutations of the RR, leading to less virulent JCV strains. These patients have lesions sparing the vital respiratory centers of the brain stem. The presence of JCV-specific CTL in these patients may translate into inflammatory infiltrates around the PML lesions in the brain, which, in turn, may produce alterations of the blood-brain barrier and marginal enhancement seen on imaging studies. JCV-specific CTL destroys infected oligodendrocytes and prevents further disease progression. JCV viral load in the CSF, therefore, drops.

Immune Response Against JC Virus

The nature of the immune response that contains JCV in immunocompetent people and fails in immunosuppressed patients is unknown. Seroconversion occurs in childhood,[10] and IgG antibodies specific for JCV can be detected in approximately

90% of the normal adult population.[11] Pregnant women in the third trimester have a measurable rise of serum JCV antibodies.[66] The humoral immune response appears to be insufficient to prevent PML. Indeed, most patients with PML have pre-existing anti-JCV IgG antibody in their serum and do not demonstrate a rise in titer at the onset of neurologic disease. Intrathecal synthesis of IgG antibodies against the JCV VP1 protein has been detected in 76% of PML patients. However, no clinical or biologic differences were noted in these patients as compared to those without detectable JCV-specific antibodies in the CSF.[11] A rise in CSF JCV-specific antibodies did not prevent a fatal outcome in two patients with PML.[67,68] In addition, IgM antibodies have not been detected in the serum or CSF of patients with PML. Finally, JCV-specific antibodies do not prevent virus excretion in the urine in immunocompetent patients.[69] These data suggest that PML occurs due to a reactivation of a latent JCV infection rather than a primary infection.

Because JCV reactivation occurs as a consequence of immune suppression and humoral immunity does not appear to be critical in controlling JCV spread, cell-mediated immunity may play a central role in the containment of JCV. However, studies of this immune response have been limited. A generalized impairment of cell-mediated immunity in PML patients has been documented, with anergy in these patients to skin tests with common antigens[27,28,70,71] and impaired lymphocyte proliferation responses to the mitogen phytohemagglutinin,[27,72] to allogeneic cells,[72] and to JCV antigen.[73,74] More recently, the major histocompatibility complex (MHC) class I and class II molecules were found to be expressed at high levels within PML lesions, indicating that an absence of antigen presentation due to decreased MHC expression could not explain the uncontrolled replication of JCV within the CNS.[75]

In a recent study, JCV antigen–stimulated PBMC of four HIV-infected patients who were survivors of PML and one HIV-negative patient with recent-onset PML lysed autologous B lymphoblastoid cell lines expressing either the JCV T regulatory gene or the VP1 major capsid gene. This lysis was mediated by CD8+ CTL and was MHC class I restricted. JCV-specific CTL could not be detected in PBMC of three HIV-infected PML patients who had progressive neurologic disease and an eventual fatal outcome. These data suggest that JCV-specific cellular

immune response may play a crucial role in the containment of PML.[57,65]

CTLs recognize virus-infected cells through the interaction of their T-cell receptor and a 9–amino acid (aa) viral epitope presented by the MHC class I molecule of the infected cells. The human leukocyte antigen (HLA)–A*0201 allele is usually chosen for immunologic studies because it is the most commonly expressed MHC class I allele, present in 46% of the white population, 30% of the black population, and 43% of the Asian population.[76] Studies aimed to characterize the JCV epitope peptides presented by HLA-A*0201 to CTL have shown that a JCV VP1 nonamer peptide ($VP1_{p100}$) elicited a CTL response in HIV-positive PML survivors but not in patients who had a progressive neurologic disease and a fatal outcome. These results indicated that the $VP1_{p100}$ was indeed an epitope recognized by the CTL of HIV-positive PML survivors. To facilitate the quantitative analysis of JCV-specific CD8+ T-cell responses in vivo, a tetrameric HLA-A*0201/JCV peptide complex was constructed, using the newly defined VP1 epitope peptide. Staining with the tetrameric HLA-A*0201/$VP1_{p100}$ complex showed that the lymphocytes of HIV-positive PML survivors had between 1–12% $VP1_{p100}$-specific CD8+ cells after in vitro peptide stimulation.[77] These data indicate that staining with the tetramer complex is a rapid and reliable method to detect JCV-specific CTL and confirm the importance of the cellular immune response to JCV in the containment of PML. This finding may also prove useful as a favorable prognostic marker in the clinical management of these patients.

JC Virus Genome

JCV, BK virus, and SV40 belong to the polyomavirus genus within the family *Papoviridae*, together with mouse polyomavirus and several others. Another genus within this family contains the papillomaviruses. JCV is a double-stranded DNA virus, with a 5,130-bp circular supercoiled genome.[78] The initial clone was called *Mad-1*, according to the University of Wisconsin (Madison), where it was initially characterized. The entire viral sequence was cloned at the EcoR1 site of the pBR322 plasmid. The JCV genome (Figure 15-3) comprises three distinct functional regions: (1) the early region, located on the proximal side of the origin of

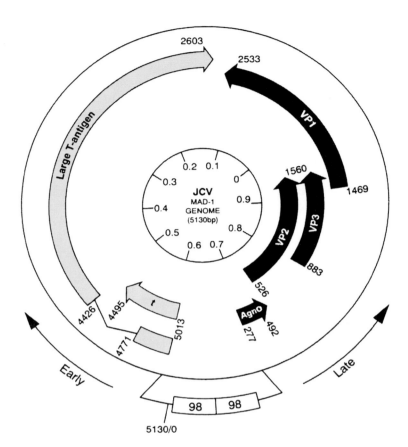

Figure 15-3. Map of the JC virus (JCV) Mad-1 genome. The numbers within the inside circle represent the map position, starting at the EcoR1 site. The early *t* and *T* genes and the late *Agno, VP1, VP2,* and *VP3* genes are depicted by arrows. The outside circle highlights the noncoding regulatory region of the viral genome, which includes two 98-bp tandem repeats. (Reprinted with permission from S Ohsumi, M Motoi, K Ogawa. Induction of undifferentiated tumors by JC virus in the cerebrum of rats. Acta Pathol Jpn 1986;36:815–825.)

replication; (2) the late region, located on the distal side of the origin of replication; and (3) the noncoding RR, located between the early and late regions, which contains the origin of replication, promoter, and enhancer regions of the virus (see Figure 15-3). Similarly to other polyomaviruses, JCV has two coding DNA strands. The early proteins T and t are transcribed counterclockwise, and the late proteins VP1, VP2, VP3, and agnoprotein are transcribed clockwise from the opposite strand.

Replication Cycle of the JC Virus

The cellular receptor for JCV is not known, although indirect evidence suggests that the JCV enters glial cells via interaction with an *N*-linked glycoprotein containing terminal α(2-6)–linked sialic acids.[79,80] This adsorption is mediated by the major viral capsid protein VP1. Entry into the cell occurs

by endocytosis, and virus-containing vesicles fuse with the nuclear membrane, delivering the virus into the nucleus. After uncoating of the virus, transcription of early messenger RNAs (mRNAs) is performed by the cell machinery and requires the presence of nuclear factor 1 (NF-1)–like proteins. NF-1 class D specifically binds to the JCV promoter. This protein is predominantly expressed in glial cells, which explains the narrow host-range of JCV in cells of glial lineage. After alternating splicing and transport to the cytoplasm, the early mRNAs are translated into the early proteins large T and small t. The large T protein is reimported into the nucleus and binds to the JCV origin of replication to initiate viral DNA synthesis. The T protein also stimulates late mRNA transcription. These mRNAs are exported into the cytoplasm and translated into the structural proteins VP1, VP2, and VP3. These capsid proteins are reimported into the nucleus and assemble around viral chromosomes to form prog-

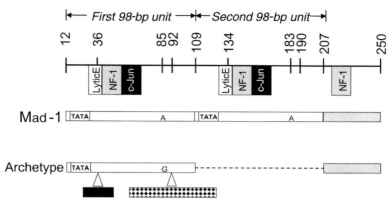

Figure 15-4. Map of the JC virus regulatory region. The numbers correspond to the nucleotide positions on the Mad-1 isolate. The known transcription regulation factor–binding sites are indicated and include the lytic control element (LyticE), nuclear factor 1 (NF-1), and c-Jun. Each 98-bp unit is represented by an open box. The TATA box is represented by TATA. The Mad-1 regulatory region found in the brain of a patient with progressive multifocal leukoencephalopathy has two identical 98-bp units, each containing a TATA box. The archetype regulatory region, found in the kidney of immunosuppressed and immunocompetent patients alike, contains only one 98-bp unit, with a 23-bp insert (*black box*) at position 36 and a 66-bp insert (*checkered box*) at position 92. The dotted lines represent deletions in the 98-bp units. (A = adenine; G = guanine.)

eny virions. The accumulation of JC virions in the nuclei of oligodendrocytes produces lysis of these cells and spread of JCV in the cerebral white matter.

JC Virus Proteins

The T protein is the main regulatory protein of JCV. It is the only JCV protein to be translated from a spliced mRNA. It is a 688-aa phosphoprotein of 83–96 kDa, which is required for the initiation of JCV DNA replication, and activates the switch from early to late gene transcription. It is also the main protein implicated in the induction of malignant cellular transformation. The function of the small t protein is less well understood. Its homolog in the SV40 appears to be a cofactor in cell transformation. It has been detected in transformed hamster cells[81] but has not been identified in infected human glial cells.[82] The 172-aa t protein shares its 5' end with the large T protein, but it is produced from an unspliced mRNA. Therefore, its 3' end is different from the T protein.

Four proteins are transcribed from the late genes sequences, clockwise and from the opposite strand as compared with the early gene sequences. The first open reading frame could encode a small protein of 71 aa. In SV40, a similar 7.9-kDa protein has been

called the *agnoprotein* because of its unknown function. The sequence of this protein is very conserved. It is able to bind DNA and appears to have a scaffolding role in viral assembly and maturation.[83] The largest open reading frame of the late region encodes a 354-aa VP1 protein of 43 kDa, which is the major capsid protein of JCV. The last two structural proteins are the 344-aa VP2 and 225-aa VP3 capsid proteins. The VP3 is a subset of the VP2 and is, therefore, identical to the 3' end of this protein. The VP1, VP2, and VP3 proteins agglomerate together to form the viral capsid. This icosahedral structure consists of 72 VP1 pentamer units containing either a VP2 or VP3 protein in their center.

JC Virus Regulatory Region

The JCV RR is a noncoding sequence located between the early and late genes and contains the origin of DNA replication, the promoter-enhancer sequences, as well as numerous binding sites for cellular factors (Figure 15-4). It is the most variable region of JCV and is also called the *ori-enhancer region*, or the *transcription control region*. The first complete JCV genome described was isolated from the brain of a patient with PML at the University of

Wisconsin (Madison) and was called the *Mad-1 strain*.[78] The nt numbers derive from this initial sequence. Its RR consists in two identical 98-bp tandem repeat sequences. As it was the first molecular clone of JCV, it has been extensively studied in vitro. Other PML isolates (called *Mad-2, -3,* and *-4*) and others were found to have a GC-rich 23-bp insertion at nt 36 and have a deleted TATA box in the second tandem repeat. They also had a 66-bp insert at nt 92. However, this 66-bp repeat was often truncated. The Mad-1 strain was, therefore, called a *type I*, and strains having the 23- and 66-bp inserts but having a deleted second TATA box, were called *type II*. Over the years, it appeared that type I strains are actually rare as compared to type II in the lesions of PML. Therefore, most of the studies performed using the Mad-1 clone have had to focus on a non-representative PML isolate. JCV genomes found in the urine of immunocompetent patients were found subsequently to have a different RR formed by a single unit without tandem repeats but with the 23-bp insert at nt 36 and the 66-bp insert at nt 92.[84] As all the elements detected in the previously described PML isolates were present in this urine-derived strain, it was presumed that all isolates were derived from this particular strain, which, as mentioned earlier, was called *the archetype*.

Since then, the archetype form of JCV RR was found worldwide to be the predominant strain isolated from the urine of immunocompetent and immunodeficient patients alike. By comparison to the archetype, tandem repeat forms have also been called *rearranged*, although it is not clear that the archetype is the strain that initially enters the body. Moreover, a recent study showed that 39% of tonsils from normal patients harbored JCV sequences. Most of the JCV RR sequences contained tandem repeats, predominantly of the Mad-1 and Mad-8 strains. These data suggest that tonsils may serve as an initial site of viral infection.[85] Therefore, a tandem-repeat strain might be responsible for primary infection via the respiratory route, whereas archetype strains are transmitted via the urine-oral route. In both cases, the immune system and selection pressure lead to the establishment of persistent infection in the kidneys with an archetype form of JCV. In any event, study of the archetype regulatory sequence in vitro has been hampered by its inability to grow in cell culture. Therefore, the apparition of mutations leading to the evolution of the archetype into a tandem repeat form has not been formally proven.

To attempt to answer this question, sequences of 198 clones from JCV RRs from blood and CNS from 16 patients were performed. These data indicate that several strains of JCV can exist in the same person. In one patient, four different JCV RRs were demonstrated, and an evolutionary gradient from archetype to tandem-repeat going from the urine to the blood and then to the CNS was apparent. In addition, patients with poor clinical outcomes have a high proportion of JCV RR clones, with both tandem-repeats in plasma and brain or CSF. In those who became survivors of PML, archetype sequences predominate in these anatomic compartments. In patients with advanced HIV infection without PML, very few of JCV RR clones obtained in the plasma contain tandem-repeats. These data suggest that the presence of tandem-repeats in plasma and in CNS JCV RR clones is associated with poor clinical outcome in patients with PML.[86]

JC Virus Regulation

A number of cis- and trans-acting factors that interact with JCV RRs have been determined.[87] These include binding sites for NF-1, NF-κB, LCP-1, c-Jun, and TFIID (reviewed in reference 88). The 23-bp insert seen in most PML isolates contains an SP1-binding site. The SP1 sites contribute to the transcription from the viral early or late promoter.[89] In addition, a region containing a pentanucleotide repeat sequence in the JCV RR, called the *lytic control element*, has been shown positively and negatively to regulate JCV early and late promoter transcription, respectively, and plays an important role in viral DNA replication.[90] Thus, the relative abundance of transcription factors, such as Tst-1, NF-1, and SP1, in glial cells may be responsible for the neurotropism of JCV.

JC Virus Coding Region

Opposite to the high variability seen in the JCV RR, the JCV coding region is highly conserved. However, several genotypes have been described, based mainly on point mutations of either the T or the VP1 genes, and correspond to the geographic origins of the patients. Types 1A and 1B are found in Europeans; types 2A, 2B, and 2C in Asians; and type 3 in Africans. In the United States, type 1 is found in patients of European origin and type 3 in those with African ancestry. Interestingly, type 2A is also found in native Americans. Minor types 4–7 have also been described.[91] The nt differences found in the coding region between different types is only approximately 1–4%, and the differences in amino acids is even smaller. Whether these small genotypic and phenotypic differences have any influence on disease pathogenesis is still unclear. Sequence analysis of strains from urine of normal people and brain of patients with PML indicate that genotype 2B is more prevalent in PML lesions (36.0% vs. 5.9%).[92] However, the urine of these patients with PML was not tested in this study.

Host Cell Range

In vivo, JCV can productively infect oligodendrocytes of immunosuppressed patients and epithelial tubular cells of the kidney in healthy subjects. Restrictive infection of astrocytes is seen within the lesions of PML. How JCV reaches the CNS from its stage of latency in the kidney remains uncertain. Hematogenous spread, however, is a likely mechanism. The type of blood cells that carry JCV in the blood has been investigated. JCV has been detected in two patients with PML in bone marrow lymphocytes bearing kappa light chains,[93] in one in CD45R-positive cells in the brain,[94] and in another in peripheral blood B-lymphocytes.[95] Between 1.0–5.9% of cells from transformed B-lymphocyte lines,[96] hematopoietic progenitor cell lines, and primary tonsillar B-lymphocytes have been infected in vitro with JCV.[95] This virus has also been detected in B-lymphocyte–depleted peripheral blood leukocytes of HIV-infected patients[97] and in brain macrophages of patients with PML.[98–100] Finally, JCV has been found in cell-free plasma of immunosuppressed patients.[18,97,101] To determine the peripheral blood cell subpopulation infected with JCV, monocytes, granulocytes, and T- and B-lymphocytes from HIV-1–infected patients and uninfected controls were purified by flow cytometry. JCV DNA could be detected by PCR amplification in all these cell subpopulations as well as in cell-free plasma, which

indicates that this virus lacks specificity in its interaction with leukocytes.[102] The receptor for JCV on cells is still unknown. In fact, it is possible that the cell-associated JCV DNA detected in this study came from viral particles sticking nonspecifically to the surface of cells and not from productively infected blood cells. Indeed, JCV seems to be present in blood during viral latency, as JCV RNA, an indicator of active viral replication, was found in the blood of only 1 of 72 HIV-infected patients.[97]

In vitro experiments using labeled JC virions and blood from a normal human volunteer indicated that JCV binds preferentially to B cells as compared to T cells. However, these experiments were not performed using the blood of an end-stage AIDS patient, which would have been more representative of the in vivo situation. In addition, JCV did bind all the cell lines tested from B or T origin as well as monkey and mouse cell lines. Treatment with trypsin of the PBMC or the B-cell line previously incubated with JCV significantly reduced the ability of these cells to transmit JCV to glial cells, indicating that the majority of transmitted virus was cell surface–associated.[103] A very low level of JCV replication was detected in the Namalwa B cell line after incubation with JCV in vitro, which was detectable only with nested reverse transcriptase PCR but not after one single round of amplification.

Contrary to glial cells, neuraminidase treatment of Namalwa B cell did not abrogate infection of these cells by JCV or the level of JCV RNA detected in these cells 24 hours after infection. It reduced only somewhat their ability to transmit virus to glial cells, indicating that the majority of virions associated with this B-cell line remain cell surface–associated and that only a minority of virus establishes infection.[103] Together with the fact that JCV can be found in cell-free plasma, these data indicate that white blood cells are likely to be innocent bystanders in the transport of JCV throughout the body but do not sustain significant viral replication in vivo.

JC Virus Culture

In vitro, JCV can be cultivated in primary human fetal glial cells and in a few transformed astroglial cell lines. The SVG cell line contains an origin-defective mutant of SV40[104] and expresses the SV40

T protein, whereas the POJ cell line has been transformed with an origin-defective mutant of JCV and expresses JCV T protein.[105] JCV could not be propagated successfully in human embryonic kidney, lung, liver, amnion, and intestine cells. To determine whether the crucial step restricting JCV replication in these cells was at the level of virion adsorption and penetration, full-length JCV circular genomic DNA was transfected in embryonic glial, lung, and kidney cells. All four isolates tested were able to induce the production of JC virions in glial cells, but only Mad-4 DNA was able to produce detectable viral proteins in non-glial cells. This indicates that cellular factors controlling early JCV transcription and replication, and not JCV entry into cells, were responsible for the narrow host-cell range of this virus. Serial passage of the Mad-1 strain in human embryonic kidney cells resulted in an adapted strain of JCV (JCV-HEK),[106] which had important mutations in the RR not found in wild-type isolates. Therefore, both the availability of cellular factors and the composition of JCV RR are the major determinants of host range in vivo and in vitro.

JC Virus Oncogenic Potential

Like other members of the polyomavirus family, JCV has oncogenic potential. Eighty-three percent of newborn Syrian hamsters inoculated intracutaneously or subcutaneously with JCV develop tumors of the CNS, including glioblastomas, medulloblastomas, primitive neuroectodermal tumor, and papillary ependymomas.[107] The type and the location of the tumor was, in part, dependent on the route of administration and the strain of JCV used. Intraocular inoculation was responsible for retinoblastomas and metastatic neuroblastoma.[108] Mad-1 and -2 tended to induce cerebellar medulloblastomas and gliomas, whereas Mad-4 was associated with pineocytomas and medulloblastomas. JCV DNA was integrated in the transformed hamster cells, and the T protein could be demonstrated in tumor cells explanted in tissue culture. Infectious virions were obtained after cocultivation with human glial cells. The T protein could bind the p53 protein as well as the retinoblastoma protein.[109,110]

JCV was found to be oncogenic in new-world monkeys as well. Two of four adult owl monkeys treated with prednisone to induce immunosuppression developed high-grade gliomas 1.5–2.0 years after inoculation. JCV T protein, but not the viral capsid proteins, were detected by immunohistochemistry, and infectious virions could not be isolated from the tumor.[111] JCV genome was integrated into the cellular DNA at a limited number of sites, and JCV T protein was not complexed with the host p53 protein.[112] One of four owl monkeys inoculated with a suspension of explanted JCV-induced glioblastoma cells developed a glioblastoma after 2 years. This tumor was again found to be T protein–positive and to harbor JCV DNA, this time both integrated and episomal. JCV virions could be isolated by successive passage, and DNA analysis revealed a 19-bp deletion in the second 98-bp repeat similar to the one found in the Mad-4 strain. This time, the T protein from this isolate was able to complex with the p53 protein of the cells.[113] Hamster brain cells could also be transformed in vitro and expressed JCV T protein but not the structural capsid proteins or infectious virions.[81] A similar phenomenon was observed after transfection of cloned Mad-1 genome into human amnion cells, suggesting that there was a block to late *JCV* gene transcription and viral DNA replication.

The oncogenic potential of JCV was also investigated in humans. JCV T antigen was not detected in 16 types of human CNS tumors, including glioblastomas, medulloblastomas, and ependymomas, using immunohistochemistry.[114] Eleven different types of CNS tumors were also negative by in situ hybridization for JCV DNA.[115] Similarly, JCV T antigen DNA sequence could not be found by PCR in 20 choroid plexus neoplasms and 11 ependymomas from pediatric patients. The absence of JCV DNA was also demonstrated in retinoblastomas.[116] Recently, JCV DNA sequences were found in 22 of 23 (95%) of human medulloblastomas by PCR, and the T antigen was detected by immunohistochemistry in 4 of 16 (25%) of these tumors.[117] However, these results were not confirmed by others, who reported the presence of JCV DNA in 0 of 17,[118] 0 of 8,[119] 0 of 15,[120] and 2 of 116[121] medulloblastomas.

JC Virus in Transgenic Mice

Further insights into JCV-associated demyelination have been brought by transgenic mice experiments.

Some of the transgenic mice containing the T protein and JCV RR display mild to severe tremor during movements, caused by dysmyelination of the CNS but not the peripheral nervous system.[122] The brain of these mice had normal axons but absence of myelin sheets and reduced levels of myelin basic protein (MBP), proteolipid protein, and myelin-associated glycoprotein. The *PLP* and *MBP* gene expression was reduced. This suggested that JCV T protein was responsible for decreasing MBP and proteolipid protein syntheses, thus hampering the maturation of oligodendrocytes in a model clearly different from the lytic infection of these cells caused by the production of mature virions in PML lesions.

Transgenic mice experiments also indicated that JCV T protein under the control of the viral early promoter was expressed primarily in cells of neural crest origin.[123] JCV early promoter, not JCV T protein, was found to be responsible for the restricted glial specificity.[124] In addition, both DNA replication and late gene transactivation have been documented in non-glial cells when the JCV early proteins were provided.[125,126] Non-glial cells may also contain cellular factors that act negatively on the JCV early promoter. Indeed, extinction of the expression of JCV early gene product was described in transformed hamster glial cells after fusion with mouse fibroblast cells.[123]

Purα is a single-stranded DNA-binding protein that binds to the GC-rich region of the MBP promoter and stimulates its expression both in vivo and in vitro.[127,128] It also binds the lytic control element of JCV RR. Purα was found to be associated with JCV T antigen in extracts from transgenic mice brains.[129] *Purα* gene expression was found to be reduced in oligodendrocytes infected with JCV in vitro. Therefore, in the early events after JCV infection of a glial cell, JCV T ag and its association with *Purα* may decrease the level of MBP expression and myelination. Interestingly, the association of *Purα* with JCV T antigen also decreases the ability of the T antigen to transactivate the JCV late promoter.[130] Thus, this early interaction between the T antigen and *Purα* also initially prevents the T antigen to trigger the late stage of the viral infection cycle and allows continuous production of the T antigen in the infected cells. In time, accumulation of T antigen in the cell will be sufficient to stimulate late gene transcription, production of vir-

ions, and lysis of the cells. These experiments indicate that the T antigen is not only a key element in the regulation of JCV lytic cycle but also may impair the normal function of oligodendrocytes by binding to cellular regulatory proteins and hampering their regulatory functions.

JC Virus and Multiple Sclerosis

Similarly to many other viruses, a possible association between JCV and MS has also been investigated.[131] However, JCV DNA was not found by PCR in the brains of MS patients.[132] In addition, excretion of JCV in the urine of MS patients was found to be similar in both genotype and frequency to that of controls and appeared to be regulated by factors unrelated to those that control CNS disease activity.[133] Therefore, there is no evidence that a direct link exists between JCV infection and MS. Recently however, the human herpesvirus 6 has been found within lesions of both PML and MS.[134,135] Although human herpesvirus 6 is a ubiquitous virus that can be found in normal brain as well, a potential synergistic activity between this virus and JCV in PML needs, therefore, to be investigated further. Similarly, the human herpesvirus 6 role in MS, if any, deserves further study.

Future Areas of Research

JCV was identified as the agent of PML 30 years ago. However, the determinants of latency, reactivation, neurotropism, and neurovirulence are still incompletely understood. Despite the fact that HAART has prolonged the average survival of HIV-infected patients with PML, there is no specific treatment for this disease, which continues to occur in patients with AIDS despite efficient antiretroviral treatment. PML remains one of the most lethal opportunistic infections in HIV disease. In addition, the incidence of PML is likely to increase in the HIV-negative population as well because of the growing numbers of organ transplant recipients.

As there is currently no specific treatment for PML, the characterization of the cellular immunity against JCV will be necessary to devise vaccination strategies aiming to enhance the immune response against this virus and prevent the development of PML in immunosuppressed patients. Understanding the molecular alterations of JCV RR implicated in the neurotropism and neurovirulence will also be particularly important. Because of its small size and circular nature, JCV genomic DNA could then become a useful tool as a vector for gene therapy targeted to oligodendrocytes, either in MS or in oligodendroglial tumors.

References

1. Astrom KE, Mancall EL, Richardson EP. Progressive multifocal leukoencephalopathy. Brain 1958;81:93–127.
2. Hallervorden J. Eigennartige und nicht rubriziebare Prozesse. In O Bumke (ed), Handbuch der Geiteskranheiten, vol. 2. Die Anatomie der Psychosen. Berlin: Springer, 1930;1063–1107.
3. Cavanaugh JB, Greenbaum D, Marshall A, Rubinstein L. Cerebral demyelination associated with disorders of the reticuloendothelial system. Lancet 1959;524–529.
4. Zu Rhein GM, Chou S-M. Particles resembling papova viruses in human cerebral demyelinating disease. Science 1965;148:1477–1479.
5. ZuRhein GM. Association of papova-virions with a human demyelinating disease (progressive multifocal leukoencephalopathy). Prog Med Virol 1969;11:185–247.
6. Padgett BL, Walker DL, ZuRhein GM, et al. Cultivation of papova-like virus from human brain with progressive multifocal leucoencephalopathy. Lancet 1971;1:1257–1260.
7. Gardner SD, Field AM, Coleman DV, Hulme B. New human papovavirus (B.K.) isolated from urine after renal transplantation. Lancet 1971;1:1253–1257.
8. Hilleman MR. Discovery of simian virus 40 (SV40) and its relationship to poliomyelitis virus vaccines. Dev Biol Stand 1998;94:183–190.
9. Holmberg CA, Gribble DH, Takemoto KK, et al. Isolation of simian virus 40 from rhesus monkeys (*Macaca mulatta*) with spontaneous progressive multifocal leukoencephalopathy. J Infect Dis 1977;136:593–596.
10. Walker DL, Padgett BL. The epidemiology of human polyomaviruses. Prog Clin Biol Res 1983;105:99–106.
11. Weber T, Trebst C, Frye S, et al. Analysis of the systemic and intrathecal humoral immune response in progressive multifocal leukoencephalopathy. J Infect Dis 1997;176: 250–254.
12. Berger JR, Kaszovitz B, Post MJ, Dickinson G. Progressive multifocal leukoencephalopathy associated with human immunodeficiency virus infection. A review of the literature with a report of sixteen cases. Ann Intern Med 1987; 107:78–87.
13. Holman RC, Janssen RS, Buehler JW, et al. Epidemiology of progressive multifocal leukoencephalopathy in the United States: analysis of national mortality and AIDS surveillance data. Neurology 1991;41:1733–1736.
14. Ammassari A, Cingolani A, Pezzotti P, et al. AIDS-related focal brain lesions in the era of highly active antiretroviral therapy. Neurology 2000;55:1194–1200.
15. Whiteman ML, Post MJ, Berger JR, et al. Progressive multifocal leukoencephalopathy in 47 HIV-seropositive patients: neuroimaging with clinical and pathologic correlation. Radiology 1993;187:233–240.
16. Chang L, Ernst T, Tornatore C, et al. Metabolite abnormalities in progressive multifocal leukoencephalopathy by proton magnetic resonance spectroscopy. Neurology 1997;48:836–845.
17. Marshall DW, Brey RL, Cahill WT, et al. Spectrum of cerebrospinal fluid findings in various stages of human immunodeficiency virus infection. Arch Neurol 1988;45: 954–958.
18. Koralnik IJ, Boden D, Mai VX, et al. JC virus DNA load in patients with and without progressive multifocal leukoencephalopathy. Neurology 1999;52:253–260.
19. McGuire D, Barhite S, Hollander H, Miles M. JC virus DNA in cerebrospinal fluid of human immunodeficiency virus-infected patients: predictive value for progressive multifocal leukoencephalopathy [published erratum appears in Ann Neurol 1995;37(5):687]. Ann Neurol 1995; 37:395–399.
20. Moret H, Guichard M, Matheron S, et al. Virological diagnosis of progressive multifocal leukoencephalopathy: detection of JC virus DNA in cerebrospinal fluid and brain tissue of AIDS patients. J Clin Microbiol 1993;31:3310–3313.
21. Finelli PF. Images in neurology. Mass effect in progressive multifocal leukoencephalopathy. Arch Neurol 1998; 55:1148–1149.
22. Thurnher MM, Thurnher SA, Muhlbauer B, et al. Progressive multifocal leukoencephalopathy in AIDS: initial and follow-up CT and MRI. Neuroradiology 1997;39:611–618.
23. Samorei IW, Schmid M, Pawlita M, et al. High sensitivity detection of JC-virus DNA in postmortem brain tissue by in situ PCR. J Neurovirol 2000;6:61–74.
24. Ueki K, Richardson EP Jr., Henson JW, Louis DN. In situ polymerase chain reaction demonstration of JC virus in progressive multifocal leukoencephalopathy, including an index case. Ann Neurol 1994;36:670–673.
25. Berger JR, Levy RM, Flomenhoft D, Dobbs M. Predictive factors for prolonged survival in acquired immunodeficiency syndrome-associated progressive multifocal leukoencephalopathy. Ann Neurol 1998;44:341–349.
26. Bauer WR, Turel AP Jr., Johnson KP. Progressive multifocal leukoencephalopathy and cytarabine. Remission with treatment. JAMA 1973;226:174–176.
27. Marriott PJ, O'Brien MD, Mackenzie IC, Janota I. Progressive multifocal leucoencephalopathy: remission with cytarabine. J Neurol Neurosurg Psychiatry 1975;38:205–209.
28. Horn GV, Bastian FO, Moake JL. Progressive multifocal leukoencephalopathy: failure of response to transfer factor and cytarabine. Neurology 1978;28:794–797.
29. Smith CR, Sima AA, Salit IE, Gentili F. Progressive multifocal leukoencephalopathy: failure of cytarabine therapy. Neurology 1982;32:200–203.
30. Hou J, Major EO. The efficacy of nucleoside analogs against JC virus multiplication in a persistently infected human fetal brain cell line. J Neurovirol 1998;4:451–456.
31. Hall CD, Dafni U, Simpson D, et al. Failure of cytarabine in progressive multifocal leukoencephalopathy associated with human immunodeficiency virus infection. AIDS

Clinical Trials Group 243 Team. N Engl J Med 1998;338: 1345–1351.

32. Aksamit AJ. Treatment of non-AIDS progressive multifocal leukoencephalopathy with cytosine arabinoside. J Neurovirol 2001;7:386–390.

33. Tarsy D, Holden EM, Segarra JM, et al. 5-Iodo-2' deoxyuridine (IUDR; NSC-39661) given intraventricularly in the treatment of progressive multifocal leukoencephalopathy. Cancer Chemother Rep 1973;57:73–78.

34. Wolinsky JS, Johnson KP, Rand K, Merigan TC. Progressive multifocal leukoencephalopathy: clinical pathological correlates and failure of a drug trial in two patients. Trans Am Neurol Assoc 1976;101:81–82.

35. Kerr DA, Chang CF, Gordon J, et al. Inhibition of human neurotropic virus (JCV) DNA replication in glial cells by camptothecin. Virology 1993;196:612–618.

36. O'Reilly S. Efficacy of camptothecin in progressive multifocal leucoencephalopathy [letter]. Lancet 1997;350: 291.

37. Vollmer-Haase J, Young P, Ringelstein EB. Efficacy of camptothecin in progressive multifocal leucoencephalopathy [letter]. Lancet 1997;349:1366.

38. Tyring SK, Cauda R, Ghanta V, Hiramoto R. Activation of natural killer cell function during interferon-alpha treatment of patients with condyloma acuminatum is predictive of clinical response. J Biol Regul Homeost Agents 1988;2:63–66.

39. Berger JR, Pall L, McArthur J. A pilot study of recombinant alpha 2A interferon in the treatment of AIDS-related progressive multifocal leukoencephalopathy. Neurology 1992;(abst):42.

40. Huang SS, Skolasky RL, Dal Pan GJ, et al. Survival prolongation in HIV-associated progressive multifocal leukoencephalopathy treated with alpha-interferon: an observational study. J Neurovirol 1998;4:324–332.

41. Geschwind MD, Skolasky RI, Royal WS, McArthur JC. The relative contributions of HAART and alpha-interferon for therapy of progressive multifocal leukoencephalopathy in AIDS. J Neurovirol 2001;7:353–357.

42. Tashiro K, Doi S, Moriwaka F, et al. Progressive multifocal leucoencephalopathy with magnetic resonance imaging verification and therapeutic trials with interferon. J Neurol 1987;234:427–429.

43. Kirsch LS, Arevalo JF, De Clercq E, et al. Phase I/II study of intravitreal cidofovir for the treatment of cytomegalovirus retinitis in patients with the acquired immunodeficiency syndrome. Am J Ophthalmol 1995;119:466–476.

44. Snoeck R, Van Ranst M, Andrei G, et al. Treatment of anogenital papillomavirus infections with an acyclic nucleoside phosphonate analogue [letter]. N Engl J Med 1995;333:943–944.

45. Van Cutsem E, Snoeck R, Van Ranst M, et al. Successful treatment of a squamous papilloma of the hypopharynx-esophagus by local injections of (S)-1-(3-hydroxy-2-phosphonylmethoxypropyl)cytosine. J Med Virol 1995;45: 230–235.

46. Meadows KP, Tyring SK, Pavia AT, Rallis TM. Resolution of recalcitrant molluscum contagiosum virus lesions in human immunodeficiency virus-infected patients treated with cidofovir. Arch Dermatol 1997;133:987–990.

47. Andrei G, Snoeck R, Vandeputte M, De Clercq E. Activities of various compounds against murine and primate polyomaviruses. Antimicrob Agents Chemother 1997;41: 587–593.

48. Al-Shahi R, Sadler M, Davies E, et al. Progressive multifocal leukoencephalopathy treatment with cidofovir. International Conference on AIDS. Geneva, Switzerland, 1998.

49. Blick G, Whiteside M, Griegor P, et al. Successful resolution of progressive multifocal leukoencephalopathy after combination therapy with cidofovir and cytosine arabinoside. Clin Infect Dis 1998;26:191–192.

50. Brambilla AM, Castagna A, Novati R, et al. Remission of AIDS-associated progressive multifocal leukoencephalopathy after cidofovir therapy [letter]. J Neurol 1999;246: 723–725.

51. De Luca A, Fantoni M, Tartaglione T, Antinori A. Response to cidofovir after failure of antiretroviral therapy alone in AIDS-associated progressive multifocal leukoencephalopathy. Neurology 1999;52:891–892.

52. Happe S, Besselmann M, Matheja P, et al. [Cidofovir (vistide) in therapy of progressive multifocal leukoencephalopathy in AIDS. Review of the literature and report of 2 cases.] Nervenarzt 1999;70:935–543.

53. Meylan PR, Vuadens P, Maeder P, et al. Monitoring the response of AIDS-related progressive multifocal leukoencephalopathy to HAART and cidofovir by PCR for JC virus DNA in the CSF. Eur Neurol 1999;41:172–174.

54. Taoufik Y, Gasnault J, Karaterki A, et al. Prognostic value of JC virus load in cerebrospinal fluid of patients with progressive multifocal leukoencephalopathy. J Infect Dis 1998;178:1816–1820.

55. De Luca A, Giancola ML, Ammassari A, et al. Cidofovir added to HAART imporves virological and clinical outcomes in AIDS-associated progressive multifocal leukoencephalopathy. AIDS 2000;14:F117–F121.

56. De Luca A, Giancola ML, Ammassari A, et al. Potent antiretroviral therapy with or without cidofovir for AIDS-associated progressive multifocal leukoencephalopathy: extended follow-up of an observational study. J Neurovirol 2001;7:364–368.

57. Du Pasquier RA, Clark KW, Smith PS, et al. JCV-specific cellular immune response correlates with a favorable clinical outcome in HIV-infected individuals with progressive multifocal leukoencephalopathy. J Neurovirol 2001;7(4): 318–322.

58. Gasnault J, Kousignian P, Kahraman M, et al. Cidofovir in AIDS-associated progressive multifocal leukoencephalopathy: a monocenter observational study with clinical and JC virus load monitoring. J Neurovirol 2001;7:375–381.

59. Levy RM, Ward S, Schalgeter K, Groothuis D. Alternative delivery systems for antiviral nucleosides and antisense oligonucleotides to the brain. J Neurovirol 1997;3:S74–S75.

60. Przepiorka D, Jaeckle KA, Birdwell RR, et al. Successful treatment of progressive multifocal leukoencephalopathy with low-dose interleukin-2. Bone Marrow Transplant 1997;20:983–987.

61. Berger JR, Pall L, Lanska D, Whiteman M. Progressive multifocal leukoencephalopathy in patients with HIV infection. J Neurovirol 1998;4:59–68.

62. Fong IW, Toma E. The natural history of progressive mul-

tifocal leukoencephalopathy in patients with AIDS. Canadian PML Study Group. Clin Infect Dis 1995;20:1305–1310.

63. Tantisiriwat W, Tebas P, Clifford DB, et al. Progressive multifocal leukoencephalopathy in patients with AIDS receiving highly active antiretroviral therapy. Clin Infect Dis 1999;28:1152–1154.

64. Richardson EP Jr., Johnson PC. Atypical progressive multifocal leukoencephalopathy with plasma-cell infiltrates. Acta Neuropathol Suppl (Berl) 1975;Suppl 6:247–250.

65. Koralnik IJ, Du Pasquier RA, Letvin NL. JC virus-specific cytotoxic T lymphocytes in individuals with progressive multifocal leukoencephalopathy. J Virol 2001;75:3483–3487.

66. Daniel R, Shah K, Madden D, Stagno S. Serological Investigation of the possibility of congenital transmission of papovavirus JC. Infect Immun 1981;33:319–321.

67. Berner B, Krieter DH, Rumpf KW, et al. Progressive multifocal leukoencephalopathy in a renal transplant patient diagnosed by JCV-specific DNA amplification and an intrathecal humoral immune response to recombinant virus protein 1. Nephrol Dial Transplant 1999;14:462–465.

68. Guillaume B, Sindic CJ, Weber T. Progressive multifocal leukoencephalopathy: simultaneous detection of JCV DNA and anti-JCV antibodies in the cerebrospinal fluid. Eur J Neurol 2000;7:101–106.

69. Coleman DV, Gardner SD, Mulholland C, et al. Human polyomavirus in pregnancy. A model for the study of defence mechanisms to virus reactivation. Clin Exp Immunol 1983;53:289–296.

70. Ellison GW. Progressive multifocal leukoencephalopathy (PML). I. Investigation of the immunologic status of a patient with lymphosarcoma and PML. J Neuropathol Exp Neurol 1969;28:501–506.

71. Mathews T, Wisotzkey H, Moossy J. Multiple central nervous system infections in progressive multifocal leukoencephalopathy. Neurology 1976;26:9–14.

72. Knight A, O'Brien P, Osoba D. "Spontaneous" progressive multifocal leukoencephalopathy. Immunologic aspects. Ann Intern Med 1972;77:229–233.

73. Willoughby E, Price RW, Padgett BL, et al. Progressive multifocal leukoencephalopathy (PML): in vitro cell-mediated immune responses to mitogens and JC virus. Neurology 1980;30(3):256–262.

74. Weber F, Goldmann C, Kramer M, et al. Cellular and humoral immune response in progressive multifocal leukoencephalopathy. Ann Neurol 2001;49:636–642.

75. Achim CL, Wiley CA. Expression of major histocompatibility complex antigens in the brains of patients with progressive multifocal leukoencephalopathy. J Neuropathol Exp Neurol 1992;51:257–263.

76. Krausa P, Barouch D, Bodmer JG, et al. Rapid characterization of HLA class I alleles by gene mapping using ARMS PCR. Eur J Immunogenet 1995;22:283–287.

77. Koralnik IJ, Du Pasquier RA, Kuroda MJ, et al. Association of prolonged survival in HLA-A2+ progressive multifocal leukoencephalopathy patients with a CTL response specific for a commonly recognized JC virus epitope. J Immunol 2002;168:499–504.

78. Frisque RJ, Bream GL, Cannella MT. Human polyomavirus JC virus genome. J Virol 1984;51:458–569.

79. Liu CK, Hope AP, Atwood WJ. The human polyomavirus, JCV, does not share receptor specificity with SV40 on human glial cells. J Neurovirol 1998;4:49–58.

80. Liu CK, Wei G, Atwood WJ. Infection of glial cells by the human polyomavirus JC is mediated by an N-linked glycoprotein containing terminal alpha(2-6)-linked sialic acids. J Virol 1998;72:4643–4649.

81. Frisque RJ, Rifkin DB, Walker DL. Transformation of primary hamster brain cells with JC virus and its DNA. J Virol 1980;35:265–269.

82. Major EO, Traub RG. JC virus T protein during productive infection in human fetal brain and kidney cells. Virology 1986;148:221–225.

83. Hou-Jong MH, Larsen SH, Roman A. Role of the agnoprotein in regulation of simian virus 40 replication and maturation pathways. J Virol 1987;61:937–939.

84. Yogo Y, Kitamura T, Sugimoto C, et al. Isolation of a possible archetypal JC virus DNA sequence from nonimmunocompromised individuals. J Virol 1990;64:3139–3143.

85. Monaco MC, Jensen PN, Hou J, et al. Detection of JC virus DNA in human tonsil tissue: evidence for site of initial viral infection. J Virol 1998;72:9918–9923.

86. Pfister L-A, Letvin NL, Koralnik IJ. JC virus regulatory region tandem repeats in plasma and central nervous system isolates correlate with poor clinical outcome in patients with progressive multifocal leukoencephalopathy. J Virol 2001;75:5672–5676.

87. Raj GV, Khalili K. Transcriptional regulation: lessons from the human neurotropic polyomavirus, JCV. Virology 1995;213:283–291.

88. Tornatore C, Amemiya K, Atwood W, et al. JC virus: current concepts and controversies in the molecular virology and pathogenesis of progressive multifocal leukoencephalopathy. Rev Med Virol 1994;4:197–219.

89. Henson J, Saffer J, Furneaux H. The transcription factor Sp1 binds to the JC virus promoter and is selectively expressed in glial cells in human brain. Ann Neurol 1992;32:72–77.

90. Tada H, Khalili K. A novel sequence-specific DNA-binding protein, LCP-1, interacts with single-stranded DNA and differentially regulates early gene expression of the human neurotropic JC virus. J Virol 1992;66:6885–6892.

91. Agostini HT, Ryschkewitsch CF, Stoner GL. Genotype profile of human polyomavirus JC excreted in urine of immunocompetent individuals. J Clin Microbiol 1996;34:159–164.

92. Agostini HT, Ryschkewitsch CF, Mory R, et al. JC virus (JCV) genotypes in brain tissue from patients with progressive multifocal leukoencephalopathy (PML) and in urine from controls without PML: increased frequency of JCV type 2 in PML. J Infect Dis 1997;176:1–8.

93. Houff SA, Major EO, Katz DA, et al. Involvement of JC virus-infected mononuclear cells from the bone marrow and spleen in the pathogenesis of progressive multifocal leukoencephalopathy. N Engl J Med 1988;318:301–305.

94. Major EO, Amemiya K, Elder G, Houff SA. Glial cells of the human developing brain and B cells of the immune system share a common DNA binding factor for recogni-

tion of the regulatory sequences of the human polyomavirus, JCV. J Neurosci Res 1990;27:461–471.

95. Monaco MC, Atwood WJ, Gravell M, et al. JC virus infection of hematopoietic progenitor cells, primary B lymphocytes, and tonsillar stromal cells: implications for viral latency. J Virol 1996;70:7004–7012.

96. Atwood WJ, Amemiya K, Traub R, et al. Interaction of the human polyomavirus, JCV, with human B-lymphocytes. Virology 1992;190:716–723.

97. Dubois V, Dutronc H, Lafon ME, et al. Latency and reactivation of JC virus in peripheral blood of human immunodeficiency virus type 1-infected patients. J Clin Microbiol 1997;35:2288–2292.

98. Boldorini R, Cristina S, Vago L, et al. Ultrastructural studies in the lytic phase of progressive multifocal leukoencephalopathy in AIDS patients. Ultrastruct Pathol 1993; 17:599–609.

99. Orenstein JM, Meltzer MS, Phipps T, Gendelman HE. Cytoplasmic assembly and accumulation of human immunodeficiency virus types 1 and 2 in recombinant human colony-stimulating factor-1-treated human monocytes: an ultrastructural study. J Virol 1988;62:2578–2586.

100. Stoner GL, Ryschkewitsch CF, Walker DL, Webster HD. JC papovavirus large tumor (T)-antigen expression in brain tissue of acquired immune deficiency syndrome (AIDS) and non-AIDS patients with progressive multifocal leukoencephalopathy. Proc Natl Acad Sci U S A 1986;83: 2271–2275.

101. Dubois V, Moret H, Lafon ME, et al. Prevalence of JC virus viraemia in HIV-infected patients with or without neurological disorders: a prospective study. J Neurovirol 1998;4:539–544.

102. Koralnik IJ, Schmitz JE, Lifton MA, et al. Detection of JC virus DNA in peripheral blood cell subpopulations of HIV-1-infected individuals. J Neurovirol 1999;5:430–435.

103. Wei G, Liu CK, Atwood WJ. JC virus binds to primary human glial cells, tonsillar stromal cells, and B-lymphocytes, but not to T lymphocytes. J Neurovirol 2000;6:127–136.

104. Major EO, Miller AE, Mourrain P, et al. Establishment of a line of human fetal glial cells that supports JC virus multiplication. Proc Natl Acad Sci U S A 1985;82:1257–1261.

105. Mandl C, Walker DL, Frisque RJ. Derivation and characterization of POJ cells, transformed human fetal glial cells that retain their permissivity for JC virus. J Virol 1987; 61:755–763.

106. Miyamura T, Jikuya H, Soeda E, Yoshiike K. Genomic structure of human polyoma virus JC: nucleotide sequence of the region containing replication origin and small-T-antigen gene. J Virol 1983;45:73–79.

107. Walker DL, Padgett BL, ZuRhein GM, et al. Human papovavirus (JC): induction of brain tumors in hamsters. Science 1973;181:674–676.

108. Varakis J, ZuRhein GM, Padgett BL, Walker DL. Induction of peripheral neuroblastomas in Syrian hamsters after injection as neonates with JC virus, a human polyoma virus. Cancer Res 1978;38:1718–1722.

109. Dyson N, Bernards R, Friend SH, et al. Large T antigens of many polyomaviruses are able to form complexes with the retinoblastoma protein. J Virol 1990;64:1353–1356.

110. Ohsumi S, Motoi M, Ogawa K. Induction of undifferentiated tumors by JC virus in the cerebrum of rats. Acta Pathol Jpn 1986;36:815–825.

111. London WT, Houff SA, Madden DL, et al. Brain tumors in owl monkeys inoculated with a human polyomavirus (JC virus). Science 1978;201:1246–1249.

112. Miller NR, McKeever PE, London W, et al. Brain tumors of owl monkeys inoculated with JC virus contain the JC virus genome. J Virol 1984;49:848–856.

113. Major EO, Vacante DA, Traub RG, et al. Owl monkey astrocytoma cells in culture spontaneously produce infectious JC virus which demonstrates altered biological properties. J Virol 1987;61:1435–1441.

114. Greenlee JE, Becker LE, Narayan O, Johnson RT. Failure to demonstrate papovavirus tumor antigen in human cerebral neoplasms. Ann Neurol 1978;3:479–481.

115. Dorries K, Loeber G, Meixensberger J. Association of polyomaviruses JC, SV40, and BK with human brain tumors. Virology 1987;160:268–270.

116. Howard E, Marcus D, O'Brien J, et al. Five DNA tumor viruses undetectable in human retinoblastomas. Invest Ophthalmol Vis Sci 1992;33:1564–1567.

117. Krynska B, Otte J, Franks R, et al. Human ubiquitous JCV(CY) T-antigen gene induces brain tumors in experimental animals. Oncogene 1999;18:39–46.

118. Huang H, Reis R, Yonekawa Y, et al. Identification in human brain tumors of DNA sequences specific for SV40 large T antigen. Brain Pathol 1999;9:33–42.

119. Hayashi H, Endo S, Suzuki S, et al. JC virus large T protein transforms rodent cells but is not involved in human medulloblastoma. Neuropathology 2001;21:129–137.

120. Kim JYH, Koralnik IJ, LeFave M, et al. Medulloblastomas and primitive neuroectodermal tumors rarely contain polyomavirus DNA sequences. Neurooncology 2002 (in press).

121. Weggen S, Bayer TA, von Deimling A, et al. Low frequency of SV40, JC and BK polyomavirus sequences in human medulloblastomas, meningiomas and ependymomas. Brain Pathol 2000;10:85–92.

122. Small JA, Scangos GA, Cork L, et al. The early region of human papovavirus JC induces dysmyelination in transgenic mice. Cell 1986;46:13–18.

123. Beggs AH, Frisque RJ, Scangos GA. Extinction of JC virus tumor-antigen expression in glial cell—fibroblast hybrids. Proc Natl Acad Sci U S A 1988;85:7632–7636.

124. Feigenbaum L, Hinrichs SH, Jay G. JC virus and simian virus 40 enhancers and transforming proteins: role in determining tissue specificity and pathogenicity in transgenic mice. J Virol 1992;66:1176–1182.

125. Feigenbaum L, Khalili K, Major E, Khoury G. Regulation of the host range of human papovavirus JCV. Proc Natl Acad Sci U S A 1987;84:3695–3698.

126. Lashgari MS, Tada H, Amini S, Khalili K. Regulation of JCVL promoter function: transactivation of JCVL promoter by JCV and SV40 early proteins. Virology 1989; 170:292–295.

127. Haas S, Gordon J, Khalili K. A developmentally regulated DNA-binding protein from mouse brain stimulates myelin basic protein gene expression. Mol Cell Biol 1993;13: 3103–3112.

128. Haas S, Thatikunta P, Steplewski A, et al. A 39-kD DNA-binding protein from mouse brain stimulates transcription of myelin basic protein gene in oligodendrocytic cells. J Cell Biol 1995;130:1171–1179.

129. Tretiakova A, Krynska B, Gordon J, Khalili K. Human neurotropic JC virus early protein deregulates glial cell cycle pathway and impairs cell differentiation. J Neurosci Res 1999;55:588–599.

130. Gallia GL, Gordon J, Khalili K. Tumor pathogenesis of human neurotropic JC virus in the CNS. J Neurovirol 1998;4:175–181.

131. Stoner GL. Implications of progressive multifocal leukoencephalopathy and JC virus for the etiology of MS. Acta Neurol Scand 1991;83:20–33.

132. Buckle GJ, Godec MS, Rubi JU, et al. Lack of JC viral genomic sequences in multiple sclerosis brain tissue by polymerase chain reaction. Ann Neurol 1992;32:829–831.

133. Agostini HT, Ryschkewitsch CF, Baumhefner RW, et al. Influence of JC virus coding region genotype on risk of multiple sclerosis and progressive multifocal leukoencephalopathy. J Neurovirol 2000;6:S101–S108.

134. Challoner PB, Smith KT, Parker JD, et al. Plaque-associated expression of human herpesvirus 6 in multiple sclerosis. Proc Natl Acad Sci U S A 1995;92:7440–7444.

135. Mock DJ, Powers JM, Goodman AD, et al. Association of human herpesvirus 6 with the demyelinative lesions of progressive multifocal leukoencephalopathy. J Neurovirol 1999;5:363–373.

Chapter 16

Guillain-Barré Syndrome and Chronic Inflammatory Demyelinating Polyneuropathy

Reinhard Kiefer

Guillain-Barré syndrome (GBS) and chronic inflammatory demyelinating polyneuropathy (CIDP) are members of a spectrum of acute and chronic polyradiculoneuropathies of presumed autoimmune origin.[1-4] *Classic GBS* refers to an acute ascending polyradiculoneuropathy that may proceed to quadriplegia and commonly involves cranial nerves. CIDP has similar clinical features but takes a slower course. Whereas GBS has been arbitrarily defined as reaching its nadir within 4 weeks, subacute GBS is defined as progressive for up to 8 weeks and CIDP as progressive beyond 2 months.[5-7] Patients with GBS spontaneously improve, but CIDP may take a chronic progressive or relapsing-remitting course. Both conditions are clinical syndromes likely comprising several entities. Careful studies of GBS in recent years led to the differentiation of a primarily demyelinating form, acute inflammatory demyelinating polyneuropathy (AIDP), and an axonal form that may be purely motor (acute motor axonal neuropathy [AMAN]) or sensorimotor (acute motor and sensory axonal neuropathy [AMSAN]).[8-12] Similarly, CIDP may have a chronic inflammatory axonal polyneuropathy as its counterpart.[13] Common to all of them are their presumed autoimmune etiology and several steps of the inflammatory cascade once the disease process has been triggered. However, there is evidence that different clinical presentations of GBS may be due to different autoimmune targets, resulting in distinct clinico-pathologic entities. It is less certain whether CIDP is triggered by mechanisms similar to those of GBS. It is also unknown whether the different clinical course merely represents one end of a disease spectrum or rather reflects a different etiology that separates CIDP from GBS. However, although GBS and CIDP share many pathologic and pathogenetic features, their clinical course, treatment, and prognosis are clearly distinct and require the clinician to separate these conditions.

Mechanisms of Immune-Mediated Injury in Guillain-Barré Syndrome and Chronic Inflammatory Demyelinating Polyneuropathy

Autoimmune injury of the peripheral nervous system (PNS)[1,14-17] resulting in demyelination or axonal damage (or both) follows a sequence of events:

1. A specific immune response directed against PNS antigens is initiated.
2. Autoantigen-specific T cells circulate and enter the PNS as part of normal immunosurveillance.
3. The autoantigen is recognized by T cells with the help of local antigen-presenting cells, leading to clonal T-cell expansion and cytokine secretion, activation of local macrophages, and activation of B cells to secrete autoantibodies.

4. The blood-nerve barrier breaks down, leading to the entrance of specific autoantibodies, macrophages, and more T cells into the nerve (Figure 16-1).

5. Destruction of the autoimmune target occurs through cytotoxic T cells, receptor-mediated phagocytosis, and complement-fixing antibodies. Nonspecific tissue damage is implemented through cytotoxic cytokines, toxic radicals, and macrophage-mediated cytotoxicity.

6. The autoimmune attack is terminated, presumably due to loss of antigenic stimulation, apoptosis of autoreactive T cells, and the action of immunosuppressive cytokines.

7. Once inflammation is subsiding, regeneration of destroyed myelin sheaths and axons may commence, leading to remyelination and axonal sprouting.

Although the basic principles are presumably identical in all forms of autoimmune polyneuropathies, the autoantigenic targets, the mechanisms of their generation, and the relative importance of T- and B-cell involvement differ among the various forms of GBS and CIDP. Also, neither form is sufficiently explained by the presence of a single autoantibody or T-cell response against a single epitope. Finally, much knowledge about effector mechanisms of demyelination in inflammatory neuropathy is gained from studies in experimental autoimmune neuritis (EAN), an animal model of GBS,[18] rather than GBS and CIDP themselves, and direct knowledge of pathogenetic pathways in human disease is limited.

Generation of Autoantibodies and Autoreactive T Cells

A multitude of autoantibodies against various targets in the PNS are found in GBS and, to a lesser degree, in CIDP. These particularly include antibodies against ganglioside moieties present on glycolipids but also against other PNS components, including various glycoproteins and the peripheral nerve myelin protein 22 (PMP22).[19] Evidence for T-cell involvement is largely derived from histologic observation of T-cell infiltrates and lessons from studies in which autoreactive T cells directed against the myelin proteins P0, P2, and others induce an inflammatory neuropathy with marked resemblance to GBS in susceptible laboratory animals.[18] An important concept of how autoimmune B and T cells are generated in patients with GBS and CIDP is that of molecular mimicry.[20] According to this concept, a normal immune response (e.g., directed against an invading microorganism) may be converted into an autoimmune response if the autoantigenic structure recognized by the immune cell is shared between the foreign antigen and normal structures of the host. An autoimmune attack against the PNS would be triggered by molecular mimicry if structures on a foreign antigen were identically present within the peripheral nerve and, as a consequence, the normal immune response were aberrantly directed against that PNS structure. Another mechanism by which autoimmune responses may be created is bystander activation, which denotes the activation of autoreactive T cells through nonspecific signals, such as cytokines secreted from other activated T-cell clones. As a consequence, with ongoing autoimmune disease, such as in CIDP, more and more autoreactive T-cell clones directed against different targets may be generated. This process of epitope spreading is further supported through tissue destruction, which may unmask novel antigens and thus trigger immune responses against additional targets. Finally, viral and bacterial superantigens may trigger autoimmune responses.

Antecedent Events

In approximately two-thirds of GBS patients, the disease is preceded by a respiratory or gastrointestinal infection, an immunization, or other events, including surgery.[21] However, among the many associations reported in the literature, only few can firmly be linked to GBS. *Campylobacter jejuni* infection is the most frequent preceding infection.[22] Although the frequency of positive serologic tests in European neurologic controls ranges from 1% to 12%, GBS is preceded by *C. jejuni* enteritis in up to 32% in Europe,[23] 45% in Japan,[24] and 66% in China.[25] Here, GBS occurs seasonally in epidemics during the summer months, as does *C. jejuni* enteritis. However, *C. jejuni* enteritis is a frequent infection throughout the world but only very rarely is followed by GBS. The most likely explanation is that GBS is triggered only by certain uncommon

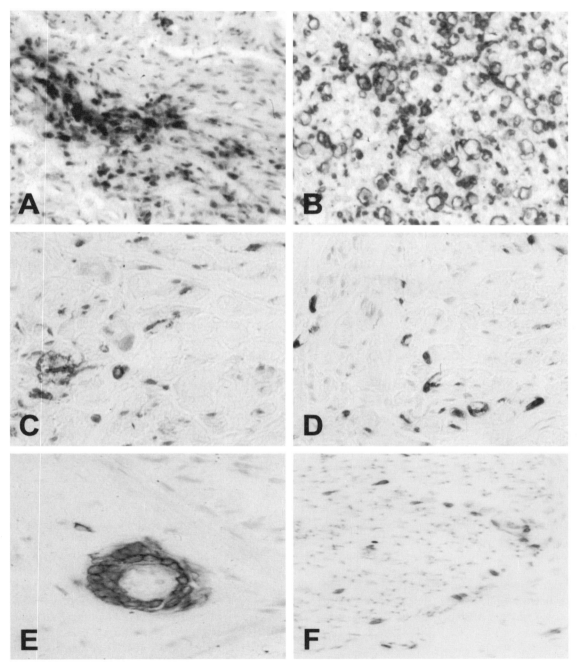

Figure 16-1. Mononuclear cell infiltration in Guillain-Barré syndrome and chronic inflammatory demyelinating polyneuropathy. **A, B.** In a postmortem case of acute Guillain-Barré syndrome, massive infiltration of lumbar roots with T-lymphocytes **(A)** and macrophages **(B)** is observed. **C, D.** In sural nerve biopsies, macrophage infiltration is typically much less severe **(C)**, but macrophages still carry inflammation-associated markers,[207] such as the calcium-binding, macrophage inhibitory factor–related protein 8 **(D)**. In sural nerves from chronic inflammatory demyelinating polyneuropathy patients, small perivascular T-cell cuffs around epineurial blood vessels **(E)** or diffuse endoneurial T-cell infiltration in low to moderate numbers may be seen **(F)**. Such changes may go undetected unless immunocytochemistry is performed.

strains, possibly in the context of immunogenetic susceptibility factors of the patient. *C. jejuni* is a highly variable bacterium, the numerous strains of which are serologically classified according to heat-stable (Penner classification) or heat-labile (Lior classification) bacterial antigens or on a genetic basis.[26] In Japan, an association of GBS with Penner serotype O:19 was found,[27,28] but this does not appear to be the case in Europe.[29,30] Strong support for a causal relationship between GBS and certain rare *C. jejuni* strains was provided by a study in South African children with GBS, where the Penner O:41 serotype was found in all patients with *C. jejuni*–associated GBS, whereas the same strain was exceedingly rare in patients with *C. jejuni* enteritis not associated with GBS.[31]

Another frequent link of GBS is with cytomegalovirus (CMV) infection. Immunoglobulin M (IgM) antibodies against CMV were significantly more frequent than in controls and found in up to 13%[23] in different series from throughout the world. An association has also been found between GBS and Epstein-Barr virus,[23] *Mycoplasma pneumoniae* infections,[23] and *Haemophilus influenzae*.[32] Reported frequencies of a preceding Epstein-Barr virus infection in GBS patients compared to controls were 10% versus 1% in one study,[23] but two other large studies found no such association.[11,33] Figures for a preceding *M. pneumoniae* infection in GBS patients are 5% versus 1% in controls.[23] There is a very slight but seemingly definite association with preceding influenza vaccination,[34] particularly if certain strain vaccines are used,[35] and another association with rabies vaccines containing myelin components.[36] Recently, an association with *H. influenzae* in the Japanese population was suggested.[32] Innumerable other preceding events have been described in single patients or small series, but their true association with GBS is unproven.[21] CIDP is not as clearly associated with a preceding infection.[37]

Autoantibodies in Guillain-Barré Syndrome and Chronic Inflammatory Demyelinating Polyneuropathy

Early studies revealed the presence of autoantibodies in patient sera against various crude peripheral nerve or myelin preparations. More detailed studies revealed autoantibodies against a large number

of glycosphingolipids, including cerebrosides, sulfatides, globosides, and, in particular, gangliosides. In addition, antibodies against myelin proteins, including P0 and P2, were occasionally found in some patients.[19,38] Antibodies against myelin-associated glycoprotein are characteristic for a chronic, primarily sensory polyneuropathy associated with an IgM monoclonal gammopathy[39] (discussed in Chapter 17). A potentially interesting autoantigen is PMP22, as it is located at the intraperiod line of compact myelin and thus potentially is accessible for antibody attachment. Indeed, immunization with a PMP22 fusion protein may cause EAN in laboratory animals.[40] In humans, autoantibodies against PMP22 were found in more than 50% of GBS and up to one-third of CIDP patients, but very rarely in controls.[41]

Glycosphingolipid antigens have attracted the most intense interest among GBS researchers, whereas investigations in CIDP were less rewarding. Glycosphingolipids are lipids based on the aminoalcohol sphingosin, with a highly variable carbohydrate side chain attached to the terminal hydroxylic group of sphingosin. Glycosphingolipids are abundantly present in nervous tissue and are classified as cerebrosides, globosides, sulfatides, and gangliosides, according to the structure of the carbohydrate side chain. The carbohydrate-free core structure of glycosphingolipids is called *ceramide*. Gangliosides carry a glycosyl backbone of four sugar residues (ceramide glucose galactose *N*-acetyl-galactosamin galactose), with one to four sialic acid residues attached. The number of sialic acid residues is denoted in the second letter of the denomination (Figure 16-2).

Autoantibodies of the IgG, IgM, or IgA subtype against ganglioside moieties are frequently found in GBS but only rarely in controls.[16] In the largest published series of unselected GBS patients participating in a large treatment trial, 22% of the patients had IgG antibodies against ganglioside GM1, 20% had IgM antibodies, and 15% had IgA antibodies.[11] In another study of GBS patients investigated for other purposes, up to 34% had IgG and 36% IgM antibodies, whereas frequencies in controls were only 12% and 6%, respectively.[42] IgA ganglioside antibodies in one study were from subclass IgA1 throughout and not of the secretory type, suggesting that they were not shed from the enteric mucosa but rather the consequence of a systemic immune reaction.[43]

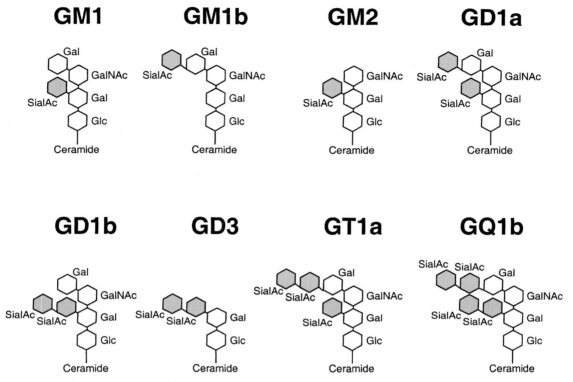

Figure 16-2. Structure of gangliosides relevant in autoimmune neuropathy. (Gal = D-galactose; GalNAc = *N*-acetyl-D-galactosamine; Glc = D-glucose; SialAc = sialic acid.)

Antibodies against ganglioside GQ1b are present in a very high number of patients with Miller-Fisher syndrome (MFS) but are rare in patients with other forms of GBS or controls.[44] Numerous reports describe further antibody responses against other ganglioside moieties in patients with various forms of GBS and rarer in CIDP. Some of the more common antibody targets other than GM1 and GQ1b in association with GBS include gangliosides GM1b, GM2, GD1a, *N*-acetyl-D-galactosamyl (GalNAc-GD1a), GD1b, GT1a, GT1b, and GM1(*N*-glycolyl-neuraminic acid [NeuGc]). Their associations with specific clinical phenotypes and putative functional implications are described in Clinicopathologic Subgroups.

The antibody responses against certain ganglioside moieties may not be specific for single gangliosides. Antibodies frequently cross-react with other ganglioside residues, and the pattern of antibody cross-reactivity may be specific for individual patients and clinical phenotypes. It may thus be that the recognition of a specific ganglioside epitope present on a set of several gangliosides rather than antibody targeting of a single ganglioside may be the relevant causative step in the pathogenesis of GBS.

Certain ganglioside antibodies occur more frequently in GBS subsequent to specific infections. In GBS cases, GM1 antibodies are more common in those cases with evidence of a preceding *C. jejuni* infection.[29,45] In Japan, GM1 antibodies are particularly associated with the Penner O:19 serotype of *C. jejuni*.[46] Similarly, antibodies against GalNAc-GD1a and GM1b are more frequent in *C. jejuni*–associated GBS cases both in Asia and in Europe.[47–50] However, ganglioside antibodies may also be frequent in GBS not associated with *C. jejuni*.[51] Autoantibodies against ganglioside GM2 have been found particularly in GBS cases after CMV infection and are present in approximately

50% of GBS cases with CMV IgM antibodies.[52–54] GM2 antibodies, however, may also be frequent in uncomplicated CMV infection not associated with GBS.[55] In CIDP, an association with ganglioside antibodies has been described, but studies are limited, and the prevalence of such antibodies is much lower than in GBS.

In addition to gangliosides, other glycosphingolipids may serve as antigens for autoantibodies.[19] The prevalence varies greatly in different studies, possibly for technical reasons. In a large series, IgG antibodies against sialosyl paragloboside were rarely found in higher titers in GBS, and IgM antibodies against sialosyl lactosaminyl paragloboside and sulfated glucuronyl paragloboside may be found in GBS and CIDP but more rarely also in neurologic and non-neurologic controls.[42] There appears to be no association of the presence of these antibodies with a preceding *C. jejuni* infection. Finally, rats immunized with myelin proteins P0 and P2 develop EAN, but evidence for a causal relationship between such antibodies and GBS or CIDP is limited.[56]

Molecular Links between Infectious Agents, Autoantibodies, and the Peripheral Nervous System

Gangliosides are abundantly present in the central nervous system (CNS) and the PNS and form integral components of various nervous structures. The Penner serotype O:19 of *C. jejuni*, which is particularly prevalent as the preceding infective organism of GBS in Japan, carries a terminal tetrasaccharide residue in its lipopolysaccharide (LPS) that is identical to ganglioside GM1[57,58] and another one that is identical to GT1a. Other ganglioside and globoside moieties found in LPS of *C. jejuni* strains include asialo-GM1, GM1b, GalNAc-GM1b, GD1a, GalNAc-GD1a, GD3, GQ1b, and sulfated glucuronyl paragloboside.[59] It was, therefore, proposed that PNS structures are attacked by antibodies primarily directed against *C. jejuni* LPS that cross-react through molecular mimicry with ganglioside structures present within the PNS. Similarly, GM2-like epitopes were detected on fibroblasts infected with CMV but not on uninfected fibroblasts, suggesting molecular mimicry between CMV-related structures and ganglioside GM2.[60] Molecular mimicry may also occur between a certain strain of *H. influenzae* and ganglioside GM1.[61] However, some *C. jejuni* strains not associated with GBS have identical LPS features and yet do not trigger a ganglioside antibody response.[62] Furthermore, ganglioside moieties are also found in LPS from bacteria not associated with GBS.[63] Finally, ganglioside antibodies may be present in patients with uncomplicated infections.[55] Additional factors of the infecting agent or the patient are, therefore, needed to cause GBS. However, therapeutic ganglioside administration is associated with a slightly increased risk of GBS,[64] and patients with GBS after parenteral ganglioside treatment had ganglioside antibodies, whereas those without GBS did not.[65]

T-Cell Responses in Guillain-Barré Syndrome and Chronic Inflammatory Demyelinating Polyneuropathy

Compared to the numerous studies of the degrees of T-cell specificity and T-cell receptor (TCR) usage in multiple sclerosis, very little is known in GBS and CIDP. Studies in laboratory animals revealed that the adoptive transfer of autoreactive T cells directed against the myelin compounds P0, P2, and myelin-associated glycoprotein may trigger EAN with a time course that excludes the secondary generation of antibodies as the causative mechanism.[66–68] In humans, these results are unconfirmed, and it is unproven whether myelin components are relevant T-cell targets in GBS and CIDP.[69,70] Nevertheless, the dense T-cell infiltrates found in the majority of AIDP cases suggest a causative role for T cells, and evidence for activation of circulating T cells in GBS was found. T cells present in peripheral nerve during GBS do not show skewing toward a preferential CD4 or CD8 phenotype. Occasional γδ T cells are found in addition to T cells in GBS peripheral nerve.[71,72] Circulating T cells during GBS show increased usage of Vβ15 TCR chains,[73] but no skewing of TCR usage was found in CIDP.[74] In a γδ T-cell line raised from a GBS sural nerve biopsy nerve, an unusual Vγ8/δ1 TCR chain usage was found, which may be related to a preceding diarrheal illness.[72]

Genetic Factors

As preceding infections and specific B- and T-cell responses cannot fully explain the evolution of GBS, and as not all infected patients experience GBS, a role for immunogenetic susceptibility factors has been proposed. Similarly, the animal model of EAN can be induced in only certain strains of rats and mice,[18] but the reasons are largely unknown. Evidence in humans is also scarce, and most studies investigating the human leukocyte antigen (HLA) system and TCR polymorphisms did not reveal any associations. When groups of patients with specific features were analyzed, some weak associations were observed. The HLA DQB1*03 haplotype was more frequent in *C. jejuni*–associated GBS patients than in GBS patients without preceding *C. jejuni* infection in the United Kingdom,[75] but two other studies in Japanese patients did not show such an association.[76,77] In such patients, an association between *C. jejuni*–associated GBS and HLA B54 and HLA Cw1 was found if compared with healthy controls.[76] In China, AIDP but not AMAN may be associated with HLA DRB1*1301.[78] The tumor necrosis factor-α2 allele associated with high tumor necrosis factor-α production was more frequent in patients with *C. jejuni*–associated GBS than in controls.[79] Immunoglobulin receptor polymorphisms may confer susceptibility to GBS, and the homozygous presence of the H131 polymorphism of IgG Fc receptor IIa was found to be associated with increased risk of GBS and more severe disease.[80] Others found an association of homozygosity for the IgG Fc receptor IIIb neutrophil antigen 1, with more severe disease.[81] In CIDP, no definitive association with any genetic features was found to date.

Immunosurveillance and Generation of a Local Immune Response in the Peripheral Nerve

Like the CNS, the PNS is regularly patrolled by T cells that can be found in very low numbers in apparently normal sural nerve biopsies.[82] Within the PNS, a population of resident macrophages exists that constitutively expresses major histocompatibility complex class II antigens besides other macrophage antigens.[17] Endoneurial macrophages activated during inflammatory neuropa-

thy upregulate major histocompatibility complex class II and newly express B7-1 costimulatory molecules.[83] Others have observed the costimulatory B7-molecule on Schwann's cells.[84] The accessory molecule CD1 may be found on macrophages and Schwann's cells during inflammatory neuropathy.[71,85] Macrophages and possibly Schwann's cells are thus equipped to act as local antigen-presenting cells to circulating T cells. Once a circulating T cell recognizes its respective antigen, it will be activated, undergo clonal expansion, and secrete proinflammatory cytokines, including interleukin-1 (IL-1), IL-2, and interferon gamma (IFN-γ).

Expansion of the Local Inflammatory Response

Once T cells are activated and secrete proinflammatory cytokines, a cascade of events is initiated, resulting in accumulation of inflammatory cells within the nerve. For T-cell and macrophage recruitment, T cells and monocytes are slowed down by rolling along the endothelium and forming loose connections with the help of selectins. Once their speed in the bloodstream is reduced, firmer adhesion is established through adhesion molecules, including vascular cell adhesion molecule-1 and intercellular adhesion molecule-1 and their respective counterligands.[86] Proteases, and matrix metalloproteases in particular, are expressed and help in opening the blood-nerve barrier,[87–91] and chemokines guide mononuclear cells through the endothelium into the peripheral nerve.[92,93] As more T cells arrive, the blood-nerve barrier breaks down,[94] and antibodies may enter the nerve from the endothelium.

Antigen-Specific Target Destruction and Antibody-Mediated Conduction Block

Antigen-specific tissue destruction may occur in several ways. Cytotoxic T cells may directly destroy their target cells through the use of granzymes and perforin, but direct evidence in GBS and CIDP is lacking. Extensive studies have been performed to clarify whether antibodies, cerebrospinal fluid (CSF), and serum components may induce conduction block and demyelination, but results are conflicting. Complement-fixing antibodies have repeatedly been demonstrated histologically in both axonal and demyelinating forms of GBS, and target destruction is likely to occur through complement-dependent cell lysis. Another mechanism by which antibodies may target subsequent tissue destruction is through Fc receptor–mediated phagocytosis of target structures by macrophages. In addition, antibodies may also exert direct neurophysiologic effects. In a series of studies using serum from patients with MFS, neuromuscular transmission was shown to be disrupted in a mouse diaphragm experimental system, and this effect was dependent on the IgG fraction of serum. However, although a causative role of GQ1b antibodies was suggested by one group, the effect was reproduced using serum without GQ1b antibodies by another.[95–97] Further support for a causative role of anti-ganglioside antibodies generated through molecular mimicry was provided by experiments in which monoclonal anti-ganglioside antibodies generated against *C. jejuni* LPS were deposited near the neuromuscular junction together with complement, causing a block of neurotransmission.[98] Finally, an endogenous pentapeptide was identified in CSF from GBS, but not control patients, that blocks sodium channels.[99] This factor is not specific for GBS, as it may occur in multiple sclerosis patients, and its importance in GBS is further questioned by the fact that it is found in only CSF, whereas GBS may affect the entire PNS.

Nonspecific Tissue Destruction

As inflammation proceeds, myriad cytokines and other regulatory mediators are secreted within the peripheral nerve.[17] Among them, several may exert direct toxic effects on myelin, Schwann's cells, and axons. The cytokine tumor necrosis factor-α found in inflammatory neuropathies[100] has been shown to promote demyelination, but studies in peripheral nerve in vivo do not consistently support this notion.[101,102] In GBS patients, circulating tumor necrosis factor-α correlates with the severity of electrophysiologic alterations.[103] Other cytokines, including IL-12[104] and IL-6,[105] may cause demyelination if injected into peripheral nerve. Macrophages secrete nitric oxide, reactive oxygen species, and prostaglandins that may be toxic to surrounding cellular structures.[106,107] Various proteases, and in particular matrix metalloproteases,

are upregulated in GBS, CIDP, and during EAN and may nonspecifically act on myelin sheaths.[87–91] Finally, the mechanical action of increased fluid pressure within the endoneurium may add to nonspecific secondary changes, particularly to secondary axonal damage.[108] In severe cases, secondary pathologic changes in the CNS may occur as a consequence of axonal degeneration.[109]

Termination of the Autoimmune Attack

Although CIDP may take a chronic progressive course, it also occurs in a relapsing-remitting form. Our understanding of the molecular basis for spontaneous remissions in GBS and in the remitting form of CIDP is only just evolving. One simple reason might be the loss of antigenic drive that may play a role in GBS. Apoptosis of inflammatory T cells is an important mechanism of T-cell elimination in rat EAN and may also occur in humans.[110] Also, a number of cytokines with predominantly anti-inflammatory actions are expressed at later stages of EAN that presumably counter-regulate inflammatory drive. Expression of transforming growth factor β1 has been documented in EAN[111] and human sural nerve biopsies, and antibodies against transforming growth factor β1 augment EAN, suggesting a potent endogenous immunosuppressive action of this cytokine. In GBS, circulating transforming growth factor β1 is depressed during disease progression and rises during recovery.[112] Similarly, immunosuppressive IL-10 was demonstrated in macrophages during EAN[113] and was shown to inhibit the disease in laboratory animals.

Remyelination and Axonal Sprouting

Recovery of function depends on the site and type of injury. Conduction block due to a direct action of immunoglobulins may improve most rapidly once antibody influx stops or existing antibodies are displaced from their targets. Remyelination of denuded internodes also occurs within a relatively short period, whereas axonal regeneration takes place at a much slower rate. Axonal growth proceeds at 1 mm per day, the speed of slow axonal transport, and axons disrupted proximally may take many months or even longer to reach their distal targets. However, if axonal damage occurs at its most distal parts near the neuromuscular junction, sprouting may be rapidly successful, with growth cones reaching their targets within a very short period. This appears to occur in some cases of AMAN, with rapid recovery.[114]

Clinical Neurology of Guillain-Barré Syndrome

Epidemiology

GBS is a rare condition with an annual incidence of approximately 1.8 cases per 100,000, ranging from 1 to 4 per 100,000 in different studies.[22,115,116] Incidence increases with age, and males are affected slightly more frequently than are females. GBS occurs in all parts of the world. There is usually no seasonal preponderance. Occasional clusters are associated with epidemic diarrhea and other infections and occur seasonally during the summer in Northern China.[117] The incidence of GBS is increased after childbirth, particularly in the first 4 weeks.

Clinical Features

Already in 1916, Guillain, Barré, and Strohl described the main clinical features of the syndrome that now carries their names, consisting of acute motor weakness, paresthesias with some sensory loss, and loss of tendon reflexes. As pointed out earlier, GBS is preceded by an antecedent event, most frequently an upper respiratory or gastrointestinal infection. Although GBS is a predominantly motor disorder, patients frequently present with paresthesias in the legs and feet and with back pain, which may be severe. Weakness then quickly develops, beginning in the feet and ascending toward proximal leg muscles, the trunk, the arms, and cranial nerves. More rarely, weakness may begin in and even remain restricted to proximal muscles. Weakness is usually symmetric, but slight asymmetries may occur. Markedly patchy muscle involvement argues against the diagnosis. One or several cranial nerves are frequently involved. Most common are unilateral or bilateral facial palsies followed by extraocular muscle involvement. Bulbar palsy with speech and swallowing difficulties is less frequent

but dangerous, owing to potential aspiration. Some degree of respiratory muscle weakness occurs frequently, and mechanical ventilation is required in up to 20% of patients. Sensory symptoms are usually less severe and may even go unnoticed by the bedridden patient, being restricted to distal impairment of position and vibration sense. Ambulatory patients may experience sensory ataxia. Deep-tendon reflexes are always diminished and usually lost early. Painful paresthesias and back pain may be severe. There may be marked involvement of autonomic nerves in up to 40% of patients, and subclinical involvement may be even more frequent.[118] Autonomic involvement may result in either loss of function or excessive activity of the sympathetic and parasympathetic nervous system, and the spectrum may change as disease progresses. As a result, hypotension and hypertension, bradyarrhythmia and tachyarrhythmia, hypohidrosis and hyperhidrosis, gastrointestinal disturbances, and pupillary dysfunction all may occur in an unforeseeable manner, but sympathetic overactivity usually predominates at the height of the disease.[119] Dysregulation of cardiac and blood pressure control is potentially dangerous and may be fatal.[120] Severity of autonomic dysfunction may not correlate with motor involvement.[121]

In addition to the classic presentation of progressive ascending tetraparesis, several clinical variants have been recognized and may overlap and share the clinical feature of generalized areflexia. The MFS is characterized by external ophthalmoplegia, ataxia, and loss of deep-tendon reflexes and accounts for approximately 5% of cases.[44] The cause of the ataxia in MFS is obscure and thought to be inappropriate input from muscle spindles. It is not a sensory ataxia due to large sensory fiber involvement, as vibration and position senses may be preserved. There may be involvement of additional cranial nerves, and an inflammatory cranial polyneuropathy, usually including the facial nerves without ophthalmoplegia, may occur and represent another variant of GBS. A purely sensory syndrome may occur[122] as may pure motor paralysis. A pharyngeal-cervical-brachial variant describes selective involvement of the arms together with oropharyngeal weakness without involvement of the legs. Acute pandysautonomia is characterized by selective involvement of sympathetic and parasympathetic nerves without motor weakness and sensory symptoms, resulting in severe autonomic failure.

There may be clinical differences, depending on the type of preceding infection. *C. jejuni* infection is more frequent in pure motor forms of the disease, which are frequently associated with GM1 antibodies.[25] Patients with preceding CMV infection are younger, have more sensory abnormalities, have more cranial nerve involvement, and more frequently require artificial ventilation as compared to those without CMV infection.[123] In another study, milder forms were less frequently associated with *C. jejuni*, CMV, Epstein-Barr virus, and *M. pneumoniae* infections than those with more severe disease.[116]

Clinicopathologic Subgroups

Acute Inflammatory Demyelinating Polyneuropathy

AIDP is the most common form of GBS in Europe and North America. The pathologic hallmark of the condition is *macrophage-mediated demyelination*. This term denotes a primary attack of macrophages on seemingly intact myelin, resulting in penetration of Schwann's cell basal lamina, with subsequent myelin stripping off its axon.[124] Consequently, electrophysiology largely demonstrates demyelination and multifocal conduction block. There is prominent lymphocytic infiltration of nerve roots and nerves, suggesting a delayed hypersensitivity type T-cell–mediated immune reaction. This view finds further support by studies in EAN, in which much of the pathology of AIDP is mimicked by passive T-cell transfer of autoreactive T cells against myelin compounds. GM1 antibodies are commonly associated with AIDP but occur even more frequently with AMAN. GM2 antibodies and a preceding CMV infection may also be associated with AIDP. A humoral autoimmune attack as an important etiologic factor is supported by morphologic studies demonstrating complement-fixing IgG antibodies at Schwann's cell surfaces and early vesiculation of myelin in AIDP.[125]

Acute Motor Axonal Neuropathy

The axonal, usually predominantly motor form of GBS occurs commonly in China, Japan, India, and South America but is rarer in Europe.[10] The pathologic hallmark is primary axonal degeneration of motor nerves, with macrophages entering the axonal space, leaving the myelin sheath intact.[9] Sensory nerves are typically spared. Activated complement components were demonstrated on the axonal surface in AMAN, suggesting a primary antibody attack followed by Fc receptor–mediated phagocytosis by macrophages.[126] T-cell infiltration is sparse in AMAN, arguing against a major involvement of T-cell–mediated autoimmunity. Axonal injury may occur near the neuromuscular junction. This might explain why affected patients sometimes recover equally quickly as AIDP patients despite the need of axonal regeneration.[114]

Patients with AMAN frequently carried antibodies against GM1 ganglioside and had a preceding infection with *C. jejuni* more frequently than patients with AIDP.[25,127] As GM1 is localized to the axolemma and paranodal myelin of motor nerves, a causative relation was suggested. Indeed, macrophage attacks are seen early at the node of Ranvier in AMAN[128] but also in AIDP associated with GM1 antibodies. Electrophysiologic studies suggest reversible conduction failure in addition to axonal degeneration in AMAN patients with GM1 antibodies.

In addition to GM1 antibodies, other ganglioside antibodies are significantly associated with AMAN. In Chinese (but not other patients studied), the syndrome is closely related to the presence of antibodies against the ganglioside GD1a.[51] GalNAc-GD1a IgG antibodies are significantly associated with a predominantly motor and axonal form of GBS, which is frequently preceded by a gastrointestinal infection.[49,129] Similarly, GM1b antibodies are associated with AMAN. Such patients frequently had a precedent gastrointestinal infection, rapid progression, and severe disease with little cranial nerve involvement.[50] In a recent study, the association of AMAN with antibodies against GM1, GD1a, GalNAc-GD1a, and GD1b was confirmed.[130] In addition to *C. jejuni*, *H. influenzae* infection appears to be associated with AMAN.[32]

Acute Motor and Sensory Axonal Neuropathy

AMSAN is an axonal variant of GBS involving both motor and sensory nerve fibers. Care must be taken not to confuse this form with demyelinating GBS and subsequent secondary axonal degeneration. Pathologic studies revealed prominent axonal degeneration. As in AMAN, macrophages entering the periaxonal space were seen leaving the myelin sheath intact.[9,12] Serologic studies revealed antibody patterns similar to AMAN, including the presence of GM1, GM1b, and GD1a antibodies.[131] Given the pathologic and serologic similarities, it thus seems likely that AMSAN and AMAN are diseases with a related etiology and pathogenesis.

Miller-Fisher Syndrome

MFS was originally described as a syndrome of ophthalmoplegia, ataxia, and loss of tendon reflexes. Subsequent studies revealed a considerable overlap between MFS and GBS[132] in that patients originally presenting with MFS may proceed to full-blown GBS with quadriplegia. MFS thus seems to be part of a continuum of clinical presentations of GBS. In such cases, where a generalized syndrome evolved, pathologic descriptions documented a multifocal demyelinating polyneuropathy resembling AIDP. However, MFS proper should be restricted to cases that conform to the original description. In such cases, there is a unique association with the presence of autoantibodies against GQ1b gangliosides, which are found in more than 90% of patients and are highly specific for MFS.[44] GQ1b antibodies in MFS frequently cross-react with GT1a, and patients with GT1a antibodies in particular may show oropharyngeal weakness. As in classic GBS, the autoimmune response is thought to be generated by molecular mimicry between an immunogenic infectious agent and GQ1b/GT1a moieties present in peripheral nerve target structures. GQ1b is present abundantly in ocular motor nerves, suggesting a cause for the peculiar involvement of extraocular muscles.[133] However, GQ1b is found in only low amounts in the lower cranial nerves frequently affected in MFS but is abundantly present in the olfactory and optic nerves not affected by the disease.[133] Careful physiologic studies located the site of action of GQ1b antibodies to the motor nerve terminal causing conduction block in a complement-dependent manner through a presynaptic mechanism.[95] Others suggested both presynaptic and postsynaptic mechanisms.[96,134] Thus, the action of GQ1b autoantibodies alone may not fully explain the disease. Conduction block was found evoked by patient sera negative for GQ1b.[134]

Other Variants

Oculopharyngeal palsy is frequently associated with GT1a and GQ1b antibodies,[135] and GT1a and GM1b antibodies are prevalent in patients with generalized GBS with prominent bulbar involvement.[136,137] Ataxic variants are frequently associated with GD1b antibodies,[138,139] and a causative role is supported by rabbit studies wherein immunization with GD1b causes severe ataxia due to neuronal sensory axonal degeneration and degeneration of DRG neurons.[140] Other cases with sensory ataxia have IgM antibodies against GQ1b-α.[141]

Clinical Differential Diagnosis

The differential diagnosis of the classic syndrome of acute GBS comprises other forms of acute polyradiculoneuropathies as well as non-neuropathic conditions that result in acute paraplegia or tetraplegia. Among the peripheral nerve disorders, neuroborreliosis may present as a rapidly progressive polyradiculoneuropathy. A history of tick bites, traveling or living in an endemic area, an episode of erythema migrans, and an asymmetric multifocal distribution may provide clues toward this differential diagnosis. Polyradiculitis due to CMV infection also follows more of a multifocal distribution, suggesting multiple nerve root involvement. Toxic neuropathies, including hexacarbon and acrylamide poisoning, are now rare and may be differentiated from GBS by associated features of intoxication, more pronounced sensory involvement, and clues from the history. Hepatic porphyrias may manifest themselves in a subacute, frequently proximal, and purely motor neuropathy that affects the arms preferentially and may involve multiple cranial nerves. Clinical diagnostic clues include preceding abdominal pain with nausea and vomiting, a positive family history, and accompanying psychiatric disturbances. Diphtheria is accompanied by a demyelinating neuropathy initially leading to palatal weakness and is now exceedingly rare.

Disorders of muscles, motoneurons, and the neuromuscular junction can usually be differentiated from GBS by their history and the complete lack of sensory symptoms. An acute attack of a periodic paralysis will be suggested by a history of previous attacks and rapid progression within minutes or hours. Subacute myasthenia gravis may occur as the primary manifestation of disease in previously undiagnosed cases but may be distinguished clinically by prominent worsening through exercise. Patients intoxicated with irreversible inhibitors of acetylcholinesterase, such as E 605, may be tetraplegic but also show autonomic signs of excessive cholinergic function, such as excessive sweating and pupilloconstriction. Botulism may be differentiated by prodromata of nausea and diarrhea, early ophthalmoplegia, descending rather than ascending paralysis, cholinergic autonomic failure, and disease in other individuals who shared the same food with the patient. Poliomyelitis, now exceedingly rare in developed countries, usually presents with prodromal fever and malaise, markedly asymmetric weakness, and absence of sensory symptoms.

Degenerative spinal conditions, such as a large median lumbosacral disk herniation, may result in acute paraplegia and may occasionally be painless. Keys toward this differential diagnosis may be sudden onset rather than progression over days, a prominent bladder dysfunction, a lumbar sensory level, positive Lasègue's sign, and absence of progression toward the arms and cranial nerves. Acute spinal cord lesions, such as infarctions or transverse myelitis, may result in flaccid paraplegia with sensory loss and loss of tendon reflexes and may be suggested by a history of sudden onset, a sensory level, and prominent bladder dysfunction. Brain stem infarction and bilateral anterior cerebral artery infarction may also occasionally lead to predominant paraplegia of the legs with loss of tendon reflexes but have other associated features that localize the lesion unequivocally toward the CNS in most cases. Psychogenic weakness can usually be differentiated by the lack of objective clinical findings, including retained tendon reflexes, inappropriate innervation with muscle strength testing, and inconsistent findings on repeated clinical examination.

Diagnostic Procedures

Diagnostic workup includes tests that positively support the diagnosis of GBS and those that are performed to exclude potential differential diagnoses. Diagnostic criteria of GBS that have been published are particularly useful for research purposes.[5]

Routine laboratory tests are usually normal. Serologic studies for *C. jejuni* and other infectious agents may elucidate the preceding infection but are still mainly of scientific interest at present. Similarly, determination of anti-ganglioside antibodies is primarily of academic interest, although the association of GQ1b antibodies with MFS is so specific that determination may be warranted in atypical cases. Once clearer associations among preceding infections, antibody patterns, and response to treatment emerge, tests for antibodies against infectious agents and gangliosides may become helpful in guiding treatment decisions.

CSF examination may be normal during the first days of disease but rarely remains normal throughout. The usual finding is a high rise in CSF protein without an accompanying rise of the CSF cell count. This is termed *albuminocytologic dissociation* and represents one of the diagnostic hallmarks of the syndrome. Pleocytosis should remain less than 10/μl, although cell counts up to 50/μl do not exclude the diagnosis and are common in patients with human immunodeficiency virus infection and GBS. Higher numbers point toward other conditions, such as viral polyradiculitis or neuroborreliosis. There may occasionally be transient oligoclonal bands.

Electrophysiologic studies are essential to confirm the diagnosis, to categorize the syndrome into its demyelinating or axonal variant, and to assess the degree of secondary axonal damage as a prognostic factor.[11] A detailed account of electrophysiologic changes in both AIDP and CIDP can be found in Chapter 7.

In AIDP, the earliest changes are prolonged distal motor latencies that may be associated with dispersed compound muscle action potentials (CMAPs) and prolonged F-wave latencies progressing toward reduced frequency or total loss of F-wave responses. These changes are due to the predilection of early demyelinating changes at sites of increased blood-nerve barrier permeability near the neuromuscular junction and at the root entry zones. It should be noted that acute spinal cord lesions may also result in absent F waves, sometimes causing diagnostic confusion.[142]

Later, multifocal conduction block as another hallmark of the condition develops, and motor conduction velocities are reduced. *Conduction block* is best defined as a reduction of CMAP amplitude by at least 50% after proximal stimulation if compared to distal stimulation, no excessive prolongation of potential duration, and near-normal conduction velocity of the remaining fibers. Focal conduction block in AIDP is the result of focal demyelination of nerve fibers, resulting in loss of impulse propagation. Excessive dispersion of the CMAP makes conduction block difficult to assess, owing to phase cancellation. Generalized and diffuse demyelination and remyelination does not result in conduction block but in reduced nerve conduction velocity. Secondary axonal damage results in reduced distal CMAP amplitudes or loss of CMAP, as do conduction blocks near the neuromuscular junction.

Definite proof of axonal degeneration is provided by the presence of fibrillation potentials and positive sharp waves on electromyography (EMG), but this is found no earlier than approximately 2 weeks from the onset of the disorder. Loss of motor unit firing on EMG without fibrillations and positive sharp waves after several weeks points toward a purely demyelinating lesion with conduction block.

Magnetic evoked potentials as used in Europe may reveal or support the finding of proximal conduction block. It should be noted that calculated central motor latencies may be prolonged in GBS. This is not due to central demyelination but rather to demyelination in proximal motor roots. Cervical and lumbar stimulation occurs at the intervertebral foramina rather than at the root entry zone, and calculated central motor latencies thus constitute both CNS and proximal motor root conduction within the spinal canal.

Changes in sensory nerve conduction studies are usually less severe and reveal reduced nerve conduction velocities and reduced sensory nerve action potential (SNAP) amplitudes if secondary axonal degeneration occurs. Somatosensory-evoked potentials may suggest proximal demyelinating lesions of sensory nerves and roots. There are no major differences in electrophysiologic findings in children as compared to adults.[143]

Primarily axonal forms of GBS produce different electrophysiologic results. Nerve conduction velocities are usually normal or near normal, but distal CMAP amplitudes are reduced early. This may be due to terminal axonal degeneration or conduction block near the neuromuscular junction. F waves may be absent, or their frequency may be reduced. Axonal degeneration is demonstrated by vivid fibrillation potentials and positive sharp waves on EMG beginning 2 weeks after onset of the disease. Although changes are restricted to the motor system in AMAN, reduced SNAP amplitudes or loss of SNAPs are additional features of AMSAN.

With recovery, electrophysiologic results gradually return to normal. However, recovery of electrophysiologic measurements is frequently delayed as compared to clinical remission and may remain pathologic for many months even after complete clinical recovery. Tests of autonomic functions are available in specialized laboratories and are useful predictors of life-threatening cardiac complications.[121,144]

Other investigations are aiming at excluding the differential diagnoses: Magnetic resonance imaging (MRI) studies of the brain may be performed in patients with prominent cranial nerve involvement and are usually normal in patients with GBS and its variants. MRI of the spinal cord may exclude acute spinal cord compression and intraspinal lesions, such as transverse myelitis and spinal infarction. MRI of the lumbar spinal cord may reveal thickening and contrast enhancement of lumbosacral roots.[145] Sural nerve biopsy usually has no place in the diagnostic workup of typical cases of GBS.

Therapy

Immunomodulatory Treatment

Therapeutic considerations can be divided into specific therapies directed at the autoimmune etiology of the disease and into supportive measures. Among the specific therapies, plasmapheresis and intravenous immunoglobulin (IVIg) treatment are of proven benefit in favorably altering the natural course of the disease.[146,147]

Plasmapheresis has been shown to be superior to sham apheresis or no treatment in several controlled trials.[148–151] The standard regimen comprises five plasma exchanges on alternating days, with exchange volumes of 30–50 ml/kg body weight per session. In a large prospective study of 556 GBS patients, four exchanges were found appropriate for patients with moderate to severe GBS who were unable to stand, and additional exchanges provided no further benefit. Two exchanges were sufficient to shorten disease in patients with mild disease and retained ability to stand alone or walk.[152] In another study, two exchanges were sufficient to reduce plasma immunoglobulin content, and further exchanges had no further effect.[153] Replacement should be with albumin rather than fresh frozen plasma, owing to fewer side effects.[150] Plasma exchange is safe if performed skillfully. The main risks arise from the placement of a central venous catheter if no appropriate peripheral venous access can be established. Specific side effects are rare and include infections, hypotension, cardiac arrhythmias, thromboembolic events, bleeding complications, and hypocalcemia.[154] Contraindications are sepsis, hemodynamic instability, thrombocytopenia, and coagulation disorders. Double-filtration plasmapheresis may be equally effective[155] but is less efficient in removing immunoglobulins and anti-ganglioside antibodies.[156] Filtration of CSF may be effective in selected patients, but randomized trials are pending.[157]

IVIg at a dose of 0.4 g/kg daily for 5 days was found to be effective in ameliorating the disease and was suggested to be even superior to plasma exchange.[158] However, the plasmapheresis group in this study showed unexpectedly poor results when compared to previous trials. A subsequent trial did not find any difference in efficacy between plasma exchange and IVIg.[159] Treatment is generally safe, with few side effects.[160] Serious complication may arise from anaphylactic reactions, particularly in patients with IgA deficiency. Occasional side effects include headache, fever and chills, back pain, tachycardia, and changes in blood pressure. These may be ameliorated by a lower infusion rate. Other rare side effects include renal failure, symptoms of volume overload, thrombotic complications, hemolytic anemia, neutropenia, and aseptic meningitis. The mechanisms of action have been reviewed[161,162] and may additionally include a reduction of circulating inflammatory cytokines.[163] Combination treatment of plasma exchange followed by IVIg is not superior to either treatment alone.[159]

As both regimens are equally effective, the choice of treatment depends on availability, costs, side effects, and specific risks for individual patients. IVIg is now preferred in most centers owing to its easy availability and applicability. In cases with preceding *C. jejuni* infections, IVIg was found to be slightly superior to plasma exchange.[45,127,164] Similarly, patients with GM1b antibodies respond better to IVIg.[165] In fewer than 10% of patients, there will be a relapse after completion of the treatment regimen independent of the treatment modality chosen, possibly indicating an ongoing immune response.[166] In such cases, reinstitution of therapy for another treatment cycle is warranted.[147] If a first treatment cycle fails to halt the disease, implementation of a second treatment cycle is controversial. However, observations in four severely affected patients treated with IVIg suggest that an additional cycle of IVIg treatment may be beneficial.[167]

Glucocorticoids alone have no place in the treatment of GBS, as two large trials did not show any benefit at regular and high doses.[168,169] The reason for the failure of the single use of glucocorticoids in GBS is unknown. However, methylprednisolone combined with IVIg may provide additional benefit.[170] Long-term immunosuppressive medication is not required, as the disease is self-limited.

In children, IVIg is generally preferred over plasma exchange, owing to greater convenience.[147] Although one retrospective study suggested a poorer response to treatment in severely affected children,[171] others found good response rates.[172]

Supportive Therapy

Supportive therapy is aimed at avoiding complications and carrying the patient safely through a phase of entire helplessness. Patients with severe or rapidly progressive disease require admission to a neurologic intensive care unit for monitoring and appropriate supportive treatment when indicated. Respiratory function needs to be monitored closely by regular determination of vital capacity at least every 4–6 hours, as respiratory insufficiency may develop rapidly and may go undetected on a regular ward. Another potential danger lies in the rapid evolution of swallowing difficulties, resulting in aspiration that may lead to suffocation or severe pneumonia. A third potential danger requiring monitoring is autonomic disturbances that may occur early during disease and may be life-threatening.

Mechanical ventilation is indicated with respiratory failure or moderate to severe swallowing disturbances with impending aspiration. Intubation should not be delayed if the vital capacity falls to less than 15 ml/kg, the PCO_2 rises beyond 50 mm Hg, the PO_2 falls to less than 65 mm Hg, or the patient is fatigued. If in doubt, early intubation after a full explanation to the patient carries fewer complications than emergency intubation in acute respiratory failure. Assisted spontaneous breathing or bilevel positive airway pressure ventilation are superior to controlled mandatory ventilation in most cases. Tracheostomy is required with prolonged intubation. Weaning from the ventilator may be achieved by the sequential reduction of positive pressure and by increased times entirely off the ventilator. Extubation should be performed only if the patient has been off the ventilator for at least 24 hours without signs of respiratory distress. Extubation performed too early causes an undue risk to the patient and should be avoided.

To avoid thromboembolic complications, tight stockings, physiotherapy, and low-molecular-weight heparins are indicated. In completely paralyzed patients, continuous intravenous heparin with a partial thromboplastin time 2.5 times normal may be warranted.

Every effort must be undertaken to avoid infections. These usually arise from pulmonary infections, skin sores, urinary catheters, and intravenous and intra-arterial lines. As a consequence, careful respiratory toilet, meticulous personal hygiene of nurses and physicians, rigorous care of all lines, and frequent turning of the patient to prevent bedsores are mandatory.

Nutrition should be by enteral route whenever possible. If prolonged artificial nutrition is required, a gastrostomy tube provides better patient comfort. Obstipation should be avoided. Cardiac monitoring is required to detect autonomic disturbances. Care must be taken when using drugs acting on the parasympathetic and sympathetic nervous system, as responses may be exaggerated. In some cases, an external or transient internal pacemaker may be necessary.

Pain must be treated symptomatically. Neuropathic pain may effectively be treated using carbamazepine,[173] phenytoin, or gabapentin. Opioids may be required for back and joint pain, particularly at early stages. Sedation with promethazine or low-dose benzodiazepines may be useful to allow endotracheal tube tolerance or relieve psychologi-cal stress but is otherwise not required. GBS patients may be severely ill being intubated, ventilated, and tetraplegic and still may be able to watch television or read the newspaper if these items are appropriately positioned.

Physiotherapy is a mainstay of supportive therapy at all stages. Passive movement of all joints during the flaccid stage is required to avoid contractures and thromboembolic complications. Active physiotherapy at later stages hastens functional recovery. Finally, psychological support is crucial. The regular presence of house staff personnel in the room, information, constant reassurance, participation of family members, and the provision of other mental inputs help in avoiding psychological deprivation and psychotic complications.[174] If such symptoms are present, neuroleptics and sedatives may be required and should not be withheld if requested by the patient.

Course and Prognosis

Natural history studies from the time before plasma exchange therapy documented that the disease progresses until reaching a plateau phase of maximum deficit, usually within 2 weeks of onset in most patients. With progression lasting for more than 4 weeks, the syndrome is arbitrarily classified as subacute GBS.[7] The plateau phase may last a few days or many weeks until gradual recovery begins. Approximately one-third of GBS patients take a mild disease course and retain their ability to walk throughout the disease course.[116] Modern treatment ameliorates the course of the syndrome. Approximately 20–25% of patients require intubation for airway protection or treatment of respiratory failure. Despite modern treatment, reported death rates still amount to 2–11%[175–178] and rise to 20% in patients requiring mechanical ventilation.[179] Besides autonomic failure, the main life-threatening complications are ventilator-associated pneumonia, sepsis, and thromboembolic events.

Most patients gain complete or nearly complete functional recovery but, in some, recovery may be prolonged or incomplete. Up to 30% of patients remain with moderately to very severe neurologic deficits.[175,176] Conversely, prognosis is excellent in children.[143] Adverse prognostic factors are older age, severe disability at the beginning of treatment, rapid progression, severe arm involvement, recent CMV infection, and preceding diarrhea[127,175,180,181] as well as inexcitable nerves,[11] the presence of GM1b antibodies,[165] and requirement for mechanical ventilation.[179] The presence of GM1 antibodies alone does not relate to a poor prognosis.[182] Even years after recovery, detectable changes in many recovered patients may be noted,[183] and continuing fatigue is a major symptom.[184]

Clinical Neurology of Chronic Inflammatory Demyelinating Polyneuropathy

Epidemiology

CIDP, defined as an inflammatory demyelinating polyneuropathy with progression for more than 2 months, is not an entirely rare condition and may account for a considerable number of patients in specialized neuromuscular centers. The prevalence has been determined as 1.0 or 1.9 in 100,000. CIDP occurs in all age groups and is slightly more frequent in males.[185,186]

Clinical Features

Classic Chronic Inflammatory Demyelinating Polyneuropathy

CIDP presents as a symmetric motor and sensory polyneuropathy. Weakness is more severe distally, but proximal weakness may also be pronounced if there is prominent radicular involvement. The legs are affected more severely than are the arms. Muscle wasting is not a prominent feature in the demyelinating form of the disease but may be prominent in the axonal form and if secondary axonal degeneration occurs. Sensory involvement usually manifests as a glove-and-stocking distribution, with hypoesthesia and impaired vibration and position senses. As in GBS, there is generalized areflexia or at least attenuation of tendon reflexes. Autonomic involvement may occur.[187] There may also be involvement of cranial nerves, particularly the facial nerves, but severe cranial nerve involvement is restricted to advanced disease. Pain is frequent and may present as burning, radicular, lancinating, or deep muscle pain.[188]

CIDP is a chronic disease. Although few patients experience a monophasic illness, approximately 40% of patients follow a progressive course, and 40–50% take a relapsing-remitting course.[185,186] The latter patients are usually younger, and remissions may be complete.

Clinical Variants of Chronic Inflammatory Demyelinating Polyneuropathy

Besides the typical presentation of CIDP, several variants have been recognized. These include pure motor and pure sensory syndromes as well as markedly asymmetric patterns.[188,189] Pure sensory syndromes may represent a transitional state developing into sensorimotor CIDP.[190] Weakness and sensory loss in patients with asymmetric involvement may manifest as a polyradicular pattern with adjacent or multiple isolated nerve roots affected, a pattern of polyneuropathy multiplex, a regional distribution pattern with preferential involvement of only one extremity, or selective involvement of arms or legs.[188,191–194] The relation between markedly asymmetric or multifocal cases and CIDP has been a matter of debate,[195] and separation of multifocal disease as a distinct entity has been suggested.[194] However, pathogenesis and response to treatment are likely to be similar, arguing against a separation.[196] Very rarely, CIDP patients have additional CNS features, with a multiple sclerosis–like picture, giving rise to speculations about common pathogenetic mechanisms of CNS and PNS inflammatory demyelination.[189,197]

Associated Conditions

Unlike GBS, CIDP is only rarely preceded by infections, and these cases account for fewer than 10%. CIDP may, however, occur concurrent with a number of medical conditions. These include monoclonal gammopathies of IgG and IgA subclass of either undetermined significance as the consequence of multiple myeloma, or in the context of a syndrome encompassing *p*olyneuropathy, *o*rganomegaly, *e*ndocrinopathy, *m*onoclonal gammopathy, and *s*kin changes (POEMS syndrome); systemic lupus erythematosus; Hodgkin's and non-Hodgkin's lymphoma; inflammatory bowel disease; active hepatitis B and C; and human immun-

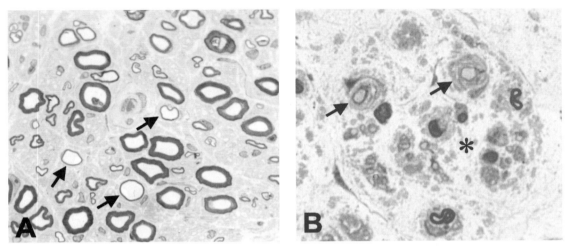

Figure 16-3. Pathology of chronic inflammatory demyelinating polyneuropathy. **A.** In mild disease, there is minimal loss of myelinated axons, but several large axons are thinly myelinated (*arrows*). **B.** In severe disease, hardly any myelinated fibers can be found. There is marked axonal loss, and retained axons are completely denuded (*arrows*) and surrounded by supernumerary Schwann's cell lamellae (onion bulbs), indicating repeated demyelination and remyelination. Note the massive endoneurial edema (*asterisk*).

odeficiency virus infection. The reasons for these associations are unknown in detail but are thought to be related to the immune deviations found in these conditions. There is an ongoing debate about whether neuropathy associated with these conditions should be regarded as CIDP or a CIDP-like illness on pathogenetic grounds. CIDP associated with most of these conditions is probably not different from ordinary CIDP in presentation and response to therapy. A recognized exception is found in cases with CIDP associated with monoclonal gammopathies, which show subtle clinical differences and a poorer response to treatment.[198] Chronic demyelinating neuropathy associated with an IgM monoclonal gammopathy and particularly with autoantibodies against myelin-associated glycoprotein has distinct clinical features with prominent sensory involvement and requires specific therapeutic considerations, as discussed in Chapter 17.[39,199] Diabetic patients may develop a demyelinating neuropathy with conduction block indistinguishable from CIDP that may respond to immuno-modulatory treatment.[200,201] However, segmental demyelination may be due to microvasculitis rather than a primary autoimmune attack on myelin.[202] Patients with hereditary neuropathies may occasionally develop secondary progression

due to an inflammatory neuropathy. This is thought to be due to unmasking of epitopes during the process of peripheral nerve breakdown and the generation of a secondary immune response. Similar observations were made in genetic animal models of these diseases.[203] Secondary CIDP in hereditary neuropathy may account for case reports of steroid-responsive hereditary neuropathies. Pregnancy may trigger CIDP, and relapses of CIDP may occur, particularly around and after the time of delivery.

Pathology

The pathologic hallmark of classic CIDP is macrophage-mediated segmental demyelination, as in AIDP.[204] In sural nerve biopsies, predominant demyelinating features (Figure 16-3) with demyelinated and remyelinated axons as well as supernumerary Schwann's cell formations (onion bulbs) are seen in only approximately one-half of the patients, whereas the remaining cases show either predominant axonal changes or a mixed picture. Autopsy studies confirmed axonal as well as motoneuron loss in CIDP.[205] Pathologic changes may be multifocal rather than evenly distributed.[206] Other features are endoneurial edema that may be marked, increased numbers of endoneurial and epineurial T cells, increased numbers of epineurial and endoneurial macrophages that may express inflammation-related antigens, and the presence of proinflammatory cytokines.[82,206–208] However, neither of these features is invariably present, and severity of changes may be from mild to very severe, with complete demyelination of all nerve fibers.

Clinical Differential Diagnosis

The list of differential diagnoses depends on the presentation and course of the disease. Relapsing-remitting CIDP has a fairly unique presentation. Hereditary neuropathy with liability to pressure palsies may be confused with asymmetric variants of relapsing-remitting CIDP and shares some electrophysiologic features. Clues toward hereditary neuropathy with liability to pressure palsies are a positive family history, a tendency toward the involvement of multiple individual nerves, precipitation of mononeuropathy symptoms by pressure and repetitive tasks, and predilection for mechanically exposed nerves. Definitive diagnosis is through genetic testing. Differentiation of the chronic-progressive, distal-symmetric, sensorimotor form of CIDP from other distal-symmetric polyneuropathies may be impossible on clinical grounds alone. Clinical categorization of the neuropathic syndrome should consider family history, age at onset, rate and character of progression, nerve fiber modalities affected, and accompanying illnesses. Clues for CIDP are a negative family history, recent onset (or at least not lifelong disease), no accompanying illnesses, proximal muscle involvement, and occasionally a stepwise progression. Clinical suspicion may be particularly difficult to entertain on clinical grounds alone in children and adolescents, in whom previously unrecognized genetic neuropathies are particularly prevalent.

Asymmetric progressive variants of CIDP are part of a different and more specific spectrum of differential diagnoses. These include vasculitis of the PNS; diabetic mononeuropathy; sarcoid neuropathy; entrapment mononeuropathy; tumors within the nerve, nerve sheath, or adjacent structures; infectious neuropathies, including borreliosis and leprosy; and lymphomatous infiltration of peripheral nerve.

Diagnostic Procedures

As in GBS, diagnostic procedures may be divided into those that support the diagnosis and those that are needed to exclude other differential diagnoses. Routine laboratory tests are usually normal but may exclude other causes of distal symmetric polyneuropathy. Serum protein electrophoresis and immune fixation are mandatory investigations and may reveal plasma dyscrasia. Patients with IgM monoclonal gammopathy and particularly those with antibodies against myelin-associated glycoprotein need to be separated from CIDP. Numerous autoantibodies can be found in serum from CIDP patients. None helps in the differential diagnosis, and routine determination is not warranted.[19] Elevated titers of antinuclear antibodies and other serologic markers of vasculitis and rheumatic disease may point toward these conditions as the cause of the neuropathy. Other serologic tests depend on the list of suspected differential diagnoses made on clinical ground. Genetic tests to exclude hereditary neuropathies should rarely be necessary if a careful history and clinical examination as well as electrophysiologic studies are performed. CSF studies reveal cytoalbuminic dissociation as in GBS. CSF cell counts should not exceed 10/µl in immunocompetent persons and 50/µl in human immunodeficiency virus–positive patients. Total CSF protein may be markedly elevated.

Electrophysiologic studies are of particular importance in supporting the diagnosis and establishing a differential diagnosis. The electrophysiologic hallmarks are similar to the findings in GBS. Thus, typical findings are prolonged distal motor latencies, prolonged F-wave latencies, reduced F-wave frequencies or total absence of F waves, multifocal conduction block, and reduced nerve conduction velocities. Sensory involvement may be more pronounced than in GBS, with marked slowing of sensory nerve conduction velocities. With secondary axonal damage, reductions in CMAP and SNAP amplitudes are observed, and EMG reveals denervation potentials. In chronic inflammatory axonal polyneuropathy, there is evidence of marked axonal damage with few or no demyelinating features. In advanced stages of the disease progressing over many years, differentiation between secondary axonal degeneration and a primary axonal neuropathy may be difficult.

MRI studies may reveal thickening and contrast enhancement of lumbosacral spinal roots, resulting in compressive injury to the affected roots due to edema.[209] Sural nerve biopsy is not indicated if clinical findings, CSF analysis, and electrophysiologic studies are typical of CIDP and other differential diagnoses are not seriously considered.[210] However, sural nerve biopsy is of considerable diagnostic value in advanced disease wherein electrodiagnostic studies are less revealing and in cases with predominant axonal involvement. The main goal is the demonstration of inflammatory infiltrates using immunocytochemistry. Although occasional endoneurial T cells and small perivascular lymphocytic cuffs of a few T cells in the epineurium are common in many forms of peripheral neuropathy, dense perivascular cuffs and numerous endoneurial T cells point toward an inflammatory cause of the condition (see Figure 16-1) and may warrant therapeutic decisions toward immunomodulatory treatment. In addition, the finding of certain inflammation-related macrophage antigens has been found to be associated with an inflammatory cause of the condition.[207] Sural nerve biopsy should be performed only if investigation in a specialized laboratory is possible. Diagnostic criteria for CIDP have been published and are widely used for research purposes.[6]

Therapy for Chronic Inflammatory Demyelinating Polyneuropathy

Immunomodulatory Therapeutic Regimens

Glucocorticoids are of proven effectiveness, as documented in numerous uncontrolled series and one controlled trial.[211] The usual dose is 1.0–1.5 mg/kg methylprednisolone, which is gradually tapered. Supplementation with vitamin D and calcium to prevent osteoporosis, appropriate peptic ulcer prophylaxis, and regular ophthalmologic examinations are recommended. The advantage of using glucocorticoids lies in its ease of application and low costs; its disadvantage is seen in side effects, particularly with prolonged treatment. Glucocorticoids are, therefore, recommended as immunosuppressive induction therapy rather than for long-term maintenance. In a small case series, high-dose pulse therapy with dexamethasone monthly for 6 months was found to induce long-lasting remissions in 6 of 10 patients studied.[212]

IVIg has been shown to be effective in CIDP in several case series and in a controlled trial.[213] There was an overall response rate of 63%, with slightly more favorable results in relapsing-remitting cases than in chronic-progressive disease. The usual dose is 0.4 g/kg daily for 5 days. Relapses after treatment may occur. The duration of a favorable response is highly variable among individual patients but usually lasts for 2–3 months. Subsequent treatments with lower doses may suffice to maintain the beneficial effect, and the interval and dosage have to be titrated individually for long-term treatment. Subsequent treatment cycles are usually given at the time of anticipated relapse or the first signs of deterioration. Advantages of IVIg as compared to other treatments are excellent tolerability in most patients, rapid effectiveness, and easy availability. The main disadvantages are occasional side effects and high costs.

Plasma exchange is another first-line standard treatment of CIDP with proven efficacy.[214,215] Response rates were up to 80% in a controlled study with newly diagnosed cases after 10 exchanges over 4 weeks. Improvement occurred rapidly but was not long-lasting in all patients, requiring additional immunosuppressive therapy or repeat exchanges. Clinical recovery was also reflected in improvements of neurophysiologic parameters.[216] The main advantage of plasma exchange is its high responder rate and efficacy, particularly in progressive, severe disease. Disadvantages are its limited availability, side effects, and high cost.

Azathioprine is used as immunosuppressive maintenance therapy to spare glucocorticoids. Combination treatment together with glucocorticoids is not superior to glucocorticoids alone.[217] However, azathioprine treatment takes some time to become effective and thus may be started together with high-dose glucocorticoids. Whereas the latter are gradually tapered, azathioprine is generally well tolerated as a long-term treatment. The standard dosage is 2–3 mg/kg daily. At effective doses, azathioprine induces lymphopenia, which has to be monitored at regular intervals. Therapy aims at moderate lymphopenia with lymphocyte counts of 600–1,000/μl, and the dose is adjusted accordingly.

Cyclophosphamide is a second-line drug if other treatments have failed. Pulse therapy appears to be superior to daily oral treatment, owing to fewer side effects. In a case series of 15 patients receiving monthly cyclophosphamide infusions at 1 g/m² for 6 months, 11 patients improved.[218] The nadir of leukopenia induced by cyclophosphamide occurs between the tenth and fourteenth day, with desired leukocyte counts of approximately 2,000/μl. With insufficient or excessive leukopenia, dose adjustments may be necessary.

Cyclosporine A may be useful as long-term treatment in selected patients if other treatments have failed.[219–221] Methotrexate at 7.5–10.0 mg weekly may alternatively be tried as long-term immunosuppressive treatment. IFN-α-2a has been shown to be effective in a proportion of patients who had CIDP unresponsive to conventional treatments in small case series or open studies.[222,223] However, IFN-α itself may lead to autoimmune disorders, possibly including CIDP.[224,225] IFN-β-1a was effective in an isolated case of severe sensorimotor CIDP[226] and provided limited benefit in another patient with pure motor CIDP, including a reduction in the degree of conduction block.[227] However, in a small double-blind randomized crossover study of 10 CIDP patients resistant to conventional therapies, no benefit of IFN-β could be demonstrated.

Pragmatic Approach to Immunomodulatory Therapy

The choice of treatment depends on the severity and progression of the disease, associated conditions, the availability and side effect profile of the various treatment modalities, and cost considerations. First-line treatments include glucocorticoids, immunoglobulins, and plasma exchange. IVIg and plasma exchange were found to be equally effective in a randomized, observer-blind study.[228] In a large retrospective series, response rates to plasma exchange, IVIg, and glucocorticoids were similar.[188] Mild disease does not warrant invasive therapy and is best treated with a single course of immunoglobulins if the costs can be afforded. Disabling disease should be aggressively treated. High-dose glucocorticoids and immunoglobulins may be used, and plasma exchange is generally reserved for patients with severe, progressive disease. If long-term immunosuppression is necessary, azathioprine is added early, as it may take several months to take its full effect. If treatment fails with one first-line treatment modality, the other first-line regimens should be tried.[188] In severe cases, combination treatment of glucocorticoids with IVIg or plasma exchange is warranted. If first-line treatment regimens fail, cyclophosphamide pulse therapy or cyclosporine A may next be tried in disabling disease, perhaps in an additive manner.

Supportive Therapy

Patients with rapidly progressive disease and severe disabilities may require hospitalization and observation in an intensive care unit, much like GBS patients. Safety measures, indications for mechanical ventilation, prophylactic treatments, and other aspects of neurologic intensive care management of severely afflicted patients are as described for GBS patients.

All patients require intensive physiotherapy throughout the course of their disease. Once discharged from the neurologic ward, most patients with residual deficits will benefit from specialized treatment in a rehabilitation unit. As relapses may occur, patients should be regularly followed up by a neurologist experienced in treating the disorder.

Course and Prognosis

Although at least two-thirds of patients experience some response to therapy,[188] improvement may not be permanent, and progressive deficits may occur.[198] In two epidemiologic studies, 13% of patients required a walking aid after a mean disease duration of 7.1 and 8.9 years, respectively.[185,186] Once secondary axonal damage has occurred, residual deficits are the rule and may be severe.[229]

References

1. Hartung HP, van der Meche FGA, Pollard JD. Guillain-Barré syndrome, CIDP and other chronic immune-mediated neuropathies. Curr Opin Neurol 1998;11:497–513.
2. Hahn AF. Guillain-Barré syndrome. Lancet 1998;352: 635–641.

3. Steck AJ, Schaeren-Wiemers N, Hartung HP. Demyelinating inflammatory neuropathies, including Guillain-Barré syndrome. Curr Opin Neurol 1998;11:311–318.

4. Ho T, Griffin J. Guillain-Barré syndrome. Curr Opin Neurol 1999;12:389–394.

5. Asbury AK, Cornblath DR. Assessment of current diagnostic criteria for Guillain-Barré syndrome. Ann Neurol 1990;27:S21–S24.

6. Research criteria for diagnosis of chronic inflammatory demyelinating polyneuropathy (CIDP). Report from an Ad Hoc Subcommittee of the American Academy of Neurology AIDS Task Force. Neurology 1991;41:617–618.

7. Hughes R, Sanders E, Hall S, et al. Subacute idiopathic demyelinating polyradiculoneuropathy. Arch Neurol 1992;49:612–616.

8. Feasby TE, Gilbert JJ, Brown WF, et al. An acute axonal form of Guillain-Barré polyneuropathy. Brain 1986;109:1115–1126.

9. Griffin JW, Li CY, Ho TW, et al. Guillain-Barré syndrome in northern China. The spectrum of neuropathological changes in clinically defined cases. Brain 1995;118:577–595.

10. McKhann GM, Cornblath DR, Griffin JW, et al. Acute motor axonal neuropathy: a frequent cause of acute flaccid paralysis in China. Ann Neurol 1993;33:333–342.

11. Hadden RD, Cornblath DR, Hughes RA, et al. Electrophysiological classification of Guillain-Barré syndrome: clinical associations and outcome. Plasma Exchange/Sandoglobulin Guillain-Barré Syndrome Trial Group. Ann Neurol 1998;44:780–788.

12. Griffin JW, Li CY, Ho TW, et al. Pathology of the motor-sensory axonal Guillain-Barré syndrome. Ann Neurol 1996;39:17–28.

13. Chroni E, Hall SM, Hughes RA. Chronic relapsing axonal neuropathy: a first case report. Ann Neurol 1995;37:112–115.

14. Ho TW, McKhann GM, Griffin JW. Human autoimmune neuropathies. Annu Rev Neurosci 1998;21:187–226.

15. Gold R, Archelos JJ, Hartung HP. Mechanisms of immune regulation in the peripheral nervous system. Brain Pathol 1999;9:343–360.

16. Hughes RAC, Hadden RD, Gregson NA, Smith KJ. Pathogenesis of Guillain-Barré syndrome. J Neuroimmunol 1999;100:74–97.

17. Kiefer R, Kieseier BC, Stoll G, Hartung HP. The role of macrophages in immune-mediated damage to the peripheral nervous system. Prog Neurobiol 2001;64(2):109–127.

18. Gold R, Hartung HP, Toyka KV. Animal models for autoimmune demyelinating disorders of the nervous system. Mol Med Today 2000;6:88–91.

19. Quarles RH, Weiss MD. Autoantibodies associated with peripheral neuropathy. Muscle Nerve 1999;22:800–822.

20. Barnett LA, Fujinami RS. Molecular mimicry: a mechanism for autoimmune injury. FASEB J 1992;6:840–844.

21. Arnason BGW, Soliven B. Acute Inflammatory Demyelinating Polyradiculoneuropathy. In PJ Dyck, PK Thomas, JW Griffin, et al. (eds), Peripheral Neuropathy. Philadelphia: WB Saunders, 1993;1437–1497.

22. Hughes RAC, Rees JH. Clinical and epidemiological features of Guillain-Barré syndrome. J Infect Dis 1997;176:S92–S98.

23. Jacobs BC, Rothbarth PH, van der Meche FG, et al. The spectrum of antecedent infections in Guillain-Barré syndrome: a case-control study. Neurology 1998;51:1110–1115.

24. Hao Q, Saida T, Kuroki S, et al. Antibodies to gangliosides and galactocerebroside in patients with Guillain-Barré syndrome with preceding *Campylobacter jejuni* and other identified infections. J Neuroimmunol 1998;81:116–126.

25. Ho TW, Mishu B, Li CY, et al. Guillain-Barré syndrome in northern China. Relationship to *Campylobacter jejuni* infection and anti-glycolipid antibodies. Brain 1995;118:597–605.

26. Moran AP, Penner JL. Serotyping of *Campylobacter jejuni* based on heat-stable antigens: relevance, molecular basis and implications in pathogenesis. J Appl Microbiol 1999; 86:361–377.

27. Kuroki S, Saida T, Nukina M, et al. *Campylobacter jejuni* strains from patients with Guillain-Barré syndrome belong mostly to Penner serogroup 19 and contain beta-*N*-acetylglucosamine residues. Ann Neurol 1993;33:243–247.

28. Nishimura M, Nukina M, Kuroki S, et al. Characterization of *Campylobacter jejuni* isolates from patients with Guillain-Barré syndrome. J Neurol Sci 1997;153:91–99.

29. Rees JH, Soudain SE, Gregson NA, Hughes RA. *Campylobacter jejuni* infection and Guillain-Barré syndrome. N Engl J Med 1995;333:1374–1379.

30. Endtz HP, Ang CW, van den Braak N, et al. Molecular characterization of *Campylobacter jejuni* from patients with Guillain-Barré and Miller Fisher syndromes. J Clin Microbiol 2000;38:2297–2301.

31. Lastovica AJ, Goddard EA, Argent AC. Guillain-Barré syndrome in South Africa associated with *Campylobacter jejuni*. J Infect Dis 1997;176:S139–S143.

32. Mori M, Kuwabara S, Miyake M, et al. *Haemophilus influenzae* infection and Guillain-Barré syndrome. Brain 2000;123:2171–2178.

33. Winer JB, Hughes RA, Anderson MJ, et al. A prospective study of acute idiopathic neuropathy. II. Antecedent events. J Neurol Neurosurg Psychiatry 1988;51:613–618.

34. Lasky T, Terracciano GJ, Magder L, et al. The Guillain-Barré syndrome and the 1992–1993 and 1993–1994 influenza vaccines. N Engl J Med 1998;339:1797–1802.

35. Langmuir AD, Bregman DJ, Kurland LT, et al. An epidemiologic and clinical evaluation of GBS reported in association with administration of swine influenza vaccines. Am J Epidemiol 1984;119:841–879.

36. Hemachudha T, Griffin DE, Chen WW, Johnson RT. Immunological studies of rabies vaccination-induced Guillain-Barré syndrome. Neurology 1988;38:375–378.

37. Vedeler CA. Inflammatory neuropathies: update. Curr Opin Neurol 2000;13:305–309.

38. Hartung HP, Kieseier RC. Antibody responses in the Guillain-Barré syndrome. J Neurol Sci 1999;168:75–77.

39. Steck AJ, Erne B, Gabriel JM, Schaeren-Wiemers N. Paraproteinaemic neuropathies. Brain Pathol 1999;9:361–368.

40. Gabriel CM, Hughes RA, Moore SE, et al. Induction of experimental autoimmune neuritis with peripheral myelin protein-22. Brain 1998;121:1895–1902.

41. Gabriel CM, Gregson NA, Hughes RA. Anti-PMP22 antibodies in patients with inflammatory neuropathy. J Neuroimmunol 2000;104:139–146.

42. Yuki N, Tagawa Y, Handa S. Autoantibodies to peripheral nerve glycosphingolipids SPG, SLPG, and SGPG in Guillain-Barré syndrome and chronic inflammatory demyelinating polyneuropathy. J Neuroimmunol 1996;70:1–6.

43. Koga M, Yuki N, Hirata K. Subclass distribution and the secretory component of serum IgA anti-ganglioside antibodies in Guillain-Barré syndrome after Campylobacter jejuni enteritis. J Neuroimmunol 1999;96:245–250.

44. Willison HJ, O'Hanlon GM. The immunopathogenesis of Miller Fisher syndrome. J Neuroimmunol 1999;100:3–12.

45. Jacobs BC, van Doorn PA, Schmitz PI, et al. Campylobacter jejuni infections and anti-GM1 antibodies in Guillain-Barré syndrome. Ann Neurol 1996;40:181–187.

46. Yuki N, Takahashi M, Tagawa Y, et al. Association of Campylobacter jejuni serotype with antiganglioside antibody in Guillain-Barré syndrome and Fisher's syndrome. Ann Neurol 1997;42:28–33.

47. Yuki N, Taki T, Handa S. Antibody to GalNAc-GD1a and GalNAc-GM1b in Guillain-Barré syndrome subsequent to Campylobacter jejuni enteritis. J Neuroimmunol 1996; 71:155–161.

48. Yuki N, Ho TW, Tagawa Y, et al. Autoantibodies to GM1b and GalNAc-GD1a: relationship to Campylobacter jejuni infection and acute motor axonal neuropathy in China. J Neurol Sci 1999;164:134–138.

49. Ang CW, Yuki N, Jacobs BC, et al. Rapidly progressive, predominantly motor Guillain-Barré syndrome with anti-GalNAc-GD1a antibodies. Neurology 1999;53:2122–2127.

50. Yuki N, Ang CW, Koga M, et al. Clinical features and response to treatment in Guillain-Barré syndrome associated with antibodies to GM1b ganglioside. Ann Neurol 2000;47:314–321.

51. Ho TW, Willison HJ, Nachamkin I, et al. Anti-GD1a antibody is associated with axonal but not demyelinating forms of Guillain-Barré syndrome. Ann Neurol 1999;45: 168–173.

52. Irie S, Saito T, Nakamura K, et al. Association of anti-GM2 antibodies in Guillain-Barré syndrome with acute cytomegalovirus infection. J Neuroimmunol 1996;68:19–26.

53. Jacobs BC, van Doorn PA, Groeneveld JH, et al. Cytomegalovirus infections and anti-GM2 antibodies in Guillain-Barré syndrome. J Neurol Neurosurg Psychiatry 1997;62: 641–643.

54. Khalili-Shirazi A, Gregson N, Gray I, et al. Antiganglioside antibodies in Guillain-Barré syndrome after a recent cytomegalovirus infection. J Neurol Neurosurg Psychiatry 1999;66:376–379.

55. Yuki N, Tagawa Y. Acute cytomegalovirus infection and IgM anti-GM2 antibody. J Neurol Sci 1998;154:14–17.

56. Khalili-Shirazi A, Atkinson P, Gregson N, Hughes RA. Antibody responses to P0 and P2 myelin proteins in Guillain-Barré syndrome and chronic idiopathic demyelinating polyradiculoneuropathy. J Neuroimmunol 1993;46:245–251.

57. Yuki N, Taki T, Inagaki F, et al. A bacterium lipopolysaccharide that elicits Guillain-Barré syndrome has a GM1 ganglioside-like structure. J Exp Med 1993;178:1771–1775.

58. Aspinall GO, Fujimoto S, McDonald AG, et al. Lipopolysaccharides from Campylobacter jejuni associated with Guillain-Barré syndrome patients mimic human gangliosides in structure. Infect Immun 1994;62:2122–2125.

59. Yuki N. Molecular mimicry between gangliosides and lipopolysaccharides of Campylobacter jejuni isolated from patients with Guillain-Barré syndrome and Miller Fisher syndrome. J Infect Dis 1997;176:S150–S153.

60. Ang CW, Jacobs BC, Brandenburg AH, et al. Cross-reactive antibodies against GM2 and CMV-infected fibroblasts in Guillain-Barré syndrome. Neurology 2000;54: 1453–1458.

61. Mori M, Kuwabara S, Miyake M, et al. Haemophilus influenzae has a GM1 ganglioside-like structure and elicits Guillain-Barré syndrome. Neurology 1999;52:1282–1284.

62. Sheikh KA, Nachamkin I, Ho TW, et al. Campylobacter jejuni lipopolysaccharides in Guillain-Barré syndrome: molecular mimicry and host susceptibility. Neurology 1998;51:371–378.

63. Sack DA, Lastovica AJ, Chang SH, Pazzaglia G. Microtiter assay for detecting Campylobacter spp. and Helicobacter pylori with surface gangliosides which bind cholera toxin. J Clin Microbiol 1998;36:2043–2045.

64. Raschetti R, Maggini M, Popoli P, et al. Gangliosides and Guillain-Barré syndrome. J Clin Epidemiol 1995;48: 1399–1405.

65. Illa I, Ortiz N, Gallard E, et al. Acute axonal Guillain-Barré syndrome with IgG antibodies against motor axons following parenteral gangliosides. Ann Neurol 1995; 38:218–224.

66. Izumo S, Linington C, Wekerle H, Meyermann R. Morphologic study on experimental allergic neuritis mediated by T cell line specific for bovine P2 protein in Lewis rats. Lab Invest 1985;53:209–218.

67. Linington C, Lassmann H, Ozawa K, et al. Cell adhesion molecules of the immunoglobulin supergene family as tissue-specific autoantigens: induction of experimental allergic neuritis (EAN) by P0 protein-specific T cell lines. Eur J Immunol 1992;22:1813–1817.

68. Weerth S, Berger T, Lassmann H, Linington C. Encephalitogenic and neuritogenic T cell responses to the myelin-associated glycoprotein (MAG) in the Lewis rat. J Neuroimmunol 1999;95:157–164.

69. Pette M, Linington C, Gengaroli C, et al. T lymphocyte recognition sites on peripheral nerve myelin P0 protein. J Neuroimmunol 1994;54:29–34.

70. Khalili-Shirazi A, Hughes RA, Brostoff SW, et al. T cell responses to myelin proteins in Guillain-Barré syndrome. J Neurol Sci 1992;111:200–203.

71. Khalili-Shirazi A, Gregson NA, Londei M, et al. The distribution of CD1 molecules in inflammatory neuropathy. J Neurol Sci 1998;158:154–163.

72. Cooper JC, Ben Smith A, Savage CO, Winer JB. Unusual T cell receptor phenotype V gene usage of gammadelta T cells in a line derived from the peripheral nerve of a patient with Guillain-Barré syndrome. J Neurol Neurosurg Psychiatry 2000;69:522–524.

73. Khalili-Shirazi A, Gregson NA, Hall MA, et al. T cell receptor V beta gene usage in Guillain-Barré syndrome. J Neurol Sci 1997;145:169–176.

74. Bosboom WM, Van den Berg LH, Mollee I, et al. Sural nerve T-cell receptor Vbeta gene utilization in chronic inflammatory demyelinating polyneuropathy and vasculitic neuropathy. Neurology 2001;56:74–81.

75. Rees JH, Vaughan RW, Kondeatis E, Hughes RA. HLA-class II alleles in Guillain-Barré syndrome and Miller Fisher syndrome and their association with preceding *Campylobacter jejuni* infection. J Neuroimmunol 1995;62:53–57.

76. Koga M, Yuki N, Kashiwase K, et al. Guillain-Barré and Fisher's syndromes subsequent to *Campylobacter jejuni* enteritis are associated with HLA-B54 and Cw1 independent of anti-ganglioside antibodies. J Neuroimmunol 1998;88:62–66.

77. Ma JJ, Nishimura M, Mine H, et al. HLA and T-cell receptor gene polymorphisms in Guillain-Barré syndrome. Neurology 1998;51:379–384.

78. Monos DS, Papaioakim M, Ho TW, et al. Differential distribution of HLA alleles in two forms of Guillain-Barré syndrome. J Infect Dis 1997;176(Suppl 2):S180–S182.

79. Ma JJ, Nishimura M, Mine H, et al. Genetic contribution of the tumor necrosis factor region in Guillain-Barré syndrome. Ann Neurol 1998;44:815–818.

80. van der Pol WL, Van den Berg LH, Scheepers RH, et al. IgG receptor IIa alleles determine susceptibility and severity of Guillain-Barré syndrome. Neurology 2000;54:1661–1665.

81. Vedeler CA, Raknes G, Myhr KM, Nyland H. IgG Fc-receptor polymorphisms in Guillain-Barré syndrome. Neurology 2000;55:705–707.

82. Schmidt B, Toyka KV, Kiefer R, et al. Inflammatory infiltrates in sural nerve biopsies in Guillain-Barré syndrome and chronic inflammatory demyelinating neuropathy. Muscle Nerve 1996;19:474–487.

83. Kiefer R, Dangond F, Mueller M, et al. Enhanced B7 costimulatory molecule expression in inflammatory human sural nerve biopsies. J Neurol Neurosurg Psychiatry 2000;69:362–368.

84. Murata K, Dalakas MC. Expression of the co-stimulatory molecule BB-1, the ligands CTLA-4 and CD28 and their mRNAs in chronic inflammatory demyelinating polyneuropathy. Brain 2000;123:1660–1666.

85. Van Rhijn I, Van den Berg LH, Bosboom WM, et al. Expression of accessory molecules for T-cell activation in peripheral nerve of patients with CIDP and vasculitic neuropathy. Brain 2000;123:2020–2029.

86. Archelos JJ, Previtali SC, Hartung HP. The role of integrins in immune-mediated diseases of the nervous system. Trends Neurosci 1999;22:30–38.

87. Hughes PM, Wells GMA, Clements JM, et al. Matrix metalloprotease expression during experimental autoimmune neuritis. Brain 1998;121:481–494.

88. Kieseier BC, Clements JM, Pischel HB, et al. Matrix metalloproteases MMP-9 and MMP-7 are expressed in experimental autoimmune neuritis and the Guillain-Barré syndrome. Ann Neurol 1998;43:427–434.

89. Creange A, Sharshar T, Planchenault T, et al. Matrix metalloproteinase-9 is increased and correlates with severity in Guillain-Barré syndrome. Neurology 1999;53:1683–1691.

90. Leppert D, Hughes P, Huber S, et al. Matrix metalloproteinase upregulation in chronic inflammatory demyelinating polyneuropathy and nonsystemic vasculitic neuropathy. Neurology 1999;53:62–70.

91. Hartung HP, Kieseier BC. The role of matrix metalloproteinases in autoimmune damage to the central and peripheral nervous system. J Neuroimmunol 2000;107:140–147.

92. Zou LP, Pelidou SH, Abbas N, et al. Dynamics of production of MIP-1alpha, MCP-1 and MIP-2 and potential role of neutralization of these chemokines in the regulation of immune responses during experimental autoimmune neuritis in Lewis rats. J Neuroimmunol 1999;98:168–175.

93. Kieseier BC, Krivacic K, Jung S, et al. Sequential expression of chemokines in experimental autoimmune neuritis. J Neuroimmunol 2000;110:121–129.

94. Spies JM, Westland KW, Bonner JG, Pollard JD. Intraneural activated T cells cause focal breakdown of the blood-nerve barrier. Brain 1995;118:857–868.

95. Plomp JJ, Molenaar PC, O'Hanlon GM, et al. Miller Fisher anti-GQ1b antibodies: alpha-latrotoxin-like effects on motor end plates. Ann Neurol 1999;45:189–199.

96. Buchwald B, Toyka KV, Zielasek J, et al. Neuromuscular blockade of IgG antibodies from patients with Guillain-Barré syndrome: a macro-patch-clamp study. Ann Neurol 1998;44:913–922.

97. Buchwald B, Bufler J, Carpo M, et al. Combined pre- and postsynaptic action of IgG antibodies in Miller Fisher syndrome. Neurology 2001;56:67–74.

98. Goodyear CS, O'Hanlon GM, Plomp JJ, et al. Monoclonal antibodies raised against Guillain-Barré syndrome-associated *Campylobacter jejuni* lipopolysaccharides react with neuronal gangliosides and paralyze muscle-nerve preparations. J Clin Invest 1999;104:697–708.

99. Brinkmeier H, Aulkemeyer P, Wollinsky KH, Rudel R. An endogenous pentapeptide acting as a sodium channel blocker in inflammatory autoimmune disorders of the central nervous system. Nat Med 2000;6:808–811.

100. Oka N, Akiguchi I, Kawasaki T, et al. Tumor necrosis factor-alpha in peripheral nerve lesions. Acta Neuropathol 1998;95:57–62.

101. Redford EJ, Smith KJ, Gregson NA, et al. A combined inhibitor of matrix metalloproteinase activity and tumour necrosis factor-alpha processing attenuates experimental autoimmune neuritis. Brain 1997;120:1895–1905.

102. Uncini A, Di Muzio A, Di Guglielmo G, et al. Effect of rhTNF-alpha injection into rat sciatic nerve. J Neuroimmunol 1999;94:88–94.

103. Sharief MK, Ingram DA, Swash M. Circulating tumor necrosis factor-alpha correlates with electrodiagnostic abnormalities in Guillain-Barré syndrome. Ann Neurol 1997;42:68–73.

104. Pelidou SH, Deretzi G, Zou LP, et al. Inflammation and severe demyelination in the peripheral nervous system induced by the intraneural injection of recombinant mouse interleukin-12. Scand J Immunol 1999;50:39–44.

105. Deretzi G, Pelidou SH, Zou LP, et al. Local effects of recombinant rat interleukin-6 on the peripheral nervous system. Immunology 1999;97:582–587.

106. van der Goes A, Brouwer J, Hoekstra K, et al. Reactive oxygen species are required for the phagocytosis of myelin by macrophages. J Neuroimmunol 1998;92:67–75.

107. van der Veen RC, Roberts LJ. Contrasting roles for nitric oxide and peroxynitrite in the peroxidation of myelin lipids. J Neuroimmunol 1999;95:1–7.

108. Berciano J, Figols J, Garcia A, et al. Fulminant Guillain-Barré syndrome with universal inexcitability of peripheral nerves: a clinicopathological study. Muscle Nerve 1997; 20:846–857.

109. Maier H, Schmidbauer M, Pfausler B, et al. Central nervous system pathology in patients with the Guillain-Barré syndrome. Brain 1997;120:451–464.

110. Gold R, Hartung HP, Lassmann H. T-cell apoptosis in autoimmune diseases: termination of inflammation in the nervous system and other sites with specialized immune-defense mechanisms. Trends Neurosci 1997;20:399–404.

111. Kiefer R, Funa K, Schweitzer T, et al. Transforming growth factor-β1 in experimental autoimmune neuritis: cellular localization and time course. Am J Pathol 1996; 148:211–223.

112. Creange A, Belec L, Clair B, et al. Circulating transforming growth factor beta 1 (TGF-β1) in Guillain-Barré syndrome: decreased concentrations in the early course and increase with motor function. J Neurol Neurosurg Psychiatry 1998;162–165.

113. Gillen C, Jander S, Stoll G. Sequential expression of mRNA for proinflammatory cytokines and interleukin-10 in the rat peripheral nervous system: comparison between immune-mediated demyelination and Wallerian degeneration. J Neurosci Res 1998;51:489–496.

114. Ho TW, Hsieh ST, Nachamkin I, et al. Motor nerve terminal degeneration provides a potential mechanism for rapid recovery in acute motor axonal neuropathy after *Campylobacter* infection. Neurology 1997;48:717–724.

115. Prevots DR, Sutter RW. Assessment of Guillain-Barré syndrome mortality and morbidity in the United States: implications for acute flaccid paralysis surveillance. J Infect Dis 1997;175:S151–S155.

116. van Koningsveld R, van Doorn PA, Schmitz PI, et al. Mild forms of Guillain-Barré syndrome in an epidemiologic survey in The Netherlands. Neurology 2000;54:620–625.

117. McKhann GM, Cornblath DR, Ho TW, et al. Clinical and electrophysiological aspects of acute flaccid paralytic disease in children and young adults in Northern China. Lancet 1991;338:593–597.

118. Flachenecker P, Wermuth P, Hartung HP, Reiners K. Quantitative assessment of cardiovascular autonomic function in Guillain-Barré syndrome. Ann Neurol 1997; 42:171–179.

119. Flachenecker P, Hartung HP, Reiners K. Power spectrum analysis of heart rate variability in Guillain-Barré syndrome. A longitudinal study. Brain 1997;120:1885–1894.

120. Pfeiffer G, Schiller B, Kruse J, Netzer J. Indicators of dysautonomia in severe Guillain-Barré syndrome. J Neurol 1999;246:1015–1022.

121. Flachenecker P, Mullges W, Wermuth P, et al. Eyeball pressure testing in the evaluation of serious bradyarrhythmias in Guillain-Barré syndrome. Neurology 1996;47: 102–108.

122. Oh SJ, LaGanke C, Claussen GC. Sensory Guillain-Barré syndrome. Neurology 2001;56:82–86.

123. Visser LH, van der Meche FGA, Meulstee J, et al. Cytomegalovirus infection and Guillain-Barré syndrome: the clinical, electrophysiologic and prognostic features. Neurology 1996;47:668–673.

124. Prineas JW. Pathology of the Guillain-Barré syndrome. Ann Neurol 1981;9(Suppl):6–19.

125. Hafer-Macko CE, Sheikh KA, Li CY, et al. Immune attack on the Schwann cell surface in acute inflammatory demyelinating polyneuropathy. Ann Neurol 1996;39:625–635.

126. Hafer-Macko C, Hsieh ST, Li CY, et al. Acute motor axonal neuropathy: an antibody-mediated attack on axolemma. Ann Neurol 1996;40:635–644.

127. Visser LH, van der Meche FG, van Doorn PA, et al. Guillain-Barré syndrome without sensory loss (acute motor neuropathy). A subgroup with specific clinical, electrodiagnostic and laboratory features. Dutch Guillain-Barré Study Group. Brain 1995;118:841–847.

128. Griffin JW, Li CY, Macko C, et al. Early nodal changes in the acute motor axonal neuropathy pattern of the Guillain-Barré syndrome. J Neurocytol 1996;25:33–51.

129. Kaida K, Kusunoki S, Kamakura K, et al. Guillain-Barré syndrome with antibody to a ganglioside, *N*-acetylgalactosaminyl GD1a. Brain 2000;123:116–124.

130. Ogawara K, Kuwabara S, Mori M, et al. Axonal Guillain-Barré syndrome: relation to anti-ganglioside antibodies and *Campylobacter jejuni* infection in Japan. Ann Neurol 2000;48:624–631.

131. Yuki N, Kuwabara S, Koga M, Hirata K. Acute motor axonal neuropathy and acute motor-sensory axonal neuropathy share a common immunological profile. J Neurol Sci 1999;168:121–126.

132. Ter Bruggen JP, van der Meche FG, de Jager AE, Polman CH. Ophthalmoplegic and lower cranial nerve variants merge into each other and into classical Guillain-Barré syndrome. Muscle Nerve 1998;21:239–242.

133. Chiba A, Kusunoki S, Obata H, et al. Ganglioside composition of the human cranial nerves, with special reference to pathophysiology of Miller Fisher syndrome. Brain Res 1997;745:32–36.

134. Buchwald B, Weishaupt A, Toyka KV, Dudel J. Pre- and postsynaptic blockade of neuromuscular transmission by Miller-Fisher syndrome IgG at mouse motor nerve terminals. Eur J Neurosci 1998;10:281–290.

135. O'Leary CP, Veitch J, Durward WF, et al. Acute oropharyngeal palsy is associated with antibodies to GQ1b and GT1a gangliosides. J Neurol Neurosurg Psychiatry 1996;61:649–651.

136. Koga M, Yuki N, Hirata K. Antiganglioside antibody in patients with Guillain-Barré syndrome who show bulbar palsy as an initial symptom. J Neurol Neurosurg Psychiatry 1999;66:513–516.

137. Yoshino H, Harukawa H, Asano A. IgG antiganglioside antibodies in Guillain-Barré syndrome with bulbar palsy. J Neuroimmunol 2000;105:195–201.

138. O'Leary CP, Willison HJ. Autoimmune ataxic neuropathies (sensory ganglionopathies). Curr Opin Neurol 1997;10:366–370.

139. Yuki N, Hirata K. Postinfection sensory neuropathy asso-

ciated with IgG anti-GD1b antibody. Ann Neurol 1998;43:685–687.

140. Kusunoki S, Hitoshi S, Kaida K, et al. Monospecific anti-GD1b IgG is required to induce rabbit ataxic neuropathy. Ann Neurol 1999;45:400–403.

141. Tagawa Y, Irie F, Hirabayashi Y, Yuki N. Cholinergic neuron-specific ganglioside GQ1b alpha a possible target molecule for serum IgM antibodies in some patients with sensory ataxia. J Neuroimmunol 1997;75:196–199.

142. Marras C, Midroni G. Transient absence of F-waves in acute myelopathy: a potential source of diagnostic error. Electromyogr Clin Neurophysiol 2000;40:109–112.

143. Delanoe C, Sebire G, Landrieu P, et al. Acute inflammatory demyelinating polyradiculopathy in children: clinical and electrodiagnostic studies. Ann Neurol 1998;44:350–356.

144. Flachenecker P, Lem K, Mullges W, Reiners K. Detection of serious bradyarrhythmias in Guillain-Barré syndrome: sensitivity and specificity of the 24-hour heart rate power spectrum. Clin Auton Res 2000;10:185–191.

145. Gorson KC, Ropper AH, Muriello MA, Blair R. Prospective evaluation of MRI lumbosacral nerve root enhancement in acute Guillain-Barré syndrome. Neurology 1996;47:813–817.

146. Hadden RD, Hughes RA. Treatment of immune-mediated inflammatory neuropathies. Curr Opin Neurol 1999; 12:573–579.

147. van der Meche FGA, van Doorn PA. Guillain-Barré syndrome. Curr Treat Options Neurol 2000;2:507–516.

148. Osterman PO, Fagius J, Lundemo G, et al. Beneficial effects of plasma exchange in acute inflammatory polyradiculoneuropathy. Lancet 1984;2:1296–1299.

149. Plasmapheresis and acute Guillain-Barré syndrome. The Guillain-Barré syndrome Study Group. Neurology 1985; 35:1096–1104.

150. Efficiency of plasma exchange in Guillain-Barré syndrome: role of replacement fluids. French Cooperative Group on Plasma Exchange in Guillain-Barré syndrome. Ann Neurol 1987;22:753–761.

151. Plasma exchange in Guillain-Barré syndrome: one-year follow-up. French Cooperative Group on Plasma Exchange in Guillain-Barré Syndrome. Ann Neurol 1992; 32:94–97.

152. Appropriate number of plasma exchanges in Guillain-Barré syndrome. The French Cooperative Group on Plasma Exchange in Guillain-Barré Syndrome. Ann Neurol 1997;41:298–306.

153. Yuki N, Tagawa Y, Hirata K. Minimal number of plasma exchanges needed to reduce immunoglobulin in Guillain-Barré syndrome. Neurology 1998;51:875–877.

154. Assessment of plasmapheresis. Report of the Therapeutics and Technology Assessment Subcommittee of the American Academy of Neurology. Neurology 1996;47:840–843.

155. Tagawa Y, Yuki N, Hirata K. Ability to remove immunoglobulins and anti-ganglioside antibodies by plasma exchange, double-filtration plasmapheresis and immunoadsorption. J Neurol Sci 1998;157:90–95.

156. Chen WH, Yeh JH, Chiu HC. Experience of double filtration plasmapheresis in the treatment of Guillain-Barré syndrome. J Clin Apheresis 1999;14:126–129.

157. Wollinsky KH, Hulser PJ, Brinkmeier H, et al. Filtration of cerebrospinal fluid in acute inflammatory demyelinating polyneuropathy (Guillain-Barré syndrome). Ann Med Interne (Paris) 1994;145:451–458.

158. van der Meche FG, Schmitz PI. A randomized trial comparing intravenous immune globulin and plasma exchange in Guillain-Barré syndrome. Dutch Guillain-Barré Study Group. N Engl J Med 1992;326:1123–1129.

159. Randomised trial of plasma exchange, intravenous immunoglobulin, and combined treatments in Guillain-Barré syndrome. Plasma Exchange/Sandoglobulin Guillain-Barré Syndrome Trial Group. Lancet 1997;349:225–230.

160. Stangel M, Hartung HP, Marx P, Gold R. Side effects of high-dose intravenous immunoglobulins. Clin Neuropharmacol 1997;20:385–393.

161. Dalakas MC. Intravenous immunoglobulin in the treatment of autoimmune neuromuscular diseases: present status and practical therapeutic guidelines. Muscle Nerve 1999;22:1479–1497.

162. Stangel M, Toyka KV, Gold R. Mechanisms of high-dose intravenous immunoglobulins in demyelinating diseases. Arch Neurol 1999;56:661–663.

163. Sharief MK, Ingram DA, Swash M, Thompson EJ. I.v. immunoglobulin reduces circulating proinflammatory cytokines in Guillain-Barré syndrome. Neurology 1999; 52:1833–1838.

164. Kuwabara S, Mori M, Ogawara K, et al. Intravenous immunoglobulin therapy for Guillain-Barré syndrome with IgG anti-GM1 antibody. Muscle Nerve 2001;24:54–58.

165. Yuki N, Ang CW, Koga M, et al. Clinical features and response to treatment in Guillain-Barré syndrome associated with antibodies to GM1b ganglioside. Ann Neurol 2000;47:314–321.

166. Visser LH, van der Meche FG, Meulstee J, van Doorn PA. Risk factors for treatment related clinical fluctuations in Guillain-Barré syndrome. Dutch Guillain-Barré study group. J Neurol Neurosurg Psychiatry 1998;64:242–244.

167. Farcas P, Avnun L, Frisher S, et al. Efficacy of repeated intravenous immunoglobulin in severe unresponsive Guillain-Barré syndrome. Lancet 1997;350:1747.

168. Guillain-Barré Syndrome Steroid Trial Group. Double-blind trial of intravenous methylprednisolone in Guillain-Barré syndrome. Lancet 1993;341:586–590.

169. Hughes RA, van der Meche FG. Corticosteroids for treating Guillain-Barré syndrome. Cochrane Database Syst Rev 2000;(3):CD001446.

170. Treatment of Guillain-Barré syndrome with high-dose immune globulins combined with methylprednisolone: a pilot study. The Dutch Guillain-Barré Study Group. Ann Neurol 1994;35:749–752.

171. Graf WD, Katz JS, Eder DN, et al. Outcome in severe pediatric Guillain-Barré syndrome after immunotherapy or supportive care. Neurology 1999;52:1494–1497.

172. Goodhew PM, Johnston HM. Immune globulin therapy in children with Guillain-Barré syndrome. Muscle Nerve 1996;19:1490–1492.

173. Tripathi M, Kaushik S. Carbamezapine for pain management in Guillain-Barré syndrome patients in the intensive care unit. Crit Care Med 2000;28:655–658.

174. Rosenlicht N, Lee K. Hallucinations in Guillain-Barré syndrome. Am J Psychiatry 2000;157:2056–2057.

175. The prognosis and main prognostic indicators of Guillain-Barré syndrome. A multicentre prospective study of 297 patients. The Italian Guillain-Barré Study Group. Brain 1996;119:2053–2061.

176. Rees JH, Thompson RD, Smeeton NC, Hughes RA. Epidemiological study of Guillain-Barré syndrome in south east England. J Neurol Neurosurg Psychiatry 1998;64:74–77.

177. Lawn ND, Wijdicks EF. Fatal Guillain-Barré syndrome. Neurology 1999;52:635–638.

178. Cheng Q, Jiang GX, Press R, et al. Clinical epidemiology of Guillain-Barré syndrome in adults in Sweden 1996–97: a prospective study. Eur J Neurol 2000;7:685–692.

179. Fletcher DD, Lawn ND, Wolter TD, Wijdicks EF. Long-term outcome in patients with Guillain-Barré syndrome requiring mechanical ventilation. Neurology 2000;54:2311–2315.

180. Rees JH, Gregson NA, Hughes RA. Anti-ganglioside GM1 antibodies in Guillain-Barré syndrome and their relationship to *Campylobacter jejuni* infection. Ann Neurol 1995;38:809–816.

181. Visser LH, Schmitz PI, Meulstee J, et al. Prognostic factors of Guillain-Barré syndrome after intravenous immunoglobulin or plasma exchange. Dutch Guillain-Barré Study Group. Neurology 1999;53:598–604.

182. Kuwabara S, Asahina M, Koga M, et al. Two patterns of clinical recovery in Guillain-Barré syndrome with IgG anti-GM1 antibody. Neurology 1998;51:1656–1660.

183. Bernsen RA, de Jager AE, Schmitz PI, van der Meche FG. Residual physical outcome and daily living 3 to 6 years after Guillain-Barré syndrome. Neurology 1999;53:409–410.

184. Merkies IS, Schmitz PI, Samijn JP, et al. Fatigue in immune-mediated polyneuropathies. European Inflammatory Neuropathy Cause and Treatment (INCAT) Group. Neurology 1999;53:1648–1654.

185. McLeod JG, Pollard JD, Macaskill P, et al. Prevalence of chronic inflammatory demyelinating polyneuropathy in New South Wales, Australia. Ann Neurol 1999;46:910–913.

186. Lunn MP, Manji H, Choudhary PP, et al. Chronic inflammatory demyelinating polyradiculoneuropathy: a prevalence study in south east England. J Neurol Neurosurg Psychiatry 1999;66:677–680.

187. Sakakibara R, Hattori T, Kuwabara S, et al. Micturitional disturbance in patients with chronic inflammatory demyelinating polyneuropathy. Neurology 1998;50:1179–1182.

188. Gorson KC, Allam G, Ropper AH. Chronic inflammatory demyelinating polyneuropathy: clinical features and response to treatment in 67 consecutive patients with and without a monoclonal gammopathy. Neurology 1997;48:321–328.

189. Rotta FT, Sussman AT, Bradley WG, et al. The spectrum of chronic inflammatory demyelinating polyneuropathy. J Neurol Sci 2000;173:129–139.

190. van Dijk GW, Notermans NC, Franssen H, Wokke JH. Development of weakness in patients with chronic inflammatory demyelinating polyneuropathy and only sensory symptoms at presentation: a long-term follow-up study. J Neurol 1999;246:1134–1139.

191. Oh SJ, Claussen GC, Kim DS. Motor and sensory demyelinating mononeuropathy multiplex (multifocal motor and sensory demyelinating neuropathy): a separate entity or a variant of chronic inflammatory demyelinating polyneuropathy? J Peripher Nerv Syst 1997;2:362–369.

192. Gorson KC, Ropper AH, Weinberg DH. Upper limb predominant, multifocal chronic inflammatory demyelinating polyneuropathy. Muscle Nerve 1999;22:758–765.

193. Saperstein DS, Amato AA, Wolfe GI, et al. Multifocal acquired demyelinating sensory and motor neuropathy: the Lewis-Sumner syndrome. Muscle Nerve 1999;22:560–566.

194. Van den Berg-Vos RM, Van den Berg LH, Franssen H, et al. Multifocal inflammatory demyelinating neuropathy: a distinct clinical entity? Neurology 2000;54:26–32.

195. Parry GJ. Are multifocal motor neuropathy and Lewis-Sumner syndrome distinct nosologic entities? Muscle Nerve 1999;22:557–559.

196. Dyck PJ, Dyck PJ. Atypical varieties of chronic inflammatory demyelinating neuropathies. Lancet 2000;355:1293–1294.

197. Butzkueven H, O'Brien TJ, Sedal L. Combined peripheral nerve and central nervous system demyelination in a patient with chronic inflammatory demyelinating polyneuropathy. J Clin Neurosci 1999;6:358–360.

198. Simmons Z, Albers JW, Bromberg MB, Feldman EL. Long-term follow-up of patients with chronic inflammatory demyelinating polyradiculoneuropathy, without and with monoclonal gammopathy. Brain 1995;118:359–368.

199. Simmons Z. Paraproteinemia and neuropathy. Curr Opin Neurol 1999;12:589–595.

200. Stewart JD, McKelvey R, Durcan L, et al. Chronic inflammatory demyelinating polyneuropathy (CIDP) in diabetics. J Neurol Sci 1996;142:59–64.

201. Gorson KC, Ropper AH, Adelman LS, Weinberg DH. Influence of diabetes mellitus on chronic inflammatory demyelinating polyneuropathy. Muscle Nerve 2000;23:37–43.

202. Dyck PJ, Norell JE, Dyck PJ. Microvasculitis and ischemia in diabetic lumbosacral radiculoplexus neuropathy. Neurology 1999;53:2113–2121.

203. Schmid CD, Stienekemeier M, Oehen S, et al. Immune deficiency in mouse models for inherited peripheral neuropathies leads to improved myelin maintenance. J Neurosci 2000;20:729–735.

204. Prineas JW, McLeod JG. Chronic relapsing polyneuritis. J Neurol Sci 1976;27:427–458.

205. Nagamatsu M, Terao S, Misu K, et al. Axonal and perikaryal involvement in chronic inflammatory demyelinating polyneuropathy. J Neurol Neurosurg Psychiatry 1999;66:727–733.

206. Rizzuto N, Morbin M, Cavallaro T, et al. Focal lesions are a feature of chronic inflammatory demyelinating polyneuropathy (CIDP). Acta Neuropathol 1998;96:603–609.

207. Kiefer R, Kieseier BC, Brück W, et al. Macrophage differentiation antigens in acute and chronic autoimmune polyneuropathies. Brain 1998;121:469–479.

208. Mathey EK, Pollard JD, Armati PJ. TNF alpha, IFN

gamma and IL-2 mRNA expression in CIDP sural nerve biopsies. J Neurol Sci 1999;163:47–52.

209. Duggins AJ, McLeod JG, Pollard JD, et al. Spinal root and plexus hypertrophy in chronic inflammatory demyelinating polyneuropathy. Brain 1999;122:1383–1390.

210. Molenaar DS, Vermeulen M, de Haan R. Diagnostic value of sural nerve biopsy in chronic inflammatory demyelinating polyneuropathy. J Neurol Neurosurg Psychiatry 1998;64:84–89.

211. Dyck PJ, O'Brien PC, Oviatt KF, et al. Prednisone improves chronic inflammatory demyelinating polyradiculoneuropathy more than no treatment. Ann Neurol 1982; 11:136–141.

212. Molenaar DS, van Doorn PA, Vermeulen M. Pulsed high dose dexamethasone treatment in chronic inflammatory demyelinating polyneuropathy: a pilot study. J Neurol Neurosurg Psychiatry 1997;62:388–390.

213. Hahn AF, Bolton CF, Zochodne D, Feasby TE. Intravenous immunoglobulin treatment in chronic inflammatory demyelinating polyneuropathy. A double-blind, placebo-controlled, cross-over study. Brain 1996;119:1067–1077.

214. Dyck PJ, Daube J, O'Brien P, et al. Plasma exchange in chronic inflammatory demyelinating polyradiculoneuropathy. N Engl J Med 1986;314:461–465.

215. Hahn AF, Bolton CF, Pillay N, et al. Plasma-exchange therapy in chronic inflammatory demyelinating polyneuropathy. A double-blind, sham-controlled, cross-over study. Brain 1996;119:1055–1066.

216. Ashworth NL, Zochodne DW, Hahn AF, et al. Impact of plasma exchange on indices of demyelination in chronic inflammatory demyelinating polyradiculoneuropathy. Muscle Nerve 2000;23:206–210.

217. Dyck PJ, O'Brien P, Swanson C, et al. Combined azathioprine and prednisone in chronic inflammatory-demyelinating polyneuropathy. Neurology 1985;35:1173–1176.

218. Good JL, Chehrenama M, Mayer RF, Koski CL. Pulse cyclophosphamide therapy in chronic inflammatory demyelinating polyneuropathy. Neurology 1998;51:1735–1738.

219. Hodgkinson SJ, Pollard JD, McLeod JG. Cyclosporin A in the treatment of chronic demyelinating polyradiculoneuropathy. J Neurol Neurosurg Psychiatry 1990;53:327–330.

220. Mahattanakul W, Crawford TO, Griffin JW, et al. Treatment of chronic demyelinating polyneuropathy with cyclosporin-A. J Neurol Neurosurg Psychiatry 1996;60:185–187.

221. Barnett MH, Pollard JD, Davies L, McLeod JG. Cyclosporin A in resistant chronic inflammatory demyelinating polyradiculoneuropathy. Muscle Nerve 1998;21: 454–460.

222. Sabatelli M, Mignogna T, Lippi G, et al. Interferon-alpha may benefit steroid unresponsive chronic inflammatory demyelinating polyneuropathy. J Neurol Neurosurg Psychiatry 1995;58:638–639.

223. Gorson KC, Ropper AH, Clark BD, et al. Treatment of chronic inflammatory demyelinating polyneuropathy with interferon-alpha 2a. Neurology 1998;50:84–87.

224. Meriggioli MN, Rowin J. Chronic inflammatory demyelinating polyneuropathy after treatment with interferon-alpha. Muscle Nerve 2000;23:433–435.

225. Lisak RP. Type I interferons and chronic inflammatory demyelinating polyneuropathy: treatment or cause? Muscle Nerve 2000;23:307–309.

226. Choudhary PP, Thompson N, Hughes RA. Improvement following interferon beta in chronic inflammatory demyelinating polyradiculoneuropathy. J Neurol 1995;242: 252–253.

227. Martina IS, van Doorn PA, Schmitz PI, et al. Chronic motor neuropathies: response to interferon-beta1a after failure of conventional therapies. J Neurol Neurosurg Psychiatry 1999;66:197–201.

228. Dyck PJ, Litchy WJ, Kratz KM, et al. A plasma exchange versus immune globulin infusion trial in chronic inflammatory demyelinating polyradiculoneuropathy. Ann Neurol 1994;36:838–845.

229. Bouchard C, Lacroix C, Plante V, et al. Clinicopathologic findings and prognosis of chronic inflammatory demyelinating polyneuropathy. Neurology 1999;52:498–503.

Chapter 17

Demyelinating Neuropathies Other Than Acute Inflammatory Demyelinating Polyneuropathy and Chronic Inflammatory Demyelinating Polyneuropathy

David M. Dawson

This chapter continues the discussion of demyelinative peripheral neuropathy begun in previous chapters. The most common of such neuropathies have already been discussed under the heading of acute and chronic inflammatory neuropathy. The distinction between chronic inflammatory demyelinating polyneuropathy (CIDP) and other demyelinative neuropathies is, however, vague and imprecise. Why this is true, and the basis for these distinctions, are important parts of this chapter.

Several investigative techniques are available to define the nature of a neuropathy. By widespread common consent of authorities, the most important feature to be decided is whether the pathologic process is primarily axonal or primarily demyelinative. That dichotomy dates back to the mid-1970s, when nerve biopsy and autopsy results first came into widespread usage. Important landmarks along the way can be listed as the papers of Waksman and Adams defining experimental autoimmune neuritis[1] and of Asbury et al.[2] defining the lymphocytic infiltration and segmental demyelination of acute inflammatory demyelinating polyneuropathy (AIDP) and the description by Dyck and colleagues[3] of CIDP in 1975. An early lesson from pathologic studies was that segmental demyelination can be found in neuropathies that are primarily axonal; this reflects the close association of

the Schwann's cells with axons. Physiologically, the processes produce fairly different results: In secondary demyelination, in which the axon is the site of the damage or degeneration, the problem is impulse generation, with additional long-term consequences in target tissues because of failure of axonal transport mechanisms. Conduction studies show loss of motor and sensory action potentials, and there is atrophy of muscle. In primary demyelinating neuropathy, the myelin sheath is the main target organ, and slow conduction and conduction block (CB) are characteristic, whereas axons are relatively spared.

In current scientific or clinical practice, it is more likely that physiologic, not pathologic, criteria will be used. It is easier and arguably more accurate to make the axonal-demyelinating dichotomy with physiologic tests. These criteria have been laid out in detail in Chapter 7. Axon loss produces a particularly characteristic set of physiologic findings: reduction of sensory amplitudes, eventually with no elicitable response; chronic neurogenic changes in motor unit morphology; and clinically visible atrophy. Criteria have been developed to indicate that a neuropathy is demyelinative; briefly stated, these criteria depend on reduction of conduction velocity of less than 75% of normal values, with or without partial CB.

The subjects covered in this chapter, therefore, are neuropathies that are demyelinating as defined by electrophysiologic criteria. AIDP and CIDP are discussed in Chapter 16.

1. Neuropathies with paraproteinemia. For the most part, this group represents neuropathies that occur with monoclonal gammopathy of undetermined significance (MGUS) (i.e., without malignant disease). There is an overlap with CIDP, and, in fact, there may be some common factor in causation.
2. Neuropathies with myeloma, Waldenström's, and other hematologic malignancies. These disorders are basically paraneoplastic neuropathies and are usually not demyelinative in character.
3. Neuropathies with antibodies to glycoproteins. The most typical among these disorders is the neuropathy found with myelin-associated glycoprotein (MAG) antibodies.
4. Multifocal motor neuropathy (MMN) with CB. Again, an overlap with CIDP and a confusing literature create problems for its accurate identification.
5. MMN without CB or with sensory loss. It resembles MMN but with features outside the boundaries of that syndrome.
6. Inherited demyelinating neuropathy. This category refers to Charcot-Marie-Tooth (CMT) disease and its variants.
7. Adrenoleukodystrophy and metachromatic leukodystrophy. In these disorders, the neuropathy is part of a generalized, inherited central nervous system and peripheral nervous system disorder of myelin.
8. Toxic neuropathy with demyelinative features. Most toxic neuropathies produce axon loss; there are a few exceptions.

Neuropathy with Paraproteinemia

Background

Immunoglobulins (Igs) consist of a heavy chain and a light chain. The heavy chain is coded on chromosome 14 and determines the Ig class (e.g., IgG or IgM). The light chain is coded either by chromosome 2 for kappa or 22 for lambda. Normally, heavy and light chain production is balanced, and

complete Igs are the only circulating proteins. If there is overproduction, it is usually a clone producing light chains so that there is a monoclonal excess. If the overproduction is marked, there will be only light chains and little complete Ig, and the excess chains will be found chiefly in the urine. Electrophoresis of serum proteins will demonstrate monoclonal proteins (M-spikes), although it will not define them; immunoelectrophoresis or immunofixation will define the protein class. Approximately 15% of all benign gammopathies are IgM monoclonal gammopathies.

Benign monoclonal gammopathy, or MGUS, is found in approximately 1% of apparently normal patients older than 50 years and in more than 3% of those older than 70 years.[4] As these patients are followed up, with time a certain proportion will "convert" to hematologic malignancy, as defined by anemia, osteolytic bone lesions, renal failure, hypercalcemia, and rising levels of monoclonal protein. Most often, the malignancy that develops is multiple myeloma, although a few patients develop osteosclerotic myeloma or Waldenström's macroglobulinemia.

In data from the Mayo Clinic,[5] the conversion to malignancy was approximately 1% per year from the time of original detection, over an interval as long as 25 years. At the time of detection of MGUS, a critical measurement is the serum level of monoclonal protein. In benign states, this is low, typically 1.7 g/dl or less. Patients with higher levels are more likely eventually to have hematologic malignancies and are probably also more likely to have symptomatic neuropathy.

However, it is clear that low levels of monoclonal protein (1 g/dl or less) can have an associated neuropathy, and if this is primarily demyelinative, there is probably a causal connection. Obviously, minimal Ig spikes are less likely to be significant.

The concept that serum paraproteins could be associated with peripheral neuropathy arose in the 1970s through the work of Kyle,[5] Kelly et al.,[6–8] Latov et al.,[9] and others.[10,11] The initial phase of this work dealt with the common issue that patients with MGUS often have another identifiable cause of neuropathy, such as diabetes, alcohol abuse, or family history of neuropathy. The Mayo Clinic workers identified 692 patients in the electromyography (EMG) laboratory over a 1-year period with a diagnosis of generalized neuropathy.[12] Approximately one-half of these had an already apparent cause, which was most often diabetes. They showed that in those without such a known cause, 10% had MGUS, whereas in the group with previously known cause, 2.5% had MGUS (a level comparable to that of age-matched community controls). This statistical association was significant and has held up with time.

In this same era, it was established that patients with malignant paraproteinemia have a comparable incidence of neuropathy; this includes multiple myeloma, osteosclerotic solitary plasmacytoma, Waldenström's macroglobulinemia, and the plasma cell dyscrasia known as POEMS syndrome (*P* for polyneuropathy; *O* for organomegaly such as liver or spleen; *E* for endocrinopathy such as gynecomastia, testicular atrophy, prolactinemia, or diabetes; *M* for M protein; and *S* for skin changes such as hypertrichosis, thickening, or fingernail changes). Clearly, a patient who is encountered with neuropathy and gammopathy may have either benign or malignant gammopathy and requires evaluation before a decision can be reached. This matter is discussed in Other Laboratory Studies.

The next step along the way was the work of Latov and colleagues[9,13,14] in the early 1980s, showing that there was a specific change in the myelin of peripheral nerves of patients with MGUS and neuropathy. They showed that immunofluorescent stains demonstrate deposition of IgM on myelin sheaths and binding of the monoclonal protein to MAG. They also showed a separation of myelin leaflets by electron microscopy. This work seemed to show a potential direct effect of the monoclonal protein on peripheral nerve structure. As this is an area of significance in the study of myelin, it is described in Other Laboratory Studies.

Since then, there has been an explosion of knowledge about this area, many hundreds of reports have been published, but areas of controversy are not difficult to find. A relatively specific clinical pattern of IgM-associated neuropathy has emerged.[15–17] Yet, there are many individual patients in whom the picture is far from clear (e.g., the patient with apparent CIDP who has MGUS, the patient with diabetes and MGUS, the patient with MGUS and very mild neuropathy which is detectable only by electrophysiologic criteria, the patient with IgA or IgG paraproteinemia, and so on). Criteria for treatment are also controversial, some authorities indicating that they find no response to treatment, whereas others advocate immunosuppression or plasma exchange.

Current Status

Clinical

The typical neuropathy found in patients with MGUS is chronic, very slowly progressive, and mainly sensory.[18–22] Approximately one-half the patients have pain, which is also distal. Mild gait ataxia is characteristic.

Sensory testing shows a symmetric polymodal loss; vibration and position senses may be the most affected. Romberg's sign is often positive. Tendon reflexes are reduced or absent. Action tremor resembling essential or familial tremor is sometimes seen in the upper extremities. The pace of the illness is often very slow, but, over the course of 5–10 years, patients will often acquire significant disability and will require canes, walkers, or other assistive devices. Most patients are elderly, and two-thirds to three-fourths are men.

Other clinical syndromes may be observed, but, in the view of most authors, they are not pathogenetically linked to the presence of the paraprotein. Various cranial nerve palsies, progressive motor neuropathies, and types of mononeuritis multiplex can be seen in patients with cryoglobulinemia, lymphocytic infiltration of nerves, or other aspects of paraproteinemia due to hematologic malignancy.[23] Chance associations between MGUS and other neuromuscular syndromes, such as amyotrophic lateral sclerosis, AIDP, and plexopathies, are occasionally encountered.

Patients with non-IgM monoclonal proteins (IgA, IgG) are much more likely to have a nonspecific symmetric sensory and motor neuropathy resembling CIDP, including the presence of proximal weakness in some patients.[24,25]

Electrodiagnostic Studies

In the great majority of patients with MGUS and neuropathy, the nerve conductions show a predominantly demyelinating sensory and motor disorder with slowing, prolongation of F waves and sometimes with CB. A disproportionate slowing of distal motor latencies, contrasting with proximal conduction velocities nearer to normal, is characteristic when found.[26,27]

Additionally, there is accentuation of the abnormality in sensory fibers, and this may help to distinguish this neuropathy from hereditary neuropathy or CIDP, which often have more obvious motor involvement.

Patients with multiple myeloma, cryoglobulinemia, and amyloidosis have primarily axonal loss, not demyelination.[28] This finding has a limited correlation with the type of paraprotein found, which tends to be IgG or IgA in these conditions. Although the neuropathy with IgM MGUS is primarily sensory EMGs show partial chronic denervation, particularly in the feet.

Serum Protein Abnormalities

The presence of an abnormal monoclonal protein can nearly always be detected by serum protein electrophoresis. Subsequent immunoelectrophoresis is then needed to characterize the M-spike, which usually runs in the gamma globulin zone. In case of a demyelinating neuropathy that seems compatible with MGUS neuropathy, an immunoelectrophoresis will rarely identify a paraprotein missed by simple electrophoresis.

An important issue is the measurement of anti-MAG antibody. MAG is concentrated in Schwann's cell membranes and apparently acts as an adhesion molecule between this membrane and axons. It contains five Ig-like domains that are exposed out of the cell membrane and are easily accessible as antigenic sites (unlike sulfated glycolipids and gangliosides, in which the exposed moieties are carbohydrate groups). MAG is found chiefly in noncompact myelin, located at incisures and nodes, along with cadherin and integrin surface molecules. By contrast, peripheral nerve myelin protein (PMP22), P_o, and myelin basic protein are located in compact myelin.[29]

Originally, anti-MAG antibodies were detected by complement fixation assays with serum or by immunohistochemistry with nerve tissue. Western blot and enzyme-linked immunosorbent assay techniques were introduced in the mid-1980s. Commercially available assays rely on both. Low baseline titers are found in the normal population.

Titers of more than a 1 to 30,000 ratio are more often correlated with neuropathy and more often found in the presence of MGUS. However, there are some patients who are MAG positive and have no detectable paraprotein. Titers may vary when followed sequentially, without evident clinical correlates, but some authors have reported that the course of the neuropathy will improve or worsen as titers rise of fall with treatment. Patients with IgA and IgG paraproteinemia usually do not have circulating anti-MAG antibodies.

Other Laboratory Studies

In many patients with paraproteinemic neuropathy, the cerebrospinal fluid (CSF) protein is elevated. Nerve biopsies are performed much less frequently that in previous years. A sural biopsy may show loss of myelinated fibers, little or no inflammatory reaction, and on teased fiber preparation will show evidence of demyelination and remyelination. A characteristic finding in the MAG-positive cases is the presence of widening of the myelin lamellae in the periphery of the nerve.[28,30] It has been found in more than 90% of biopsies from MAG-positive patients. Nevertheless, the meaning of the abnormality is still in doubt. The lack of inflammation in the nerve is in marked contrast to the findings in CIDP. Some authors have detected complement in addition to deposits of IgM, but if the nerve is responding immunologically to the presence of the paraprotein, it must be a very-low-grade or blunted response. Some think that it is the physical presence of the bound paraprotein that is sufficient to separate the myelin lamellae. Evidence that antibody is directly linked to neuropathy has been furnished by studies of intraneural injection of serum and by passive transfer experiments, both of which have shown experimental evidence of demyelinating neuropathy in recipient animals.[31,32]

Patients who are known to have neuropathy and paraproteinemia need to have an evaluation for hematologic malignancy. Multiple myeloma is a systemic malignancy in which a clone of plasma cells produces an Ig in excess. Usually, these cells are widespread throughout the marrow; rarely they are solitary. Patients have symptoms of systemic malignancy, with bone pain, anemia, and renal failure. A skeletal bone survey is indicated and will be positive for osteolytic lesions in more than one-half of the cases; bone marrow aspiration is indicated if there is gammopathy and symptoms of myeloma and the skeletal survey is unrevealing. Overall, only a small percentage of myeloma patients have neuropathy and, of those, only a small percentage is clearly demyelinative in nature.[26]

The situation is fairly different in the osteosclerotic variant of myeloma.[23] For one thing, neuropathy is much more common, occurring in approximately one-half of the patients. Additionally, the myeloma variant with osteosclerosis rather than osteoporosis is often accompanied by other systemic disorders, such as the so-called POEMS syndrome (as defined earlier) or Crow-Fukase syndrome. The motor weakness of POEMS syndrome patients is often rather severe, often leading to wheelchair or bed confinement, and this stands in contrast to the mild sensory neuropathy of patients with MAG positivity.[23]

Waldenström's macroglobulinemia is a chronic lymphoproliferative disease, typically involving B-lymphocytes and associated with the production of large amounts of IgM protein. Hyperviscosity and cryoglobulinemia are common. One-half of the patients are positive for MAG when tested. The neuropathy that develops is very similar to that seen in the benign MAG-positive MGUS patients (i.e., a chronic ataxic sensory neuropathy with distal accentuation).

Other Antibody Studies

Several other antibodies in addition to anti-MAG have been described and associated with peripheral neuropathy of a demyelinative type. These are included here because they are thought to have a comparable pathophysiology. Most of the work in this field has come from the laboratories of Pestronk et al.[33] and Lopate et al.[34]; the antibody tests are commercially available and therefore have been widely measured, although published data are limited.

Antisulfatide antibodies have been described. Sulfatides are ceramide lipids, with a sulfated galactose presumably serving as the antigen to which an IgM antibody response is directed. Patients have a distal symmetric sensory neuropathy, and 50% have a gait disorder. Nerve conduction studies resemble those seen in anti-MAG neuropathy, with some axon loss and slowing of conduction in distal segments. The titer of anti-sulfatide antibody is clearly important. In one study,[35] 15% of normal controls had detectable antibody, and the antibody was also found in 65% of AIDP and 87% of CIDP cases.

In a report from Dabby et al.,[36] several subtypes of neuropathy were observed. It must be presumed that some of the associations observed were chance relationships. Of 25 patients with anti-sulfatide antibody, the majority had distal axonal loss with sensory findings on clinical examination, and three patients were indistinguishable from CIDP patients. Neither a defined clinical picture, electrophysiologic pattern, nor a direct relationship to these highly elevated antibodies could be found consistently in this study. The authors commented that much further work in this area will be required.

A syndrome associated with an autoantibody to a central myelin antigen has been described, under the acronym of GALOP syndrome (*G* for gait disorder, *ALO* for late age onset, and *P* for polyneuropathy).[37] Patients with presumed GALOP and concomitant presence of M-protein may also exhibit conduction velocity slowing. Again, further work in this area is needed to establish this syndrome as an entity.

Treatment

Treatment of patients with paraproteinemic neuropathy has been attempted by a number of ways, usually with a goal of lowering the serum level of the abnormal protein or, if MAG positive, reducing the titer of this antibody. In patients with hematologic malignancy (myeloma, Waldenström's syndrome), there are additional goals of controlling plasma cell proliferation or bone destruction or reducing levels of circulating cryoglobulins.

Immunosuppressive regimens have most often been used, consisting of high-dose steroids and cytotoxic agents.[9,38,39] Plasma exchange has been attempted as well and is effective in rapidly lowering serum IgM levels, but its effects are usually too transient to be useful unless supplemented by other forms of therapy.[40]

In anti-MAG neuropathy patients, it has been consistently observed that a maintained reduction of anti-MAG titer of 50% is associated with clinical improvement, however that is achieved.[41] However, this fact needs to be placed in perspective;

anti-MAG neuropathy is inherently very slowly progressive. In a study of 25 treated patients followed up for a minimum of 24 months, 12% were asymptomatic, and another 60% had only minimal or minor symptoms.[41] It should be noted that sensory testing, in itself, is a major impediment in these kinds of studies, as it is so difficult to measure in an objective manner.

An additional obstacle in the interpretation of studies of therapy in MGUS neuropathy, including MAG-positive neuropathy, is that most series of patients have been retrospective, uncontrolled, and unblinded. A double-blind, placebo-controlled study of pheresis (pheresis vs. sham pheresis) was carried out; there was improvement only in a subgroup of IgG and IgA MGUS patients, and even that was not statistically significant.[42]

A study of intravenous immunoglobulin in 11 patients with IgM MGUS neuropathy was blinded, placebo-controlled, and crossover: In this setting, only two patients had improvement in strength and one patient in sensory impairment.[43]

The group from Milan, led by Nobile-Orazio,[44] has led the way in treatment of these patients. Their program has usually consisted of chlorambucil, with or without oral steroids, at a dose sufficient to reduce the total lymphocyte count to 500–1,000, alone or in combination with plasma exchange. This program is maintained for 6 months; if the cytotoxic agent appears to be ineffective, plasma exchange alone every 2–3 weeks is continued. A more intense immunosuppressive program[38] is more effective but is more toxic.

A valuable recent publication from the Italian group summarizes their experience with 25 patients with anti-MAG neuropathy who were treated in the era from 1984 to 1994.[45] By the time of death or last follow-up, 44% of the patients were disabled by tremor, gait ataxia, or both. In no case was neuropathy the direct cause of death. Nineteen patients were treated for periods of 0.5–11.0 years with various immune therapies. Of these 19 patients, 5 reported a consistent and 4 a slight improvement at some point during treatment. Only one patient steadily improved to the time of the last follow-up. In 10 of these patients (more than one-half), there were severe adverse effects of treatment, and three patients were considered to have died of iatrogenic causes.

With these data available, a degree of caution in treating MGUS patients obviously is indicated.

Many patients are elderly. The neuropathy—especially in those with MAG antibodies—is often very slowly progressive. To achieve a treatment effect, relatively major degrees of immunosuppression must be maintained. Many authorities observe patients for months before embarking on a course of treatment, and, if treatment is begun, it is discontinued if the results are not encouraging.

Relationship to Chronic Inflammatory Demyelinating Polyneuropathy

The neuropathies associated with MGUS, however, have vague and indistinct boundaries. When a patient has a slowly progressive sensory neuropathy with gait disorder and high-titer anti-MAG antibodies, there are no arguments. Such patients probably constitute one-half of the MGUS neuropathies. However, there are many situations that are far less clear:

1. A patient may have the clinical picture of CIDP with MGUS. Findings such as subacutely progressing proximal weakness, widespread loss of reflexes, or marked motor rather than sensory loss are all characteristic of CIDP. As CIDP and MGUS are both relatively common, it should be assumed that they can occasionally be comorbid but unrelated conditions.

2. A few patients with MGUS have primarily axon-loss sensory neuropathy. This is the common neuropathy of elderly persons, and again one must assume that it and the paraproteinemia are not directly related. For instance, in the survey of anti-sulfatide neuropathy from the Columbia group, 8 of 25 patients would have fit this description.[36] However, it is possible that in some cases, axon-loss neuropathy and IgM paraproteinemia are directly related in some, as yet, unknown manner.

3. The neuropathies associated with multiple myeloma, amyloidosis, and cryoglobulinemia are primarily axon-loss in type. Usually, they are present rather late in the course of the illness but, in the rarer situation wherein paraproteinemia and neuropathy both occur early in the course of the malignancy, there can be confusion. It would be commoner for the excess Ig to be IgG or IgA in these kinds of cases.

In many texts and monographs, the subjects of CIDP and paraproteinemic neuropathy are discussed together, and some authors include a number of disorders under the general title of CIDP, including typical CIDP, paraproteinemic neuropathy, MMN (see Multifocal Motor Neuropathy), multifocal demyelinating motor and sensory neuropathy, and others. A common assumption in classification is that all these disorders involve an immune system causation and, therefore, should be grouped together. There are strong arguments against this practice. AIDP and CIDP are certainly related and appear to have an inflammatory autoimmune pathogenesis. The other neuropathies listed earlier seem different in a number of important ways, and until more is known about their cause, splitting, rather than lumping, is to be recommended. IgM antibodies derived from patients with neuropathy can be shown to bind directly to nerve and, in some experiments, can cause experimental neuropathy in vivo by passive transfer.[31,32] However, the cascade of a typical autoimmune pathogenesis, with complement, proinflammatory cytokines, and deposition of chronic inflammatory cells, may not exist in the IgM neuropathies.

Multifocal Motor Neuropathy

Clinical Features

Although MMN has a relatively well-defined clinical presentation, it was not until the advent of well-designed motor and sensory electrodiagnostic tests that it was recognized as a distinct entity. The first report by Lewis et al.[46] emphasized multifocal CB as a pathophysiologic explanation; in fact, those patients had some sensory abnormalities too and would nowadays be titled *multifocal motor and sensory neuropathy* (see later under Multifocal Demyelinating Motor and Sensory Neuropathy). Early reports render it clear that distinction from motor neuron disease was the problem faced by those investigators.[47–49] Although rare, MMN is now well known and is detected in large EMG laboratories many times each year. One estimate gives a ratio of 50 patients with motor neuron disease to every case of MMN.[50] Males are affected three times as often as females. The onset is usually in midlife.

MMN is a chronic disease that may go on for many years. It usually begins in the upper extremities, presenting with painless asymmetric weakness. There may be a resemblance to a specific nerve deficit, and the pattern may resemble a posterior interosseous palsy or a proximal median neuropathy. Patients usually do not have sensory symptoms. One or the other lower extremity may be affected at a later time. The resemblance to motor neuron disease derives from the atrophy that eventually develops, accompanied by fasciculations. Sometimes, especially in areas that have recently become weak, there is the very characteristic finding of marked weakness without atrophy; this is a clue to the pathophysiology, which involves CB. Sensory testing is normal even although patients may present with stiffness, tightness, or numbness. Reflexes are absent or reduced only in relation to weakness of the effector muscles.

Electrodiagnostic Features

The hallmark of MMN is the presence of multifocal CB at areas where there is no site for nerve entrapment or compression.[47,48,51,52] There are no fully accepted criteria for the presence of CB. A totally absent motor response with proximal stimulation and preserved response with distal stimulation, persisting for many days, is firm evidence for block. Temporal dispersion, block of more than 50% of amplitude, and a preserved distal amplitude would be acceptable as well. However, in chronic axon loss, there may be reinnervation producing large and complex motor units, phase cancellation, and other artifacts that lead to pseudo-block; however, pseudo-block is most commonly found in amyotrophic lateral sclerosis, a disease in which clarifying the diagnosis is clinically of the greatest significance.[53]

In some patients who otherwise seem typical, CB cannot be found. Other features of demyelination may be present, specifically temporal dispersion, slow velocity, or prolonged distal motor latency. Patients with these features may respond identically to treatment.

Sensory nerves characteristically are normal in all respects. Important is that the same nerve (e.g., median) in which there is motor CB will have normal sensory conduction and amplitude. EMG shows abnormalities that correlate with the degree of muscle atrophy, although not necessarily with the degree of clinical weakness.

Pathologic Findings

Many authorities hold the belief that MMN is a variant of CIDP. The best support for that view comes from the pathologic studies that have been carried out on nerves in a few cases of MMN. Demyelination, remyelination in the form of onion bulb formation, and perivascular inflammation have all been observed. Biopsy of sensory nerves does show some evidence of inflammation and demyelination but, according to one study, these findings were "never extensive."[54]

The disparity between motor and sensory nerve involvement obviously suggests that an immune attack is directed against an antigen present in motor nerves but not in sensory nerves. The nature of such an antigen has remained unknown. Serum from patients with MMN injected into rat sciatic or tibial nerves can produce CB either in vitro or in vivo, indicating possible transferable autoimmunity.[55–57] As many patients with MMN have elevated serum levels of anti-ganglioside antibodies, ganglioside is an obvious candidate. Against that theory is the fact that not all patients have anti-ganglioside antibodies.

Serum Anti-Ganglioside Antibody

Serum antibodies to the ganglioside GM1 are frequently found in patients with MMN.[58–61] Reports of the prevalence of antibody vary from 20% to 80% and seem to be highly dependent on technique. Most data have been based on standard enzyme-linked immunosorbent assay technique, using passive adsorption binding. The use of a covalently bound "spacer" may improve accessibility to antigen and has recently been claimed to increase sensitivity and specificity. However, not all authors agree, and the matter continues to be vigorously debated.[62–64]

Surveys of patients with CIDP, amyotrophic lateral sclerosis, and other neuropathies show that some of these patients have GM1 antibodies as well, usually in relatively low titer and, in nearly all reports, in a small percentage of the patients.

However, the issue of the specificity of the GM1 antibodies has remained unaddressed.

Gangliosides are glycoconjugates that are transmembrane in location; the antigenic component is the oligosaccharide "tail" composed of galactose moieties. In some patients, antibodies are found directed against asialo-GM1, a molecule lacking one sialic acid residue.

The clinical usefulness of GM1 testing continues to be a matter of debate.[62,63] Most authorities at this time rely on clinical examinations and detailed neurophysiologic testing to establish a diagnosis of MMN and to distinguish it from amyotrophic lateral sclerosis and other lower motor neuron syndromes. A high titer of GM1 could be considered confirmatory evidence of the presence of MMN. Efforts to produce MMN by passive transfer have not succeeded, the titer may not change with successful therapy, and a consistent relatively high percentage of patients are GM1-negative; for these reasons, the testing, at this time, has limited value.

Treatment

One of the compelling reasons for separating MMN as an entity from CIDP and from motor-sensory neuropathies is the distinct therapeutic responses observed in these patients. It is clear that high-dose steroids have no role to play, the opposite of what is seen with CIDP.[48,49,51,65] Therapy depends mainly on the use of intravenous IgG.[66,67] Dosage regimens vary; 0.4 g/kg repeated five times over the course of several weeks (thus, 100–140 g total) has been an accepted standard form of therapy. However, simpler schedules often suffice, such as 30–50 g once every 2–4 weeks. Maintenance programs are usually needed. Side effects of the infusion, such as headache, may require that dosages be lowered, split into successive days, or individually titered.

Immunosuppressive drugs also may play a role in MMN treatment. Oral azathioprine, low-dose oral cyclophosphamide, and plasma exchange all appear to be ineffective. Monthly bolus cyclophosphamide treatment, in the range of 1.0–1.5 g per month, has been reported to be effective in more than one-half the patients.[61] However, dosage at this level is associated with hemorrhagic cystitis, alopecia, and other complications and is not to be undertaken lightly.

Multifocal Demyelinating Motor and Sensory Neuropathy

Patients with MMN, by definition, do not have clinical or electrophysiologic evidence of impairment of sensory nerve fibers. In fact, a hallmark of the disease is the presence of normal sensory function in the very nerve trunk in which motor loss has developed.

Nevertheless, there are patients with multifocal neuropathy in which sensory loss is a component. They range all the way from patients with typical MMN who present with slight numbness to patients with marked focal tingling and loss of sensation. This is one of the reasons why some authorities believe that all the acquired demyelinating neuropathies should be grouped together and considered to be variants or subcategories of CIDP. However, there may be substantial differences in the pace of the illness, in certain characteristic features, and especially in the response to treatment. MMN is known not to respond to steroids. When a patient with apparent MMN is found to have significant sensory loss, that prediction will not apply; such patients may well be steroid-responsive.

Saperstein et al.[68] have coined the term *multifocal acquired demyelinating sensory and motor* (MADSAM) neuropathy. This term has not been accepted everywhere but does describe the patients well. Others[69–71] merely indicate that the patients are MMN cases, with sensory loss. As mentioned earlier, the cases reported by Lewis et al.[46] were probably examples of MADSAM; some of them had focal sensory loss and ophthalmoparesis.

Clinical Features

MADSAM is a chronic illness, with features of a multifocal neuropathy. Some patients (including some of those in the original description by Saperstein et al.) have had cranial neuropathies, including ophthalmoparesis. The usual age of onset is in middle age, and it is commoner in men by a 2 to 1 ratio. Pain is not a typical feature.

An unusual variant of MADSAM affects the brachial plexus primarily.[72–74] Some of these patients have only merely a localized area of proximal CB in the plexus (e.g., affecting ulnar nerve fibers).

Others have a florid plexopathy, with inflammatory and demyelinating aspects, onion bulb formation, and enlargement of trunks and cords of the plexus. Several patients have been operated on with the assumption that Schwannoma or fibrosarcoma was present, only to have the pathologic diagnosis be that of demyelinating neuropathy.

Laboratory Aspects

The CSF protein is elevated in more than one-half the MADSAM patients; elevated CSF protein occurs in fewer than 10% of MMN cases. Few patients have anti-GM1 antibodies. One survey indicated that 1 of 40 patients had detectable anti-GM1 (A. A. Amato, personal communication, 1999).

The nerve conduction testing shows, as it does in MMN, evidence of multifocal CB, which is persistent. Sensory fibers are probably affected in the same way but, for technical reasons, this is very difficult to show (sensory action potentials usually decrease normally when comparing distal to proximal segments because of phase cancellation).

Treatment

Patients with MADSAM neuropathy have been treated with a wide variety of approaches, including steroids, plasma exchange, and intravenous Ig. They appear to respond to these modalities in a manner comparable to CIDP patients. Their response to high-dose oral steroids is very distinct from that of the MMN neuropathy patients, who are known to have no response; the MADSAM patients respond in at least 50% of cases.[74,75]

Hereditary Demyelinating Neuropathies

The title of this section is chosen deliberately. Hereditary demyelinating neuropathies form a group of neuropathies sharing only two features: hereditary cause and demyelinating pathology. Their clinical abnormalities, course, and genetic associations are very divergent. The number of types of neuropathy in this field is growing very rapidly, with new genetic loci and correspondingly new clinical features being described almost each month. Although the name *CMT disease* can be criticized on several grounds, it is now the term most widely used for the most common versions of hereditary neuropathy. Hereditary neuropathy with pressure palsies (HNPP) is another relatively common adult form of hereditary neuropathy. The term *hereditary motor and sensory neuropathy*, although logical, is not widely used, nor is this an uncommon problem. Although the names of these illnesses are fairly unfamiliar to the medical world in general and often provoke blank stares and raised eyebrows from nonneurologists, they are actually very common. In many referral-based neuromuscular clinics, they constitute the largest single group of neuropathies. For example, in a survey of 402 neuropathy patients referred to two clinics in Texas, hereditary neuropathy accounted for 30%, idiopathic sensory neuropathy (usually in the elderly) for 23%, diabetic neuropathy for 15%, and CIDP for 13% (A.A. Amato, personal communication, 2000). A recent review quotes an estimate of prevalence of CMT in one of its versions as 1 per 2,500 patients,[76] which is approximately one-third as common as multiple sclerosis and five times as common as myasthenia gravis.

Charcot-Marie-Tooth Neuropathy Type 1

The CMT neuropathy type 1 syndrome accounts for approximately 75% of all the hereditary neuropathy patients. It presents in the first or second decade of life, often because of abnormal gait or foot deformity. Approximately 75% of patients have the classic hammer toes and high arched foot; it is rare to see the inverted champagne bottle legs that Charcot emphasized.[77] The autosomal dominant nature of the disease is usually apparent, although as many as 20% of patients appear to represent new mutations.

Examination shows distal weakness affecting intrinsic foot muscles, dorsiflexors, and everters— hence the name *peroneal muscle atrophy*. Approximately two-thirds of patients will eventually develop significant hand weakness due to intrinsic muscle atrophy. Pain is not a feature. In most patients, the loss of muscle strength is fairly symmetric. There are no sensory symptoms, although mild sensory loss may be apparent on testing. The disease progresses through life, and patients may develop

significant disability in gait or hand strength, even in the last few decades of life. Enlargement of peripheral nerve trunks (ulnar, peroneal, greater auricular) due to hypertrophic changes in the nerves is present in one-half the patients if sought.[77]

Electrophysiologic features of CMT-1 are characteristic[78,79] and often will allow for precise clinical diagnosis even when the history and physical examination are not clear. As opposed to acquired demyelinating polyneuropathy, the studies show uniform slowing of peripheral velocities, without evidence of partial CB or asymmetry. Longitudinal studies show that there is no real change in the electrophysiologic data after the first decade or two, even although the patient worsens clinically.[80,81] In one study of patients with documented chromosomal CMT-1 abnormalities, all the subjects had slowing of median motor velocities of less than 43 m/second, reaching the criterion of more than 25% reduction in velocity.[78]

The pathology in the nerves of CMT patients shows striking evidence of remyelination. There is Schwann's cell proliferation and a loose reduplication of cell membranes producing the well-known onion-skin pattern. Teased nerve fiber preparations show segmental and paranodal demyelination. There is no inflammatory infiltrate.

Three genetic abnormalities are now known to cause CMT-1. The first discovered was linked to the Duffy blood group on chromosome 1 (now titled *CMT-1B*), but in fact more than 70% of CMT-1 patients have a duplication of a large segment of chromosome 17, encompassing 1.5 megabases. This chromosome locus codes for the *PMP22* gene and is now known as *CMT-1A*. Because the net effect of the duplication is to produce trisomy at this locus,[82] the disease is thought to result from overexpression of PMP22; however, in a minority of patients, there is a point mutation and, in these, it is assumed that an abnormal PMP22 protein is expressed.

CMT-1B has its genetic locus on chromosome 1, and the relevant protein is known as P_o, an integral myelin protein. CMT-1C has no known genetic marker or chromosome localization. It may be that more than one condition is subsumed under this title. There is sufficient overlap in the clinical and pathologic features of all three types of CMT-1 such that they are not distinguishable except by DNA analysis.[77] These tests are available in a number of research laboratories and are commercially available as well. The decisions about which patients and which apparently unaffected family members should be tested can be complex and may involve genetic counseling as well as clinical examinations. This is true in many other diseases of autosomal dominant nature, of course.

The molecular mechanism of the demyelinative neuropathy of CMT-1A is of great interest. The *PMP22* gene encodes for a membrane-associated protein, which is located in the compact portions of peripheral nerve myelin. The protein is highly conserved through evolution. It has four apparent transmembrane domains connected by loops. Four demyelinative neuropathies are associated with these transmembrane domains: CMT-1A, the *trembler* mouse mutation, Dejerine-Sottas disease, and HNPP. The latter two of these are human diseases.

To reconcile the fact that either duplication and gene overexpression or point mutation (less commonly) may produce the clinical picture of CMT-1A, the theory has been proposed that there needs to be strict stoichiometry in content of these myelin proteins, and either deficit or excess of PMP22 will cause abnormal function of Schwann's cells.[83–85]

The molecular mechanism of CMT-1B depends on P_o, an important myelin protein, accounting for approximately 50% by weight of the proteins of peripheral nervous system myelin. This protein, containing 284 amino acids, has a single large transmembrane domain and large intracellular and extracellular segments. The protein is a member of the Ig superfamily of cell adhesion molecules. At the time of this writing, 13 different point mutations associated with pedigrees of CMT-1B families have been described[76]; all of these have been found in the glycosylated segment containing a disulfide bond and none in the transmembrane domain.

Other Types of Charcot-Marie-Tooth Disease

A total of four types of CMT are now recognized. They will be mentioned only briefly, particularly as this a field in which rapid changes are occurring and current concepts are liable to be replaced soon.

CMT-2 comprises a group of autosomal dominant neuropathies in which the primary damage is axonal. Clinically, the patients may be indistinguishable from the commoner CMT-1.[77] Nerve

conduction testing does not show the prominent slowing found in CMT-1; the motor and sensory action potentials are reduced in a manner typical of axon loss. Chromosome localizations are known in some instances.

CMT-3, by contrast, is a demyelinating neuropathy, although it bears no resemblance to CMT-1. These patients present in childhood, often before the age of 5, and have a severe paralytic motor and sensory neuropathy. Nerve conduction velocities are severely reduced, often less than 10 m/second and, in nerve biopsies, there is a marked loss of large myelinated fibers. The disease is also known as *Dejerine-Sottas disease* and was originally thought to be an autosomal recessive condition, as there is no family history. It is now known that most are due to sporadic point mutations; either the PMP22 or P_o protein may be affected; if the latter, the domain affected is the transmembrane segment of the protein.

CMT-4 is a poorly understood condition. The patients who have been studied most intensively are of Tunisian background, have a severe neuropathy with onset before age 2 years and have evidence of demyelination on biopsy and nerve conduction study. Little is now known about the genetic basis.

Hereditary Neuropathy with Pressure Palsies

HNPP is autosomal dominant and has gone by a number of different names. It was originally recognized as a cause of recurrent familial pressure palsies, with a very distinctive clinical picture and characteristic changes on nerve biopsy.[86,87] These features are still found, but the syndrome has been expanded and now constitutes a relatively common form of inherited neuropathy presenting in a number of ways. *Hereditary neuropathy with liability to pressure palsies* is now the accepted name.

The original descriptions emphasized recurrent, painless, multifocal neuropathies, typically as acute pressure palsies of large nerves (radial, peroneal, median, or others) occurring with far less trauma or pressure than that required to affect nerves in normal individuals. With time, the patient might accumulate neurologic deficits if the recovery was incomplete. Nerve biopsies in some cases showed focal thickenings of the myelin sheaths, termed *tomacula*.[88]

Identification of a segment of chromosome 17, corresponding to the same exact segment that is usually duplicated in CMT-1A, was the next step.[89–91] All the markers known to be duplicated in CMT1A, including those associated with the *PMP22* gene, are known to be deleted in nearly all patients. The concept that underexpression of PMP22 is causally related to HNPP is supported by rare patients in whom a 2-bp deletion, causing early codon termination, led to lack of PMP22 expression.[76]

Having found the deletion, it was then possible to survey patients with this abnormality to search for other clinical and electrophysiologic expressions. An example is the report of Mouton et al.[92] from Paris. They surveyed 99 persons known to have the 17p11.2 deletion; these represented data from 34 families. Twenty-five of the patients were apparently isolated cases, although screening of their relatives uncovered additional asymptomatic subjects.

Six clinical phenotypes were found in these 99 persons. The largest group, totaling 70, had the commonly recognized HNPP version. Five had recurrent, very brief sensory symptoms induced by movement, sometimes over the trunk. Ten had various forms of symmetric distal motor and sensory neuropathy, sometimes with high arched feet, or peroneal muscular atrophy reminiscent of CMT. Finally, 14 patients with the characteristic chromosomal deletion were asymptomatic.

All subjects, regardless of clinical phenotype, had a relatively characteristic pattern on nerve conduction testing. This pattern consisted of relatively normal motor nerve conduction velocities, slowed distal motor latencies, reduction in sensory action potentials in many nerves, and multiple areas of focal slowing at typical sites of entrapment. These authors believed that a typical presentation would consist of bilateral carpal tunnel syndrome accompanied by slowed distal motor conduction in one or both peroneal nerves.[92] A recent comparison of nerve conduction data from nine HNPP patients, compared to inflammatory and axonal forms of neuropathy, reached the same conclusions.[93]

The close relationship of CMT-1A and HNPP provides a possibility of some knowledge of the function of myelin proteins. Patients with one normal copy of the gene for PMP22 and deletion of the other have a relatively mild disease (HNPP). Two copies is the normal circumstance. Three cop-

ies causes CMT-1A. Four copies causes a severe paralytic neuropathy resembling Dejerine-Sottas disease (this has occurred when two patients with CMT-1A had such an offspring). As Chance[76] has pointed out, complete deletion of PMP22 (no copies) would likely also produce a severe neuropathy. That has been seen in knockout mice, although not in humans.

HNPP is not the only inherited focal neuropathy. Although HNPP may present with an apparent brachial plexopathy (usually painless), there is another condition, genetically fairly distinct, known as *hereditary neuralgic amyotrophy* or *familial brachial plexus palsy*. It is usually painful. The gene, although mapping to chromosome 17, is at a different location: 17q23-25.

Other Genetic Neuropathies

A number of rare genetic diseases cause peripheral neuropathy, in most instances of axonal type. These are merely listed here, and the reader is referred to other sources for descriptions of their characteristics:

- Congenital hypomyelinating neuropathy has occurred in a few families. In two families, it has been associated with a mutation in the gene coding for P_o.
- Adrenoleukodystrophy is an X-linked illness, the main features of which are adrenal insufficiency and severe progressive encephalopathy. Very-long-chain fatty acids are elevated in serum. A neuropathy with demyelinating features is also present.
- Two mitochondrial diseases affect nerves: combined neuropathy, ataxia, and retinitis and mitochondrial nerve gastrointestinal encephalomyopathy.
- Refsum's disease, Tangier disease, and metachromatic leukodystrophy may also be listed under this group.

Toxic Neuropathies

Most toxic neuropathies in the modern era are due to prescribed drugs. In previous decades, exposure to lead, mercury, hexacarbons, and industrial chemicals was far more common; an inquiry into possible chemical exposure is still a useful approach but not often productive.

Most toxic neuropathies due to prescribed drugs are axonal in type, subacute in onset, and related to total dose and duration of treatment. Vincristine, paclitaxel, cisplatin, and dideoxycytidine are examples that are encountered frequently in clinical practice. Most are chiefly sensory in onset and then, if severe, involve motor fibers. A few, such as high-dose pyridoxine, are nearly exclusively sensory.

Some, such as gold, used for rheumatoid arthritis, involve a fair degree of secondary segmental demyelination, so that there may be considerable slowing of nerve conduction values, although not into the true demyelinative range.

Amiodarone is an antiarrhythmic agent, an iodinated benzofuran. A potentially severe peripheral neuropathy may occur,[94] presenting with aching pain in proximal and distal muscles. Myopathy, tremor, altered mental status, and ataxia may occur. There may be signs of systemic toxicity, including dermatitis, gastrointestinal toxicity, and bone marrow suppression. Nerve conduction studies show a combination of axonal and demyelinative features. Lysosomal dense bodies can be identified in Schwann's cells in nerve biopsies.

Perhexiline is a drug prescribed for angina, although its usage is very limited at this time. After some months of treatment, patients may show distal pain and paresthesias, followed by distal and proximal weakness and sometimes by postural hypotension.[95] Additional toxic effects may include papilledema, elevated CSF protein, weight loss, and abnormal liver function test results. There may be marked slowing on nerve conduction testing. On biopsy, the largest fibers may show segmental demyelination, and lipid inclusions may be found in Schwann's cells as well as in other tissues, such as muscle fibers, fibroblasts, and sweat glands.

Tacrolimus (FK 506) is an immunosuppressant used in solid-organ transplantation patients. Marked central nervous system toxicity has been noted in a few patients, apparently due to a posterior leukoencephalopathy. Mutism, visual agnosia, bizarre emotional behavior, tremor, and apraxia have been noted. In some patients, there has been a reversible motor neuropathy that cleared with discontinuation of the drug.[96] However, in others, another mechanism seems to play a role. Some patients have a subacute demyelinating neuropathy, resembling AIDP or subacute CIDP; it has been observed that improvement may occur after plasma exchange or intravenous Ig therapy, strongly suggesting an immunologic mechanism.[97] In fact, this same sequence of events has been seen after immunotherapy with killed cell lysates.[98] Tacrolimus can apparently have either a toxic or vasculopathic effect or an autoimmune pathogenesis. In the latter instance, demyelinative features would be expected and have been seen.

Conclusions

This survey of demyelinative neuropathies other than AIDP and CIDP has identified three main categories of disease: paraproteinemic, hereditary, and toxic. Some of these have distinct clinical pictures, such as anti-MAG neuropathy with its late age of onset, slow progression, and predominance of sensory findings. Others are easily recognizable by their electrophysiologic data; the best example of this would be CMT-1A. Some neuropathies, as experiments of nature, have provided valuable information about the structure of myelin. This is particularly true of CMT-1 and HNPP, two related genetic diseases with considerable clinical variation within a family. Knowledge of their modifier genes seems sure to tell us why one patient with a deletion or another with a duplication differs from another patient from the same family.

References

1. Waksman BH, Adams RD. Allergic neuritis: an experimental disease of rabbits induced by the injection of peripheral nervous tissue and adjuvants. J Exp Med 1955;102:213–236.
2. Asbury AK, Arneson BG, Adams RD. The inflammatory lesion in idiopathic polyneuritis. Medicine 1969;48:173–215.
3. Dyck PJ, Lais AC, Ohta M, et al. Chronic inflammatory polyradiculoneuropathy. Mayo Clin Proc 1975;90:621.
4. Latov NR, Hays AP, Sherman WH. Peripheral neuropathy and anti-MAG antibodies. Crit Rev Neurobiol 1988;3:301.
5. Kyle RA, Therneau TM, Rajkumar V, et al. A long term study of prognosis in monoclonal gammopathy of undetermined significance. N Engl J Med 2002;346:564–569.
6. Kelly JJ, Kyle RA, Miles JM, et al. The spectrum of peripheral neuropathy in myeloma. Neurology 1981;31:24–31.

7. Kelly JJ, Kyle RA, O'Brien PC, et al. Prevalence of monoclonal protein in peripheral neuropathy. Neurology 1981; 31:1480–1483.

8. Kelly JJ. Polyneuropathies Associated with Malignancies and Plasma Cell Dyscrasias. In WF Brown, CF Bolton (eds), Clinical Electromyography. Boston: Butterworth, 1987;305–319.

9. Latov N, Sherman WH, Nemni R, et al. Plasma cell dyscrasia and peripheral neuropathy with monoclonal antibody to peripheral nerve myelin. N Engl J Med 1980;303:618–621.

10. McLeod JG, Walsh JC, Pollard JC. Neuropathies Associated with Paraproteinemias and Dysproteinemias. In PJ Dyck, PK Thomas, EH Lambert, R Bunge (eds), Peripheral Neuropathy, 2nd ed. Philadelphia: WB Saunders 1984; 1847–1865.

11. Nobile-Orazio E, Marmiroli P, Baldini L, et al. Peripheral neuropathy in macroglobulinemia: incidence and antigen specificity of M-protein. Neurology 1987;37:1506–1514.

12. Kelly JJ. Prevalence of monoclonal protein in peripheral neuropathy. Neurology 1981;31:1480–1483.

13. Abrams GR, Latov N, Hays AP, et al. Immunocytochemical studies of human peripheral nerve with serum from patients with polyneuropathy and paraproteinemia. Neurology 1982;32:821–826.

14. Braun PE, Frail DE, Latov N. Myelin associated glycoprotein is the antigen for monoclonal IgM in polyneuropathy. J Neurochem 1982;39:1261–1265.

15. Latov N. Evaluation and treatment of patients with neuropathy and monoclonal gammopathy. Semin Neurol 1994;14: 118–122.

16. Bosch EP, Smith BE. Peripheral neuropathies associated with monoclonal proteins. Med Clin North Am 1193;77: 125–139.

17. Smith IS. The natural history of chronic demyelinating neuropathy associated with benign IgM paraproteinemia. A clinical and neurophysiological study. Brain 1994;117:949–957.

18. Kissel JT, Mendell JR. Neuropathies associated with monoclonal gammopathies. Neuromusc Disord 1996;6:3–18.

19. Nobile-Orazio E. Neuropathies Associated with Anti-MAG Antibodies and IgM Monoclonal Gammopathies. In N Latov, JHJ Wolke, JJ Kelly Jr. (eds), Immunological and Infectious Diseases of the Peripheral Nerves. Cambridge: Cambridge University Press, 1998;168–189.

20. Nobile-Orazio E, Manferdini E, Carpo E, et al. Frequency and clinical correlates of antineural-IgM antibodies in neuropathy associated with IgM monoclonal gammopathy. Ann Neurol 1994;36:416–424.

21. Gosselin S, Kyle RA, Dyck PJ. Neuropathy associated with monoclonal gammopathies of undetermined significance. Ann Neurol 1991;30:54–61.

22. Yeung KB, Thomas PK, King RHM, et al. The clinical spectrum of peripheral neuropathies associated with benign monoclonal IgM, IgG, and IgA paraproteinemia: comparative clinical, immunological and nerve biopsy findings. J Neurol 1991;238:383–391.

23. Kelly JJ Jr. Epidemiology of Autoimmune Polyneuropathies. In N Latov, JHJ Wolke, JJ Kelly Jr. (eds), Immunological and Infectious Diseases of the Peripheral Nerves. Cambridge: Cambridge University Press, 1998;29–35.

24. Suarez GA, Kelly JJ Jr. Polyneuropathy associated with monoclonal gammopathy of undetermined significance: further evidence that IgM-MGUS neuropathies are different from IgG-MGUS. Neurology 1993;43:1304–1308.

25. Notermans NC, Wokke JHJ, Lokhorst HM, et al. Polyneuropathy associated with monoclonal gammopathy of undetermined significance: a prospective study of the prognostic value of clinical and laboratory abnormalities. Brain 1994;117:1385–1393.

26. Shields RW, Wilbourn AJ. Demyelinating Disorders of the Peripheral Nervous System. In CG Goetz, EJ Papper (eds), Textbook of Clinical Neurology. Philadelphia: WB Saunders, 1999;990–1006.

27. Kaku DA, England JD, Sumner AJ. Distal accentuation of conduction slowing in polyneuropathy associated with antibodies to myelin-associated glycoprotein and sulphated glucuronyl paragloboside. Brain 1994;117:941–947.

28. Ropper AH, Gorson KC. Neuropathies associated with paraproteinemia. N Engl J Med 1998;338:1601–1607.

29. Scherer SS. The biology and pathobiology of Schwann cells. Curr Opin Neurol 1997;10:386–397.

30. Mendell JR, Sahenk Z, Whitaker JN, et al. Polyneuropathy and IgM monoclonal gammopathy: studies on the pathogenetic role of anti-myelin-associated glycoprotein antibody. Ann Neurol 1985;17:243–254.

31. Hays AP, Latov N, Takatsu M, Sherman WH. Experimental demyelination of nerve induced by serum of patients with neuropathy and an anti-MAG IgM M-protein. Neurology 1987;37:242–256.

32. Tatum AH. Experimental paraprotein neuropathy, demyelination by passive transfer of human IgM anti-myelin-associated glycoprotein. Ann Neurol 1993;33:502–506.

33. Pestronk A, Li F, Griffin JW. Polyneuropathy syndromes associated with serum antibodies to sulfatide and MAG. Neurology 1991;41:357–362.

34. Lopate G, Parks BJ, Goldstein JM, et al. Polyneuropathies associated with high titre antisulfatide antibodies: characteristics of patients with and without serum monoclonal proteins. J Neurol Neurosurg Psychiatry 1997;62:581–585.

35. Fredman P, Vedeler CA, Nyland H, et al. Antibodies in sera from patients with inflammatory demyelinating polyradiculopathy react with ganglioside LM1 and sulphatide of periipheral nerve myelin. J Neurol 1991; 238:75–79.

36. Dabby R, Weimer LH, Hays AP, et al. Antisulfatide antibodies in neuropathy. Neurology 2000;54:1448–1452.

37. Pestronk A, Choksi R, Bieser K. Treatable gait disorder and polyneuropathy associated with high serum IgM binding to antigens that co-purify with myelin-associated glycoprotein. Muscle Nerve 1994;17:293–300.

38. Kelly JJ, Adelman LS, Berkman E, Bhan I. Polyneuropathies associated with IgM monoclonal gammopathies. Arch Neurol 1988;45:1355–1359.

39. Nobile-Orazio E, Baldini L, Barbieri S, et al. Treatment of patients with neuropathy and anti-MAG IgM M-proteins. Ann Neurol 1988;24:93–97.

40. Ernerudh JH, Brotbkorb E, Olsson T, et al. Peripheral neuropathy and monoclonal IgM with antibody activity against peripheral nerve myelin: effects of plasma exchange. J Neuroimmunol 1986;11:171–178.

41. Simmons Z, Albers JW, Bromberg MB, et al. Long term followup of patients with chronic inflammatory polyradiculoneuropathy without and with monoclonal gammopathy. Brain 1995;118:359–68.

42. Dyck PJ, Low PA, Windebank AJ, et al. Plasma exchange in polyneuropathy associated with monoclonal gammopathy of undetermined significance. N Engl J Med 1991; 325:1482–1486.

43. Dalakas MC, Quarles RH, Farrer RG, et al. A controlled study of intravenous immunoglobulin in demyelinating neuropathy with IgM gammopathy. Ann Neurol 1996; 40:792–795.

44. Nobile-Orazio, E. Neuropathies Associated with Anti-MAG Antibodies and IgM Monoclonal Gammopathies. In N Latov, JHJ Wolke, JJ Kelly Jr (eds), Immunological and Infectious Diseases of the Peripheral Nerves. Cambridge: Cambridge University Press, 1998;168–189.

45. Nobile-Orazio E, Meucci N, Baldini L, et al. Long-term prognosis of neuropathy associated with anti-MAG IgM-proteins and its relationship to immune therapies. Brain 2000;123:710–717.

46. Lewis RA, Sumner AJ, Brown MJ, et al. Multifocal demyelinating neuropathy with persistent conduction block. Neurology 1982;32:958–964.

47. Chad DA, Hammer K, Sargent J. Slow resolution of multifocal weakness and fasciculation: a reversible motor neuron syndrome. Neurology 1986;36:1260–1263.

48. Feldman EL, Bromberg MB, Albers JW, Pestronk A. Immunosuppressive treatment in multifocal motor neuropathy. Ann Neurol 1991;30:397–401.

49. Parry GJ, Clarke S. Multifocal acquired demyelinating neuropathy masquerading as motor neuron disease. Muscle Nerve 1988;11:103–107.

50. Chaudry V. Multifocal motor neuropathy. Semin Neurol 1998;18:73–81.

51. Krarup C, Stewart JD, Sumner AJ, et al. A syndrome of asymmetric limb weakness with motor conduction block. Neurology 1990;40:118–127.

52. Parry GJ. Motor neuropathy with multifocal conduction block. Semin Neurol 1993;13:269–275.

53. Cornblath DR, Sumner AJ, Daube J, et al. Conduction block in clinical practice. Muscle Nerve 1991;14:869–871.

54. Corse AM, Chaudry V, Crawford TO, et al. Sensory nerve pathology in multifocal motor neuropathy. Ann Neurol 1996;39:319–325.

55. Arasaki K, Kusunoki S, Kudo N, et al. Acute conduction block in vitro following exposure to antiganglioside sera. Muscle Nerve 1993;16:587–593.

56. Roberts M, Willison HJ, Vincent A, et al. Multifocal motor neuropathy human sera block distal motor nerve conduction in mice. Ann Neurol 1995;38:111–118.

57. Santoro M, Uncini A, Corbo M, et al. Experimental conduction block induced by serum from a patient with anti-GM1 antibodies. Ann Neurol 1992;31:385–390.

58. Pestronk A, Cornblath DR, Ilyas AA, et al. A treatable multifocal motor neuropathy with antibodies to GM1 gangliosides. Ann Neurol 1988;24:73–78.

59. Pestronk A, Chauddhry V, Feldman EL, et al. Lower motor neuron syndromes defined by patterns of weakness, nerve conduction abnormalities, and high titers of antiglycolipid antibodies. Ann Neurol 1990;27:316–326.

60. Sadiq SA, Thomas FP, Kilidireas K, et al. The spectrum of neurologic disease associated with anti-GM1 antibodies. Neurol 1990;40:1067–1072.

61. Tan E, Lynn DJ, Amato AA, et al. Immunosuppressive treatment of motor neuron syndromes. Attempts to distinguish a treatable disorder. Arch Neurol 1994;51:194–200.

62. Parry GJ. Antiganglioside antibodies do not necessarily play a role in multifocal motor neuropathy. Muscle Nerve 1994;17:97–99.

63. Holloway RG, Feasby FE. To test or not to test? That is the question. Neurology 1999;53:1905–1907.

64. Pestronk A, Choksi R. Multifocal motor neuropathy serum IgM anti-GM1 ganglioside antibodies in most patients detected using covalent linkage of GM1 to ELISA plates. Neurology 1197;49:1289–1292.

65. Donaghy M, Mills KR, Boniface SJ, et al. Pure motor demyelinating neuropathy; deterioration after steroid treatment and improvement with intravenous immunoglobulin. J Neurol Neurosurg Psychiatry 1994;57:778–783.

66. Azulay J-P, Blin O, Pouget J, et al. Intravenous immunoglobulin treatment in patients with motor neuron syndromes associated with anti-GM1 antibodies: a double-blind, placebo-controlled study. Neurology 1994;44:429–432.

67. Azulay J-P, Rihet P, Pouget J, et al. Long term followup of multifocal motor neuropathy with conduction block under treatment. J Neurol Neurosurg Psychiatry 1997;62:391–394.

68. Saperstein DS, Amato AA, Wolfe GI, et al. Multifocal acquired demyelinating sensory and motor neuropathy. The Lewis-Sumner syndrome. Muscle Nerve 1999;22:560–566.

69. Van den Berg-Vos, RM, Van den Berg LH, Franssen H, et al. Multifocal inflammatory demyelinating neuropathy. A distinct clinical entity? Neurology 2000;54:26–32.

70. Kaji R, Noboyuki O, Tsuji T, et al. Pathological findings at the site of conduction block in multifocal motor neuropathy. Muscle Nerve 1994;17:108–110.

71. Oh SJ, Claussen GC, Dae SK. Motor and sensory demyelinating mononeuropathy multiplex (multifocal motor and sensory demyelinating neuropathy): a separate entity or a variant of chronic inflammatory demyelinating polyneuropathy. J Peripher Nerv Syst 1997;2:362–369.

72. Thomas PK, Claus D, Jaspert A, et al. Focal upper limb demyelinating neuropathy. Brain 1996;119:765–774.

73. Cusimano MD, Bilbao JM, Cohen SM. Hypertrophic brachial plexus neuritis: a pathological study of two cases. Ann Neurol 1988;24:615–622.

74. Amato AA, Jackson CE, Kim JY, et al. Chronic relapsing brachial plexus neuropathy with persistent conduction block. Muscle Nerve 1997;20:1303–1307.

75. Thomas PK, Lascelles RG, Hallpike JF, et al. Recurrent and chronic relapsing Guillain-Barré polyneuritis. Brain 1987;110:53–76.

76. Chance PF. Inherited Demyelinating Neuropathy: Charcot-Marie-Tooth Disease and Related Disorders. In RN Rosenberg, SB Prusiner, S DiMauro, RL Barchi (eds), The Molecular and Genetic Basis of Neurological Disease. Boston: Butterworth–Heinemann, 1997;807–816.

77. Mendell JR. Charcot-Marie-Tooth neuropathies and related disorders. Semin Neurol 1998;18:41–48.

78. Kaku DA, Parry GJ, Malamut R, et al. Uniform slowing of conduction velocities in Charcot-Marie-Tooth polyneuropathy type 1. Neurology 1993;43:2664–2667.

79. Yudell A, Pyck PJ, Lambert EH. A kinship with Roussy-Levy syndrome: a clinical and electrophysiologic study. Arch Neurol 1965:13:432–440.

80. Gutmann L, Fakadej A, Riggs J. Evolution of nerve conduction abnormalities in children with dominant hypertrophic neuropathy of the Charcot-Marie-Tooth type. Muscle Nerve 1983;6:515–519.

81. Killiam JM, Tiwari PS, Jacobson S, et al. Longitudinal studies of the duplication form of Charcot-Marie-Tooth polyneuropathy. Muscle Nerve 1996;19:74–78.

82. Chance PF, Bird TD, Matsunami N, et al. Trisomy 17p associated with Charcot-Marie-Tooth neuropathy I phenotype: evidence for gene dosage as a mechanism in CMT 1A. Neurology 1992;42:2295.

83. Lupski JR, Chance PF, Garcia CA. Inherited primary peripheral neuropathies. Molecular genetics and clinical implications of CMT 1A and HNPP. JAMA 1993;270: 2326–2330.

84. Lupski JR, Wise CA, Kuwano A, et al. Gene dosage is a mechanism for Charcot-Marie-Tooth disease type 1A. Nat Genet 1992;1:29–33.

85. Rosa BB, Garcia CA, Pentao L, et al. Evidence for a recessive PMP22 point mutation in Charcot-Marie-Tooth disease type 1A. Nat Genet 1993;5:189–94.

86. Earl CJ, Fullerton PM, Wakefield GS, Schutta HS. Hereditary neuropahty with liability to pressure palsies: a clinical and electrophysiological study of four families. QJM 1964;33:481–498.

87. Behse F, Buchthal F, Carlsen F, Knappeis GG. Hereditary neuropathy with liability to pressure palsies. Electrophysiological and histopathological aspects. Brain 1972;95: 777–794.

88. Madrid R, Bradley WG. The pathology of neuropathies with focal thickening of the myelin sheath (tomaculous neuropathy): studies on the formation of the abnormal myelin sheath. J Neurol Sci 1975;25:415–448.

89. Chance PF, Alderson MK, Leppig KA, et al. DNA deletion associated with hereditary neuropathy with liability to pressure palsies. Cell 1993;72:143–151.

90. Mariman EC, Gabreels-Festen AA, van Beersum SE, et al. Prevalence of the 1.5 Mb 17p deletion in families with hereditary neuropathy with liability to pressure palsies. Ann Neurol 1994;36:650–655.

91. LeGuern E, Goudier R, Lopes J, et al. Constant rearrangement of the CMT 1A-REP sequences in HNPP patients with a deletion of 17p11.2: a study of 30 unrelated cases. Hum Mol Genet 1995;4:1673–1674.

92. Mouton P, Tardieu BS, Goudier R, et al. Spectrum of clinical and electrophysiologic features in HNPP patients with the 17p11.2 deletion. Neurology 1999;52:1440–1446.

93. Andersson P-B, Yuen E, Parko K, et al. Electrodiagnostic features of hereditary neuropathy with liability to pressure palsies. Neurology 2000;54:40–44.

94. Jacobs JM, Costa-Jussa FR. The pathology of amiodarone neurotoxicity in man. Brain 1985;108:753–769.

95. Wijesekera R, Critchley EM, Fahim Y, et al. Peripheral neuropathy due to perhexiline maleate. J Neurol Sci 1980; 46:303–309.

96. Grimbert P, Azema C, Pastural M, et al. Tacroilimus (FK506)-induced severe and late encephalopathy in a renal transplant recipient. Nephrol Dialysis Trans 1999;14:2489–2491.

97. Wilson JR, Conwit RA, Eidelman BH, et al. Sensorimotor neuropathy resembling CIDP in patients receiving FK506. Muscle Nerve 1994;17:528–532.

98. Fuller GN, Spies JM, Pollard JD, McLeod JG. Demyelinating neuropathies triggered by melanoma immunotherapy. Neurology 1994;44:2185–2186.

Chapter 18

From Genetics to Genomics and Proteomics: New Fields and Technologies and Their Application to Myelin Research

Fernando Dangond

The completion and release of the draft nucleotide sequence of the human genome by the Human Genome Project participants[1,2] in 2001 was received with great enthusiasm and praise by the general public and the scientific community, as the Project provided researchers with remarkable new tools for exploring the functional intricacies of complex biological systems, including the nervous system. Researchers are now occupied with a great and challenging task: elucidate the function and biological interactions of the proteins encoded by the genome. Neurologists practicing in the decade of the brain (1990–2000) witnessed unprecedented advances in the understanding of many brain disorders, with most of the impetus fueled by the revolution in molecular biology. This revolution began within the field of genetics, which focused on establishing the hereditary bases for human diseases. A new field— functional genomics—applies newer technologies and our expanding knowledge of the human genome to examine the functional expression of thousands of genes simultaneously. DNA microarray technology, an extraordinary new approach that examines the expression of genes on a large scale, is beginning to provide an integrated view of metabolic and transcriptional regulatory pathways that control cell growth, differentiation, and survival mechanisms. These pathways assume a greater importance when analyzed at the protein level, as proteins but not messenger RNAs (mRNAs) are the effector molecules that, when dysregulated, may lead to disease causation. The field of proteomics is, therefore, a logical next step in the scientific quest that will complement and clarify questions raised by the genomics revolution. The application of the new technologies brought on by these new research tendencies will ensure a greater understanding of how the nervous system works at the molecular level, and this includes the elucidation of major questions related to the physiology of myelin during development and its vulnerability to disease.

Impact of Genetics

Mendel first postulated a hereditary basis for common traits based on his studies of plants. The characterization of hereditary disorders as mendelian in nature (i.e., dominant, recessive, X-linked, with a strong genotype-phenotype correlation) or non-mendelian (the more common complex-trait; polygenic; due to polymorphic variants) has been under an intense research focus for the last 100 years. Fueled by the advent of the polymerase chain reaction (PCR) in 1985 and other techniques of gene cloning and rapid, automated DNA sequencing, the field of genetics grew at an unprecedented rate, with the discovery of a great number of gene defects (i.e., mutations, deletions) that lead to human hereditary diseases. In fact, accurate chro-

Table 18-1. Some Neurologic Diseases Due to Mutations in Genes That Have Been Positionally Cloned

Disease	Gene Symbol
X-linked adrenoleukodystrophy	*ALD*
Amyotrophic lateral sclerosis	*SOD1*
Ataxia telangiectasia	*ATM*
Neuronal ceroid lipofuscinosis	*INCL*
Duchenne's muscular dystrophy	*DMD*
Emery-Dreifuss muscular dystrophy	*STA*
Fragile X syndrome	*FMR1*
Friedreich's ataxia	*FRDA*
Huntington's disease	*HD*
Lissencephaly	*LIS1*
Machado-Joseph disease	*MJD1*
Menkes' syndrome	*MNK*
Myotonic dystrophy	*DM*
Neurofibromatosis, type 1	*NF1*
Neurofibromatosis, type 2	*NF2*
Niemann-Pick disease, type C	*NPC*
Progressive myoclonus epilepsy	*EPM1*
Spinal muscular atrophy	*SMA*
Spinocerebellar ataxia 1	*SCA1*
Spinocerebellar ataxia 2	*SCA2*
Spinocerebellar ataxia 7	*SCA7*
Tuberous sclerosis	*TSC*
von Hippel-Lindau disease	*VHL*
Wilson's disease	*WND*
CADASIL	*NOTCH3*
Hyperekplexia	*GLRA2*
Early-onset torsion dystonia	*DQ1*

CADASIL = cerebral autosomal dominant arteriopathy with subcortical infarcts, dementia, and leukoencephalopathy.

mosomal localizations for inherited diseases now number in the thousands. The realization of the fact that two alleles from different loci occurring (segregating together) in the same individual more often than would be predicted by random chance (linkage disequilibrium) would give clues to disease gene localization helped to transform the field of population genetics. Restriction fragment length polymorphisms were identified by Gusella and collaborators[3] as size patterns of DNA fragmentation after enzymatic digestion that suggested interindividual polymorphic variations and supported linkage hypotheses. Botstein and collaborators[4] used restriction fragment length polymorphisms to construct the first genetic linkage maps of the human genome.

Thus, identification and isolation of disease-associated genes were tasks performed by adopting two traditional methods: The first involved using an "educated guess" approach to cloning, based on known or presumed function of a DNA sequence (this function could also be inferred based on the sequence homology to other known DNAs); the second was cloning by screening for abnormalities on candidate genes based on chromosome localization. These candidate genes were selected based on their localization to the region presumed to be implicated in the phenotype, and this method of isolation was termed *positional cloning*. Both approaches have been known to be laborious and depend highly on chance and on the ability of the existing databases, before the human genome project completion, to provide homology information to deduce function.

When PCR and positional cloning approaches to gene discovery became widespread, the rapid expansion of the field of molecular biology resulted in a revolutionary and exponential growth in biomedical approaches to human disease (see Table 18-1 for some neurologic diseases, the genes of which were identified by positional cloning methods). Within two decades, the genetic abnormalities underlying various central nervous system (CNS) disorders were revealed at the molecular level. Examples include the discovery of the DNA repeats responsible for Huntington's disease[5] and the gene mutations responsible for familial forms of amyotrophic lateral sclerosis,[6] Alzheimer's dementia,[7] and Parkinson's disease.[8] In addition, the precise identification of infectious disorders of the nervous system by techniques such as PCR has also had a profound impact on the practice of neurology. These discoveries have been translated into new diagnostic tests, treatment algorithms, and prognostic indicators.

Human Genome Project

The U.S. Human Genome Project, sponsored by the U.S. federal government, was launched as a 15-year endeavor with the ultimate aim of determining the complete sequence of the human DNA subunits and rendering them accessible to further scientific inquiry. Such a project required access to computer-based methods that helped to obtain, analyze, and store data; instrumentation for high-throughput sequencing-screening; and coordination of major international efforts to avoid repetition and expedite completion. The feasibility of the Human Genome Project had been highlighted by the completion of the sequencing of genomes of multiple organisms, including *Haemophilus influenzae*, *Escherichia coli*, *Bacillus subtilis*, *Helicobacter pylori*, *Mycoplasma genitalium*, the yeast *Saccharomyces cerevisiae*, *Mycobacterium tuberculosis*, *Treponema pallidum*, the archeal thermobacteria *Methanococcus jannaschii* and *Archeoglobus fulgidus*, and the nematode *Caenorhabditis elegans*, among others. The new challenge of the postgenomic era is to integrate the information of gene expression with our growing knowledge of the function of each gene in the human genome. Newer technologies examine the expression of all genes simultaneously, under various experimental conditions, to attempt to correlate dysfunctional pathways with disease phenotype (the differential expression approach).

Differential Gene Expression

The first wave of expansion triggered by the advent of PCR was followed by the introduction of techniques of differential gene expression. Newer techniques that include subtractive hybridization, mRNA differential display, electronic DNA sequence subtraction, and serial analysis of gene expression[9,10] have allowed the rapid identification and cloning of multiple differentially expressed genes in various biological systems.[11] However, the pace of discovery had been somewhat slowed by our limited understanding of the structure of the human genome and our inability to examine the functionally expressed genes in parallel.

DNA Microarrays: A Newer Technique for Detecting Differentially Expressed Genes

A new and powerful methodology that allows an investigator to examine all expressed genes in a single experiment—high-density oligonucleotide array analysis—has come of age under the term *DNA chip* or *DNA microarray* technology and was pioneered by Southern[12] and Fodor.[13] This technology allows natural fragments of genomic or complementary DNA libraries or newly, chemically synthesized complementary DNA oligomer probes to be attached microscopically (by electrochemical copolymerization, by robotic microspotting, by photolithography technology from the semiconductor industry, or by ink-jetting) in arrays to solid supports (i.e., silicon,[14] glass, or fiber-optic sensors[15]) that serve as highly parallel screening "platforms" or complementary hybridization targets for entire mRNA populations to be analyzed. This RNA is dually labeled with fluorescent markers, and its differential hybridization to the small nucleic acid "platform" (after washing out the noncomplementary strands) will be revealed as a strong fluorescent signal at any place of the array, accurately reflecting its expression, in comparison to control RNA. The sample rows are scanned by a confocal device (laser and pinhole detection combined) for fluorescence emission after independent wavelength laser excitation of the fluors used. Gene chips can contain thousands of different small oligonucleotides representing defined sequences in an area of less than 2 cm². This technique has had ample validation and offers a rapid, robust, reproducible, miniaturized, and quantitative approach to examining the expression of genes in large scale, providing an integrated view of the changing mRNA concentrations of cells in a biological system. Furthermore, the technique can detect as low abundance transcripts as those represented in a 1 to 1,000,000 ratio sequences of total mRNA.[16,17]

Once synthetic complementary DNA fragments can be arrayed at will and with precision on platforms, it is clear that examination of single nucleotide polymorphisms (also known as *SNPs*) responsible for any polygenic traits can also be analyzed using a single gene chip. This has also been demonstrated as feasible, efficient, and highly specific and sensitive[18] (see Table 18-2 for neurologic diseases thought to be triggered by the unfavorable presence of polymorphic gene variants). Other applications include the examination of mutations[19]; sequence analysis and identification of viral[20] or bacterial strains and their resistance to drugs (e.g., human immunodeficiency virus resistance to retroviral therapy); the molecular staging and classification of tumors[21]; and the effect of mutagenic drugs on DNA and of teratogenic drugs

Table 18-2. Non–Human Leukocyte Antigen Polymorphisms Implicated in Multiple Sclerosis*

Gene	Polymorphism	Association
Interleukin-4	IL-4 B1 allele	Age of disease onset[38]
Interleukin-6	A5 allele	Disease severity[39]
γ-Aminobutyric acid A3R	GABRA3 16-repeat	Disease susceptibility[40]
Monocyte chemotactic protein 3	A2 and A4 alleles	Disease risk[41]
Immunoglobulin G Fc receptor (FcγR)	IIA and IIIB	Disease severity[42]
CTLA4	G49 allele	Disease susceptibility[43]
CTLA4	G49 allele	Disease severity[44]
Vitamin D receptor	Bsm1 restriction site	Disease susceptibility[45]
Tumor necrosis factor-α	TNFA-376	Disease susceptibility[46]
Tumor necrosis factor-α	a11 Allele	Disease susceptibility[47]
Glutathione-S-transferase	GSTM1 and GSTP1	Disease severity[48]
Plasminogen activator inhibitor-1	5G5G	Disease susceptibility in women[49]
Chemokine receptor CCR5	CCR5Δ32	Age of onset[50]
Apolipoprotein E	Epsilon 2 allele	Remyelination capacity[51]
Estrogen receptor	PvuII restriction site	Disease susceptibility[52]
Estrogen receptor	XbaI restriction site	Age of disease onset[52]
SCA2	22 Repeat length allele	Disease susceptibility[53]
Interferon alpha	IFNA 17 nonfunctional	Disease susceptibility[54]

CTLA4 = cytotoxic T lymphocyte–associated antigen 4.
*An unfavorable combination of polymorphic common variants may lead to susceptibility to multiple sclerosis. Multiple allelic variants have been investigated, especially for cytokine or cytokine pathway–related genes. Tumor necrosis factor-α polymorphisms may be linked due to their proximity to human leukocyte antigen genes in a region on the short arm of chromosome 6, which has, so far, the most reliable polymorphic association with multiple sclerosis. This table summarizes results from different populations studied, and several of these results await confirmation. Human leukocyte antigen polymorphisms are not included.

on development. This technology will have an impact on our understanding of the etiology of brain tumors and demyelination and suggest targets for the treatment of CNS infections, inflammation, degeneration, and autoimmunity.

Examples of the diverse uses of microarrays include the examination of the effects of starvation, heat shock, differentiation inducers, and oxygen deprivation on diverse cell types and organisms, including yeast[22,23] and plants.[24] The study of human populations and the effect of polymorphisms on susceptibility to CNS infections, autoimmunity, neurodegenerative illnesses, and tumors will be underscored by these new techniques. The study of behavior-controlling genes will have an impact on our views of gender, sexual orientation, and psychiatric illness. Likewise, genes that, as a set, cooperate in maintaining cell viability and genetic integrity will be pursued as targets of aging studies. Furthermore, DNA chip technology will help in "filling the gaps" in our knowledge of important metabolic pathways that directly or indirectly affect

the nervous system. Finally, identification of small-molecule drugs that specifically alter the expression of the "deleterious" gene or "block" the function of its protein product, the ultimate goal of molecular medicine,[25] will be helped by these techniques. In summary, DNA microarrays have the advantage of providing massive amounts of data while simultaneously allowing high-throughput screening of small samples. The integrated acquisition of data and their analysis, however, remain some of the greatest challenges for the next decade.

Genes of known similar function can be arrayed on chips. On the other hand, it is possible to identify these clusters of functionality with the DNA chips themselves, using computer algorithms. For example, it has been possible to determine which clusters of genes exhibit temporally grouped expression during CNS development in rat spinal cord.[26,27]

Significant efforts have been devoted to create expression profile libraries of diseased tissue, including pancreatic cancer.[28] Remarkably, there has been little effort to represent the normal human gene expression, information that is crucial for interpreting and determining truly altered gene expression in a given tissue. We have generated, under a Merck Genome Research Institute–funded initiative, a comprehensive data set of normally expressed human RNA that includes nervous system tissue[29] and is available through the internet as a free service to investigators around the world (http://www.hugeindex.org). The data has been generated using DNA chip technology. For genomic studies, there is a need for appropriate tissue banks and accuracy in the collection, timing, and categorization of the samples to be used as controls. These tissue banks must be accessible to the general scientific community to ensure universality and reproducibility. With the expanding knowledge of the function of the approximately 30,000 human genes, novel experimental investigations addressing fundamental questions about the nervous system can be launched.

The repertoire of expressed genes reflects the cell's physiology. Genes with altered expression may represent the diseased genes or, indirectly, the secondary effect of a diseased gene. Gene chips may allow the detection of the variability in gene expression of such diseases as Tay-Sachs, Huntington's, myotonic dystrophy, multiple sclerosis, amyotrophic lateral sclerosis, and many forms of CNS cancer. Studies of the effects of metabolic (hyperosmolarity, heat shock) dysregulation in mouse cells[30] can be translated to similar human disorders.

Model Organisms and Large-Scale Genome Expression Studies

Knowledge of the complete mouse genome will allow mutagenesis experiments that up to the present could be performed only in yeast, *Drosophila*, *C. elegans*, or zebrafish, providing a more direct correlation with human diseases. For instance, the discovery of the mutation in *jimpy* mice[31] led to isolation of the gene defective in human Pelizaeus-Merzbacher disease,[32] and superoxide dismutase 1–transgenic animal models of amyotrophic lateral sclerosis that mimic the human disease are now commercially available to investigators. DNA microarrays can now be applied

to study various stages of disease in brain or spinal cord tissues from these animal models.

Such techniques as saturation mutagenesis allow the screening of defective genes in model organisms. New techniques that attempt to create mutations in embryonic stem cells will allow the generation of whole genome-spanning embryonic stem libraries that can be used by researchers to create transgenic mutant mice at will and are already being developed.[33]

Single Nucleotide Polymorphisms

Different individuals have a different nucleotide or base at a given location on their genome. These variations, termed *SNPs* and pronounced "snips," may predispose the individual to various disorders. SNPs occur in the approximately 2.9-billion-base human genome approximately once in every 1,000–2,000 bases. Although a *mutation* is defined as a rare difference that occurs in less than 1% of the population, a polymorphism is the least common allele occurring in 1% or more of the general population.[34] A potential difficulty with the elucidation of the association of SNPs with human disease is the fact that, as only approximately one-third of SNPs may be applicable to all human populations, the medical importance of the remainder may vary among ethnic groups.

The ability to predict the response of a given patient to a drug and the potential side effects that the patient may experience will be commonplace in the not-so-distant future. Optimization of drug treatment will be possible based on the knowledge of susceptibility genes in a given patient with a given symptomatology (which may or may not deviate from the norm). Different types of the same syndrome or disease (i.e., relapsing-remitting vs. primary-progressive multiple sclerosis) may be better characterized and the likely response to a given treatment better determined. SNPs may also be inherited in "linkage disequilibrium," which means that genetic regions that are physically close to each other in a chromosome will more likely segregate together during the process of genetic recombination. Maps of these SNPs and their heritability will be of great aid in establishing individual predispositions to migraine, Alzheimer's, subtypes of multiple sclerosis, and many other disorders.

Proteomics

Proteomics can be defined as the study of proteins on a large scale as they interact functionally in cellular regulatory or metabolic pathways. The development of the field of proteomics complements genomics, as there is no strict correlation between the number of genes in an organism and the number of proteins that are expressed and functional. It is now estimated that at least 60% of proteins exist in different versions (i.e., different mRNA splice variants of the same DNA, which result in different protein isoforms). It is expected that this wide variation will explain the great complexity of humans, as compared to most other species, despite the limited number of genes in the human genome. In addition, modification of the protein molecules by phosphorylation, glycosylation, sulphation, myristylation, ubiquitination, acetylation, and other chemical reactions has an impact on pathway regulation that cannot be studied using DNA microarrays. The study of body fluids wherein mRNA cannot be obtained for analysis will also require proteomic techniques. The techniques used in proteomics include a shift from using two-dimensional polyacrylamide gel electrophoresis to more elaborate and large-scale protein chips (using immobilized proteins or antibodies in a concept analogous to DNA chips described earlier) and mass spectrometry (matrix-assisted laser desorption ionization, electrospray, and tandem) technologies that allow accurate identification of proteins. These biochemical techniques can be adapted to investigate proteins that are differentially expressed or present in a given tissue or body fluid (protein differential display). Finally, protein-protein interactions can be investigated using techniques such as yeast or mammalian two-hybrid assays, phage display techniques, or purification of multi-protein complexes by affinity-based methods (immunoprecipitation with antibodies against the native protein or against a tagged epitope).

Impact of Genetics and New Technologies on Treatment of Myelin Disorders

An unprecedented explosion of knowledge has occurred in the last 50 years, generating new questions about what we are made of and how finite our molecular variability really may be. Localization of gene defects in disorders of myelin, such as Pelizaeus-Merzbacher disease in humans and its *jimpy* homolog in mice, attest to the power of methods used in genetics. Another implication of the genetics revolution was the realization of the potential for gene therapy, as it has been demonstrated that gene delivery to the nervous system is feasible and can be readily achieved in experimental animal models.

Although the treatment of most neurologic disorders has lagged behind the described, rapid expansion in our knowledge of DNA sequences, it is becoming increasingly clear that the next revolution in biomedical science will be triggered by the understanding of disease pathways and the large-scale screening of multiple pharmaceutical compounds that modify these pathways. The advent of newer, more efficient high-throughput techniques that dramatically simplify the drug screening process, allowing a genome-wide view of the expression pathways, will signal the beginning of the twenty-first century's medical revolution. Large libraries of small molecules will be designed specifically to block defects in pathways that lead to disease. These large libraries will be screened under multiple assay conditions that will determine likelihood of drug treatment success. In addition, DNA microarrays and proteomic techniques can be applied to the study of lineage determination in neural stem cells, helping researchers to harness the potential of these cells for treatment. For instance, understanding the gene expression profile behind the phenotype of neural progenitor cells with the capacity to remyelinate may facilitate the search for drugs that enhance this phenotype in vivo. The application of DNA microarrays to myelin disorders, such as Sandhoff's disease[35] and multiple sclerosis,[36] has already begun revealing target pathways potentially implicated in the pathogenic mechanisms of these diseases.

A New Paradigm of Research: The Study of Human Biology on a Massive Scale

Genetics brought to researchers the tools to correlate phenotype with genotype at the DNA level. From the study of chromosomes to gene mapping, followed by the molecular genetics revolution, scientists were able to pinpoint the gene defects for many hereditary conditions, one at a time. In the postgenomic era, a brave new world now exists in which massive amounts of information must be handled by researchers to comprehensively study gene function. Therefore, new high-throughput technologies are now being developed and implemented to facilitate our exploration of biology and physiology on a large scale, with the obvious potential applications to the study of disorders of the nervous system in humans. In addition, miniaturization and speeding of chemical reactions is becoming a reality with the merging of powerful analytic measurement formats. For instance, microchip capillary electrophoresis, which integrates small sample handling and automated analysis capabilities all in a miniaturized space ("lab-on-a-chip" concept) has great potential value for laboratory diagnosis. Fabrication of multiparallel channels on a chip platform will allow the sequential chemical reactions (as in PCR) to take place in an automated fashion.[37]

Functional genomics will help us understand the interaction, modulation, and organization of human genes and will provide a framework for the emerging fields of proteomics (the study of the function and interactions of proteins and protein pathways on a massive scale), structural genomics (identification of the three-dimensional configuration of proteins at the atomic level by high-throughput methods), and bioinformatics (the science of analyzing, storing, and interpreting biological data). The data generated in these new fields of research will be complementary to biological studies with knockout or transgenic model organisms, including animal models of autoimmunity or demyelination.

Thus, in a century that began with the growth of nervous system histopathology and anatomy and the application of chromosomology and cytogenetics to the study of nervous system disorders, neurologists witnessed the advent of molecular neurobiology and neurobiochemistry, the application of transgenic technology to experimental models of human neurologic diseases, and, more recently, the birth of structural and functional neurogenomics and proteomics, the creation of massive DNA databases, and the expansion of globally interconnected computer-based (virtual) research.

Need for Public Education, Protective Legislation, and Scientific Exchange

Information extracted from the functional genomics initiative will have to be examined in the context of the environmental factors that alter our physiology and behavior and the legal, social, and ethical implications of implementing gene therapy for humans. Discussions regarding these subjects must be included in scientific meetings (governmentally or privately funded), encouraging the public's input into the debate. These massive efforts will lead to successful outcomes only if neurologists and neuroscientists throughout the world join forces to share resources, maintain scientific openness, support legislation banning discriminatory practices based on genetic testing, and cooperate in educating the general public about the fundamental value of understanding the complex physiologic neuronal and genetic circuitry that sets us apart as human beings. The public also needs to be informed of the distinctions between rare genetic diseases (traditional mendelian or mitochondrial inheritance for which traditional genetic counseling methods have been set in place) and common complex diseases, the latter related to SNPs or susceptibility genes, for which new approaches to patient information and privacy protection have to be designed.

References

1. Venter JC, Adams MD, Myers EW, et al. The sequence of the human genome. Science 2001;291:1304.
2. Lander ES, Linton LM, Birren B, et al. Initial sequencing and analysis of the human genome. Nature 2001;409:860.
3. Gusella JF, Wexler NS, Conneally P, et al. A polymorphic DNA marker genetically linked to Huntington's disease. Nature 1983;306:234.
4. Botstein D, White RL, Skolnick M, Davis RW. Construction of a genetic linkage map in man using restriction fragment length polymorphism. Am J Hum Genet 1980;32:314.
5. The Huntington's Disease Collaborative Research Group. A novel gene containing a trinucleotide repeat that is expanded and unstable on Huntington's disease chromosomes. Cell 1993;72:971.
6. Rosen DR, Siddique T, Patterson D, et al. Mutations in Cu/Zn superoxide dismutase gene are associated with familial amyotrophic lateral sclerosis. Nature 1993;362:59.
7. Sherrington R, Rogaev EI, Liang Y, et al. Cloning of a gene bearing missense mutations in early-onset familial Alzheimer's disease. Nature 1995;375:754.

8. Polymeropoulos MH, Lavedan C, Leroy E, et al. Mutation in the alpha-synuclein gene identified in families with Parkinson's disease. Science 1997;276:2045.

9. Velculescu VE, Zhang L, Vogelstein B, Kinzler KW. Serial analysis of gene expression. Science 1995;270:484.

10. Powell J. Enhanced concatemer cloning-a modification to the SAGE (Serial Analysis of Gene Expression) technique. Nucleic Acids Res 1998;26:3445.

11. Dangond F, Hafler DA, Tong JK, et al. Differential display cloning of a novel human histone deacetylase (HDAC3) cDNA from PHA-activated immune cells. Biochem Biophys Res Commun 1998;242:648.

12. Maskos U, Southern EM. A novel method for the analysis of multiple sequence variants by hybridisation to oligonucleotides. Nucleic Acids Res 1993;21:2267.

13. Fodor SP, Read JL, Pirrung MC, et al. Light-directed, spatially addressable parallel chemical synthesis. Science 1991;251:767.

14. Livache T, Fouque B, Roget A, et al. Polypyrrole DNA chip on a silicon device: example of hepatitis C virus genotyping. Anal Biochem 1998;255:188.

15. Ferguson JA, Boles TC, Adams CP, Walt DR. A fiberoptic DNA biosensor microarray for the analysis of gene expression. Nat Biotechnol 1996;14:1681.

16. Schena M, Shalon D, Heller R, et al. Parallel human genome analysis: microarray-based expression monitoring of 1,000 genes. Proc Natl Acad Sci U S A 1996;93:10614.

17. Schena M. Genome analysis with gene expression microarrays. Bioessays 1996;18:427.

18. Hacia JG, Brody LC, Chee MS, et al. Detection of heterozygous mutations in BRCA1 using high density oligonucleotide arrays and two-colour fluorescence analysis. Nat Genet 1996;14:441.

19. Cronin MT, Fucini RV, Kim SM, et al. Cystic fibrosis mutation detection by hybridization to light-generated DNA probe arrays. Hum Mutat 1996;7:244.

20. Kozal MJ, Shah N, Shen N, et al. Extensive polymorphisms observed in HIV-1 clade B protease gene using high-density oligonucleotide arrays. Nat Med 1996;2:753.

21. Golub TR, Slonim DK, Tamayo P, et al. Molecular classification of cancer: class discovery and class prediction by gene expression monitoring. Science 1999;286:531.

22. DeRisi J, Penland L, Brown PO, et al. Use of a cDNA microarray to analyse gene expression patterns in human cancer. Nat Genet 1996;14:457.

23. DeRisi JL, Iyer VR, Brown PO. Exploring the metabolic and genetic control of gene expression on a genomic scale. Science 1997;278:680.

24. Schena M, Shalon D, Davis RW, Brown PO. Quantitative monitoring of gene expression patterns with a complementary DNA microarray. Science 1995;270:467.

25. Denison C, Kodadek T. Small-molecule-based strategies for controlling gene expression. Chem Biol 1998;5:R129.

26. Wen X, Fuhrman S, Michaels GS, et al. Large-scale temporal gene expression mapping of central nervous system development. Proc Natl Acad Sci U S A 1998;95:334.

27. Michaels GS, Carr DB, Askenazi M, et al. Cluster analysis and data visualization of large-scale gene expression data. Pac Symp Biocomput 1998;42.

28. Gress TM, Muller-Pillasch F, Geng M, et al. A pancreatic cancer-specific expression profile. Oncogene 1996;13:1819.

29. Hsiao LL, Dangond F, Yoshida T, et al. A compendium of gene expression in normal human tissues. Physiol Genomics 2001;7:97–104.

30. Chevaile A, Santos B, Randall J, et al. Approaches to identifying cell volume-regulated genes. Contrib Nephrol 1998;123:110.

31. Dautigny A, Mattei MG, Morello D, et al. The structural gene coding for myelin-associated proteolipid protein is mutated in jimpy mice. Nature 1986;321:867.

32. Hudson LD, Puckett C, Berndt J, et al. Mutation of the proteolipid protein gene PLP in a human X chromosome-linked myelin disorder. Proc Natl Acad Sci U S A 1989;86:8128.

33. Friedrich G, Soriano P. Promoter traps in embryonic stem cells: a genetic screen to identify and mutate developmental genes in mice. Genes Dev 1991;5:1513.

34. Marez D, Legrand M, Sabbagh N, et al. Polymorphism of the cytochrome P450 CYP2D6 gene in a European population: characterization of 48 mutations and 53 alleles, their frequencies and evolution. Pharmacogenetics 1997;7:193.

35. Wada R, Tifft CJ, Proia RL. Microglial activation precedes acute neurodegeneration in Sandhoff disease and is suppressed by bone marrow transplantation. Proc Natl Acad Sci U S A 2000;97:10954.

36. Whitney LW, Becker KG, Tresser NJ, et al. Analysis of gene expression in multiple sclerosis lesions using cDNA microarrays. Ann Neurol 1999;46:425.

37. Colyer CL, Tang T, Chiem N, Harrison DJ. Clinical potential of microchip capillary electrophoresis systems. Electrophoresis 1997;18:1733.

38. Vandenbroeck K, Martino G, Marrosu M, et al. Occurrence and clinical relevance of an interleukin-4 gene polymorphism in patients with multiple sclerosis. J Neuroimmunol 1997;76:189.

39. Vandenbroeck K, Fiten P, Ronsse I, et al. High-resolution analysis of IL-6 minisatellite polymorphism in Sardinian multiple sclerosis: effect on course and onset of disease. Genes Immun 2000;1:460.

40. Gade-Andavolu R, MacMurray JP, Blake H, et al. Association between the gamma-aminobutyric acid A3 receptor gene and multiple sclerosis. Arch Neurol 1998;55:513.

41. Fiten P, Vandenbroeck K, Dubois B, et al. Microsatellite polymorphisms in the gene promoter of monocyte chemotactic protein-3 and analysis of the association between monocyte chemotactic protein-3 alleles and multiple sclerosis development. J Neuroimmunol 1999;95:195.

42. Myhr KM, Raknes G, Nyland H, Vedeler C. Immunoglobulin G Fc-receptor (FcgammaR) IIA and IIIB polymorphisms related to disability in MS. Neurology 1999;52:1771.

43. Ligers A, Xu C, Saarinen S, et al. The CTLA-4 gene is associated with multiple sclerosis. J Neuroimmunol 1999;97:182.

44. Fukazawa T, T Yanagawa, S Kikuchi, et al. CTLA-4 gene polymorphism may modulate disease in Japanese multiple sclerosis patients. J Neurol Sci 1999;171:49.

45. Fukazawa T, Yabe I, Kikuchi S, et al. Association of vitamin D receptor gene polymorphism with multiple sclerosis in Japanese. J Neurol Sci 1999;166:47.

46. Fernandez-Arquero M, Arroyo R, Rubio A, et al. Primary association of a TNF gene polymorphism with susceptibility to multiple sclerosis. Neurology 1999;53:1361.

47. Lucotte G, Bathelier C, Mercier G. TNF-alpha polymorphisms in multiple sclerosis: no association with -238 and -308 promoter alleles, but the microsatellite allele a11 is associated with the disease in French patients. Mult Scler 2000;6:78.

48. Mann CL, Davies MB, Boggild MD, et al. Glutathione *S*-transferase polymorphisms in MS: their relationship to disability. Neurology 2000;54:552.

49. Luomala M, Elovaara I, Ukkonen M, et al. Plasminogen activator inhibitor 1 gene and risk of MS in women. Neurology 2000;54:1862.

50. Barcellos LF, Schito AM, Rimmler JB, et al. CC-chemokine receptor 5 polymorphism and age of onset in familial multiple sclerosis. Multiple Sclerosis Genetics Group. Immunogenetics 2000;51:281.

51. Carlin C, Murray L, Graham D, et al. Involvement of apolipoprotein E in multiple sclerosis: absence of remyelination associated with possession of the APOE epsilon2 allele. J Neuropathol Exp Neurol 2000;59:361.

52. Niino M, Kikuchi S, Fukazawa T, et al. Estrogen receptor gene polymorphism in Japanese patients with multiple sclerosis. J Neurol Sci 2000;179:70.

53. Chataway J, Sawcer S, Coraddu F, et al. Evidence that allelic variants of the spinocerebellar ataxia type 2 gene influence susceptibility to multiple sclerosis. Neurogenetics 1999;2:91.

54. Miterski B, Jaeckel S, Epplen JT, et al. The interferon gene cluster: a candidate region for MS predisposition? Multiple Sclerosis Study Group. Genes Immun 1999;1:37.

Index

Note: Page numbers followed by *f* indicate figures; page numbers followed by *t* indicate tables.